# METHODS IN MOLECULAR BIOLOGY™

*Series Editor*
**John M. Walker**
**School of Life Sciences**
**University of Hertfordshire**
**Hatfield, Hertfordshire, AL10 9AB, UK**

For further volumes:
http://www.springer.com/series/7651

# Molecular Methods for Evolutionary Genetics

Edited by

**Virginie Orgogozo**

*CNRS UMR7592, Université Paris VII, Paris, France*

**Matthew V. Rockman**

*Department of Biology and Center for Genomics and Systems Biology, New York University, New York, NY, USA*

Humana Press

*Editors*
Virginie Orgogozo
CNRS UMR7592
Université Paris VII
15 rue Hélène Brion
75013 Paris
France
orgogozo@ijm.univ-paris-diderot.fr

Matthew V. Rockman
Department of Biology and
Center for Genomics and Systems Biology
New York University
New York, NY 10003-6688, USA
mrockman@nyu.edu

ISSN 1064-3745 e-ISSN 1940-6029
ISBN 978-1-61779-227-4 e-ISBN 978-1-61779-228-1
DOI 10.1007/978-1-61779-228-1
Springer New York Dordrecht Heidelberg London

Library of Congress Control Number: 2011934052



Printed on acid-free paper

Humana Press is part of Springer Science+Business Media (www.springer.com)

# Preface

Rapid technological progress is transforming the investigation of genetic variation within and between species. We are entering a particularly fruitful period in evolutionary genetics, as two of its main goals – reconstruction of population histories and identification of the mutations responsible for evolutionary changes in phenotypes – have now turned into tractable problems.

This book is a collection of molecular biology protocols and general overviews intended to represent the essential methods currently bringing evolutionary genetics to fruition. It begins with methods for the basic characterization of an unknown genome and ends with the functional dissection of individual allelic variants. We chose to focus on protocols that are widely applicable to all species and that require, when possible, little money and equipment. Part I includes two essential traditional methods for characterizing genomes, genome size determination and chromosomal analysis. It also describes the construction, screening and sequencing of genomic libraries, a classic tool for genome walking and for obtaining the DNA sequence of a genomic region of interest. Part II describes various approaches to enrich DNA for subsets of the genome prior to sequencing, including methods for isolating and sequencing the transcriptome. Even as next-generation sequencing technologies are rapidly improving in terms of efficiency and cost, sequencing targeted regions of the genome is likely to remain a compelling strategy, particularly in non-model organisms and population samples. Part III contains five powerful protocols for sampling genetic variation for genetic mapping studies and for population genetic studies. Many evolutionary studies aiming at identifying the mutations responsible for evolutionary change converge on genomic regions containing one or several candidate genes that must be tested and validated. The last three parts of this book focus on such candidate gene studies. Part IV describes three molecular biology methods that can be used to obtain the DNA sequence of a region of interest: degenerate PCR, circular RACE and inverse PCR. Part V includes protocols for measuring gene expression, including two allele-specific methods that can identify cis-regulatory changes. In part VI, two general strategy chapters outline the main steps for testing the functional import of candidate cis-regulatory and protein-coding mutations. Testing a candidate mutation usually involves the construction of artificial DNA sequences. Part VI includes several powerful methods for making these constructs, Gateway cloning, PCR stitching, homologous recombination using yeast and fosmid recombineering in liquid culture. A functional assay applicable to many species, RNAi injection, is described in the last chapter of our book.

It has been a real pleasure for us to work with the authors of this book. They have shown an admirable willingness to share their knowledge and expertise. We deeply appreciate their efforts to make their protocols widely accessible to our readers. We thank them all for their work and their dedication.

We hope that this volume will provide a rich resource for biologists interested in evolution, whether they are specialists or beginners in molecular biology.

*Paris, France* — *Virginie Orgogozo*
*New York, NY, USA* — *Matthew V. Rockman*

# Contents

## Contributors

PETER AHLFELD • *Max Planck Institute of Molecular Cell Biology and Genetics, Dresden, Germany*
ERIK C. ANDERSEN • *Lewis-Sigler Institute for Integrative Genomics, Princeton University, Princeton, NJ, USA*
JOSÉ A. ANDRÉS • *Department of Biology, University of Saskatchewan, Saskatoon, SK, Canada*
SUSAN BASSHAM • *Center for Ecology and Evolutionary Biology, University of Oregon, Eugene, OR, USA*
SIMON W. BAXTER • *Department of Zoology, University of Cambridge, Cambridge, UK*
HELEN BEASLEY • *Sequencing, DNA Pipelines, Wellcome Trust Sanger Institute, Cambridge, UK*
JOSÉ BESSA • *Centro Andaluz de Biología del Desarrollo (CABD), CSIC-Universidad Pablo de Olavide, Seville, Spain*
STEVEN M. BOGDANOWICZ • *Department of Ecology and Evolutionary Biology, Cornell University, Ithaca, NY, USA*
MARIA BOGDANZALIEWA • *Max Planck Institute of Molecular Cell Biology and Genetics, Dresden, Germany*
MARTINA BRADIĆ • *Department of Biology, New York University, New York, NY, USA*
ADRIAN W. BRIGGS • *Department of Genetics, Harvard Medical School, Boston, MA, USA*
KAREN L. CARLETON • *University of Maryland, College Park, MD, USA*
AMY A. CAUDY • *Lewis-Sigler Institute for Integrative Genomics, Princeton University, Princeton, NJ, USA*
IVO M. CHELO • *Instituto Gulbenkian de Ciência, Oeiras, Portugal*
JOÃO COSTA • *Instituto Gulbenkian de Ciência, Oeiras, Portugal*
WILLIAM A. CRESKO • *Center for Ecology and Evolutionary Biology, University of Oregon, Eugene, OR, USA*
RADOSLAW KAMIL EJSMONT • *Max Planck Institute of Molecular Cell Biology and Genetics, Dresden, Germany*
PAUL D. ETTER • *Institute of Molecular Biology, University of Oregon, Eugene, OR, USA*
DAVID H. A. FITCH • *Department of Biology, New York University, New York, NY, USA*
RYO FUTAHASHI • *Bioproduction Research Institute, National Institute of Advanced Industrial Science and Technology (AIST), Tsukuba, Ibaraki, Japan*
JOSÉ LUIS GÓMEZ-SKARMETA • *Centro Andaluz de Biología del Desarrollo (CABD), CSIC-Universidad Pablo de Olavide, Seville, Spain*
JEFFREY M. GOOD • *Division of Biological Sciences, University of Montana, Missoula, MT, USA*

DAVID GRESHAM • *Department of Biology and Center for Genomics and Systems Biology, New York University, New York, NY, USA*
FRANK GRUTZNER • *School of Molecular & Biomedical Science, The University of Adelaide, SA, Australia*
EMILY E. HARE • *Locus of Development, Inc., San Francisco, CA, USA*
PAUL A. HOHENLOHE • *Center for Ecology and Evolutionary Biology, University of Oregon, Eugene, OR, USA*
ERIC A. JOHNSON • *Institute of Molecular Biology, University of Oregon, Eugene, OR, USA*
J. SPENCER JOHNSTON • *Department of Entomology, Texas A&M University, College Station, Austin, TX, USA*
MICHAEL LANG • *CNRS, Institut Jacques Monod, Paris, France*
SHU LY LIM • *School of Molecular & Biomedical Science, The University of Adelaide, SA, Australia*
KAMIL ANDRZEJ LIPINSKI • *Max Planck Institute of Molecular Cell Biology and Genetics, Dresden, Germany*
CHRISTINE LLYOD • *Sequencing, DNA Pipelines, Wellcome Trust Sanger Institute, Cambridge, UK*
LUCY MATTHEWS • *Sequencing, DNA Pipelines, Wellcome Trust Sanger Institute, Cambridge, UK*
PATRICK T. MCGRATH • *The Rockefeller University, New York, NY, USA*
MATTHEW D. NELSON • *Department of Biology, New York University, New York, NY, USA*
VIRGINIE ORGOGOZO • *CNRS UMR7592, Université Paris VII, Paris, France*
ANASTASIOS PAVLOPOULOS • *Department of Zoology, University Museum of Zoology, Laboratory for Development and Evolution, University of Cambridge, Cambridge, UK*
BENJAMIN N. PHILIP • *Department of Biology, Rivier College, Nashua, NH, USA*
ANDREI POZNIAKOVSKY • *Max Planck Institute of Molecular Cell Biology and Genetics, Dresden, Germany*
MIKE A. QUAIL • *Sequencing Research and Development, Wellcome Trust Sanger Institute, Cambridge, UK*
MARK REBEIZ • *Department of Biological Sciences, University of Pittsburgh, Pittsburgh, PA, USA*
SCOTT A. RIFKIN • *Division of Biological Sciences, Section of Ecology, Behavior and Evolution, University of California, San Diego, CA, USA*
MATTHEW V. ROCKMAN • *Department of Biology and Center for Genomics and Systems Biology, New York University, New York, USA*
DAVID M. ROWELL • *Department of Evolution, Ecology and Genetics, Research School of Biology, Australian National University, Canberra, ACT, Australia*
MIHAIL SAROV • *Max Planck Institute of Molecular Cell Biology and Genetics, Dresden, Germany*
SARAH SIMS • *Sequencing, DNA Pipelines, Wellcome Trust Sanger Institute, Cambridge, UK*
A. FRANCIS STEWART • *Max Planck Institute of Molecular Cell Biology and Genetics, Dresden, Germany*

JAY F. STORZ • *School of Biological Sciences, University of Nebraska, Lincoln, NE, USA*
PAVEL TOMANCAK • *Max Planck Institute of Molecular Cell Biology and Genetics, Dresden, Germany*
YOSHINORI TOMOYASU • *Department of Zoology, Miami University, Oxford, OH, USA*
HEIKO VOGEL • *Department of Entomology, Max Planck Institute for Chemical Ecology, Jena, Germany*
CHRISTOPHER W. WHEAT • *Department of Biological and Environmental Sciences, University of Helsinki, Helsinki, Finland;Centre for Ecology and Conservation, School of Biosciences, University of Exeter, Cornwall Campus, UK*
THOMAS M. WILLIAMS • *Department of Biology, University of Dayton, Dayton, OH, USA*
PATRICIA J. WITTKOPP • *University of Michigan, Ann Arbor, MI, USA*
SHOZO YOKOYAMA • *Emory University, Atlanta, GA, USA*
ANTHONY J. ZERA • *School of Biological Sciences, University of Nebraska, Lincoln, NE, USA*

# Abbreviations

| | |
|---|---|
| aDNA | Ancient DNA |
| Ara | Arabinose |
| BAC | Bacterial artificial chromosome |
| BSA | Bovine serum albumin |
| CHEF | Clamped homogeneous electric field |
| Cm | Chloramphenicol |
| CRE | Cis-regulatory element |
| ddH2O | Double-distilled water |
| DMSO | Dimethylsulfoxide |
| DSN | Duplex-specific nuclease |
| EDTA | Ethylene diamine tetraacetic acid |
| EGFP | Enhanced green fluorescent protein |
| FCS | Foetal calf serum |
| FRT | Flippase recombination target |
| HBSS | Hank's balanced saline solution |
| HCS | Head capsule slippage |
| HMP | High melting point |
| iPCR | Inverse PCR |
| LB | Luria-Bertani broth |
| LMP | Low melting point |
| OTE | Off-target effect |
| PBS | Phosphate-buffered saline |
| PCR | Polymerase chain reaction |
| PFGE | Pulse-field gel electrophoresis |
| PI | Propidium iodide |
| RISC | RNA-induced silencing complex |
| RT-PCR | Reverse transcription-polymerase chain reaction |
| SDS | Sodium dodecyl sulfate |
| SEM | Scanning electron microscopy |
| SOC | Super optimal broth with catabolite repression |
| SRD | Sequencing reaction diluent |
| ss | single stranded |
| SSC | Saline-sodium citrate |
| SSH | Sonic hedgehog |

| | |
|---|---|
| TBE | Tris/borate/EDTA |
| TE | Tris/EDTA |
| UV | UltraViolet |
| qRT-PCR | Quantitative reverse transcription-polymerase chain reaction |
| siRNA | Small interfering RNA |
| YENB | Yeast extract, nutrient broth |
| v | Volume |
| vol | Volume |
| w | Weight |

# Part I

## Characterizing the Genome

# Chapter 1

## Genome Size Determination Using Flow Cytometry of Propidium Iodide-Stained Nuclei

**Emily E. Hare and J. Spencer Johnston**

### Abstract

With the rapid expansion of whole-genome sequencing and other genomic studies in nonmodel organisms, there is a growing demand for robust and user-friendly methods for estimating eukaryotic genome sizes across a broad range of taxa. Propidium iodide (PI) staining with flow cytometry is a powerful method for genome sizing because it is relatively fast, works with a wide variety of materials, and provides information on a very large number of nuclei. In this method, nuclei are stained with PI, which intercalates into the major groove of DNA. Unknown samples are typically costained with standard nuclei of a known genome size, and the relative fluorescence is used to calculate the genome size of the unknown.

**Key words:** Genome size, Propidium iodide, Flow cytometry, *C*-value

## 1. Introduction

With the availability of genome sizes for thousands of eukaryotic organisms determined during the last 50 years, a fascinating picture is emerging regarding the function of and constraints on genome size. Genome size has been shown to correlate with numerous organismal characteristics, including egg size and developmental patterning mechanisms (1), cell size, mitotic and meiotic cell division rates, deletion rate, developmental rate, and body size (reviewed in (2)). However, the full spectrum of functional constraints on genome size is not yet understood and closely related taxa can have significantly different genome sizes, as in the *Drosophila melanogaster* subgroup species, *D. simulans* and *D. orena*, with 150 and 275 Mb genomes, respectively (3, 4). Lynch (5) has suggested that correlations may be due, not to direct genome size effects, but rather to differential responses to the

Virginie Orgogozo and Matthew V. Rockman (eds.), *Molecular Methods for Evolutionary Genetics*,
Methods in Molecular Biology, vol. 772, DOI 10.1007/978-1-61779-228-1_1, 

mutational hazard of mobile elements that is associated with species level effective population size differences. Ongoing research is addressing these and other questions in the field of genome-size evolution: What is the origin of noncoding DNA in eukaryotes, and what are the mechanisms for its expansion and reduction during evolution? What are the functions of this noncoding DNA, and why do some taxa have vast amounts of it while others have relatively little?

The substantial variation in genome sizes across even closely related taxa has significant implications for the rapidly expanding field of whole-genome sequencing and other genomic techniques, including the screening of whole-genome libraries. An accurate measurement of genome size is a necessary prerequisite for estimating clone coverage in shotgun sequencing and library screening and is essential for estimating the necessary read coverage for next-generation sequencing technologies. Thus, there is a high demand for robust and user-friendly methods for estimating genome sizes across a broad range of eukaryotic taxa.

The most commonly used methods for current genome sizing in eukaryotes are densitometry and flow cytometry. The first method utilizes Feulgen staining, in which nuclei are stained with Schiff's reagent, which stains DNA magenta. The intensity of magenta stain is measured with a densitometer, thus quantifying the amount of DNA in the nuclei. In the second method, nuclei are stained with propidium iodide (PI), which intercalates into the major groove of DNA and RNA without sequence preference, with one dye molecule per 4–5 bp (6). This binding enhances the fluorescence of PI by 20- to 30-fold, and the excitation and emission maxima are shifted (6). Unknown samples are typically costained with standard nuclei of a known genome size, RNA is removed by RNase, and the relative fluorescence of the DNA in the unknown and standard is used to calculate the genome size of the unknown. Relative fluorescence is quantified in a flow cytometer with a laser tuned to 488 or 514 nm (see Fig. 1).

PI staining with flow cytometry has the advantage that it is relatively fast, works with a wide variety of materials and provides information on a very large number of nuclei. A potential limitation of PI staining is that inhibitors and possibly chromatin condensation can bias the result (7). This limitation can be minimized by suitable choice of run conditions, the most important of which is the use of an internal standard that is coprepared with the sample. Attempts to use an external standard have led to estimates as low as 30% of the true genome size value (7). Feulgen densitometry, because it uses acid hydrolysis, is less sensitive to inhibitors and to chromatin condensation, but is not entirely free from inhibitor bias. Good practice, as described in (7, 8), remains the best protection against bias.

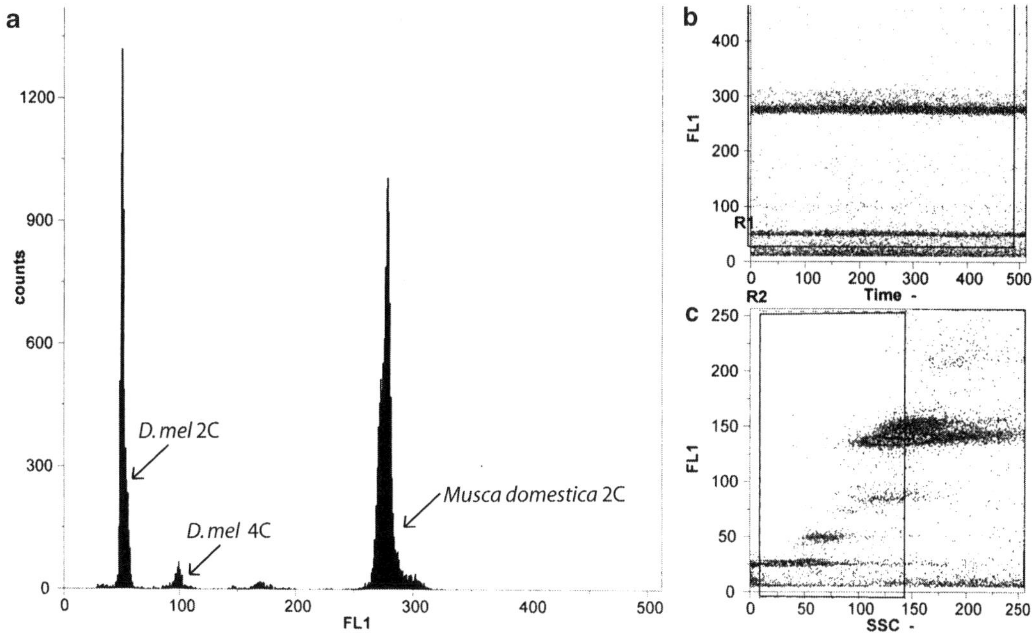


| Region | Gate | Ungated | Count | Count/ml | %Gated | Mean-x | CV-x% | Mean-y | CV-y% |
|---|---|---|---|---|---|---|---|---|---|
| R1 | <None> | 36720 | 36720 | - | 72.56 | 235.62 | 57.59 | 182.38 | 63.17 |
| R2 | <None> | 19861 | 19861 | - | 39.25 | 93.91 | 49.84 | 92.81 | 59.71 |

**d**

$$GS_{M.\ dom} = GS_{D.\ mel} \times \text{PI-fluor}_{M.\ dom} / \text{PI-fluor}_{D.\ mel}$$
$$= 175 \text{ Mb} \times 271.0/49.9$$
$$= 950.4 \text{ Mb}$$

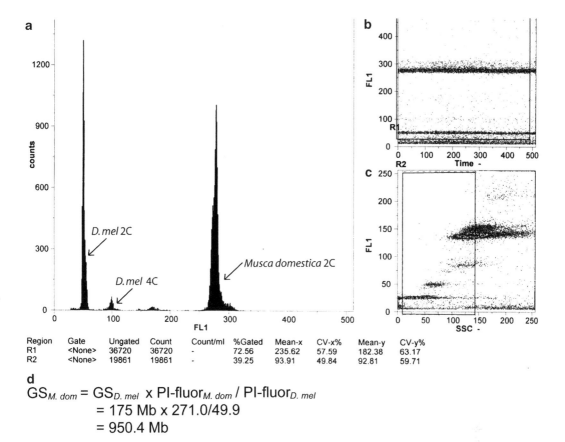

Fig. 1. Flow cytometry of propidium iodide-stained *Drosophila melanogaster* and *Musca domestica* nuclei. (**a**) A histogram showing the red fluorescence peaks of *D. melanogaster* 2C (channel 49.9) and 4C (channel 98.8) and *M. domestica* 2C (channel 271.0) nuclei. Note that the channel for the *D. melanogaster* 4C peak is twice that of the 2C peak, confirming linearity of the fluorescence measurements. (**b**) A cytogram showing red fluorescence (FL1) against time. A gate that selects only the perfectly flat portion of the run (R1) will produce usable data should a problem occur during the run. (**c**) A cytogram showing red fluorescence (FL1) against scattered light (SSC). Arthropod nuclei display a tight low-scatter pattern, while broken cells/nuclei with cytoplasmic tags scatter light broadly; therefore a gate (R2) that selects only the low-scatter nuclei can be used to eliminate not only debris, but also potential bias due to nuclei with adherent fluorescent tags. (**d**) The calculation of the *M. domestica* genome size (1C = 950.4 Mb) is based on the known *D. melanogaster* genome size and the relative red fluorescence in coprepared samples [175 Mb × (271.0/49.9)].

A new method that has been suggested for genome size estimation uses quantitative real-time PCR (qPCR) (9). Although a more time-consuming method than flow cytometry, qPCR would appear to have the advantage that it does not require nuclear isolation and can be conducted in a molecular laboratory, which typically will not have a flow cytometer or densitometer. However, to date, the qPCR method has provided estimates that are very much smaller than those from Feulgen densitometry and flow cytometry. The house fly, *Musca domestica*, for example, was estimated by this method to have a genome size of 295 Mb (9). Estimates from more conventional methods range from 870 to 1,017 Mb (10). An estimate of 950.4 Mb is shown using the methods presented here

(Fig. 1). Caution is thus suggested in use of a qPCR approach without corroboration from densitometry or flow cytometry.

The first step of genome sizing by PI staining is to isolate nuclei from a tissue sample of the organism of interest and a suitable standard. There is substantial variation in the methods for nuclear isolation depending on the organism and tissue type, so a single method optimized for arthropod samples is presented here. Suggestions for adapting the method to other organisms are provided. The purified nuclei are then stained with PI and run on a flow cytometer to measure the relative fluorescence of the unknown and internal standard samples, from which the genome size can be calculated. Detailed instructions for setting up the flow cytometer and troubleshooting the method are also included.

## 2. Materials

1. Fresh or frozen tissue samples for unknown(s) and standard(s) (see Notes 1–2 and Table 1).
2. Galbraith buffer: Dissolve 4.26 g $MgCl_2$, 8.84 g sodium citrate, 4.2 g 3-[*N*-morpholino] propane sulfonic acid ("MOPS"), 1 ml Triton X-100, and 1 mg boiled ribonuclease A into 1 l of $ddH_2O$. Adjust the pH to 7.2 with HCl and filter through a 0.22-μm filter. Store at 4°C.
3. A 2-ml or 7-ml glass Dounce tissue grinder with the A pestle (large-clearance pestle).
4. 20-μm nylon mesh filters.
5. 5-ml round bottom tubes (Falcon Cat# 352063). These tubes are compatible with Beckman-Coulter EPICS XL-MCL flow cytometers. See the manufacturer's instructions to determine the appropriate tubes for other instruments.

**Table 1**
**Suggested eukaryotic genome sizing standards**

| Sizing standard (see Note 12) | Suggested tissue source and starting amount | C-value (1C) |
|---|---|---|
| *Drosophila melanogaster* female | 1 adult head | 175 Mb |
| *Drosophila virilis* | 1 adult head | 328 Mb |
| *Gallus gallus domesticus* (white leghorn rooster) | 50 μl of freshly drawn or fresh frozen blood stored at −80°C in citrate buffer | 1,140 Mb |

6. Propidium iodide stock: Dissolve PI into $ddH_2O$ at a final concentration of 1 mg/ml (20×). PI is light-sensitive and once diluted should be stored at −20°C and wrapped in foil.
7. Flow cytometer with excitation between 488 and 530 nm and a long-pass filter to detect fluorescence above 590 nm.

## 3. Methods

The first step of the protocol (Subheading 3.1) is the isolation of intact nuclei from a tissue sample of the organism of interest. The tissue source and details of this step must be optimized for each organism, taking into consideration the ease of homogenization and the cell and nuclear diameters of different tissues. The goal is to isolate a significant number of nuclei whose DNA is unreplicated (G1 phase of the cell cycle) from soft tissue that is free of DNAase. For insects, this typically means neural tissue and blood cells from the head of an adult. The following protocol is optimized for nuclear isolation from arthropods (11), but Note 2 provides suggestions for other organisms. See also (10, 12, 13) for published tissue sources for diverse eukaryotic taxa. Prior to starting the procedure, appropriate standards should be obtained (see Note 1 and Table 1 for suggested standards).

Each time a new unknown and/or standard is used, an initial experiment must be performed to determine the nuclear yield from the chosen tissues and the appropriate ratio of unknown to standard (see Note 3). This process is described starting from Subheading 3.1, step 1a. After the individual samples have been optimized once, the protocol should be repeated starting from Subheading 3.1, step 1b to determine the genome size(s) of the unknown(s).

### *3.1. Isolation and Propidium Iodide Staining of Nuclei from Fresh or Frozen Tissue Samples*

1. Start at step 1a if using a new combination of unknown and standard samples. Proceed to step 1b if the individual samples have already been optimized.
   (a) Place each individual tissue sample into 1 ml of cold Galbraith buffer on ice (see Notes 3–6).
   (b) Place each pair of tissue samples (unknown + standard) into 1 ml of cold Galbraith buffer on ice. When possible, at least five technical replicates should be performed for each experimental sample.
2. Place each sample in a Dounce tissue grinder and stroke 15 times with an A pestle (see Note 7). Wash the Dounce thoroughly with filtered (0.2 μm) deionized water between samples.

3. Filter ground nuclear suspension through 20-μm nylon mesh to remove cellular debris and recover flow-through into a 5-ml round-bottomed tube on ice.
4. Add PI to samples to a final concentration of 50 μg/ml and cover samples with aluminum foil.
5. Allow samples to stain in the dark at 4°C for up to 24 h. The duration of staining must be determined empirically for each organism, but 30 min can be used as a starting point (see Note 8).

### 3.2. Instrumentation Setup Procedure for Flow Cytometry

Instrument setup can be problematic for operators used to running immunological samples. Rather than scoring all cells using scatter detection, DNA flow cytometry counts only red fluorescent nuclei, and the cytometer must be set to activate only on red fluorescence (>590 nm). Scatter (both forward and/or side) is used to gate out anything except whole, intact nuclei, which scatter very little light. Linearity is essential for accurate DNA determinations. The following guidelines will allow you to set up an appropriate protocol file for the flow cytometer and to make the necessary adjustments during sample runs to ensure reliable data.

1. Open a new parameter file according the manufacturer's instructions of the flow cytometer.
2. Set the cytometer to activate only on red fluorescence (>590 nm).
3. Set the flow rate to low (see Note 9).
4. During each sample run, it is essential to confirm the linearity of fluorescence measurements. To confirm linearity, check that the mean channel number of 4C (G2 phase) nuclei is exactly twice that of the 2C (G1-phase) nuclei of the standard (see Fig. 1). Often, this requires that voltage to the photomultiplier measuring red fluorescence be adjusted so that sample and standard means fall between 200 and 800.
5. During each sample run, confirm that the 2C peaks are symmetric about the mean. When the sample is skewed, it suggests overlap with another peak or degradation. If this is unavoidable, then the statistical gate should be set around the symmetric portion of the peak (see Fig. 1).

### 3.3. Flow Cytometry of PI-Stained Samples and Data Analysis

1. After following the manufacturer-recommended start-up procedures for the flow cytometer, load the PI genome sizing protocol generated in Subheading 3.2.
2. Invert samples several times to resuspend and then load the first tube onto the cytometer.
3. Initiate the protocol and run each sample until approximately 1,000 counts are collected under each of the unknown and standard 2C peaks (see Note 9 and Fig. 1).

4. If performing the initial experiment on individual samples (from Subheading 3.1, step 1a), proceed to step 4a. If sizing combined experimental samples (from Subheading 3.1, step 1b), proceed to step 4b.
   (a) Use the unknown-alone and standard-alone samples to determine the locations of the unknown and standard 2C peaks. If the unknown and standard peaks overlap or are too far apart, it will be necessary to choose another standard. If the peak separation is acceptable, use the peak heights for the unknown and standard 2C peaks to estimate the appropriate initial amounts of sample and standard for the combined experimental sample, and repeat the protocol starting from Subheading 3.1, step 1b to determine the unknown genome size.
   (b) Use the tools in the flow cytometer to set the statistical gates for the unknown and standard 2C peaks within each sample. This can often be done while the data are being collected (see Fig. 1 and Note 10).
5. Calculate the genome size of unknowns from the channel numbers of the 2C peaks using the following formula:

$$GS_{\text{unknown}} = GS_{\text{standard}} \times \text{PI - fluor}_{\text{unknown}} \,/\, \text{PI - fluor}_{\text{standard}}$$

where GS = genome size and PI-fluor = the channel number of red PI fluorescence (see Fig. 1 and Note 11).

### 3.4. Troubleshooting

Table 2 includes common problems encountered during this procedure and recommendations for remedying the problems.

## 4. Notes

1. Choosing an appropriate standard for genome sizing can be challenging due to the extensive evolution of genome size even in fairly closely related organisms. *C*-values (1C = the genome size of a "hypothetical" gamete) for related taxa should be used as a starting point for selecting a standard, but the standard may need to be revised after initial sizing experiments. There are several databases available online that compile genome size data for various eukaryotic phyla (2, 10).
2. For genome sizing, choose cells with a low mitotic index and a large proportion of 2C nuclei. Typically, blood cells and neural adult brain tissue meet these criteria. In insects, it can be a challenge to identify 2C nuclei if the levels of endoreduplication and possible under-replication are high. Additionally, DNA synthesis can skew the 2C peak, inflating the mean.

**Table 2**
**Troubleshooting PI staining and flow cytometry**

| Symptom | Likely cause | Suggested actions |
|---|---|---|
| The calculated size of the positive control does not agree with the published value | The standard for the positive control lies outside of the linear range<br>One of the samples did not stain completely with PI | Repeat experiment with two samples with more similar genome sizes<br>Perform a saturation curve to ensure that both samples are stained completely |
| There is a broad peak at low fluorescence channel numbers | The samples were ground too forcefully, resulting in sheared nuclei | Repeat nuclear prep, being sure to grind the samples gently (stirring vs. grinding) |
| There is only a single tall peak | Too much of one of the samples was added, swamping the signal from the other peak | Dilute the concentrated sample before PI staining |
| The genome size estimate based on separate preparations of sample and standard (external standard) is significantly lower that the estimate based on a copreparation of sample and standard (internal standard) | The tissue used for the unknown sample likely contained inhibitors that prevent PI binding | Use a different tissue type |

Insect sperm is not a good choice for flow cytometry. Insect sperm DNA, unless treated with acid hydrolysis as in Feulgen densitometry, does not take up PI well, which will result in gross underestimates of genome size with flow cytometry.

3. Although it is recommended that sample and standard be prepared, stained, and run as a combined sample for estimates of DNA content, it is always good practice to run at least a portion of the sample first without the standard. This best allows one to identify all the different diploid and endoreduplicated peaks in the unknown sample. Failure to take this step with a new unknown can result in the misidentification of the sample 2C peak, as it may not be the dominant peak, or may be obscured by a standard peak.

4. Use Table 1 as a starting point for the type and amount of tissue for the suggested standards. The relative amounts of unknown and standard sample tissue may need to be adjusted

after initial sizing experiments so that the PI fluorescence peaks are of similar heights. A single dissected head is optimal for most *Drosophila* species. For organisms of different sizes, the tissue amount or volume of Galbraith buffer should be adjusted accordingly.

5. Accurate sizing experiments have been performed with samples frozen and stored at –80°C (14). If fresh samples are unavailable, try the same procedure with frozen samples.
6. The sex of the sample should be reported with the genome size estimate. There can be substantial differences in genome sizes between males and females (15), which may need to be taken into account depending on the application.
7. The technique during the grinding step is important. Too much grinding will destroy nuclei, creating debris that can obscure the smallest 2C peak; too little grinding will result in poor yields. The material should be crushed at the bottom of the Dounce before beginning the grinding. Strokes should be performed at a rate of one per second – the motion feels more like stirring than grinding.
8. To determine the appropriate length of staining, a saturation curve should be run to ensure that both the unknown and standard samples reach similar levels of saturation. The optimal stain time is determined by comparing the ratio of the mean fluorescence of the unknown 2C and standard 2C peaks from nuclei that were stained for increasing lengths of time. The appropriate staining time is a time period after which this ratio has plateaued. An initial run with stain times of 20, 40, 60, and 120 min should be sufficient to determine the best stain time.
9. For best results, samples should be run as slowly as possible. This can mean that a single sample may take 5–10 min to run, a much longer run time than used for immunological samples. A typical run for well-prepared samples is approximately 5 min and 6,000 total counts. There is no hard and fast rule on the number of nuclei that must be counted; typically, the 2C peak of the unknown and the standard will not change after 1,000 nuclei are scored in each.
10. If the samples are badly skewed, the peak rather than the mean may be most appropriate. It is recommended to estimate the genome size using both the average and the peak, and then use the estimator that gives the lower standard error.
11. This calculation assumes that the PI fluorescence is linear across the range of the unknown and standard. Thus, a standard should be chosen that is close in size to the unknown sample. If the original standard choice is too far from the unknown, choose a more appropriate standard to repeat the experiment.

12. To verify a new standard, choose an available organism with a known genome size based on a reliable source (whole-genome sequence, published PI staining). Run this sample in the same way as you would an unknown, first individually and then in combination with another standard. Calculate the genome size of the new standard based on the copreparation and compare this value to the published genome size. If the two are in agreement, then (and only then) should the new standard be used for subsequent experiments.

## References

1. Schmidt-Ott U, Rafiqi AM, Sander K, Johnston JS (2009) Extremely small genomes in two unrelated dipteran insects with shared early developmental traits. Dev Genes Evol **219**: 207–210.
2. Gregory TR (2005) The C-value enigma in plants and animals: a review of parallels and an appeal for partnership. Annals of Botany **95**:133–146.
3. Gregory TR, Johnston JS (2008) Genome size diversity in the family Drosophilidae. Heredity **101**:228–238.
4. Bosco G, Campbell P, Leiva-Neto JT, Markow TA (2007) Analysis of Drosophila species genome size and satellite DNA content reveals significant differences among strains as well as between species. Genetics **177**:1277–1290.
5. Lynch M (2006) The origins of eukaryotic gene structure. Mol Biol Evol **23**:450–468.
6. Waring M (1965) Complex formation between ethidium bromide and nucleic acids. Journal of Molecular Biology **13**:269–282.
7. Bennett MD, Price HJ, Johnston JS (2008) Anthocyanin inhibits propidium iodide DNA fluorescence in *Euphorbia pulcherrima*: implications for genome size variation and flow cytometry. Annals of Botany **101**: 777–790.
8. Dolezel J (2005) Plant DNA flow cytometry and estimation of nuclear genome size. Annals of Botany **95**:99–110.
9. Gao J, Scott JG (2006) Use of quantitative real-time polymerase chain reaction to estimate the size of the house-fly *Musca domestica* genome. Insect Mol Biol **15**:835–837.
10. Gregory T (2010) The Animal Genome Size Database. http://www.genomesize.com.
11. Bennett MD, Leitch IJ, Price HJ, Johnston JS (2003) Comparisons with *Caenorhabditis* (100 Mb) and *Drosophila* (175 Mb) using flow cytometry show genome size in *Arabidopsis* to be 157 Mb and thus 25% Larger than the *Arabidopsis* Genome Initiative estimate of 125 Mb. Annals of Botany **91**:547–557.
12. Kullman B, Tamm H, Kullman K (2005) The Fungal Genome Size Database. http://www.zbi.ee/fungal-genomesize.
13. Bennett M, Leitch I (2005) The Plant DNA C-values Database. http://data.kew.org/cvalues.
14. Hare EE, Peterson BK, Iyer VN et al (2008) Sepsid even-skipped enhancers are functionally conserved in *Drosophila* despite lack of sequence conservation. PLoS Genetics **4**:e1000106.
15. Johnston JS, Ross LD, Hughes DP et al (2004) Tiny genomes and endoreduplication in Strepsiptera. Insect Mol. Biol **13**:581–585.

# Chapter 2

# Chromosome Analysis in Invertebrates and Vertebrates

David M. Rowell, Shu Ly Lim, and Frank Grutzner

## Abstract

The revolution in molecular techniques over the last 30 years detracted from many traditional cytological techniques for examining basic biological problems. One of these casualties is the preparation of karyotypes and analysis of chromosomal structure, behaviour, and variation. Recent technology permitting the full sequencing of organisms has highlighted (but does not replace) the importance of understanding chromosomal constitution and karyotype structure, which underpin genome organisation. This chapter provides simple and straightforward protocols for the preparation of chromosome spreads from animals, and more advanced techniques for cell culture and chromosomal banding and hybridisation.

**Key words:** Chromosomes, Invertebrate genetics, Cytological techniques, Karyology, Cell culture, Fluorescence in situ hybridisation

## 1. Introduction

### *1.1. Background*

Much of the early work in genetics focussed on chromosomal variation and chromosomal behaviour. However, with the advent of techniques focussing on single genes (initially allozyme electrophoresis) and more recently microarray technology and mass DNA sequencing of entire genomes, the focus of pure genetic research shifted away from cytogenetics, leaving unsolved many problems that could only be answered using chromosomal techniques. These included questions revolving around genome organisation in the nucleus, sex chromosome constitution, coadapted gene complexes, and evolutionary problems such as chromosomal speciation. Indeed, whole-genome sequencing projects are already in progress on species for which even basic karyotypic information is lacking.

In recent years, there has been a resurgence of interest in chromosome structure, behaviour, evolution, and the organisation of the genome in the context of the nucleus. In these studies, the use

Virginie Orgogozo and Matthew V. Rockman (eds.), *Molecular Methods for Evolutionary Genetics*,
Methods in Molecular Biology, vol. 772, DOI 10.1007/978-1-61779-228-1_2, © Springer Science+Business Media, LLC 2011

of modern molecular techniques has been a valuable addition to the range of tools available. Nevertheless, most chromosomal studies still require basic chromosomal preparation and microscope use. Ironically, with the decline of traditional cytology, rather than taking the obvious approach of simply looking at the chromosomes themselves, many recent studies have used complex molecular tools to ask simple questions regarding chromosome number and sex determining systems – "If your only tool is a hammer, every problem looks like a nail."

With the surge of sequencing capacity at dramatically declining cost, we see many species being fully sequenced, but often at low coverage (for example, cat and tammar wallaby (1)) or using short read sequencing technology (2). This often leads to patchy assemblies and little or no information on the chromosomal position of sequence contigs. Physical maps can help assemblies and provide additional information (for example, gene order), and it is surprising that in many species already sequenced basic cytogenetic information is not available. In turn the wealth of genomic information and clones provided by genome projects provide fantastic resources for further cytological research and ambitious plans to sequence 10,000 vertebrate species will open great opportunities for cytological research (3). However, even in species where we do not have the luxury of a genome sequence, cytogenetic information, including karyotypes, banding patterns and markers (rDNA clusters, telomeres, centromeres, and blocks of heterochromatin), and identification of sex chromosomes can provide invaluable information on genome organisation and evolution.

In biodiversity studies, chromosomal analysis has also revealed a wealth of cryptic species that are otherwise indistinguishable from one another (see Figs. 1–4) (4–6). As chromosomal variation often corresponds with or directly causes reproductive isolation, conservation management plans that fail to consider chromosomal variation risk wasted expenditure and species extinction.

Amongst well-studied model organisms such as humans, mice, and *Drosophila*, well-established protocols have been developed (7), and "kits" are available for carrying out simple karyotyping and more complex techniques such as fluorescence in situ hybridisation (FISH) and chromosome banding. However, different organisms require unique variations to these standard protocols, requiring an understanding of the basic principles behind chromosomal preparation and analysis. We have worked on basic and molecular karyology in various disparate species including velvet worms, spiders, insects, fish, reptiles, and mammals. For each new species, we have adapted protocols for direct preparation of chromosomes and culturing of cells, as well as chromosome spreading, banding, and hybridisation procedures. This chapter discusses the main steps in chromosomal preparation for the light microscope and outlines protocols that are successful in invertebrates and vertebrates.

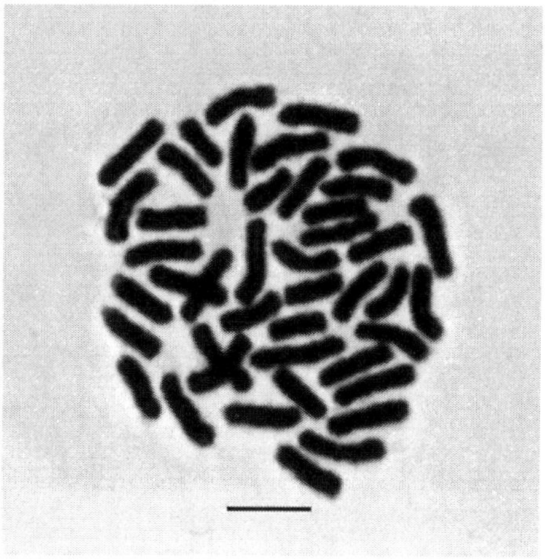

Fig. 1. Giemsa-stained mitosis from an Australian huntsman spider, prepared from embryonic material. Males of this species have 43 chromosomes, which are rod shaped, as their centromere is located at one extreme end of each chromosome. This is the ancestral karyotype for endemic Australian huntsman spider genera. The separate sister chromatids are not clearly discernible in this preparation. Scale bar = 5 μm.

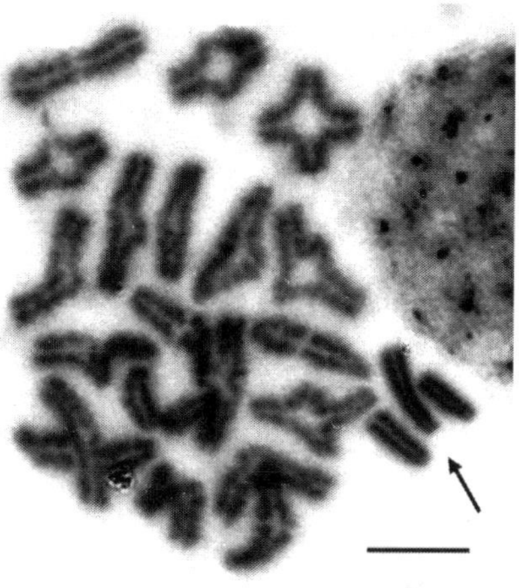

Fig. 2. Giemsa-stained meiosis from the same species as Fig. 1, prepared from testis material. This preparation shows 20 bivalents and three unpaired X-chromosomes (*arrow*). From this, it can be deduced that sex is determined by three X-chromosomes in the male and six in the female. This is borne out by comparison with mitosis from female embryos, where 46 chromosomes are visible. Scale bar = 5 μm.

The methods described here provide a set of tools that only require access to biological material and basic lab equipment and basic microscopy. More complex protocols may require access to a basic molecular laboratory, advanced microscopy (epifluorescence), and tissue culture facilities. With these protocols as a starting point, researchers can develop protocols specific to their organism and troubleshoot any difficulties they may have.

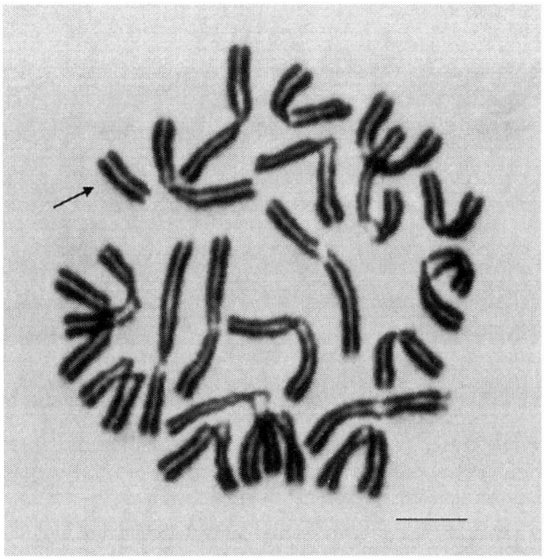

Fig. 3. Giemsa-stained mitosis from an Australian huntsman spider closely related to those in Figs. 1 and 2, prepared from testis material. This karyotype is derived from the ancestral karyotype (Fig. 1) by multiple centric fusions whereby each telocentric chromosome in the ancestral form has fused to another chromosome at the centromere (centric fusion), resulting in telocentric chromosomes twice the length of those in Fig. 1. As the number of chromosomes in the ancestral male karyotype is odd, one unfused chromosome remains in this karyotype (*arrow*). In this karyotype, the individual sister chromatids of each chromosome are clearly visible. Many populations of huntsman spider have been shown to differ in the presence of these fusions, despite the absence of any morphological variation (26). Scale bar = 5 μm.

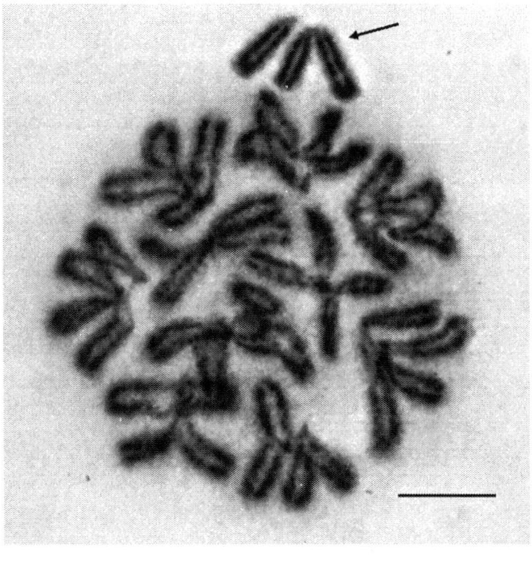

Fig. 4. Giemsa-stained meiosis prepared from testis material from the same individual as in Fig. 3. The wholesale fusion of the karyotype results in ten large bivalents (cf. (20) in Fig. 2). Two of the three X-chromosomes seen in Fig. 2 have fused, and the remaining, unfused chromosome arrowed in Fig. 3 is the third X-chromosome. Scale bar = 5 μm.

### 1.2. Chromosomal Banding

Numerous treatments have been developed to visualise characteristics of chromatin structure and density variation along the length of a chromosome. These techniques include G-, C-, and R-banding, each of which highlights different aspects of chromatin differentiation, and NOR staining. G- and R- banding is indirectly associated with variation in AT and GC richness, while C-banding highlights heterochromatin-rich regions on chromosomes, and NOR staining permits the visualisation of ribosomal gene clusters (7). In larval Diptera and some other insect groups, endoreduplication in polytene chromosomes permits direct visualisation of variations in chromosome density. Banding techniques permit the identification of homologues, and the visualisation of major chromosomal rearrangements such as fusions, fissions, or inversions (8). Banding techniques are highly dependent on the organism of study – for example, G-banding is only reliable in higher vertebrates – and the development of these techniques for new taxa is very much a process of trial and error. As a starting point for the development of banding techniques, the reader is referred to the protocols given in Czepulkowski (7).

### 1.3. Tissues Used for Chromosome Preparation

While chromosomes exist as discrete entities throughout the cell cycle, in most species it is only at cell division that they can be observed visually and their morphology and behaviour analysed. Thus, chromosomal preparation requires the use of living cells (not frozen), and samples for chromosomal preparation must be derived from tissues in which cells are actively dividing, such as gut lining, digestive gland, spleen, and embryonic tissue (9) (see Fig. 1). Testis tissue yields mitotic and meiotic cells (see Figs. 2–4). Meiotic metaphase spreads can be used for chromosome counting (counting bivalents in meiotic metaphase I) and characterisation of sex chromosome systems (e.g. by detection of unpaired DNA in heteromorphic sex chromosomes) (see Figs. 2 and 4). Ovary tissue can yield meiotic and mitotic preparations in some species; however, cell division in ovaries is much slower and success is reduced proportionally. Plant tissues most commonly used for chromosome preparation are root tips and anthers (the latter yielding meiotic preparations). Material from cell culture is also suitable. This chapter does not discuss the preparation of plant chromosomes, as this is dealt with in considerable detail elsewhere (10, 11).

Direct preparation of chromosomes using the tissues described above is by far the simplest means of visualising chromosomes. However, if available tissue is limited, cell division can be stimulated through *in vitro* cell culture, including short-term stimulation of lymphocytes or establishment of fibroblast cell lines. Some cell culture techniques are straightforward and robust; we have established fibroblast cell lines (see Fig. 5 for an example of an explant culture) from various tissues (skin, heart tip, eye, toe web) from road-killed animals (mammals and birds) and from biopsies that have been stored in culture medium (at room temperature) for almost two weeks before culturing. Culture protocols for lymphocytes have been published elsewhere (12–14).

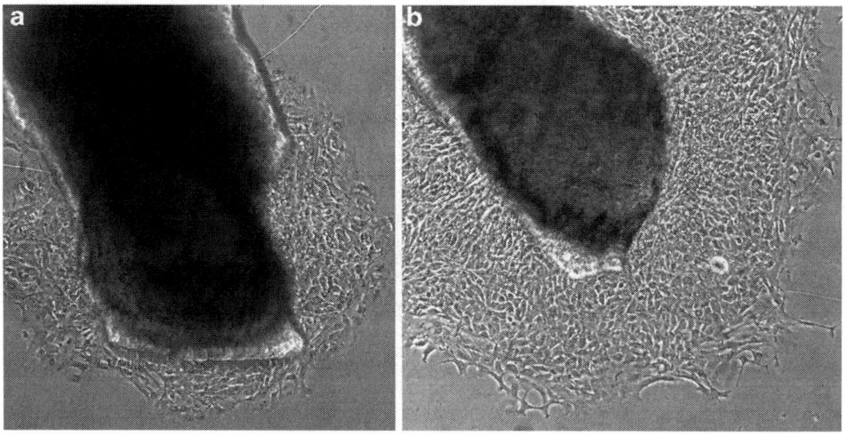

Fig. 5. Fibroblasts growing from platypus toe-web tissue (×100). (**a**) After about 1 week of culturing a ring of fibroblast cells grows around the planted tissue piece. (**b**) Same culture after another 2 weeks culturing. If there are several pieces showing a growth like this, the cells can be harvested and split into passage 1.

### 1.4. Basic Principles of Chromosomal Preparation and Troubleshooting Tips

Chromosome preparation techniques for karyotyping, chromosome banding or FISH usually involve three common steps. With an understanding of the significance of these steps, it is possible to troubleshoot problems and make appropriate modifications to suit the particular species under analysis.

1. The enrichment of metaphase plates by inhibition of microtubule polymerisation (15). When cells are exposed to colchicine, microtubules fail to form and mitosis is arrested at metaphase. Thus, colchicine treatment of tissue *in vitro* or *in vivo* results in an accumulation of metaphase cells (see Fig. 6). Different species respond differently to colchicine, so it may be necessary to vary concentrations as appropriate (for example, we have found that colchicine, even at extremely low concentrations, is lethal to onychophoran cells). Although colchicine arrests the progress of meiosis, chromosomes will continue to contract. Thus, if tissue is treated with colchicine for too long, the chromosomes will appear as very short, squat structures, with little clear morphology. If treatment is too short, few spreads will be visible. In particular, it is important in cell culture to identify when cells divide to decide when to add the colchicine to obtain high frequency of metaphase plates (see Fig. 6).
2. Hypotonic treatment before fixation to swell the cells, leading to spreading of the metaphase plate. The introduction of the hypotonic step revolutionised karyology (16). The basic principle behind this is that if cells are exposed to a solution that is hypotonic to their internal electrolyte concentration, water will move into the cell by osmosis, resulting in swelling, leading to even spreading of chromosomes, reducing clumping and overlaps. Hypotonic solutions specific to particular species are given

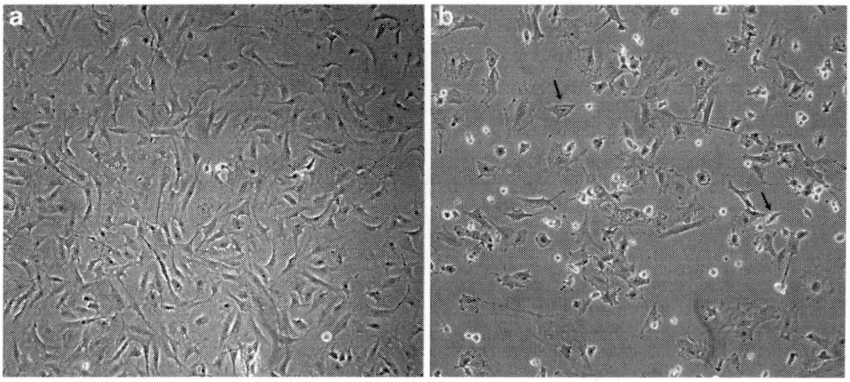

Fig. 6. Metaphase chromosome preparation from fibroblasts after Colcemid treatment. (**a**) Phase-contrast image of normal growing fibroblasts (×100). (**b**) 2 h Colcemid-treated fibroblasts (×100). Under normal culturing condition, fibroblasts are long and spindle-shaped. After Colcemid treatment, fibroblasts rounded up (*arrows*) as cells enter metaphase.

in the protocols below. A general rule of thumb is that hypotonic solution should be approximately half the concentration of the standard saline used for that species. If there is no standard, some experimentation may be necessary. In the case of marine invertebrates (which tend to be internally isotonic with seawater), a saline that is isotonic with seawater, or seawater itself, may be appropriate. For vertebrates, Hank's balanced saline solution may be a good starting point, and for terrestrial or aquatic invertebrates, insect saline is a good choice. If the hypotonic solution is too dilute, cells will burst, and loose chromosomes will be visible on slides. If the hypotonic solution is too concentrated, clumps of overlapping chromosomes will be visible, making it impossible to obtain accurate counts or to prepare karyograms.

3. Fixation, usually by freshly prepared methanol (or ethanol) acetic acid. Fixation prevents tissue degradation through the action of biologically active molecules and preserves the morphology of the chromosomes during preparation. Poor fixation results in a lack of clear definition to the chromosomes – such as fuzzy edges and chromosomes that appear contorted rather than relatively straight. In our experience, poor fixation usually results from fix that is not freshly made, an unidentified problem with the acetic acid (some batches of acetic acid simply do not work, even though they may be adequate for other purposes), or insufficient fixation time.

In animals, the main technique for preparing chromosomes is direct preparation from actively dividing tissue. However, improved cell culture techniques have made it possible to establish short- or long-term cell cultures in many vertebrates, and these are routinely used in birds, reptiles, and mammals.

The first three protocols presented below are for direct preparation from dividing tissue and can be carried out in the field. Subsequent protocols involve the use of cell culture techniques. Information about viewing of chromosomal preparations is provided after preparation protocols.

All of the protocols below result in the production of a layer of air-dried chromosomes over the surface of a glass slide. Before use, commercial glass microscope slides usually need to be treated by washing (even if the manufacturer claims they are prewashed). Slides can be pretreated in large numbers and stored indefinitely before use. Commonly, slides are pretreated with washes in 0.01 N HCl or 1% SDS for 6 h, and thoroughly washed in filtered water. In many cases, a vigorous cleaning using ethanol and lint-free wipes (Kimwipes) will suffice. Note that there are different quality slides and changing your supplier may affect the spreading of the cells.

## 2. Materials

### *2.1. Direct Preparation of Meiotic and Mitotic Chromosomes from Vertebrates and Invertebrates*

1. Washed slides.
2. Crystal glasses or watch glasses with flat glass covers.
3. 3-mm diameter brass rod. This can be bought at hardware stores or metal shops. The end must be flattened and smoothed with a grinding stone or equivalent. Its length should be sufficient to hold it easily for tapping out tissues (ballpoint pen length is appropriate).
4. Pasteur pipettes.
5. 37°C hotplate.
6. Coplin jar or equivalent container in which slides can be placed and immersed in liquid.
7. 60% Acetic acid.
8. Fixative: 3:1 methanol–acetic acid (fresh).
9. Insect saline: 7.0 g NaCl, 0.2 g $CaCl_2$ per litre of solution (see Note 1).
10. Phosphate buffer: 1.0 g $KH_2PO_4$, 2.0 g $NaH_2PO_4.12\ H_2O$ per litre of solution. Adjust pH to 6.8 with NaOH or HCl.
11. Giemsa stain. This is a compound stain that can be purchased as a powder, but we recommend purchasing it in liquid form (dissolved in methanol). Manufacturers rarely list ingredients or concentrations, but all commercial solutions appear to be of roughly the same concentration. In our experience, there is considerable variation in the results achieved using different

brand products, and some give better results with certain species. We have found Giemsa stain lasts indefinitely and may even improve with age.

12. 0.002% Colchicine in insect saline (powder, also sold as Colcemid (trademark of Ciba Geigy AG) and Demecolcine (Sigma-Aldrich)).

### *2.2. Direct Preparation of Metaphase Chromosomes from Kidney, Gills or Spleen (Fish)*

1. Centrifuge.
2. Glass pipettes.
3. Ice.
4. Colchicine (10 μg/ml in HBSS).
5. Hypotonic solution: 0.075 M KCl or 50% foetal calf serum (FCS) in water.
6. Fixative: 3:1 methanol–glacial acetic acid. Freshly made and stored at −20°C.
7. Hank's balanced saline solution (HBSS), purchased from suppliers.

### *2.3. Direct Preparation from Bone Marrow (Mouse)*

1. 0.1 mg/ml Colcemid solution.
2. 2-ml Syringe.
3. Each of the items listed in Subheading 2.2.

### *2.4. Chromosome Preparation from Cultured Fibroblast Cells*

1. 500 ml DMEM supplemented with 15% FCS, penicillin, streptomycin, and l-glutamine. Alternatively, combine 500 ml AmnioMAX C-100 (GibcoBRL) and 50 ml AmnioMAX C-100 supplement.
2. Medium for cell culture from fish (prepared according to Collodi and Barnes (17)). This medium is a variation from routinely used media. The basic medium is 80% DMEM/F12 and 20% Leibovitz's L15. This is then supplemented to 15% FCS, l-glutamine (2 mM), penicillin–streptomycin (final concentration is 100 U/ml penicillin, 100 μg/ml streptomycin), HEPES buffer (final concentration 5 mM), and MEM non-essential amino acids (final concentration 50 μM). Several growth factors are added: bovine insulin (final concentration 10 μg/ml), β-mercaptoethanol (final concentration 50 μM), human epidermal growth factor (final concentration 20 ng/ml, dissolve in PBS), human fibroblast growth factor, basic (final concentration 2 ng/ml, dissolve in PBS), and sodium selenite (final concentration 2.5 nM, dissolve in sterile water). Because of the growth factors, this medium should be made up only in small quantities and used only for up to a week.
3. Phosphate-buffered saline (PBS; cell culture grade).
4. 1× Trypsin solution (0.25%, 2.5 g/l) (cell culture grade).

5. Medium for collecting material (high concentration of antibiotic and antifungal agents): In 100 ml plain DMEM (HEPES), add 2 ml of kanamycin (50 mg/ml), 4.7 μl of chloramphenicol (34 mg/ml), 100 μl of penicillin–streptomycin (our solution contains 10,000 U/ml penicillin and 10,000 μg/ml streptomycin). In addition to the antibiotics, fungicide is added: 160 μl of amphotericin B (250 μg/ml) and 50 μl of tetracyclin (20 mg/ml).
6. Medium for freezing cells: 10% DMSO, 10%, FCS, and 80% DMEM. After mixing the ingredients, cool the medium down in a 4°C fridge until used, and prepare fresh for each experiment.

### 2.5. Fluorescence In Situ Hybridisation

1. Metaphase spreads on slides prepared using any of the protocols described.
2. Genomic DNA (male/female) from different species isolated using standard procedures. The DNA can be isolated by basic phenol chloroform isolation or kit spin column and tested on an agarose gel.
3. Saline sodium citrate (20× SSC) (pH 7.0): 175.3 g sodium chloride (NaCl) (3 M), 88.2 g sodium citrate ($Na_3C_6H_5O_7{\cdot}2H_2O$) (0.3 M) per 1 L of water. Adjust pH to 7.0 with 10 N NaOH and sterilise by autoclaving.
4. Phosphate-buffered saline (10× PBS): 79.5 g sodium chloride (NaCl) (1.4 mM), 1.5 g potassium chloride (KCl) (20 mM) 15 g sodium phosphate, dibasic ($Na_2HPO_4$) (106 mM), 2 g potassium phosphate, monobasic ($KH_2PO_4$) (15 mM) in 1 L distilled water. Adjust pH to 7.2–7.4 and autoclave.
5. RNAse (100 mg/ml): 1 g RNAse A (powder) (100 mg/ml), 33 μl 3 M sodium acetate (10 mM) in distilled water to 10 ml. Boil for 10 min to inactivate DNAse.
6. 10% Pepsin in water, final concentration 0.005% pepsin/0.001 M HCl.
7. Formaldehyde.
8. 1 M $MgCl_2$.
9. Formamide.
10. Rinsing solution 1 (50 mM $MgCl_2$/1× PBS): 2.5 ml 1 M $MgCl_2$ in 47.5 ml 1× PBS.
11. Rinsing solution 2 (50 mM $MgCl_2$/1% formaldehyde/1× PBS): 2.5 ml 1 M $MgCl_2$, 1.25 ml 40% formaldehyde in 46.25 ml 1× PBS.
12. Denaturing solution (70% formamide/2× SSC): 35 ml formamide and 15 ml 2× SSC.
13. Washing solution 1 (50% formamide/2× SSC): 75 ml formamide and 75 ml 2× SSC.

14. Formamide (deionised).
15. Hybridisation mixture (20% dextran sulphate/4× SSC). Use High Molecular Weight Dextran Sulphate (Sigma).
16. Ethanol (methylated and unmethylated).
17. DAPI solution. Make a 0.2 μg/ml working solution by dissolving 10 μl of a 1 mg/ml stock in 50 ml 2× SSC.
18. Mounting medium (Vectashield).
19. Rubber cement (e.g. tyre glue from the bike shop).

*Labelling materials and solutions as follows*:

20. Salmon sperm DNA (Sigma).
21. 9-mer random primer.
22. MQ water.
23. Exonuclease-free Klenow Polymerase (5 U/μl) and 5× Klenow buffer (New England Biolabs).
24. Fluorescent-Dye (Spectrum Orange and Spectrum Green dUTPs, Vysis). The 50 nmol pellet is diluted in 50 μl water, aliquoted, and stored at −20°C.

## 3. Methods

### 3.1. Direct Preparation of Meiotic and Mitotic Chromosomes from Vertebrates and Invertebrates

The technique as described below was developed for visualising spider meiosis and spermatogonial mitosis, and alternative tissues and modifications are described under Notes. The authors have had success using this protocol with minor modification on a range of invertebrate and vertebrate species for mitotic and meiotic preparations (for example, see Figs. 1–4). A protocol involving the surface spreading technique outlined here (steps 5–8) was published by (18).

1. Dissect testes into insect saline at room temperature (see Note 2).
2. Add an equal volume of distilled water and leave to stand for 5–10 min (hypotonic treatment) (see Note 3).
3. Remove hypotonic saline/water mixture and replace with freshly made 3:1 ethanol:acetic acid fixative and cover to prevent evaporation.
4. Replace the fixative every 15–30 min for 2–3 h (try 2 h initially) (see Note 4).
5. Place a small piece of tissue (~1 mm) in three drops of 60% acetic acid and tap with the end of the 3-mm brass rod until the tissue has formed a rough cell suspension.

6. Add another drop or two of acetic acid if necessary, and tilt the slide back and forth so the droplet of cell suspension spreads over the whole surface of the slide (see Note 5).
7. Place the slide on hotplate (37°C) for 2 min then tilt the slide to spread the remaining liquid over the slide (see Note 6).
8. Repeat step 7 until all of the liquid has evaporated.
9. Slides can be stored indefinitely in at room temperature before staining and viewing. In humid regions, if the slides are to be kept for long periods (months) the box should be sealed and a desiccant (e.g. silica gel) is included in the box.
10. Stain in a Coplin jar in 5% Giemsa stain in phosphate buffer for 3 min (5% stain cannot be stored).
11. Rinse with phosphate buffer in a Coplin jar or sprayed from a squeeze bottle.
12. Tilt slides upright on a piece of tissue to drain.
13. Once dry, stained slides can be stored indefinitely as per step 9 above.

### *3.2. Direct Preparation of Metaphase Chromosomes from Kidney, Gills, or Spleen (Fish)*

This protocol applies the same principles as Subheading 3.1, but tissue is converted to a cell suspension at the beginning of the fixation process. The later steps are common to many other published protocols, including those involving blood samples.

1. Dissect gills, cephalic kidney, or spleen and place the tissue into 10 ml Hank's balanced saline solution (HBSS).
2. Macerate clean tissue using a pin and forceps in 5–8 ml fresh HBSS. Hold a piece of tissue and use forceps to pull the tissue apart. This will rupture the connective tissue and release cells that can be arrested in metaphase and spread on a glass slide. In some cases it can also help to resuspend the tissue with a glass pipette to free more cells.
3. Add 100 μl colchicine to the tissue solution and leave for 15 min at 37°C.
4. Centrifuge at 276 × *g* for 10 min in a 15-ml tube.
5. Discard all but 0.5 ml of supernatant and resuspend the pellet in the remaining liquid.
6. Add 5–7 ml of 37°C hypotonic solution and mix gently. Leave for 20–40 min at 37°C (see Note 7).
7. Add 4–5 drops of freshly made ice-cold fixative on top of the hypotonic solution and mix thoroughly with a Pasteur pipette. (This is crucial, as lumps will not resolve later on.) Add about 4 ml of fixative and mix again.
8. Centrifuge at 276 × *g* for 10 min. Discard the supernatant and resuspend the pellet in fresh fixative. Leave the cells to fix overnight at –20°C. These cell suspensions keep for many years.

9. Centrifuge at 276×*g* for 10 min (if solutions are stored in smaller 1.5-ml tubes, at 4,024×*g* for 5 min) and resuspend in fresh ice-cold fixative. The volume of fixative depends on the size of the cell pellet. 200–500 μl is a good starting point, but if the cells are too crowded or sparse on the slide, modify the concentration. Cell suspension and fixative should always be kept on ice (see Note 8).
10. Using a Pasteur pipette, apply one drop of the cell suspension to a dry slide from a height of about 5 cm. Air-dry the slide. Getting the best possible metaphase spread may require adjustments to the environment, fixative and slide preparation as discussed (see Note 9).
11. For extended storage, dehydrate the slides (80, 90, and 100% ethanol series at room temperature) and keep at −20°C or store in a Coplin jar in ethanol at 4°C.

### 3.3. Direct Preparation from Bone Marrow (Mouse)

1. Inject mouse with 200 μl of 0.1 mg/ml Colcemid solution (intraperitoneal).
2. After 1–2 h, kill the mouse and remove the femurs.
3. Cut femurs at both ends and use a syringe of hypotonic solution (0.075 M KCl) to flush out bone marrow into a 10-ml tube.
4. Incubate for 20 min at 37°C in the hypotonic solution. Continue from step 7 of Subheading 3.2.

### 3.4. Chromosome Preparation from Cultured Fibroblast Cells

Improved cell culture techniques allowing short- or long-term culturing of fibroblasts of different species are increasingly used in research in wild species. These culture techniques offer the advantage that cells can be cryopreserved for years, thawed, and propagated for 15–20 passages. The technique described below was developed for short-term culture from fin tissue of pufferfish, as we discovered that there is a first wave of rapidly dividing cells that can be utilised for metaphase preparation (19), while subsequent establishment of stable fibroblast cell lines is difficult. Incubation time, temperature, and hypotonic solution can vary between species as discussed below.

1. Cut off fin tips and place them in a petri dish with tissue culture medium.
2. Cut the tissue into 0.5-mm pieces in medium using two scalpel blades. Then, use a plugged (and sterilised) glass Pasteur pipette to carefully suck in a piece and transfer it into a in 25-ml tissue culture flasks. Often the tissue will float in a droplet. It is important that excess liquid is removed around the tissue so the tissue makes contact with the surface of the flask. The tissue pieces should be planted in rows of 3–4 pieces and 4–5 rows. Also avoid any contact with the tissue culture flask as residual medium can increase chances of infection of the culture. Change the pipette after transferring a few pieces.

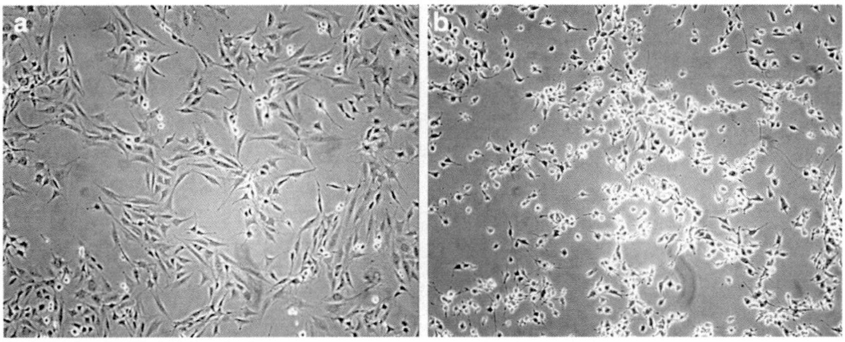

Fig. 7. Trypsin treatment. (**a**) Normal growing fibroblast culture. (**b**) Minutes after trypsin has been added the cell start to become round with many detaching from the culture dish surface. Gentle tapping will detach all cells.

3. Add 5 ml of medium to the bottom of the flask, taking care not to wash the tissue off the side of the flask.
4. Keep the flasks capped and upright for 1–3 h to allow the tissue to attach. The flasks are then carefully tilted to immerse the tissue with medium. Culture temperature should be similar to body temperature of the animal (see Note 10), with 5% $CO_2$ supply (standard of all cell culture).
5. Within days, a pale area around the fin tissue is clearly visible (similar to the outgrowth seen in Fig. 5). In pufferfish, extended culturing leads to structural changes, so cells are harvested 4–7 days after planting (20).
6. Before harvesting, add colchicine (final concentration, 0.1 mg/ml of medium).
7. To harvest, remove the medium and wash the cells with 1× PBS to remove FCS (which inactivates trypsin). Remove PBS.
8. To the 25-ml flask, add 2 ml of trypsin and incubate for 5 min. Once cells have contracted (see Fig. 7b) they can be detached by gently tapping the flask.
9. Inactivate trypsin by adding 5 ml of medium (with FCS) to the cells. This is only to inactivate the trypsin, so normal DMEM/15%FCS can be used.
10. Spin the cell suspension for 10 min at 276 ×*g* in a 10-ml plastic centrifuge tube and resuspend the pellet in 1–4 ml hypotonic solution for 20 min (see Note 7).
11. Fixation and slide preparation as for Subheading 3.2.

### 3.5. Establishment of Fibroblast Cell Line

Tissue from most vertebrates can be cultured using today's refined media and commercially available supplements. Tissue can be collected easily post mortem (even from reasonably fresh road kill) or as a minor invasive skin biopsy and stored in medium for some days before planting. The establishment of cell lines allows the living cells to be stored frozen as a source for chromosome preparations and DNA for many years.

Tissue for culturing can be taken from internal and external tissues. External tissues are usually more prone to contamination and pieces of tissue should be wiped carefully with 70% ethanol before transferring into a medium enriched with antibiotics and fungicide (see Subheading 2). The tissue should not be kept in antibiotic medium for more than 48 h.

1. Follow steps 1–4 of Subheading 3.4 for setting up primary cultures.
2. Cells in exponential growth (about 70% confluent, i.e. the cells take up 70% of the surface area in the tissue culture) are lifted using trypsin and transferred to a centrifuge tube as described at Subheading 3.4.
3. Spin the cells (276 × *g* for 10 min), aspirate the supernatant, and resuspend the cells in 2 ml freezing medium containing 10% DMSO.
4. Place the tube in a cryostat and transfer into −80°C to freeze at a rate of 1°C/min. Leave overnight and transfer into liquid nitrogen for long-term storage.
5. To thaw, place the tube containing the frozen cells in 2 ml of freezing medium containing 10% DMSO into a 37°C water bath. As soon as the medium in the tube is thawed, transfer cells to a 15-ml tube containing 10 ml fresh 10% DMEM cell culture medium to dilute the toxic effect of DMSO on the cells.
6. Spin cells at 276 × *g* for 10 min. Resuspend the pellet in 5–10 ml of 10% DMEM and transfer into a 25-ml or 75-ml flask depending on the size of the pellet.
7. Change the medium the next day to remove dead cells (see Notes 11 and 12). For a medium change simply aspirate the old medium and add new medium to the tissue culture flask.
8. Once larger patches of cells are visible on a number of tissue pieces (see Fig. 5), cells can be removed with a gentle trypsin treatment (see Subheading 3.4, Fig. 7) and transferred in to new flasks as passage 1 cells. These newly established early passage cells are best for chromosome preparation. It is important to check the cells regularly and split them before they are confluent (i.e. the fibroblasts have formed a monolayer and ceased cell division) to keep exponential growth. Cells prepared for further cryopreservation should be actively dividing.
9. Fixation and slide preparation as for Subheading 3.2, and see Note 13.

### 3.6. Fluorescence In Situ Hybridisation

For several decades, basic chromosome morphology (chromosome number, fundamental number, and centromere index) was the only way of characterising and comparing karyotypes of different species.

In the 1970s, a wide range of structural banding and replication banding allowed the identification and comparison of individual chromosomes. The hybridisation of DNA or RNA molecules onto cells on slides (in situ hybridisation) has revolutionised the field of cytogenetics. Now, we have a range of different techniques, probes to identify DNA or RNA on extended chromatin fibres (fibre FISH), metaphase chromosomes, or the interphase nucleus (21). There is a growing range of probes and variations of the FISH procedure described in several books and numerous reviews. One of the more recent techniques used in tumour cytogenetics is the comparative hybridisation of two different genomes labelled with different fluorophores onto reference chromosomes. The comparative genome hybridisation (CGH) technique originally used to identify large deletions and amplifications in tumours (22) has been modified and used to detect blocks of heterochromatin (20) and cryptic sex chromosomes (23) and to highlight species-specific repeat structures (24) in various species. Here, we describe a CGH protocol that can be used for basic characterisation of a new chromosome complement. Figure 8 shows an example of how comparative hybridisation in two bovine subspecies highlights bulk blocks of centromeric heterochromatin. In addition, the hybridisation of

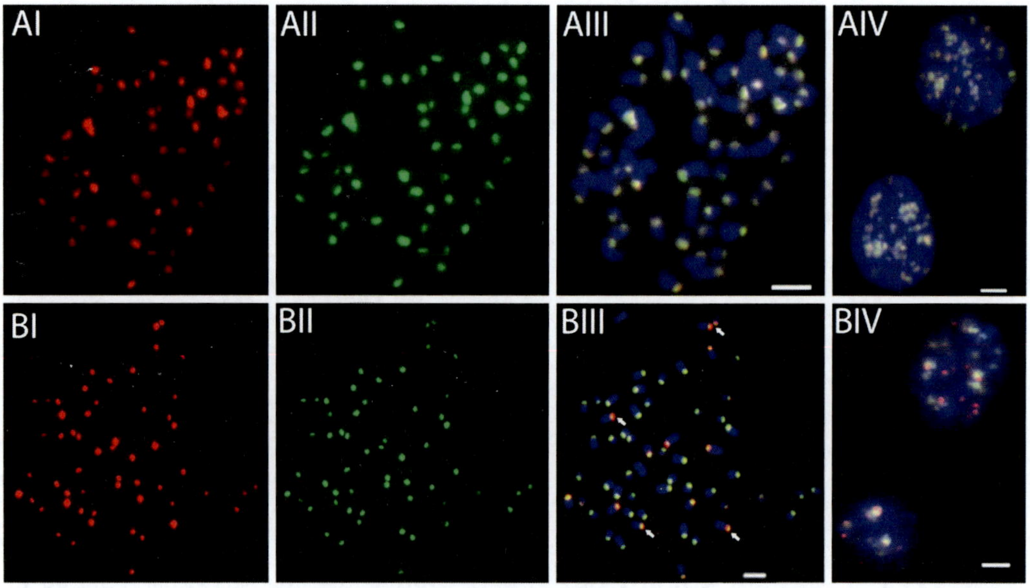


Fig. 8. Comparative genome hybridisation (CGH) to detect centromeric heterochromatin and species-specific repeat amplification. In this example, equal amounts of DNA from two different bovine subspecies were labelled with different fluorophores and hybridised onto chromosomes of both subspecies. In this case, DNA from *Bos taurus* and *Bos indicus* was hybridised back onto *Bos taurus* (AI-AIII) and *Bos indicus* (BI–BIII) metaphase chromosomes and interphase cells (AIV, BIV). Centromeric regions of all autosomes are hybridised with similar intensity of both red and green probes in *Bos taurus* (AIII), whereas in *Bos indicus* a number of chromosomes have a stronger red signal (BIII, *arrow*). Scale bar = 5 μm. This suggests repeat amplification and possibly divergence of these repeats in the *Bos indicus* lineage.

DNA from two closely related species revealed a set of chromosomes showing differentiation in repeat content and sequence (see Fig. 8). This procedure is almost identical to methods used to map genomic clones or large cDNA clones. Labelling of the DNA is done the same way as a clone. The main differences in this approach are the lack of competitor DNA and a pre-annealing step after the denaturation of the probe DNA, which are usually used to reduce hybridisation of repetitive elements.

The FISH procedure involves (A) the labelling of the probe (in this case genomic DNA), (B) preparation of the metaphase slide, and (C) setting up of the hybridisation mixture. After the hybridisation (usually overnight), excess probe is washed off (D) and the slides are ready to be analysed under an epifluorescence microscope.

A. Labelling:

Fluorophores labels can be attached to the probe directly (fluorophores such as Cy dyes, FITC, TRITC, and Alexa dyes are directly attached to the nucleotide incorporated) or indirectly (biotin- or digoxigenin-carrying nucleotides are incorporated). We describe direct labelling, which simplifies the FISH procedure and leads to cleaner signal.

1. For the labelling mix 300 ng of genomic DNA, 5 μl 9-mer random primer (1 μg/ml) and add MQ water (so the whole reaction volume is 25 μl) in a PCR tube. Spin down and denature at 95°C for 10 min followed by a 5-min incubation on ice.
2. Add 0.3 μl fluorescent dye (Spectrum orange or Spectrum green), 4.6 μl Klenow enzyme buffer, 1 μl Klenow enzyme to the reaction, mix (short vortex), spin down, and incubate overnight at 37°C (keep dark). Labelled probes can be kept at –20°C and can be used for months.

B. Pretreatment of the metaphase slides:

3. Slides can be stored in 100% ethanol or frozen (after dehydrating in ethanol series). Fresh slides are best. If frozen slides are used, they should be dehydrated in 100% ethanol for 3 min and air-dried before the RNAse treatment. The pretreatment of the slides includes an RNAse digest to reduce background and pepsin treatment to improve accessibility and background if antibodies are used.
4. Check the quality of the slides under the microscope (phase contrast). Mark the hybridisation area on the back of the slide with a diamond pen (see Note 14).
5. RNAse treatment: Rinse slides for 5 min in 2× SSC (at room temperature, no shaking required). Take the slides and place them in a moist chamber. Then, pipette 200 μl RNAse (100 μg RNAse A per ml in 2× SSC) onto the slides, cover with a coverslip, and incubate for 30 min at 37°C.

6. Tilt the slides to remove coverslips and wash the slides three times in 2× SSC.
7. Pepsin treatment: Add 25 μl of 10% pepsin to 50 ml 37°C pre-warmed 0.01N HCl solution and mix well. Incubate the slides for exactly 10 min at 37°C in pepsin solution.
8. After the pepsin treatment wash the slides twice in 1× PBS for 5 min (room temperature).
9. Rinse the slides in rinsing solution 1 for 5 min (room temperature).
10. Transfer the slides into rinsing solution 2 (room temperature) to fix cells after the pepsin treatment for at least 10 min.
11. Wash the slides once with 1× PBS for 5 min (room temperature).
12. Dehydrate the slides in 70, 85, and 100% ethanol for 3 min each and air-dry. The slides are now ready for denaturation.
13. For denaturation, place the slides in Coplin jar with pre-warmed (at 70°C) Denaturing solution for 1.5–3 min. Rinse briefly in 2× SSC to wash off the formamide. Then, dehydrate the slides in 70, 85, and 100% ethanol for 3 min each (agitate gently) and air-dry. The slides are now ready for hybridization.

C. Preparation of hybridisation probe:

14. For a two-colour FISH experiment mix 12.5 ml of each probe (one labelled with Spectrum green and one with Spectrum orange) with 5 ml of 10 mg/ml salmon sperm (carrier). Add 2.5 volumes of ice-cold 100% ethanol (we use non-methylated ethanol for the precipitation), mix well, and precipitate DNA in –80°C for 30 min (or at –20°C overnight) (see Note 15).
15. Centrifuge the probe at 21,912 × g for 30 min at 4°C. A yellow pellet should be visible.
16. Carefully remove the supernatant. Make sure that residual ethanol in the lid or around the pellet is removed (tap the tube opening on a towel). Air-dry the pellet at room temperature for 10 min.
17. Add 5 ml of deionised formamide and let the pellet dissolve for at least 15 min in a heated shaker at 37°C.
18. Add 5 ml of hybridisation mixture (dextran sulphate/4× SSC, see Subheading 2) and shake at 37°C for another 15 min. The hybridisation mix is viscous and needs to be mixed thoroughly before using.
19. Denature the probes at 80°C for 10 min and cool them on ice for 2 min (see Note 16).

20. Without delay, quick-spin the pellet and add 10 ml of the probes onto the pretreated chromosome slides (from step 13) (see Note 17).
21. Carefully add a coverslip (22 mm×22 mm). Press the coverslip gently to disperse the hybridisation mix and to remove bubbles. Seal the coverslip with rubber cement. Incubate the slides at 37°C overnight in a moist chamber.

D. Washing of the slides:

22. Gently peel the rubber cement off with tweezers. Often the coverslip will come off with the rubber cement. If not, soak the slides in 2× SSC for a few minutes and gently push off the cover slip.
23. Wash the slides three times for 5 min in Washing solution 1 at 42°C and agitate. Then, wash once for 5 min in 0.1× SSC at 60°C (no agitating).
24. Dip the slides in 1 mg/ml DAPI solution in for 1 min. Transfer the slides from DAPI into a fresh Coplin jar with MQ water and rinse them 3–4 times. Tap the slides on a towel to remove excess water (or air-dry). Add two drops of mounting medium (Vectashield) and cover with 22 mm×50 mm coverslips. Press gently to remove bubbles.

### 3.7. Viewing Slides

A. General slide viewing:

1. Microscope magnification is calculated as product of the magnification of the eyepieces and the magnification of the objective. Thus, if a microscope has 10× eyepieces (which is usual), a 10× objective gives an overall magnification of 100×. Some microscopes may also have an inbuilt magnifying lens (usually 1–2 times).
2. For most species, 100× magnification is sufficient for initial slide scanning to find dividing cells. However, chromosome number and detail can rarely be established without at least a 63× objective, and preferably 100×.
3. The protocols given above all produce slides coated with a thin layer of cells. These can be viewed directly with dry objectives. If oil immersion is used, oil can be applied directly to the slide surface; however, over 2–3 days the oil de-stains the slides and disrupts the preparations.

B. Making preparations permanent:

4. If slides are to be stored or repeatedly viewed by oil immersion, they should be coverslipped. Commonly used mounting media are Eukitt Mounting Medium (Electron Microscopy Sciences, PA, USA) and Euparal (ANSCO Laboratories, Manchester, UK). Coverslips commonly

come in two sizes (22 mm round or square, and 22 mm × 64 mm). To apply a 22-mm coverslip, place one drop of mounting medium on the slide in the centre of the area to be covered and gently drop the coverslip onto the slide. The weight of the coverslip will slowly spread the medium over a few minutes and most bubbles will disperse. Leave the slide on a hotplate at ~37°C for at least 24 h, or longer if at room temperature. The process is the same for a 22 mm × 64 mm coverslip, but use three drops spaced evenly across the slide.

C. Viewing slides using fluorescence:

5. To view FISH slides, an epifluorescence microscope with appropriate filter sets is required. Excitation and emission spectra of the fluorescent dyes are provided with the chemical.
6. A standard dye combination is DAPI, Texas Red (TRITC), and FITC (GFP, green).
7. Additional dyes and combinations of dyes can be used for multi-colour FISH experiments where all chromosomes in human and mouse karyotypes can be marked with a specific colour. Black and white pictures of each channel are taken using high-powered charge-coupled device (CCD) cameras and then false coloured. This is often done automatically by the software provided.

## 4. Notes

1. Insect saline (Subheading 2.1, item 9) has been successful for a range of terrestrial invertebrates. Other solutions (e.g. HBSS – see Subheading 2.2, item 7) may give better results for vertebrates, and seawater or equivalent isotonic saline for marine invertebrates.
2. If embryonic tissue is used, it should be dissected from eggs, separated from all yolk material, and placed in 0.002% colchicine in insect saline for 30 min before hypotonic treatment.
3. If chromosomes appear clumped with many overlaps, trial a more dilute hypotonic (e.g. two parts water to one part saline).
4. If fixation is poor (chromosomes deformed with poor definition), a longer period in fixative may help. However, fixation of over 3 h tends to make many tissues brittle and difficult to break up for spreading. If fixation is good, the number of changes of fixative (step 4) may be reduced.

5. The moving droplets of cell suspension (steps 6 and 7) leave a trail of cells on the slide surface in their wake, and these become firmly attached to the slide surface on drying.
6. The use of a ~37°C hotplate is desirable; but if it is not available (e.g. in the field), acceptable preparations can still be obtained by drying at room temperature.
7. If chromosomes appear clumped with many overlaps, other hypotonic treatments can be tried (e.g. 50% FCS in water). In pufferfish, a hypotonic solution of 0.05 M KCl is used instead of the usual 0.075 M.
8. The quality of the slides and metaphase spreads may be improved by repeated rounds of spinning down and fixative replacement, as this reduces debris from cells in the suspension.
9. There are a number of factors affecting chromosome spreading on slides (see (25) for further discussion). Chromosome spreading can be affected by humidity of the environment. In very dry environments, chromosome spreading can be challenging and many cytogenetics labs have chambers with constant humidity. In our experience, a combination of drying and exposing the slide with the cells to hot steam can produce better spread cells as well as less debris on the slide. In this protocol, the slide is quickly run over a boiling kettle to moisten the slide surface. The cell suspension is then dropped on the slide. As soon as drying on the outside of the drop is observed (or after 2–3 s), hold the slide for 1–2 s over a steaming water bath or boiling kettle (keep a distance in case of a kettle as the hot steam might damage the chromosome structure). The slide can then be dried on a hotplate (for banding, ageing at 65°C over night may improve results). Spreading may be also be improved by adding a few drops of acetic acid to the fixative before dropping on the slide.
10. Cell culture temperature: In most mammals and birds, this will be 37°C with the exception of monotreme mammals, which will grow at 32°C. Reptile and fish cells will be cultured at room temperature or up to 27°C.
11. The risk of bacterial or fungal infection is the largest in the first 1–2 weeks of the primary culture, so it is vital to carefully check the cultures daily. Often, fungal infections can be prevented from spreading by removing tissue pieces with beginning fungal growth. Also, floating tissue needs to be removed. If no infections occur and no rapid growth has commenced, medium can be changed once or twice a week. Bacterial infection if detected early can be suppressed with higher dose of antibiotics. Often, these latent infections can flare up again when the cells are thawed for further culturing.

12. Do not change medium too soon, as growing cells will provide growth signals to other cells.
13. Timing of the colchicine treatment is vital when preparing chromosome from growing fibroblast. It is important to monitor cell lines. Cells undergoing division and in metaphase will become round and are clearly distinct from the flat fibroblast (Fig. 2.6b). With new cell lines, it is best to check growing cells every few hours and determine the time when the frequency of round cells peaks. Colchicine should then be added 1 h earlier to capture cells in metaphase. After colchicine is added, the frequency of round cells should increase (see Fig. 6a, b as an example).
14. A good slide is vital for FISH and it is disappointing to find out after this long procedure that the slide was not good. Are there too many cells (and lumps) or too few? Are there enough metaphases and are the chromosomes well spread? Is the slide littered with debris? Rather, make a new slide with fresh fixative than proceed with a low-quality slides.
15. Precipitation: Some protocols use 1/20 volume of 3 M sodium acetate or other salts to help with the precipitation. We recommend trying to precipitate without additional salt to avoid excess salt in the hybridisation mix. If salt is used, an additional 70% ethanol wash can be done.
16. Denaturation: in our experience the denaturation time has to be optimised in different species. In some species, denaturation may be less efficient due to differences in chromatin compaction and GC content. In humans, denaturation times of 1 min at 70°C work. In the case of monotremes, we routinely use 3 min. It is important not to over denature as this damages chromosome structure. Over-denatured chromosomes are puffed up and three dimensional, so it is often impossible to see specific signals.
17. Timing: It is important that the slides are ready for hybridisation once the probe has been denatured, particularly in this type of CGH experiment where there is no pre-annealing of repeats in the probe. Probes can easily be stored in formamide or as a hybridisation mix.

## Acknowledgements

We thank Professor Stefan Hiendleder (The University of Adelaide) for providing samples from bovine species. F. Grutzner is an ARC Australian Research Fellow.

## References


1. Pontius JU, Mullikin JC, Smith DR et al (2007) Initial sequence and comparative analysis of the cat genome. Genome Res **17**:1675–1689
2. Li R, Fan W, Tian G et al (2010) The sequence and de novo assembly of the giant panda genome. Nature **463**:311–317
3. Genome 10K Community of Scientists (2009) Genome 10K: a proposal to obtain whole-genome sequence for 10,000 vertebrate species. J Hered **100**:659–674
4. Tait NN, Briscoe DA, Rowell DM (1995) Onychophora–Ancient and modern radiations. Memoirs of the Association of Australian Palaeontologists **18**:21–30
5. Rowell DM, Higgins AV, Tait NN et al (1995) Chromosomal evolution in viviparous onychophorans from Australia (Onychophora: Peripatopsidae). J Linn Soc Lond **114**: 139–153
6. Rowell DM, Rockman MV, Tait NN (2002) Extensive Robertsonian Rearrangement: Implications for the radiation and biogeography of Planipapillus Reid (Onychophora: Peripatopsidae). J Zool Lond **257**:171–179
7. Czepulkowski B (2001) Analyzing chromosomes. Oxford, UK
8. Yunis JJ, Prakash O (1982) The origin of man: a chromosomal pictorial legacy. Science **215**: 1525–1530
9. Wolf K, Quimby MC (1976) Procedures For subculturing fish cells and propagating fish cell lines. Tissue Culture Assoc Manual **2**:471–474
10. Anamthawat-Jonsson K (2003) Preparation of chromosomes from plant leaf meristems for karyotype analysis and in situ hybridization. Methods Cell Sci **25**:91–95
11. Armstrong SJ, Sanchez-Moran E, Franklin FC (2009) Cytological analysis of *Arabidopsis thaliana* meiotic chromosomes. Methods Mol Biol **558**:131–145
12. Rohilla MS, Rao RJ, Tiwari PK (2006) Use of peripheral blood lymphocyte culture in the karyological analysis of Indian freshwater turtles, *Lissemys punctata* and *Geoclemys hamiltoni*. Curr Sci **90**:1130–1134
13. Spowart G (1994) Mitotic metaphase chromosome preparation from peripheral blood for high resolution. Methods Mol Biol **29**:1–10
14. Benn P, Delach J (2008) Human lymphocyte culture and chromosome analysis. Cold Spring Harb Protoc. doi:10.1101/pdb.prot5035
15. Brinkley HJ, Norton HW, Nalbandov AV (1964) Role of hypophysial luteotrophic substance in the function of porcine corpora lutea. Endocrinology **74**:9–13
16. Hsu TC (1952) Tissue culture studies on human skin. III. Some cytological fractures of the outgrowth of epithelial cells. Tex Rep Biol Med **10**:336–352
17. Collodi P, Barnes DW (1990) Mitogenic activity from trout embryos. Proc Natl Acad Sci USA **87**:3498–3502
18. Crozier RH (1968) An acetic acid dissociation, air-drying technique for insect chromosomes, with aceto-lactic orcein staining. Stain Technol **43**:171–173
19. Grutzner F, Himmelbauer H, Paulsen M et al (1999) Comparative mapping of mouse and rat chromosomes by fluorescence in situ hybridization. Genomics **55**:306–313
20. Grutzner F, Lutjens G, Rovira C et al (1999) Classical and molecular cytogenetics of the pufferfish *Tetraodon nigroviridis*. Chromosome Res 7:655–662
21. Haaf T (2006) Methylation dynamics in the early mammalian embryo: implications of genome reprogramming defects for development. Curr Top Microbiol Immunol **310**:13–22
22. Kallioniemi A, Kallioniemi OP, Sudar D et al (1992) Comparative genomic hybridization for molecular cytogenetic analysis of solid tumors. Science **258**:818–821
23. Ezaz T, Valenzuela N, Grutzner F et al (2006) An XX/XY sex microchromosome system in a freshwater turtle, *Chelodina longicollis* (Testudines: Chelidae) with genetic sex determination. Chromosome Res **14**:139–150
24. Hardt T, Himmelbauer H, Mann W et al (1999) Towards identification of individual homologous chromosomes: comparative genomic hybridization and spectral karyotyping discriminate between paternal and maternal euchromatin in *Mus musculus* x *M. spretus* interspecific hybrids. Cytogenet Cell Genet **86**:187–193
25. Henegariu O, Dunai J, Chen XN et al (2001) A triple color FISH technique for mouse chromosome identification. Mamm Genome **12**:462–465
26. Sharp HE, Rowell DM (2007) Unprecedented chromosomal diversity and behavior modify linkage patterns and speciation processes: structural heterozygosity in an Australian spider. J Evol Biol **20**:2427–2439

# Chapter 3

## Genomic Libraries: I. Construction and Screening of Fosmid Genomic Libraries

**Mike A. Quail, Lucy Matthews, Sarah Sims, Christine Lloyd, Helen Beasley, and Simon W. Baxter**

### Abstract

Large insert genome libraries have been a core resource required to sequence genomes, analyze haplotypes, and aid gene discovery. While next generation sequencing technologies are revolutionizing the field of genomics, traditional genome libraries will still be required for accurate genome assembly. Their utility is also being extended to functional studies for understanding DNA regulatory elements. Here, we present a detailed method for constructing genomic fosmid libraries, testing for common contaminants, gridding the library to nylon membranes, then hybridizing the library membranes with a radiolabeled probe to identify corresponding genomic clones. While this chapter focuses on fosmid libraries, many of these steps can also be applied to bacterial artificial chromosome libraries.

**Key words:** Genome library, Vector, Fosmid, BAC, T1 bacteriophage, *Pseudomonas*, Nylon membrane, Hybridization

## 1. Introduction

Genome libraries hold an important role in biology as they can be utilized to assemble eukaryote genomes, characterize sequence repeats, and gene duplications, as well as facilitate gene discovery, particularly in nonmodel organisms. Constructing a genomic DNA library can be achieved through first shearing DNA to a suitable size, ligating fragments into a vector, and introducing these circularized genome fragments into a suitable host, usually bacterial cells. The bacteria are then plated onto agar and individual colonies picked and grown in microtitre plates. To identify a clone containing a sequence of particular interest, colonies are gridded (and DNA fixed) to nylon membranes, then hybridized with a labeled

Virginie Orgogozo and Matthew V. Rockman (eds.), *Molecular Methods for Evolutionary Genetics*, Methods in Molecular Biology, vol. 772, DOI 10.1007/978-1-61779-228-1_3, © Springer Science+Business Media, LLC 2011

single-stranded DNA probe and result is visualized through exposing the membrane to film or a phosphorimager screen.

Bacterial artificial chromosome (BAC) libraries were first developed in the early 1990s, and are capable of maintaining genomic DNA inserts of up to 300 kilobase pairs (kbp) (1). Due to their relative stability and large insert size, BAC libraries have become the standard library type for genome sequencing. BAC library construction is generally outsourced to private companies or genome centers, for efficiency, quality, and reliability. However, producing genome libraries with smaller insert sizes is entirely possible within a standard molecular laboratory. Fosmid genome libraries have a restricted insert size range of approximately 38–42 kb, making them particularly useful for scaffolding genome assemblies in sequencing projects. Furthermore, as fosmids are generally more stable than BACs, they are more representative of a genome, making fosmid libraries an extremely useful tool for covering sequence gaps. Fosmids have a cosmid vector backbone with the F factor origin of replication, which restricts the vector to typically one copy per cell. This limits the potential for cells to be intolerant to toxic or repetitive sequences, limits recombination that may occur if multiple copies of a sequence were present and therefore creates a stable genomic library.

Aside from whole genome sequencing, BAC or fosmid libraries are particularly useful for sequencing a targeted genome region, analyzing promoters, or comparing haplotypes of polymorphic variants. Linkage mapping is often used to identify molecular markers associated with genomic regions controlling major phenotypic effects. Genome libraries can be screened using markers linked to a phenotype and therefore facilitate the discovery of genes that underlie phenotypic change. This approach has been applied to identifying loci controlling polymorphic wing color patterns in butterflies (2), disease resistance loci in lettuce (3), and armor plate patterning in three-spine stickleback fish (4) to name a few. Fosmid construction as described herein uses random physical shearing to fragment DNA to the correct size range, resulting in the least biased and most representative large insert libraries currently available. Furthermore, genome libraries are now being used to develop constructs for fosmid-based reporter genes to examine *cis*-regulatory expression patterns ((5) and see Chapters 25 and 26).

This chapter describes a method for constructing a fosmid library, testing for common contaminants and gridding library clones to a nylon membrane. We also describe how to screen the library with a radiolabeled probe to identify clones containing genomic regions of interest. Chapter 4 outlines methods to isolate DNA from a clone, sequence and then assemble the product into a single finished contig.

## 2. Materials

### *2.1. Random Sheared Fosmid Library Construction*

1. Sterile 1-ml syringe and 23-gauge needle.
2. CopyControl Fosmid library construction kit (EPICENTRE).
3. 20 μg of Genomic DNA in a volume of 200 μl or less of water and with an average size of 40 kb or above (see Note 1).
4. DNA markers: Lambda genomic DNA (NEB); Lambda *Hin*dIII marker (NEB); Low range PFGE marker (NEB).
5. Phenol chloroform:chloroform:isoamyl alcohol (25:24:1, v/v).
6. Glycogen (10 mg/ml).
7. 96% Ethanol.
8. 1 M NaCl.
9. T0.1E buffer: 10 mM Tris–HCl, 0.1 mM EDTA, pH 8.0.

### *2.2. Size Selection of Genomic DNA by CHEF*

1. High melting point (HMP) agarose for electrophoresis, for example, UltraPure™ Agarose (Invitrogen).
2. Low melting point (LMP) agarose for preparative electrophoresis gels, for example, UltraPure™ Low Melting Point Agarose (Invitrogen).
3. CHEF gel electrophoresis apparatus.
4. SYBR Green (Sigma).
5. CopyControl Fosmid library construction kit (EPICENTRE).
6. Dark Reader (Clare Chemical Research).
7. 1× TBE: 90 mM Tris–borate, 2 mM EDTA, pH 8.3.
8. Ficoll loading dye: 0.1% (w/v) bromophenol blue, 10% (w/v) Ficoll 400, 1× TBE.
9. 30-ml Sterilin tubes.
10. TE5 buffer: 10 mM Tris–HCl, pH 8.0, 0.5 mM EDTA.

### *2.3. Recovery of DNA and Ligation into pCC1Fos Vector*

1. Saran wrap.
2. Dialysis tubing (Spectra/Por 7, MWCO 3500, Cat. No. 132110).
3. Dialysis clip (Spectrapor Cat. No. 132736).
4. 0.5× TE: 5 mM Tris–HCl, 0.5 mM EDTA, pH 8.0.
5. 5× TBE: Dissolve 54 g of Tris base and 27.5 g of boric acid in approximately 900 ml of deionized water. Add 20 ml of 0.5 M EDTA, pH 8.0, and adjust the solution to a final volume of 1 l. This solution can be stored at room temperature but a precipitate will form in older solutions. Store the buffer in glass bottles and discard if a precipitate has formed.

6. 3 M Sodium acetate, pH 5.2.
7. 96 and 70% Ethanol.
8. Pellet paint (VWR).
9. T0.1E buffer: 10 mM Tris–HCl, 0.1 mM EDTA, pH 8.0.
10. 30-ml Sterilin tubes.
11. High melting point (HMP) agarose for electrophoresis, for example, UltraPure™ Agarose (Invitrogen).
12. T4 DNA ligase (and 10× ligase buffer) (Roche).
13. Proteinase K (Roche).
14. Phenol chloroform:chloroform:isoamyl alcohol (25:24:1, v/v).

### 2.4. Introducing Fosmids into Escherichia coli by Phage Infection

1. TYE agar plate: 1.0% Tryptone, 0.8% sodium chloride, 0.5% yeast extract, 0.1% glucose, and 1.5% agar. Autoclave to sterile. Cool to 50°C before adding any antibiotics, then pour into 9-mm agar dishes.
2. LB: 1% tryptone, 0.5% yeast extract, 0.5% sodium chloride. Autoclave to sterilize.
3. 1 M and 10 mM $MgSO_4$.
4. Maxplax packaging extract (EPICENTRE).
5. Phage dilution buffer: 10 mM Tris–HCl, 10 mM $MgCl_2$, pH 7.4.
6. 80% Glycerol.
7. Chloramphenicol (Sigma). 500× stock solution is 50 mg/ml in ethanol. Filter sterilize before use.

### 2.5. Estimating the Fosmid Library Insert Size

1. GTE: 50 mM Glucose, 25 mM Tris–HCl, 10 mM EDTA.
2. RNAse A (Sigma). 1,000× stock solution is 100 mg/ml in water.
3. 0.2 M NaOH + 1% SDS solution. Make fresh by mixing 0.5 ml of 4 M NaOH (BDH), 1 ml of 10% SDS (BDH), and 8.5 ml of water.
4. 3 M potassium acetate (KOAc), pH 5.5 (Fisher).
5. Isopropanol.
6. 70% Ethanol.
7. T0.1E buffer: 10 mM Tris–HCl, 0.1 mM EDTA, pH 8.0.
8. *NotI*, 10× Buffer and 100× BSA (NEB).
9. 10 mg/ml Ethidium bromide (Sigma).
10. Phage dilution buffer: 10 mM Tris–HCl, pH 7.4, 10 mM $MgCl_2$.
11. TE5: 10 mM Tris–HCl, pH 8.0, 0.5 mM EDTA.

12. Ficoll 10% (w/v) and Ficoll loading dye.
13. Low range PFG marker (NEB).
14. Seakem GTG agarose (Lonza).
15. Low melting point (LMP) agarose for preparative electrophoresis gels, for example, UltraPure™ Low Melting Point Agarose (Invitrogen).

#### 2.6. Preparing Assay Plates to Test for Library Contamination

Items 1–15 are required for T1 bacteriophage assay plates and items 16–24 are required for *Pseudomonas* assay plates.

1. LB agar.
2. LB agarose: Mix 4 g of agarose into 500 ml of LB. Prepare two bottles containing 500 ml of LB agarose each.
3. LB broth.
4. Boiling water bath.
5. DH10B cells streaked so a single colony may be picked.
6. 250-ml sterile conical flask.
7. Shaking incubator at 37°C.
8. 50°C and 42°C water baths.
9. Pouring plates rectangular, 86 mm × 128 mm (Nunc http://www.nuncbrand.com).
10. Lamina flow hood.
11. Proceine 40 (Agma).
12. Azowipes.
13. Sterile pipette tip.
14. Power pipette.
15. Sealable bag.
16. 500-ml sterile glass bottle.
17. Oxoid Pseudomonas agar base.
18. Power pipette.
19. 100% Glycerol.
20. Milli-Q water.
21. 50°C water bath.
22. Oxoid SR102E C-N supplement.
23. 50% Ethanol.
24. Pouring plates rectangular, 86 mm × 128 mm (Nunc).

#### 2.7. Picking Clones, Replicating the Library, and Testing for Contaminants

1. Laminar flow hood.
2. Sterile 96-pin disposable replicators (Thermo).
3. Library source plates, defrosted.

4. Destination 96-well plates (Falcon) containing LB, chloramphenicol (20 μg/ml) and 8% v/v of 100% glycerol.
5. Phage and *Pseudomonas* testing plates (see Subheading 2.6).
6. Virkon solution (Russell Mainstream Supply) in a bucket.
7. A 35°C incubator and a 37°C incubator.

### 2.8. Gridding a Library to a Nylon Membrane

1. Gridding Robot.
2. Nylon Membranes for library filters (Amersham).
3. LB plates with 1.5% agar and 20 μg/ml chloramphenicol, poured into trays that have the same dimensions as a library filter.
4. Two trays plus two sealable containers large enough for the library filter.
5. 10% SDS.
6. Milli-Q water.
7. Denaturation solution (5 l): 438 g Sodium chloride, 100 g sodium hydroxide dissolved in Milli-Q water to 5 l.
8. 20× SSC (5 l): 876.5 g Sodium chloride, 441 g sodium citrate, dissolve in Milli-Q water to make 5 l. Dilute stock 1/10 with Milli-Q water for 2× SSC.
9. Neutralization solution (5 l) : 604.5 g Tris–HCl, 438.3 g sodium chloride. Bring the pH to 7.5 using concentrated hydrochloric acid. Make up to 5 l with Milli-Q water.
10. Tris–HCl 1 M (pH 7.5). Dilute 1/20 with Milli-Q water.
11. Whatman paper.
12. UV transilluminator.

### 2.9. Preparing a Radiolabeled Probe

1. Prime-a-Gene Labeling System (Promega).
2. PCR Purification Kit (Qiagen).
3. 0.2-ml PCR tube.
4. Phosphorus-33 Radionuclide, deoxycytidine 5′-triphosphate [a-$^{33}$P]dCTP (10 mCi/ml) (PerkinElmer).
5. Heat block or thermal cycler.

### 2.10. Screening a Genome Library

1. Hybridization oven (e.g., Techne Hybridiser Oven HB-1D).
2. Hybridization tubes or box.
3. SSC (20×): Add 88.23 g of Tri-sodium citrate and 175.32 g of NaCl to 800 ml of water and dissolve. Ensure that pH is 7–8 and make up to 1 l. Store up to 3 months at room temperature.
4. 10% SDS.

5. 50× Denhardt's solution: Mix 1 g of bovine serum albumin, 1 g of Ficoll 400, and 1 g of polyvinylpyrrolidone. Add 50 ml of distilled water to dissolve and then complete to a final volume of 100 ml. Store at −20°C.
6. Denhardt's buffer (hybridization buffer): 5× SSC, 5× Denhardt's solution, 0.5% (w/v) SDS. Store at −20°C.
7. 10 mg/ml Salmon Sperm DNA solution (Invitrogen).
8. Low stringency wash solution: 2× SSC, 0.1% (w/v) SDS.
9. Medium stringency wash solution: 1× SSC, 0.1% (w/v) SDS.
10. Stripping solution: 0.1% (w/v) SDS.
11. Flat-tip tweezers for handling filters.
12. X-ray Film and Processor (e.g., Xograph) or a phosphorimager and phosphor screen.
13. When a library screen is complete, the library membrane should be covered in plastic wrap while still damp, and stored inside an autorad cassette at room temperature.

## 3. Methods

### 3.1. Random Sheared Fosmid Library Construction

The 8.1-kb pCCfos vector (supplied in the EPICENTRE kit) contains cos sites for packaging, antibiotic resistance for clone selection, and the ability to propagate as a circular extrachromosomal element. The user should begin with high molecular weight DNA (>50 kb) and obtain DNA fragments ranging between 38 and 42 kb following gentle physical shearing. DNA from different organisms and from different preparations can give vastly different outcomes. It is therefore recommended that one should first use test DNA, for example, ultrapure human genomic DNA (Promega), before committing and then potentially wasting the DNA of interest (see Note 2).

1. Prepare about 20 μg of your genomic DNA and adjust volume to 200 μl with double distilled water. DNA should have an average size higher than 50 kb and can be prepared by a large range of methods including silica-based ion exchange columns, such as those included in Qiagen kits, or by traditional organic extraction and spooling approaches.
2. Shear the DNA by sucking through a 23-gauge needle into a 1-ml syringe and rapidly extruding it again into a 1.5-ml Eppendorf tube. Repeat this 10–20 times.
3. Run 0.5 μl on a 0.5% agarose gel alongside 50 ng of lambda *Hind*III and intact lambda DNA markers. The sheared DNA should run *between* the lambda *Hind*III and intact lambda

*DNA* markers. If sheared DNA is higher than the intact lambda DNA then repeat steps 2 and 3.

4. Extract with phenol chloroform: Add an equal volume of phenol chloroform. Mix by gently inverting the tube for 1 min (do not vortex, as this can break up DNA fragments), place on ice for 5 min, and separate phases by centrifugation at 16,000 × *g* at room temperature for 5 min. Carefully pipette off the upper layer leaving behind approximately 10% without disturbing the interface of lower layer and pipette into a fresh Eppendorf tube. Add 1 μl of 10 mg/ml glycogen, 1/10th volume of 1 M NaCl and 2.5 volumes of ice-cold 96% ethanol. Incubate overnight at −20°C.
5. Pellet DNA by centrifugation at 16,000 × *g* at 4°C for 30 min, wash with 500 μl of ice-cold ethanol and air-dry (place the tube with lid open in an empty tip box at room temperature for 15 min).
6. Add 20 μl of T0.1E buffer to the pellet and leave on ice for at least 1 h to resuspend DNA. If needed, mix gently by pipetting up and down with a sterile pipette tip.
7. End Repair the DNA to make it suitable for ligation using the EPICENTRE CopyControl Fosmid or through our preferred method (see Note 3).
8. Add 150 μl of T0.1E. Extract with phenol chloroform (as in step 4 of Subheading 3.1), mix by gently inverting the tube for 1 min, and ethanol precipitate.
9. Pellet DNA by centrifugation at 16,000 × *g* at 4°C for 30 min, wash with 500 μl of ice-cold 96% ethanol and dry.
10. Add 20 μl of T0.1E to the pellet and leave on ice for at least 1 h to resuspend DNA. If needed mix gently with a sterile pipette tip.

### *3.2. Size Selection of Genomic DNA by CHEF*

Clamped homogenous electric field (CHEF) electrophoresis is used to give good resolution and separation of large DNA fragments for cloning.

1. Add 2.0 g of HMP agarose into 200 ml of 0.5× TBE. Melt in a microwave and equilibrate to 50°C.
2. Prepare the gel casting assembly and comb with large wells at 4°C. Pour gel and leave at 4°C to set for at least 1 h.
3. After rinsing the CHEF gel bed, pour 4 l of 0.5× TBE in it and let it circulate and chill to 14°C.
4. Load the gel in the following manner: Control, Marker, Blank, Sample(s), Blank, Marker, Control.
5. Put a sliver of low range PFG marker, approximately 1-mm thick, in the two marker wells as indicated above. Seal marker

wells by pipetting molten LMP agarose on top (1% LMP made using TBE). Leave to set. Add 20 μl of 2× loading dye solution containing 1×TBE to each 20 μl sample and pipette slowly up and down to mix.

6. Take 3 μl of T7 Fosmid Control DNA (40 kb) and make up to 40 μl with Ficoll loading dye (see Note 4).
7. Remove the gel casting box and gently slide the gel with black plate into the gel bed.
8. Load the Fosmid Control DNA and the samples as indicated in step 4 of Subheading 3.2.
9. Close lid and run CHEF at 6 V/cm, 0.1–40 s pulse for 16 h at 14°C (angle 120°, linear ramping factor).
10. Prepare a gel staining box (approximately 30 cm square) containing 50 ml of 0.5× TBE running buffer and 50 μl of SYBR Green.
11. Carefully remove the gel from the CHEF apparatus and place in the staining box for 30 min (agitation not required).
12. View the gel on a Dark Reader and cut out a gel slice that corresponds to the desired 38–42 kb DNA fraction and place in a fresh, labeled 30-ml Sterilin tube. (Gel slices that are not immediately used can be stored in TE5).

### 3.3. Recovery of DNA and Ligation into pCC1Fos Vector

The 35–45 kb DNA fraction is now recovered from the gel slice by electroelution.

1. Cover area of bench with Saran wrap and then put gel slices in well-rinsed dialysis tubing that has been presoaked in molecular biology grade water for at least 30 min. Add 400 μl of sterile 0.5× TE and close with rinsed dialysis clips. When closing the second clip try to remove all air bubbles and to get the gel slice at a right-angle to the clips.
2. Lay the tubing so that gel slices lie horizontally in the gel bed near the anode (black pole). Fill the gel bed with sterile 0.5× TBE until just covering the tubing.
3. Electroelute for 2 h at 60 V. When the run is complete change plugs around in power pack to reverse polarity and run for 45 s.
4. *Dialysis and concentration.* Into a 1-l beaker pour 500 ml of ice-cold 0.5× TE and add the dialysis bags and a magnetic flea.
5. Leave this spinning gently in the cold room for 1 h then replace with fresh chilled 0.5× TE and leave to stir for another hour. Dialysis removes borate and other contaminants from the DNA contained within the tubing.

6. Recover solution from dialysis bag using a pipette and put into a 1.5-ml Eppendorf tube. Add 0.1 volumes of 3 M sodium acetate, pH 5.2 (typically ~40 μl), add two volumes of ice-cold 96% ethanol (typically ~900 μl) and 1 μl of pellet paint. Leave at −20°C overnight.
7. Keep the tubing and gel slice suspended in 1 ml of T0.1E in 30-ml Sterilin tubes and store at 4°C in case there was a problem with electroelution and the DNA is still in the gel or attached to the tubing. This can be discarded at the end of step 9 in Subheading 3.3.
8. Pellet the DNA using a microfuge at 16,100 × *g* for 30 min at 4°C. Remove the supernatant carefully using a pipette, then wash the pellet with 1 ml of 70% ethanol, remove the supernatant and air-dry.
9. Resuspend in 5 μl of T0.1E and run 0.5 μl (with 4.5 μl of Ficoll loading dye) on a 0.8% HMP gel next to a quantitative marker to ascertain DNA concentration and to ensure that DNA of approximately the right size has been recovered.
10. *Ligation of DNA into pCC1Fos vector.* Approximately 100 ng of DNA insert is required per ligation (use 25 ng if DNA smearing below 23 kb is visible on the check gel).
11. Set up ligations on ice for the genomic library DNA and two controls, (1) test insert DNA and (2) no DNA as follows:

| | |
|---|---|
| DNA | 100 ng |
| 10× ligase buffer | 1 μl |
| pCC1Fos (200 ng) | 1 μl |
| Ligase | 1 μl |
| DDW | Up to 10 μl |

12. Incubate overnight at 16°C.
13. Next morning stop the ligation. For genomes above 40% G/C composition incubate at 70°C for 10 min; for high A/T genomes add 40 μl of T0.1E and 1 μl of proteinase K, incubate at 37°C for 1 h, extract carefully with phenol chloroform (as in step 4 in Subheading 3.1), ethanol precipitate, and resuspend in 10 μl of T0.1E.
14. Use the ligation straight away or store at −20°C.

### 3.4. Introducing Fosmids into E. coli by Phage Infection

Introducing fosmids into *E. coli* can be achieved by virtue of the cos recognition sequence in the fosmid vector. Practically, this is done by mixing the fosmid ligation mixture with a commercially available "packaging extract" that contains the proteins necessary to restrict DNA at the cos site and assemble infective phage particles around DNA molecules between approximately 47 and 52 kb that contain that cos site (see Note 5). The phage particles created are very infective and will transfect *E. coli* cells that have the phage receptor on their surface at very high efficiency. With the pCC1Fos vector we use the EPI300 $^{T1R}$ *E. coli* strain that requires magnesium in the growth medium to induce the phage receptor. This strain is also T1 bacteriophage resistant and contains the genes necessary for fosmid copy number induction (see Note 6).

1. *Preparation of plating cells.* Streak 20 µl of EPI300 cells (EPICENTRE) from glycerol stock, or single colony from a recent plate, onto a TYE plate.
2. Incubate overnight at 37°C.
3. Inoculate a single colony into a 250-ml flask containing 50 ml of LB and 0.5 ml of 1 M $MgSO_4$. Incubate at 37°C at 200 rpm for 4–5 h (until OD 600 is approximately 0.8). If all colonies have similar appearance you can use multiple colonies to inoculate enabling a faster culture time.
4. Transfer the cell culture to a 50-ml Falcon tube and pellet cells by centrifugation at 500×*g* for 12 min. Remove all supernatant.
5. Slowly resuspend the cells in 1 ml of ice-cold 10 mM $MgSO_4$ and then make up to a cell density at OD 600 nm of 1.0 (approximately 40 ml). Keep these plating cells on ice.
6. *Packaging.* To prepare the packaging reaction take up to 4 µl of ligation, add 25 µl of MaxPlax packaging extract and mix gently with a pipette, ensuring that there are no bubbles. Archive remaining ligation in a −20°C freezer.
7. Incubate on a heat block at 30°C for 90 min, then add a further 25 µl of MaxPlax packaging extract, gently mix again, and incubate for a further 90 min.
8. To stop the packaging reaction add 300 µl of phage dilution buffer.
9. *Preparative transfection.* This is generally preferred as the packaged phages do not have a long shelf-life and the preparative transfection process results in glycerol stocks of infected cells that can be stored at −80°C for at least 1 year. Small-scale transfection where 1 µl packaged phages are incubated with 200 µl of plating cells can give higher total efficiencies than larger scale transfection, and may be useful as a quick test before proceeding to preparative transfection as described below.
10. In 50-ml Falcon tubes, add 100–200 µl of packaged ligations to 10 ml of plating cells (from step 5) and gently mix by inversion.

11. Incubate at 37°C for 30 min.
12. Add 40 ml of LB and incubate at 37°C for 1 h.
13. Pellet cells by spinning at 500×*g* for 12 min. Remove all supernatant.
14. Resuspend cell pellets in 1 ml of LB.
15. Transfer into labeled cryovial (labeled with date and library name). Add 330 μl of 80% glycerol, mix, and place on dry ice and ethanol. Remove 10 μl and plate on TYE chloramphenicol (25 μg/ml) agar with 50 μl LB.
16. Transfer cryovial to storage box in −80°C freezer as soon as possible and record position.
17. Incubate plates overnight at 37°C.
18. In the morning count the colonies and record the titre of stored glycerol stock.

### 3.5. Estimating the Fosmid Library Insert Size

It is recommended to grow up, miniprep, and analyze fosmid DNA from 12 separate colonies in order to ensure that clones have inserts of the correct size (38–42 kb). Once library insert size has been validated, the desired number of colonies can be picked, grown in plates, tested for contaminants, and replicated (Subheadings 3.6 and 3.7).

1. Inoculate 6 ml of LB with 12.5 μg/ml chloramphenicol (in 20-ml Sterilin tube or similar) with a single colony (see Note 7).
2. Incubate in a shaker overnight at 37°C and 250 rpm.
3. Pour the contents into 50-ml Falcon tubes and centrifuge at 500×*g* at 4°C for 12 min.
4. Pour off the supernatant fluid and resuspend the cell pellet in 200 μl of ice-cold GTE containing 0.1 mg/ml RNAse, pipette into a 1.5-ml tube, and place on ice.
5. Add 400 μl of fresh 0.2 M NaOH + 1% SDS solution, mix by inversion several times, and place on ice for 5 min.
6. Add 300 μl of ice-cold 3 M potassium acetate (KOAc) and invert several times.
7. Centrifuge at 16,000×*g* for 15 min.
8. Transfer 750 μl of the supernatant fluid to a fresh 1.5-ml tube, without disturbing the pellet.
9. Add 480 μl of isopropanol to precipitate, invert several times then centrifuge at 16,000×*g* for 15 min.
10. Remove the supernatant, rinse the pellet with 1 ml of cold 70% ethanol and dry.
11. Resuspend in 10 μl of T0.1E.

12. Minipreps are digested with *NotI* to free the insert from vector and thereby ascertain the average insert size of the library. For each miniprep prepare the following in a 0.5-ml Eppendorf tube:

| | |
|---|---|
| DNA | 4 μl |
| DDW | 4.4 μl |
| 10× NEBuffer 3 | 1 μl |
| 100× BSA | 0.1 μl |
| *NotI* | 0.5 μl |

For 12 digests make the following premix:

| | |
|---|---|
| DDW | 61.6 μl |
| 10× NEBuffer 3 | 14 μl |
| 100× BSA | 1.4 μl |
| *NotI* | 7 μl |

Pipette 6 μl of this mixture into each tube. Add 4 μl of miniprep DNA to each tube.

13. Incubate at 37°C for 3–4 h.
14. Add to each tube 10 μl of a 1:1 mixture of Ficoll loading dye and Ficoll (10% w/v).
15. Prepare a 1% Seakem GTG agarose CHEF gel in 0.5× TBE, pour, and use 27-well-comb.
16. Add low range PFE marker gel and seal in with LMP agarose and put the gel in the CHEF gel bed, containing 4 l of cooled 0.5× TBE.
17. Load the samples (along with 5 μl of 1 kb extension ladder if possible) and run the gel at 6 V/cm, 0.1–40 s pulse for 16 h at 14°C (angle 120° linear ramping factor).
18. Recover the gel in 500 ml of running buffer and add 25 μl of ethidium bromide. Stain the gel for 30 min and destain for 30 min before photographing. Ideally, all lanes should have a vector band of 8.1 kb and at least one insert band of around 40 kb (or several smaller bands adding up to 40 kb in total).

### 3.6. Preparing Assay Plates to Test for Library Contamination

Under good laboratory practice, clone libraries are tested for the two most common contaminants; *Pseudomonas aeruginosa* and T1 bacteriophage. *P. aeruginosa* can be found in various environmental habitats such as water, air soil, feces, vegetation, and the gut of 10% of healthy people. It has broad resistance to antibiotics including ampicillin, tetracycline, chloramphenicol, and kanamycin.

Infection with *P. aeruginosa* is rare in healthy adults, although it is capable of infecting almost all types of tissue, particularly the urinary tract, cystic fibrosis patients (6), and burns injuries. T1 bacteriophage can exist in research laboratories and is very hardy and highly virulent to *E. coli* strains. It spreads easily, can be airborne and can survive desiccation. For further information see http://bacpac.chori.org/phage_testing_protocol.htm.

Preparation of approximately 30 T1 bacteriophage assay plates is described in steps 1–14, while preparation of approximately 12 *Pseudomonas* assay plates is described in steps 15–24:

1. On day 1, put 1 l of LB agar and two bottles containing 500 ml of LB agarose each to melt overnight in the boiling water bath.
2. Take a 250-ml sterile conical flask, aseptically add 100 ml of LB broth. Inoculate with a single colony of DH10B. Grow at 37°C for 16 h at 200 rpm in a shaking incubator with the flask lid slightly loose. The seeded DH10B in the LB agarose will grow overnight, causing the top layer to become opaque.
3. On day 2, remove the culture of DH10B from the shaking incubator and keep at room temperature until ready to use.
4. Transfer the melted bottle of LB agar from the boiling water bath to a 50°C water bath and allow to cool for at least 30 min.
5. Remove bottles of melted LB agarose from the boiling water bath, mix well, and transfer to a 42°C water bath. *This temperature is crucial – if too hot the DH10B will be killed, if too cool and the agar will set.* Cool for at least 2 h with gentle mixing for every 30 min.
6. Use the cooled LB agar to pour "thin" plates in a lamina flow hood. Allow to cool and set before replacing lids. Keep at 37°C until ready to pour the LB agarose, or if not to be used the same day, store plates inverted at 4°C.
7. Thoroughly clean lamina flow hood with Proceine 40, leave for 10 min, wipe dry then wipe with Azowipe.
8. Lay out the agar plates and remove lids.
9. To one 500-ml bottle of LB agarose, use a power pipette to add 11.25 ml of DH10B culture (made on day 1, step 2). Mix gently but thoroughly by rocking and rolling the bottle, without introducing air bubbles.
10. Pour a layer of LB agarose plus DH10B onto the set LB agar plates. Use a sterile pipette tip to push any air bubbles to the side of the plate.
11. Allow plates to cool and set before replacing lids. This step takes about 15 min in hood.

12. Repeat steps 6–11 with the second bottle of top agar.
13. Once phage assay plates are cool and set, they can be used for stamping fosmid library clones (see Subheading 3.7). Include an unused plate as a negative control.
14. Once plates have been stamped, incubate 37°C overnight in a sealed bag. Do not invert the plates. If T1 bacteriophage is present in the sample being tested, it will infect the DH10B resulting in a clear plaque in the DH10B lawn.
15. Weigh 24.2 g of Oxoid Pseudomonas agar base into bottle.
16. Warm a bottle of 100% glycerol in a microwave for a few seconds to make pipetting easier. Pipette 5 ml of glycerol into the bottle containing agar base.
17. Add 500 ml of Milli-Q water, shake to mix.
18. Autoclave the bottle for 20 min at 120°C. Use on same day, do not allow to set.
19. Cool to 50°C for at least 30 min in a water bath.
20. Take one vial of Oxoid SR102E C-N supplement. Resuspend the contents in 2 ml of 50% ethanol (gently, without causing frothing).
21. Add the supplement to the cooled agar base. Mix very gently but thoroughly. Take care not to generate too many air bubbles which are very difficult to remove.
22. Pour the agar into plates, with approximately 40 ml per plate. Gently push bubbles to the edge of the plate using a sterile pipette tip.
23. Once set, put the lids on the plates, invert, and store at 4°C until use.
24. Once plates have been stamped with fosmid library clones (Subheading 3.7), incubate at 35°C for 48 h. Include an unused plate as a negative control. Do not invert the plates.

If *Pseudomonas* contamination is present, colonies appear pale yellow in color. For confirmation, store plates at 4°C for 2 days. Colony color should change to blue-green and they will also glow under ultraviolet light. No growth in the assay plate confirms no *Pseudomonas* contamination.

### 3.7. Picking Colonies, Replicating the Library, and Testing for Contaminants

Once fosmid libraries have been created, it is necessary to pick individual colonies into 96-well (or 384-well) plates, test for *Pseudomonas* or T1 bacteriophage contamination and replicate the library to protect and maintain the resource for future use. The number of colonies picked is dependent on genome size and required coverage. Due to the large number of colonies required for genome libraries, it is recommended to use a colony picking robot, for example, a QPix (Genetix), although colonies can be picked manually. If picking by hand, use sterile toothpicks to stab and transfer single colonies.

In order to create identical copies of the original (archive) library, a hand replication tool such as a 96-pin hedgehog is used. These copies are then grown and frozen in glycerol and stored at –70°C in separate freezers for each copy. It is good practice to keep a score sheet to mark any wells without growth, to ensure that subsequent copies of library plates are identical to the original archive copy.

1. Grow the fosmid library overnight at 37°C on LB plates containing 20 μg/ml chloramphenicol.
2. Working in the hood, prepare 96-well destination plates containing 200 μl of LB, chloramphenicol (20 μg/ml) and 8% v/v of 100% glycerol, as well as assay plates for common contaminants as described in Subheading 3.6.
3. Place the replicating tool gently into the library source plate for 1 s with careful agitation, then gently stamp it onto the destination plate, then back into the source plate, then into the *Pseudomonas* assay plate and finally into the phage assay plate. It is very important to stamp in this exact order, as stamping the phage assay plate before the *Pseudomonas* assay plate will lead to false positives in the *Pseudomonas* assay plate.
4. Discard the replicator into a bucket containing virkon solution.
5. Repeat steps 3–4 for every plate requiring replication.
6. Seal plates. Grow phage plates for 16 h at 37°C, *Pseudomonas* plates for 48 h at 35°C, and destination plates for 16 h at 37°C.
7. After growth period has elapsed, examine test plates for evidence of contamination (clear plaques on T1 bacteriophage plate, yellow colonies on *Pseudomonas* plate).
8. Discard plates containing contamination (see Note 8).
9. Place replicated library plates in flow hood, remove lids, allow to cool for 10 min then score the missing wells, if desired.
10. Store replicated library plates in a separate –70°C freezer for each copy.

### 3.8. Gridding a Library to a Nylon Membrane

The clones are arrayed onto filters robotically so that a small amount of DNA from every clone in a library is present on the filter, or set of filters; these are then used in hybridization experiments in order to choose clones of interest for sequencing. Gridding protocols are machine-specific, so the manufacturer's instructions should be followed for creating filters. A general outline of the protocol for gridding is as follows.

1. Defrost library source plates and load on the robotic gridder.
2. Fill destination plates with LB agar plus antibiotic (20 μg/ml chloramphenicol).
3. Label filters and place them onto the agar destination plates. The grid pattern and clone DNA density should be selected to suit the preferred screening method. Run the automated gridding program.
4. Place the plates in a 37°C incubator for growth, inverted, for 16 h. After small colonies have grown on the filter, the bacterial cells are broken open using alkaline lysis, to release the DNA. Cell debris is removed during this stage.
5. Place a sheet of Whatman paper in a large tray and cover with 10% SDS. Pour off excess solution. Remove library filter(s) from LB agar plate and place colony side up onto the SDS saturated Whatman paper. Leave at room temperature for 5 min.
6. Remove filters and blot on clean Whatman paper to absorb any excess 10% SDS liquid.
7. Place filters in a second tray and cover with denaturation solution, and leave for 10 min.
8. Place filters on a clean sheet of Whatman paper and air-dry for 20 min.
9. Add neutralization solution to a new container (preferably with sealable lid to prevent splashing when rocking) then add the filter. Rock briefly for a few seconds to remove some cellular debris, pour off the liquid, then refill the box with fresh neutralization solution. Leave the box for 5 min on a rotating or rocking platform. Pour off the liquid.
10. Prepare a 1/10 dilution of neutralization solution with Milli-Q water, add to the box containing a filter, and rock again for 5 min, then pour off the liquid.
11. Pour 1 l of 2× SSC into a new container and add 1 ml of 10% SDS. Add the library filter and rock for 5 min. Pour off solution and add a second liter of 2× SSC, with no SDS, and place on rocker for 5 min. Pour off liquid.
12. Prepare a 1/20 dilution of Tris–HCl 1 M stock with Milli-Q water.
13. Add 1 l of 1/20 Tris–HCl solution to the container and rock for 5 min. Pour off solution and add a second liter for 1/20 Tris–HCl and rock for 5 min. Pour off solution.
14. Air-dry library filter for 24 h.
15. Fix DNA to the filters by placing them DNA side down on a UV transilluminator for 2 min.

### 3.9. Preparing a Radiolabeled Probe

To sequence a genome region of particular interest, a genome library must be screened to identify the few target clones containing the correct insert. Two common methods to screen a BAC of fosmid library are (1) using PCR-based technique of amplifying structured pools and superpools of clones and (2) hybridizing a labeled probe to a nylon membrane containing thousands of gridded clones. Both methods have advantages and disadvantages. The PCR pooling process can be used to screen thousands of probes, but is costly when purchased from a commercial source. As this method relies on PCR, amplification can fail if there are polymorphic differences between primers and the library. With the hybridization method, each nylon membrane can only be reused 3–10 times, however, a nylon membrane can be screened with multiple probe products simultaneously. The method outlined here requires the use of radiolabeled probes and follows the traditional screening technique of nylon membrane hybridization. For information on clone pool and superpool techniques, refer to commercial suppliers (e.g., Amplicon Express).

Probes are usually made from a purified PCR product. If the desired sequence to be used as a probe was previously cloned into a plasmid vector, it may well be easier to PCR amplify a product directly from the plasmid. The simplest method to create a probe for hybridization is to use a commercial kit, using random priming of a denatured PCR template to incorporate radiolabeled nucleotides with Klenow DNA Polymerase I. However, the process is quite straightforward and can also be achieved using standard molecular biology methods. Generally, PCR products of about 200–1,000 bp can be used to make suitable probes for library screening, although it is possible to use shorter fragments. Products containing repetitive sequences within intronic or noncoding DNA regions often identify many false positives, making detection of correct clones extremely difficult. If screening the library for a specific expressed gene, it is useful to PCR amplify a product from cDNA, thus avoiding introns that may contain sequence repeats. It is possible to screen a filter with multiple probes simultaneously, and then to test all the identified clones by PCR using primers specific for each probe.

1. Purify PCR product (e.g., Qiagen spin column) and quantify using a spectrophotometer (e.g., NanoDrop).
2. Denature 25 ng of probe in a volume of 10 μl of water for 2 min at 95°C using a 0.2-ml tube in a thermal cycler, then chill in an ice bath for 2 min.
3. Pulse spin to collect reaction in the bottom of the tube and return to ice.

4. Add the following reaction components:

| | |
|---|---|
| Labeling 5× buffer | 10 μl |
| dNTP (A/G/T, 500 μM each) | 2 μl |
| Denatured DNA | 25 ng |
| BSA (10 mg/ml) | 2 μl |
| Water | (To a final volume of 50 μl) |
| [a-$^{33}$P]dCTP (10 mCi/ml) | 1 μl (depending upon number of half-lives) |
| Klenow | 1 μl (5 U) |
| Total | 50 μl |

5. Mix reaction components and incubate at room temperature for 1 h.
6. Denature at 95°C for 2 min and chill in an ice bath for 2 min. At this point the probe is ready for hybridization (see Note 9).

### *3.10. Screening a Genome Library*

Hybridization can be carried out in tubes or boxes. The advantage of using tubes include (1) less buffers are required and (2) multiple hybridizations may be performed in the same oven using different tubes.

1. While the probe is being labeled, turn on the hybridization oven and preheat to 65°C.
2. With the nucleic acid uppermost, prewet the membrane in water, then in 5× SSC. Roll the blot lengthways, with nucleic acid side innermost. Place inside a hybridization tube and add 5× SSC. Unroll the membrane, so that it is evenly set around the glass tube, with no air bubbles (see Note 10).
3. Drain excess of 5× SSC and add hybridization buffer. Preheat for 30 min at 65°C, taking care to place the tube in the correct orientation so that the membrane does not roll upon itself.
4. Add denatured probe (Subheading 3.9, step 6) to the hybridization tube containing hybridization buffer, and 100 μl of salmon sperm DNA (10 mg/ml) per 10 ml of buffer.
5. Hybridize overnight at 65°C.
6. Prewarm low stringency wash buffer (2× SSC, 0.1% SDS) to 65°C. This can be done using a microwave, and checking the temperature with a thermometer (overheating may cause overflow).
7. Drain hybridization buffer containing probe (check local guidelines for disposal) and add an excess of low stringency buffer. Wash for 10 min. During this time prewarm the medium stringency buffer (1× SSC, 0.1% SDS) to 65°C. Drain low stringency buffer, add medium stringency buffer and wash for 10 min. Drain medium stringency buffer (see Note 11).

8. Remove the filter from the hybridization tube and unroll onto a suitable platform. Using a Geiger counter, check signal strength. Some background is required to help orientate clones that contain the probe. If excessive wash steps are performed and no background is present, positive clones will be identified but it will be virtually impossible to locate the grid position.
9. Wrap filter in plastic wrap and expose to film or a phosphorimager screen (Fig. 1).
10. Hybridized probe can be stripped from the membrane placing a still damp filter into the box, and immersing in boiling 0.1% (w/v) SDS. Allow to cool to room temperature, rinse in 2× SSC. Check the membrane with a Geiger counter and re-expose to a phosphorimager screen to ensure that the probe has been removed.

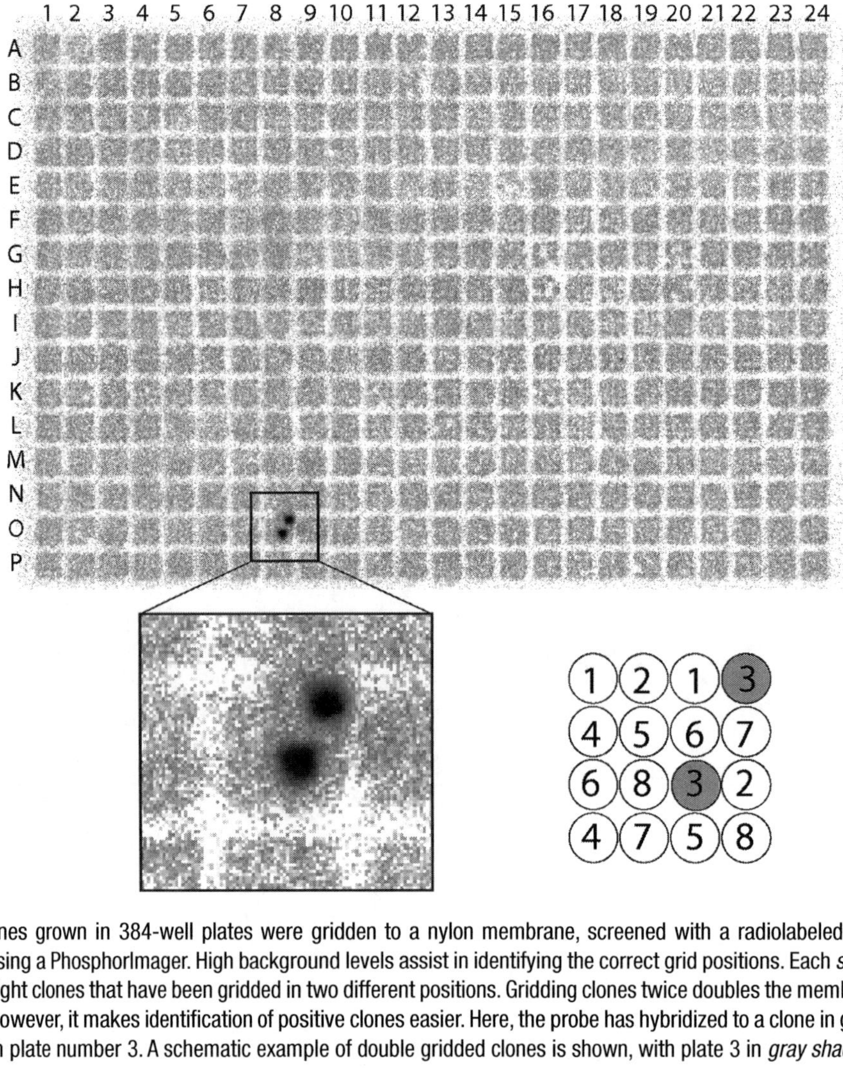


Fig. 1. Clones grown in 384-well plates were gridden to a nylon membrane, screened with a radiolabeled probe, and scanned using a PhosphorImager. High background levels assist in identifying the correct grid positions. Each *small square* contains eight clones that have been gridded in two different positions. Gridding clones twice doubles the membrane space required, however, it makes identification of positive clones easier. Here, the probe has hybridized to a clone in grid position "O-8" from plate number 3. A schematic example of double gridded clones is shown, with plate 3 in *gray shading*.

## 4. Notes

1. The best way to assess genomic DNA quality and quantity is to run 1 μl of a 10× dilution of the genomic DNA on a 0.8% high melting point agarose gel alongside quantitative markers and an aliquot of intact T7 phage DNA from the EPICENTRE CopyControl Fosmid library construction kit. After electrophoresis and staining with ethidium bromide the genomic DNA should migrate at or above the T7 phage control and can be quantified by comparing with the fluorescence of the quantitative markers.
2. Once mastered, fosmid library construction is a relatively robust process. However, there are several steps (particularly, the electroelution of DNA from the CHEF gel; Subheading 3.3) and the packaging and transfection of ligations (Subheading 3.4) that if not performed properly will result in a library with very low titre. DNA from different organisms and from different preparations can give vastly different outcomes. It is therefore recommended that one should perform a first run with test DNA (e.g., ultrapure human genomic DNA, Promega, Cat. No. G3041) before committing and then potentially wasting the DNA of interest. There are several steps in the protocol that can be quality control checked to ensure all is going well, for example, viewing the stained preparative CHEF gel (step 12 in Subheading 3.3), gel analysis of eluted DNA fraction (step 9 in Subheading 3.3), and performing a scaled down (1/100) test transfection first before committing all your material.
3. Preferred DNA end repair method.

   In a 1.5-ml Eppendorf tube mix:

| | |
|---|---|
| DNA | 20 μl |
| Water | 60 μl |
| 10× NEB buffer 2 | 10 μl |
| 100× BSA | 0.5 μl |
| 10 mM ATP | 5 μl |
| 5 mM dNTPs | 1.5 μl |
| T4 Polynucleotide kinase (NEB) | 1 μl |
| Klenow polymerase (NEB) | 1 μl |
| T4 Polymerase (NEB) | 1 μl |

Incubate at 37°C for 45 min and continue protocol at step 8 of Subheading 3.1.

4. Do not load the control DNA in the lane next to your sample as any spill over will result in contamination of your library with T7 phage inserts. Running some of the EPICENTRE CopyControl Fosmid kit test insert on the CHEF gel together with the experimental DNA gives a good indication of the size of DNA that is required and therefore which region of the DNA smear should be excised.
5. Before using a new pack of packaging extract determine its packaging efficiency using the tester phage supplied.
6. While fosmid ligations are stable when stored at –20°C, packaged fosmids do not keep very well. When stored at 4°C, however, they are stable for up to 1 month.
7. When necessary test minipreps and digestions may be performed; this is only needed if there are very few colonies, if it is a difficult genome, or if there is a doubt about the results.
8. Although it is important to discard plates which contain even one well with phage in, it is possible to clean out wells which have tested positive for *Pseudomonas*: evacuate the well using a pipette, refill the well with 70 μl of Virkon. Remove the Virkon using a pipette, then refill using 70% ethanol. Remove this and then allow to dry before freezing the plate. Keeping a score sheet of empty wells allows accurate records of library copies to be maintained.
9. For additional information on making probes, see the technical bulletin for Prime-a-Gene Labeling System, Promega.
10. Flat-Tip Tweezers can be used to pick up the membrane by the corners to avoid damaging gridded clones.
11. For additional information on hybridization, see Hybond-N + instructions, Amersham Biosciences.

## References


1. Shizuya H, Birren B, Kim UJ et al (1992) Cloning and stable maintenance of 300-kilobase-pair fragments of human DNA in *Escherichia coli* using an F factor based vector. Proceedings of the National Academy of Sciences of the United States of America **89**:8794–8797
2. Baxter SW, Papa R, Chamberlain N et al (2008) Convergent evolution in the genetic basis of Müllerian mimicry in Heliconius butterflies. Genetics **180**:1567–1577
3. Meyers BC, Chin DB, Shen KA et al (1998) The major resistance gene cluster in lettuce is highly duplicated and spans several megabases. Plant Cell **10**:1817–1832
4. Colosimo P, Hosemann K, Balabhadra S et al (2005) Widespread parallel evolution in sticklebacks by repeated fixation of Ectodysplasin alleles. Science **307**:1928–1933
5. Tursun B, Cochella L, Carrera I et al (2009) A Toolkit and Robust Pipeline for the Generation of Fosmid-Based Reporter Genes in C. elegans. PLoS ONE **4**:e4625
6. Musken M, Di Fiore S, Romling U et al (2010) A 96-well-plate-based optical method for the quantitative and qualitative evaluation of *Pseudomonas aeruginosa* biofilm formation and its application to susceptibility testing. Nature Protocols **5**:1460–1469

# Chapter 4

## Genomic Libraries: II. Subcloning, Sequencing, and Assembling Large-Insert Genomic DNA Clones

**Mike A. Quail, Lucy Matthews, Sarah Sims, Christine Lloyd, Helen Beasley, and Simon W. Baxter**

### Abstract

Sequencing large insert clones to completion is useful for characterizing specific genomic regions, identifying haplotypes, and closing gaps in whole genome sequencing projects. Despite being a standard technique in molecular laboratories, DNA sequencing using the Sanger method can be highly problematic when complex secondary structures or sequence repeats are encountered in genomic clones. Here, we describe methods to isolate DNA from a large insert clone (fosmid or BAC), subclone the sample, and sequence the region to the highest industry standard. Troubleshooting solutions for sequencing difficult templates are discussed.

**Key words:** Genome library sequencing, Sequence assembly, Subclone, Contig, Phrap, Phred, Finishing standards, Short insert library, Transposon library

## 1. Introduction

Genome libraries offer the ability to close sequencing gaps in eukaryotic genomes, particularly in euchromatin regions, and can act as a valuable reference to verify genome assemblies generated with next-generation sequencing technologies. Sequencing large genomic clones can produce a >100 kbp haplotype, compared to the shorter and often polymorphic contigs generated through next-generation approaches (e.g. (1)). When sequencing a genome, or a specific genome region, generating a "tile path" of genomic clones is a particularly useful strategy to identify the minimum number of clones required. To achieve this, a restriction digest of each library clone is performed and banding pattern, known as a "fingerprint," is analyzed with electrophoresis. Overlapping clones share some

Virginie Orgogozo and Matthew V. Rockman (eds.), *Molecular Methods for Evolutionary Genetics*, Methods in Molecular Biology, vol. 772, DOI 10.1007/978-1-61779-228-1_4, © Springer Science+Business Media, LLC 2011

common band patterns, enabling this method to predict the minimum number of clones required for sequencing a genome. The maize genome, for example, was sequenced from the minimum tile path of 16,910 overlapping BAC and fosmid clones (2).

In order to sequence a fosmid (38–42 kb) or a BAC (100–300 kb), the clone DNA is isolated and sheared into smaller fragments (often 100–800 bp), subcloned into a vector and transformed into competent cells. DNA from the subclones is purified using a miniprep, sequenced with BigDye terminator chemistry, and assembled into contigs. Sequencing gaps can often occur when attempting to assemble a genomic clone into a single contiguous sequence. Gaps may be caused by a variety of reasons including low sequence coverage, poor quality data caused by simple sequence repeats, or complex secondary structures that are extremely difficult to sequence through.

The Sanger DNA sequencing method has been a routine molecular laboratory technique for more than two decades, yet problematic templates can be common. Here, we provide a robust and cost-effective strategy for sequencing large insert genomic clones, plus methods to assemble and finish clones as single contiguous regions. Examples of the most commonly encountered sequencing problems are described, alongside the best strategy to overcome such difficulties. These protocols follow on from Chapter 3, which describes construction and screening of fosmid genomic libraries.

## 2. Materials

### *2.1. DNA Isolation from Large Insert Clones (e.g., Fosmid or BAC)*

1. 2× TY: 1.6% Bactotryptone, 10% bacto-yeast extract, 0.5% NaCl. Autoclave to sterilize.
2. Chloramphenicol (Sigma). 500× stock solution is 50 mg/ml in ethanol. Filter sterilize before use.
3. 15- and 50-ml Falcon tubes.
4. Benchtop centrifuge that can spin 50-ml Falcon tubes at 15,200 × *g*, for example, Thermo Scientific Heraeus Multifuge 3/3R plus.
5. 10 mM EDTA, pH 8.0.
6. 20% SDS dissolved in water.
7. 4 M NaOH (BDH).
8. 3 M potassium acetate, pH 5.5 (Fisher).
9. Isopropanol (BDH).
10. TE buffer: 10 mM Tris–HCl, 50 mM EDTA, pH 8.0.
11. 7.5 M potassium acetate (not pHed).

12. 50 mM Tris–HCl, 50 mM EDTA, pH 8.0.
13. RNAse A (Sigma). 1,000× stock solution is 100 mg/ml in water.
14. UltraPure™ phenol:chloroform:isoamyl alcohol (25:24:1, v/v) (Invitrogen).
15. Chloroform (Applied Biosystems).
16. 96% Ethanol.
17. T0.1E buffer: 10 mM Tris–HCl, 0.1 mM EDTA, pH 8.0.
18. Electrophoresis gel system.

### 2.2. Subcloning DNA from a Fosmid or BAC Clone

1. Mung bean nuclease and 10× buffer (NEB).
2. Sonicator, for example, Branson digital sonifier model S-250D with cup horn probe http://www.bransonultrasonics.com/.
3. 10× TBE: 900 mM Tris–borate, 20 mM EDTA, pH 8.3.
4. 10× TAE: 400 mM Tris–acetate, 10 mM EDTA, pH 8.2.
5. High gelling temperature (HGT) agarose for electrophoresis, for example, UltraPure™ Agarose (Invitrogen).
6. Low melting point (LMP) agarose for preparative electrophoresis gels, for example, UltraPure™ Low Melting Point Agarose (Invitrogen).
7. *Hin*dIII and *Bst*NI (NEB).
8. Lambda DNA and pBR322 (NEB).
9. SYBR Green (Sigma).
10. Dark Reader (Clare Chemical Research; http://www.clarechemical.com/).
11. Ficoll loading dye: 0.1% (w/v) bromophenol blue, 10% (w/v) Ficoll 400, 1× TBE (90 mM Tris–borate, 2 mM EDTA, pH 8.3).
12. T0.1E buffer: 10 mM Tris–HCl, 0.1 mM EDTA, pH 8.0.
13. 1 M NaCl.
14. Buffered phenol solution, pH 8.0 (Sigma).
15. AgarACE (Promega).
16. Pellet paint (VWR).
17. 70 and 96% ethanol.
18. Microfuge capable of reaching 4°C.
19. 30°C, 42°C, and 65°C water baths or incubators.
20. T4 DNA ligase and 10× ligase buffer (Roche).
21. 40 ng/ml pUC19 *Sma*I digested and dephosphorylated (Fermentas).
22. phiX174 DNA digested with *Hae*II (NEB).
23. Proteinase K (Roche).
24. *Escherichia coli* Electromax DH10B electrocompetent cells (Invitrogen).

25. Gene Pulser cuvettes with 0.1-cm electrode gaps (Bio-Rad).
26. Electroporation equipment, for example, Micropulser (Bio-Rad).
27. SOC medium: 2% (w/v) Bactotryptone, 0.5% (w/v) yeast extract, 0.05% (w/v) NaCl, 2.5 mM KCl, 10 mM $MgCl_2$, 20 mM glucose, pH 7.0.
28. Bactoagar TYE plates: 1% (w/v) Bactotryptone, 0.5% (w/v) yeast extract, 0.8% NaCl, 0.1% glucose, 1.5% agar. Autoclave to sterile. Cool to 50°C before adding any antibiotics (e.g., ampicillin to a final concentration of 50 μg/ml) then pour into 9-mm agar dishes.
29. 2% Xgal: Dissolve in formamide.
30. 10% IPTG: Dissolve in water.
31. Ethidium bromide, 10 mg/ml (Sigma).

### 2.3. Growing Fosmid or BAC Subclones for Library Stock

1. Chloramphenicol (Sigma) stock solution (125 mg/ml). Add 5 g of chloramphenicol to 40 ml of methanol.
2. Circle grow growth media containing 12.5 μg/ml chloramphenicol (add 100 μl of chloramphenicol stock solution per liter of growth media).
3. 96-Well 2-ml boxes (Corning).
4. 100% glycerol.
5. Gas permeable seal (Abgene).

### 2.4. Growing Subclones for Sequencing

1. Circle grow growth media containing 12.5 μg/ml chloramphenicol.
2. 96-Well-ml boxes (Corning).
3. Gas permeable seal (Abgene).
4. Mylar nongas permeable seals.
5. 96-Pin stamping tool.
6. 96% Ethanol in trough that is large enough to hold a 96-pin stamping tool.
7. Bunsen flamer.
8. Double distilled water ($ddH_2O$) in a trough that is large enough to hold a 96-pin stamping tool.

### 2.5. Purifying DNA from Subclones for Sequencing

1. Double distilled water ($ddH_2O$).
2. RNAse A (20 mg/ml): Mix 1 g of RNAse A, 500 μl of 1 M Tris–HCl, pH 7.4 and 750 μl of 1 M NaCl into 48.75 ml of deionized water, mix well, store in 1-ml aliquots in Eppendorf tubes at −20°C.
3. GTE: In 828 ml of $ddH_2O$, add 46 ml of 20% glucose, 100 ml of 0.1 M EDTA, and 26 ml of 1 M Tris–HCl, pH 8.0. Store at room temperature until RNAse A is added, then store at 4°C.

4. NaOH/SDS: In 900 ml of $ddH_2O$, add 50 ml of 4N NaOH and 50 ml of 20% SDS. Store at room temperature. In cold weather salt may come out of solution. Place the bottle in warm water to redissolve before use.
5. 3 M potassium acetate: In 14 ml of $ddH_2O$, add 14 ml of concentrated glacial acetic acid and 75 ml of 5 M potassium acetate.
6. 70% Ethanol.
7. 100% Isopropanol.
8. Plate seals.
9. HPLC water.
10. 96-Well, 360-μl storage plates (Costar 3365 serocluster, Cat. No. DPS-136-030R).
11. 96-Well, 0.2-μm filter plate (Costar 3504 filter plate, Cat. No. DPS-148-010E).
12. A centrifuge able to hold 96-well plates.

### 2.6. Sequencing Subclones

1. Sequencing reaction diluent: Mix 160 ml of 1 M Tris base, pH 9.0, 3 ml of 1 M $MgCl_2$, 0.9 ml of Tween-20, 60 ml of 50% glycerol, and 5.5 ml of formamide into 224 ml of $ddH_2O$. Add 50 ml of tetramethylene sulfone and mix. Then add 0.8 g of potassium glutamate and 2 ml of bovine serum albumin. Prepare the day before and store at 4°C.
2. 96- or 384-well thermocycling plates, for example, half-skirted 96-well-plates (Greiner Bio One) or 384-well plates (Eppendorf).
3. Big Dye™ Terminator v3.1 Cycle Sequencing Kit and dGTP Big Dye™ V3.0 Terminator mix (Applied Biosystems).
4. Sequencing primers (120 pmol/μl): M13/pUC forward 5′-GTAAAACGACGGCCAGT-3′ and M13/pUC reverse 5′-AGCGGATAACAATTTCACACAGGA-3′.
5. Double distilled water ($ddH_2O$).
6. Precipitation mix: Mix 80 ml of 96% ethanol, 1.6 ml of 3 M sodium acetate, and 3.2 ml of 0.1 mM EDTA into 17 ml of $ddH_2O$.
7. 70% Ethanol.
8. Thermoheat seals (Bio-Rad).
9. Tissue or blotting pad (Pal).

### 2.7. Sequence Assembly and Finishing

1. Database assembly software.
2. Data viewing and manipulation package.
3. Internet access or database for BLAST search.
4. Custom primers to close sequencing gaps.
5. dGTP BigDye™ Terminator (PE Applied Biosystems).
6. SequenceR$_X$ Enhancers (Invitrogen).

7. Dimethylsulfoxide (DMSO).
8. Sequence Finishing Kit (TempliPhi).
9. EZ-Tn5 < Kan-2 > insertion kit (EPICENTRE).

## 3. Methods

### *3.1. DNA Isolation from Large Insert Clones (e.g., Fosmid or BAC)*

DNA isolated for sequencing should be prepared from a high-quality alkaline lysis miniprep. The purified DNA can have high levels of contamination from the *E. coli* host genome, which will carry through to sequencing. To minimize *E. coli* contamination when isolating DNA from large insert clones, there are several commercial options, such as the Large-Construct Kit (Qiagen) or the BACmax DNA Purification Kit (EPICENTRE). While these kits are excellent, if expensive when doing large numbers of samples, high quality preparation of BAC, PAC, or Fosmid DNA can be achieved using an inexpensive protocol that we describe here, which relies on two precipitations with potassium acetate to remove cellular debris and *E. coli* genomic DNA.

1. Inoculate 200 ml of 2× TY containing 12.5 μg/ml chloramphenicol with a single colony and incubate overnight at 37°C at 250 rpm.
2. Transfer 50 ml of each culture into Falcon tubes. Centrifuge in a benchtop centrifuge at 5,500 × *g* for 7 min.
3. Decant the supernatant and drain the pellet. Resuspend in 5 ml of 10 mM EDTA, pH 8.0. Leave on ice for 5 min.
4. Make the NaOH/SDS solution by mixing 120 ml of water with 6 ml of 20% SDS and 6 ml of 4 M NaOH.
5. Add 10 ml of NaOH/SDS, do not mix. Stand on ice for 5–10 min.
6. Add 7.5 ml of cold 3 M potassium acetate. Do not mix. Leave on ice for 15 min.
7. Centrifuge at 15,200 × *g* for 40 min. Decant the supernatant to a fresh Falcon tube and repeat centrifugation.
8. Decant into a fresh Falcon tube and add 11.25 ml of isopropanol. Centrifuge at 4,500 × *g* for 20 min.
9. Discard the supernatant and resuspend the pellet in 2 ml of TE buffer.
10. Transfer to 15-ml Falcon tubes.
11. Add 1 ml of 7.5 M potassium acetate (not pHed). Leave at −70°C for 30 min.
12. Thaw, then centrifuge at 4,500 × *g* for 15 min.
13. Add 6 ml of ethanol to separate 15-ml Falcon tubes. Decant the supernatant into these tubes. Mix.

14. Centrifuge at 2,500 × *g* for 10 min. Discard the supernatant and resuspend the pellet in 175 μl of 50 mM Tris–HCl, 50 mM EDTA.
15. Transfer to 1.5-ml Eppendorf tubes. Add 2.5 μl of DNAse-free RNAse. Incubate at 37°C for 60 min.
16. Phenol:Chloroform extract twice, then chloroform extract (add an equal volume of phenol:chloroform or chloroform). Mix by gently inverting the tube for 1 min. Do not vortex, as this can break up DNA fragments. Place on ice for 5 min and separate phases by centrifugation at 16,000 × *g* at room temperature for 5 min. Carefully pipette off the upper layer leaving behind approximately 10% without disturbing the interface of lower layer and pipette into a fresh Eppendorf tube.
17. To aqueous layer add 700 μl of isopropanol and centrifuge for 5 min.
18. Wash pellet with 500 μl of ethanol and dry.
19. Resuspend in 40 μl of TE buffer.
20. Take a 1-μl aliquot and dilute to 20 μl with T0.1E. Run 1 μl of this dilution on an agarose gel alongside quantitative lambda *Hin*dIII markers (NEB). Each prep should have a visible band that migrates above the 23-kb marker fragment. Estimate concentration relative to intensity of markers.

### 3.2. Subcloning DNA from a Fosmid or BAC Clone

In order to shotgun sequence a genomic clone, the DNA is routinely subcloned into a suitable sequencing vector (e.g., pUC19). This typically involves random shearing of purified DNA prepared from individual clones, gel purification of the desired size (generally, fractions from within the range 100–800 bp), DNA end-repair, and blunt-end ligation into vector.

1. *Shearing purified DNA.* Pipette 5 μg of DNA (or less, down to a minimum of 1 μg), into a fresh 1.5-ml tube. Add 6 μl of 10× mung bean buffer followed by water to a final volume of 60 μl.
2. *Assemble sonicator.* Put prechilled water in the sonicator cup.
3. Microfuge samples to settle contents. Place first tube in clip centrally and about 1 mm from the face of the probe. Sonicate for 15 s on number 3 checking the output and that movement or cavitation can be seen in the cup. Repeat for the other tubes. Microfuge samples once more to settle contents and sonicate samples for a second time.
4. Intensity of sonication will depend upon the concentration and G/C composition of the DNA. A/T-rich DNA is more fragile. Typically, sonicate at setting of 3 for two pulses of 10 s each. For A/T-rich DNA use a lower power and/or raise tube to be approximately 15 mm away from probe.

5. Briefly microfuge samples to settle contents then run a 1-µl aliquot of each sample through a 0.8% high gelling temperature agarose gel in TBE buffer. Run the gel at 70 V for 40 min alongside a 5-µl loading of marker (lambda DNA digested with *Hin*dIII and pBR322 digested with *Bst*NI (NEB)). Stain with ethidium bromide for 30 min and view on a UV transilluminator.
   There are three possible outcomes:
   (a) Complete sonication (no sign of high molecular weight DNA, smear between 4 kb and 500 bp).
   (b) Near complete sonication (smear and faint high molecular weight DNA).
   (c) Unsonicated (faint smear and substantial high molecular weight DNA).

   In the case of (b) resonicate for 5 s, further checking optional. In the case of (c) resonicate again for 2× 10 s and recheck on a minigel before proceeding.
6. *End-repair*. To the sonicated DNA add 0.3 µl (45 U) of mung bean nuclease and incubate at 30°C for 10 min. Place the samples on ice, then add T0.1E to bring the volume of the sample up to 200 µl.
7. Add 20 µl of 1 M NaCl, 2 ml of pellet paint, and 550 µl of 96% ethanol to each sample. Precipitate the DNA at −20°C overnight or at −70°C for 30 min.
8. Pellet the DNA in a microfuge at 16,000 ×*g* for 30 min at 4°C. Wash the pellet with 500 µl of 70% ethanol and respin for 15 min. Dry the DNA pellet in a desiccator for 15 min.
9. Dissolve the sonicated end-repaired DNA in 6.25 µl of T0.1E, 0.75 µl of 10× TAE, and 2 µl of Ficoll loading dye.
10. Load the samples onto a 0.8% LMP agarose gel in 1× TAE, leaving a blank lane between each sample. Electrophorese at 20 V for 2 h. Visualize the DNA by staining with SYBR Green for 20 min and viewing on a Dark Reader. By reference to the 100-bp marker, cut out gel slices corresponding to 100–300, 300–500, and 500–800 bp.
11. *AgarAce digestion and phenol extraction*. Melt the appropriate gel slice at 65°C for 5 min, then equilibrate at 42°C for 5 min.
12. Add 4 µl of AgarAce and continue the incubation at 42°C for 20 min. Transfer the samples to ice and add T0.1E to 200 µl. Add 200 µl of buffered phenol solution on ice. Equilibrate the samples for 5 min on ice and separate the phases by centrifugation at 16,000 ×*g* for 2 min.
13. Remove the upper aqueous phase carefully. Add 20 µl of 1 M NaCl, 2 µl of pellet paint and 550 µl of 96% ethanol. Precipitate the DNA at −20°C overnight or −70°C for 30 min.

14. Pellet the DNA in a microfuge at 16,000 × *g* for 30 min at 4°C. Wash the pellet with 500 μl of 70% ethanol and respin for 15 min. Dry the DNA pellet in a desiccator for 15 min.
15. *Ligations into pUC19* (see Note 1). Dissolve the DNA pellet in 4 μl of T0.1E. In a 0.5-ml tube, ligate 2 μl of sonicated, gel-purified DNA to 0.25 μl of pUC19 in a 4-μl reaction containing 0.4 μl of 10× ligase buffer, 0.3 μl of T4 DNA ligase, and 1.05 μl of water. Incubate the ligations at 16°C for 16 h. Set up also three control reactions using phiX174 DNA digested with *Hae*II as a control DNA (1) control DNA without ligase, (2) no DNA and no ligase, and (3) control DNA and ligase.
16. Add 1 μl of proteinase K (0.47 U) and 46 μl of T0.1E and incubate at 50°C for 1 h.
17. For transformations of pUC ligations, electroporate 40 μl of *E. coli* DH10B electrocompetent cells with 0.5 μl of the ligation (1,900 V; 200 Ω; 25 μF). Immediately, add 0.5 ml of SOC medium to the cells and mix gently.
18. Transfer the cells to a clean tube and incubate at 37°C for 1 h with shaking at 300 rpm. Meanwhile allow TYE plates containing 50 μg/ml ampicillin to equilibrate to room temperature and spread 40 μl of 2% *Xgal* and 20 μl of 10% IPTG over the surface of each plate. Dry plates.
19. Plate out 25 and 100 μl of the transformed cell mix onto separated plates and incubate at 37°C overnight.
20. Next morning count the number of colonies on the plates.

    Expect:

| Ligation | Blue colonies per plate | White colonies per plate |
|---|---|---|
| Experimental ligation | No more than 2× control 2 | >50 and at least 8× no. of blues |
| Control 1: phiX174 DNA, no ligase | 0–100 | 0–10 |
| Control 2: no phiX174 DNA, no ligase | 0–100 | 0–10 |
| Control 3: phiX174 DNA with ligase | 100s | Approximately 3× no. of blues |

### 3.3. Growing Fosmid or BAC Subclones for Library Stock

Prior to sequencing, subclones are first picked and grown in stock plates. The stock plates may then be replicated to generate material for sequencing.

1. To 925 ml of circle grow growth media add 75 ml of 100% glycerol giving a final concentration of 7.5% glycerol.

2. Fill a 96-well growth box with 1.5 ml of circle grow medium. This can be done manually using a multichannel pipette or multidispensing liquid handling equipment.
3. Each well is then inoculated by picking a colony using a sterile cocktail stick or using automation such as the Genetix platform.
4. Seal all growth boxes with a gas permeable seal. It is a good idea to produce a control box containing just growth media and to grow the control box at the same time under the same conditions. If there is subsequent growth in the control box this may indicate contamination.
5. Place boxes in an incubator for 22 h at 37°C at a speed of 320 rpm (see Note 2).
6. After growth, remove gas permeable seal and reseal completely with a mylar (or similar) seal. Proceed with Subheading 3.4 then place a lid on the sealed plate and store at –70°C.

### 3.4. Growing Subclones for Sequencing

1. Fill 96-well growth boxes with 1.5 ml of circle grow containing chloramphenicol. This can be done manually using a multichannel pipette or multidispensing liquid handling equipment.
2. Inoculate each well using the following method (NB: disposable 96-pin picking tools may also be used):
   (a) Place the 96-pin picking tool in the trough containing 96% ethanol.
   (b) Flame the picking tool using the Bunsen flamer, then allow to cool.
   (c) Place the picking tool into the glycerol stock plate and inoculate the new 96-well growth box.
   (d) Remove from the plate and place into a water trough until ready to inoculate the next growth box. Dab picking tool on tissue to remove excess water and repeat steps (a)–(d) for the remaining plates.
3. Seal all growth boxes with a gas permeable seal. It is a good idea to produce a control box containing just growth media and grow the control box at the same time under the same conditions. If there is subsequent growth in the control box this may indicate contamination.
4. Place boxes in an incubator for 22 h at 37°C at a speed of 320 rpm (see Note 2).

### 3.5. Purifying DNA from Subclones for Sequencing

1. Prior to performing this protocol add 5 ml of RNAse A to 1 l of GTE (shake well).
2. Growth boxes must be spun to pellet the cells for 2–3 min at 2,147 × $g$, then the supernatant decanted for appropriate disposal. The growth boxes must then be inverted and tapped gently on tissue to remove any residual supernatant.

3. At this stage, it is useful to prepare the corresponding number of 96-well storage plates. Using a multichannel pipette or semi-automated liquid dispenser, add 140 μl of isopropanol each well of the empty storage plates. These isopropanol filled plates are required at step 9 in Subheading 3.5.
4. Add 120 μl of GTE/RNAse solution to each pellet and resuspend by vortexing for 2 min. It is important to make sure that the cells are completely resuspended.
5. Add 120 μl of NaOH/SDS solution to each well. The box now needs to be sealed (e.g., by using a 3-M scotch plate sealer) and then mixed by slow inversion ten times.
6. Leave the plate at room temperature for 2 min. Do not leave longer than 5 min (see Note 3).
7. Add 120 μl of 3 M potassium acetate to each well. Seal the plate and then mix by slow inversion ten times.
8. Transfer 140 μl of this solution to the corresponding wells of a 96-well 0.2-μm filter plate.
9. Place the 96-well filter plate on top of the corresponding isopropanol-filled storage plate. Centrifuge for 20 min at 2,147 × *g* and 4°C.
10. Discard the filter plate and the supernatant. Gently tap the inverted storage plate on paper towels to remove any residual isopropanol.
11. Add 100 μl of 70% ethanol to the storage plate.
12. Centrifuge for 5 min at 2,147 × *g* and 4°C.
13. After centrifugation, invert the plate to remove the ethanol, and gently tap the plate on paper towels.
14. Place the inverted plate on tissue or filter paper in the centrifuge and spin for 10 s at 8.4 × *g*.
15. Leave to dry covered with tissue (to prevent debris from falling in) on bench for at least 1 h. Alternatively, leave in a vacuum dryer for 30 min.
16. Resuspend with 40–60 μl of HPLC water and leave to stand overnight at 4°C. Mix before performing next stage.
17. At this point it is ideal to quantify the DNA in a few random samples.

### 3.6. Sequencing Subclones

1. To each well of a thermocycling plate, add 4 μl of sequencing enzyme mix that contains: 0.125 μl of BigDye™ V3.1 Terminator mix, 2.335 μl of Sequencing reaction diluent, 0.04 μl of dGTP Big Dye™ V3.0 Terminator mix, 1.475 μl of $ddH_2O$, 0.025 μl of one sequencing primer (concentration of 120 pmoles/μl). Subclone sequencing is commonly performed in both the forward and reverse directions to assist in DNA assembly.

2. To each 96-well add 4–6 μl of purified DNA (200 ng).
3. Spin the plate briefly and seal with heat sealing lid or mat.
4. Amplify the DNA on a thermocycler using the following program:
   (a) 96°C 45 s
   (b) 92°C 10 s
   (c) 52°C 10 s
   (d) 60°C 2 min
   (e) Go to step (b) another 59 times
   (f) 10°C forever.
5. Centrifuge the plate briefly before adding 60 μl of precipitation mix to each well. This can be done with a multichannel pipette or semi-automated using liquid handling equipment.
6. Centrifuge the plate for 20 min at 1,610 × *g* and 4°C.
7. Invert the plate onto a blotting pad (Whatman) or tissue and spin for 1 min at 16 × *g*.
8. Discard the blotting pad or tissue in a suitable container.
9. To each well add 70 μl of 70% ethanol (kept at –20°C), again using a multichannel pipette or semi-automated using liquid handling equipment.
10. Centrifuge the plate for 5 min at 1,610 × *g* and 4°C.
11. Invert the plate onto a fresh blotting pad (Whatman) or tissue and spin for 1 min at 16 × *g*.
12. Discard the blotting pad or tissue.
13. Dry the plate (not inverted) overnight at room temperature in dark conditions, or for 2 h in a vacuum chamber.
14. Ensure that all ethanol has evaporated before loading on a ABI 3730 (see Note 4).

### 3.7. Sequence Assembly and Finishing

Sequence assembly is the process of aligning the reads generated by shotgun sequencing. If using trace files from ABI 3730 or similar, data are base called and quality values are assigned using phred (3). The reads can be clipped according to quality and screened for sequencing and cloning vector sequence and contamination such as *E. coli* and bacterial transposon sequences using computer programs such as those available as part of the Staden package (4). Reads are assembled into contigs using software such as phrap (3) and data can be viewed and manipulated using packages such as gap4 (5, 6) and consed (7).

Generally, the most cost-effective level of read coverage is 6–8×. At levels lower than 6×, there will be several gaps and regions of low quality in the fosmid or BAC sequence, ultimately causing increased costs and delays in achieving a final assembly. At levels greater than 8× there will be extra redundancy, and some sequence gaps may still remain, caused for example, by structural elements of the DNA that could not be obtained with standard sequencing methods. Following the first round of shotgun sequencing, if the coverage is less than 6× the number of extra shotgun reads needed to attain the desired coverage can be calculated using the following equations:

$$\frac{\text{Coverage acquired}}{\text{Coverage required}} \times 100 = \%\ \text{coverage gained}$$

$$\frac{\text{Contigs} > 2\text{kb}}{\%\ \text{Coverage gained}} \times (100 - \%\ \text{coverage gained})$$
$$= \text{number of reads required for desired coverage}$$

The percentage failure rate of the first round of shotgun sequencing should be calculated and used to predict the failure rate in the next round. This then needs to be factored into the estimate of how many more reads need to be sequenced.

The sequence of the contigs can be BLAST searched against sequences submitted to the public databases, such as the EMBL nucleotide sequence database (8), to confirm that it is the expected species and to check for matches with any expected overlapping clones. If a restriction digest has been performed before sequencing the clone, then this can be used to check the expected size against the total length of contigs in the assembly. Once these checks have been carried out work can begin to close gaps and verify ambiguous and low quality sequence. This process is known as finishing.

The definition of finishing and finishing standards for large genome projects, such as the Human Genome Project, were agreed at the Second International Strategy Meeting in Bermuda in 1997 (9). The finishing standards for smaller projects may vary depending on funding and project requirements. Guidelines for data submission to public sequence databases using the High Throughput Genomic Sequences (HTGS) scheme have been set out by GenBank, EMBL, and DDBJ (10) (Table 1, see Note 5).

**Table 1**
**Guidelines for data submission to public databases using the High Throughput Genomic Sequences scheme (http://www.ncbi.nlm.nih.gov/HTGS/)**

| Status | Definition |
|---|---|
| Phase 0 | One-to-few pass reads of a single clone (not contigs) |
| Phase 1 | Unfinished, may be unordered, unoriented contigs, with gaps |
| Phase 2 | Unfinished, ordered, oriented contigs, with or without gaps |
| Phase 3 | Finished, no gaps (with or without annotations) |

The following methods described below can be employed to achieve the desired level of sequence gap closure from noncontiguous draft to fully finished depending on the project objective (Fig. 1a, b). Although a contiguous assembly can occasionally be achieved from shotgun sequencing a BAC or fosmid, in general there will be gaps in the assembly for a variety of reasons. The sequence of a particular region may have a structure that has a detrimental effect on the sequencing reaction, causing it to stop at that point in the sequence. Some regions may contain genes that affect growth of the subclones, leading to under-representation or absence of subclones covering these regions. There may also be

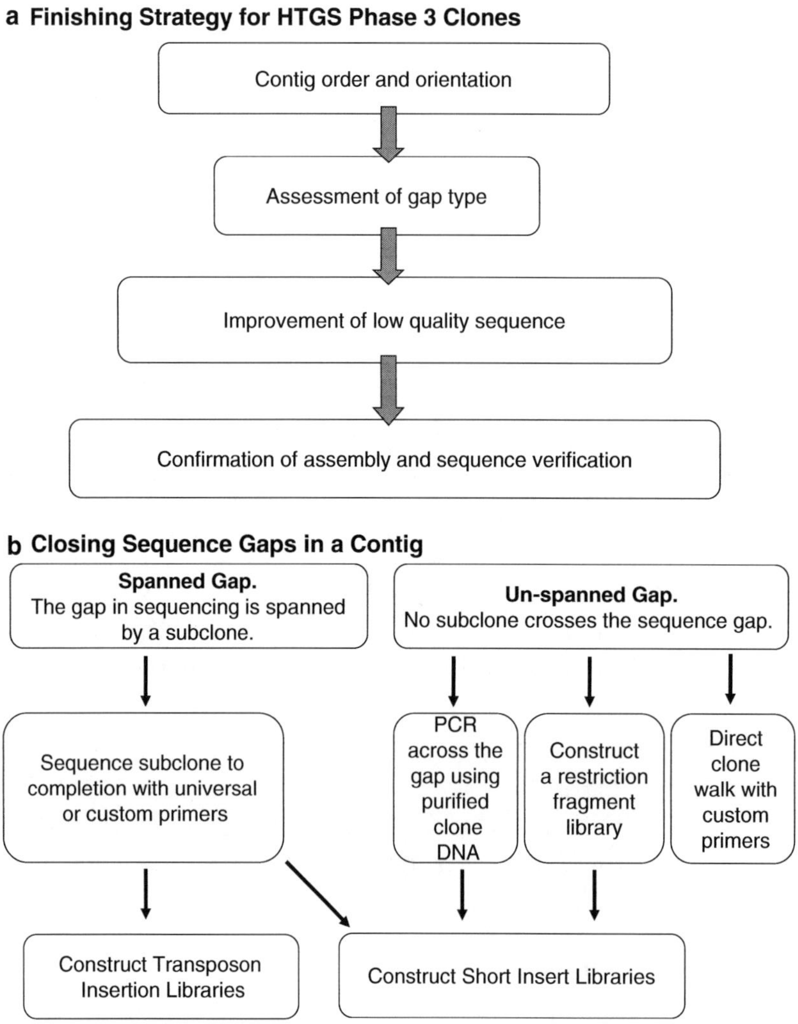


Fig. 1. (**a**) Flowchart for finishing assemblies to HTGS Phase 3 standards. (**b**) Flowchart for closing sequencing gaps. If a subclone spans a sequencing gap, custom primers can be designed to sequence the region. If the gap is not spanned by a subclone, PCR from clone DNA across the gap may be necessary. Alternatively, walks using custom primers can be carried out from the clone DNA (Direct clone walks), or new restriction fragment libraries can be made.

repeat sequences that the assembler fails to put together. Gaps may also occur purely by chance.

When determining the most appropriate method to close each gap, it is helpful to ascertain whether the gaps are spanned or unspanned and to order and orientate each contig in the assembly. Whether gaps are spanned or unspanned in the assembly will depend on the choice of sequencing vector used in the original shotgun sequencing. If single stranded M13 vectors have been used then all gaps are technically unspanned, and PCR will be required to elicit the reverse strand of the M13. Further PCR on clone DNA may be necessary in multiple combinations to establish contig order and orientation from shotgun libraries derived solely from M13 vectors. If double stranded plasmid vectors are used for sequencing, then mate pairs derived from sequencing a single plasmid in both directions (also referred to as subclones) can be used to order and orientate contigs (Fig. 2a).

The contig at each end of the BAC or fosmid insert can be identified by the presence of cloning vector sequence, then the relative positions of the other contigs to each end contig can be assessed using mate pairs. When working with an assembly consisting of mate pairs from double stranded plasmid subclones, the order and orientation of the majority of contigs can usually be identified by finding the positions of mates for reads that sequence from the ends of the contigs into each gap. Gap4 and consed have in-built read pair finding tools, assuming that each subclone has a unique identifier, and the forward and reverse strands for each subclone are also identifiable. Gaps which have mate pairs sequencing in from each contig are said to be spanned; further work to capture the sequence missing in the gap can be carried out using the spanning subclone as a template (Fig. 2b).

If there are reads sequencing into a gap, but their mate pairs are absent from the assembly, this may be because the assembly software has failed to incorporate them. A search for the identifying read name can be made for the missing mate pair in the original file of shotgun reads so that it can then be manually added to the assembly. Alternatively, the mate pair may be absent because the sequencing reaction failed, because of a random event or because of sequence structure. Another attempt at sequencing can be made, and it may be worthwhile using alternative sequencing chemistries (Table 2, Fig. 3, Note 6).

If there are no mate pairs across a gap then it is said to be unspanned. A direct walk using a custom primer may be tried from the BAC or fosmid DNA, but more commonly a PCR using the BAC or fosmid DNA is performed to generate a template from which further sequencing can be carried out. In order to assess the most appropriate parameters for the PCR reaction it may be helpful to determine the size of the gap using restriction enzymes. If several gaps are unspanned and the contigs cannot therefore be ordered,

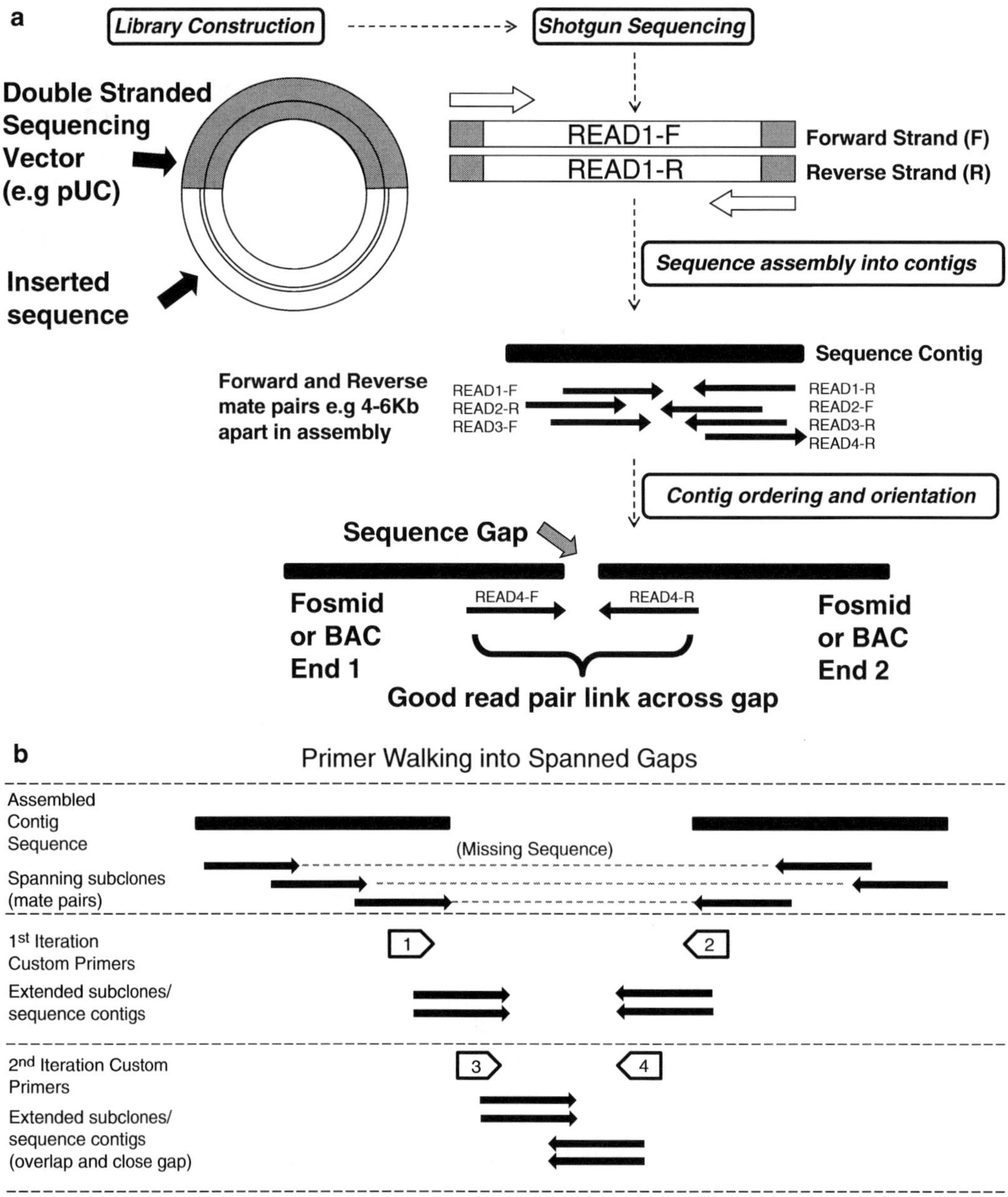


Fig. 2. (**a**) Double stranded sequencing vectors and their uses in ordering and orienting assembled sequence contigs. (**b**) Primer walking into spanned gaps. The assembled contig sequence contains a gap spanned by mate paired subclones (represented by *arrows*). Custom primers (1 and 2) are designed off the end of assembled contigs. The spanning mate pairs may not have sequenced this far but the assumption is made that these will contain the primer sequence and the sequence up to and beyond the end of the existing contigs. This process is repeated (e.g., primers 3 and 4) until the gap has been completely closed.

combinatorial PCRs will be needed. Custom primer sequences for direct walks from the fosmid DNA and for PCRs should be confirmed for uniqueness within the entire fosmid. Sequence searches can be performed in gap4 or consed to check the primer

**Table 2**
**Troubleshooting sequencing reactions**

| Problem type | Suggested chemistry usage |
|---|---|
| General | 4:1 Mix ratio of ABI BigDye Terminator: ABI dGTP BigDye Terminator |
| Di-nucleotide runs (especially TA runs) e.g., TATATATA$^n$, CGCGCGC$^n$ | ABI dGTP BigDye Terminator |
| Inverted repeats/sequence trace stops | ABI dGTP BigDye Terminator<br>Sequence Finishing Kit (SFK) (aka TempliPhi – Amersham) |
| Mono-nucleotide runs e.g., GGGGGGGGG$^n$ | Combination of SequenceRx Enhancer Solution A (Invitrogen) + dimethylsulfoxide (DMSO) + dGTP |

sequence is unique. Web-based tools are also available that allow sequence comparison checks to be made.

Once the appropriate template for each gap has been determined, custom primers can be designed at the ends of each contig in order to sequence into the gap. Primer design tools such as Primer3 (11, 12) or the tools within gap4 can be used to select primers in good quality data approximately 100–200 bp from the contig end, allowing primer walks to be anchored to the original sequence while giving extension. Primer design parameters should include annealing temperatures of 50–60°C, GC content 40–60% with a GC clamp. These parameters will depend on the GC content of substrate and cycling conditions used in sequencing. Primer length may need to be extended to increase chances of the sequence being unique. Primer sequences should be confirmed for uniqueness within the subclone or PCR template. This first round of sequencing may extend the contigs but not fully close the gap, in which case further custom primers should be designed using the extended sequence and subsequent rounds of sequencing carried out until the gap is closed (Fig. 1b).

Occasionally, the structure of the sequence in the gap is such that attempts at sequencing fail or give poor quality reads which provide little or no extension. In these cases, short insert libraries generated from subclones, PCRs, or restriction fragments can be effective (13). The template DNA spanning the problem region is broken up into small fragments by extensive sonication, then the required size fractions are isolated and recloned into plasmid vector for sequencing. For extreme GC or AT biased regions subcloning in M13 may be necessary (14). Each of these short insert subclones contains such a small region of the sequence that structures are not formed within them and therefore can more easily be sequenced.

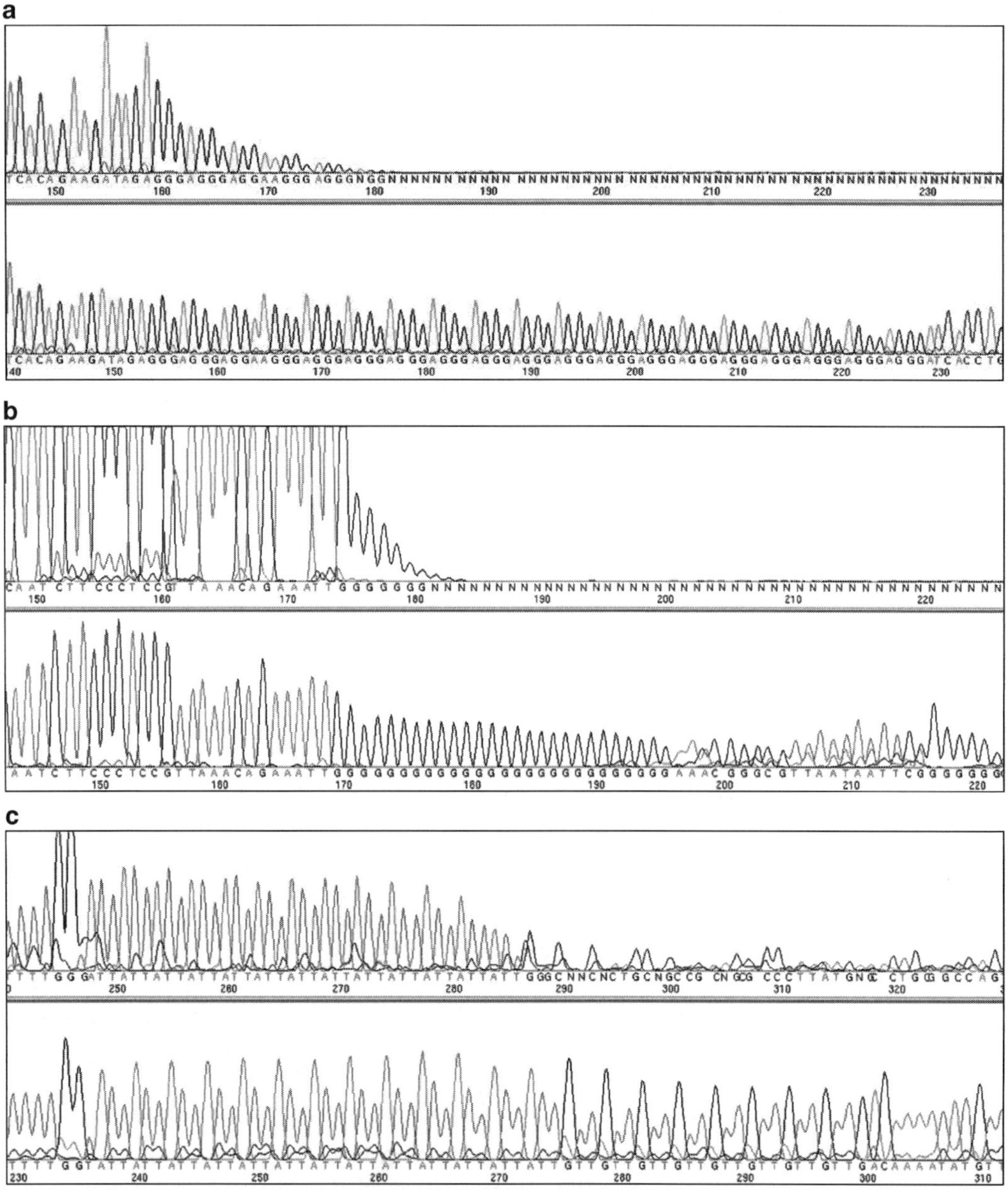

Fig. 3. Sequencing through complex repeat structures. (**a**) Example of sequencing through a complex AGG repeat region using ABI BigDye Terminator chemistry (*upper trace*) compared with ABI dGTP BigDye Terminator chemistry (*lower trace*). (**b**) Example of sequencing through a mono-nucleotide run with ABI BigDye Terminator chemistry (*upper trace*) compared with a combination of ABI dGTP BigDye Terminator, SequenceR$_x$ Enhancer A and DMSO (*lower trace*). (**c**) Example of sequencing through an ATT$^n$/GTT$^n$ repeat using ABI BigDye Terminator chemistry (*upper trace*) with the Sequence Finishing Kit (TempliPhi) (*lower trace*).

Transposon insertion libraries can also be generated from plasmid subclones (15). Transposon insertions are introduced into the insert DNA and the resulting library is then sequenced using transposon-specific primers. Therefore, new priming sites are generated within the plasmid clone in order to sequence through the problem structure. Transposon insertion libraries are particularly helpful in assembling regions of repeat sequence, as mate pairs sequence away from each other, with a short overlap at the transposon insertion site.

If the gap has resulted because of a large tandem or inverted repeat that has proved too difficult for the assembly software to put together, then larger insert libraries (6,000–8,000 bp) may be needed to provide long range information across these repeat structures. Regions of tandemly repeated sequence may prove impossible to assemble accurately. In these cases, a decision will need to be made as to whether the cost of further rounds of sequencing can be justified depending on the biological significance of the repeat region. If a decision is made not to fully finish the region, while still aiming to submit the sequence of the BAC or fosmid as Phase 3, then a miscellaneous feature tag can be employed to indicate that the region has been put together by forcing the join. Attempts should be made to prove that there is no nonrepeat sequence missing from the join by searching in the database for all contigs which contain repeat sequence but have not been joined to the main contig. Such contigs should then be scrutinized to ensure they do not contain any nonrepeat sequence. Restriction digests should be carried out, using restriction enzymes which do not have a cut site in the repeat sequence, in order to estimate the gap size.

Confirmation of assembly for contiguous sequence, or the estimation of gap sizes or repeats can be achieved by carrying out electronic virtual digests on consensus sequence, for example, using restriction enzyme map in gap4 or other tools such as restriction mapper (16). These virtual digests can then be compared with fragments produced from the original clone fingerprint data if available. Alternatively, specific restriction enzymes may be chosen and new digests performed so that any regions under question can be sized.

If restriction digest information is unavailable, and the assembly is based on a paired end library then sequence gaps and repeat sizes can be estimated by sizing spanning subclone templates on a gel. Alternatively, PCR products across a problem region can be sized, but this may be misleading if repetitive sequence or a structure leads the PCR to collapse or delete.

Sequence can be checked for repeat structures using comparison tools such as dotter (17). Special attention should be paid to regions of inverted repeat, using mate pair information and base differences between repeat arms, to ensure that the unique central loop of the repeat is anchored in the correct orientation to the unique region outside the repeat. Occasionally, restriction digest data can be helpful in orienting inverted repeats if the sequence at one of the ends of the central loop has a cut site. If the shotgun has been derived from double stranded subclones, then mate pair information can be used to check the assembly throughout the clone.

Phred quality scores can be used to assess the accuracy of the sequence. Quality values from 1 (lowest) to 99 (highest) are calculated using:

$$Q = -10 \log_{10}(P_e)$$

where $Q$ is the quality value and $P_e$ is the estimated error probability derived from various parameters of the trace, such as peak spacing and resolution (18). A decision should be made as to the quality threshold for the finished sequence; for example, a Q30 base call has a probability of 0.1% of being incorrect. Then search tools, for example in the gap4 browser, can be employed to search for bases where the combined quality scores of sequence reads at that point fall below the threshold. An experienced finisher may decide to edit the base by raising the confidence value if the traces are reasonably clear, or alternatively extra sequencing reactions may be carried out to provide good quality data over the region. Search tools should also be used to detect high quality discrepancies between reads so that again a decision can be made whether to edit the region or carry out extra sequencing reactions. High quality discrepancies between reads may also be an indication that the region has been mis-assembled, though SNPs and haplotype issues may also cause regions of high quality divergence and can be investigated further using PCR.

The finished assembly should ideally have coverage from at least two subclones throughout to reduce the possibility of errors due to chimaerism or subclone deletions. Extra checks should also be carried out where sequencing chemistry issues are likely to increase the likelihood of errors in the sequence. For example, dGTP BigDye Terminator chemistry is prone to GC compressions, so if the only reads across a region have been sequenced using this chemistry in one direction, then sequencing the opposite strand or on the same strand with alternative chemistry will reduce the possibility of error. Bases after a mono-nucleotide run sequenced with BigDye Terminator chemistry can sometimes be mis-called, so these regions should be scrutinized, ideally using reads sequenced on the opposite strand.

Once the assembly has achieved the desired level of finishing according to the project aim, then the data can be submitted to one of the public sequence databases, the European Molecular Biology Laboratory (EMBL) (19), GenBank (20), or the DNA DataBank of Japan (DDBJ) (21). These three organizations form the International Nucleotide Sequence Database Collaboration with an agreed data sharing policy (22). Once submitted, sequence data can be updated and annotation added.

## 4. Notes

1. Some preparations of pUC19 (cut with *Sma*I and dephosphorylated with calf intestine phosphatase) sequencing vector have a high background of nonrecombinants and require prepurification. Batches should be tested prior to use by setting up control ligations and observing the results following transformation and plating. If there is a high background of nonrecombinants then linearized vector should be purified prior to use. To do this, load 5 μg of vector across several 1-cm wide wells of a low-melting point agarose gel and run as described in step 10 in Subheading 3.2. After running stain gel with SYBR Green, excise linearized vector (approximately 2.7 kb) and extract DNA from gel as described previously. Resuspend in T0.1E and determine the vector concentration by running a small aliquot on an agarose gel alongside quantitative markers.
2. Growing BAC/Fosmid subclones is a fairly robust process, but issues may arise from lack of growth/low growth in some or all wells. There may be a number of reasons for this which are relatively easy to check:
   (a) Boxes may not have been sealed correctly.
   (b) Incubator may not be working correctly.
   (c) Contamination may have occurred, phage may be checked for and if this is a problem all equipment and areas need to be thoroughly cleaned using Procine, followed by ethanol to eliminate all possible contamination. If picking from glycerols the source may be contaminated, in which case this will need to be reselected.
   (d) The wrong concentration of antibiotic selective agent may have been used.
   (e) The size of the recombinant growth could be due to the length of growth time, low growth could be due to growing the cells for too long or not long enough.
3. When purifying DNA from subclones for sequencing, problems that occur with the DNA preparation will appear on the agarose QC gel. The main ones being: the processes outlined here maybe more automated using liquid handling robots and may also be produced in 384-well format.
   (a) A smear will be seen if RNA remains. To ensure this does not happen the RNAse A must be made up correctly and added to the GTE.
   (b) Large inserts may be visible, which could be due to vortexing too long at the lysing stage and disrupting the cell

membrane too much, or leaving the experiment too long at the lysing stage causing irreversible denaturation to occur.

4. A number of problems may occur when sequencing BAC or fosmid subclones including:
   (a) Reads may be top heavy giving short read lengths. This could be due to excessive amounts of template DNA. Quantifying your DNA beforehand will prevent this. Also the extension step in cycling may be too short.
   (b) Reads may be noisy/messy, this could be due to the annealing temperature being too low, the template DNA may have too much salt remaining or primers may have been mixed.
   (c) If the ethanol is not entirely removed after sequencing, while the instrument is running a yellow tinge may be visible.

   The processes outlined here maybe more automated using liquid handling robots and may also be produced in 384-well format.
5. With the advent of comparative genomics and new sequencing technologies, alternative finishing standards are described by Chain et al. (23).
6. If insufficient pUC subclone DNA is available more can be prepared by transforming a small aliquot of what remains into electrocompetent *E. coli*, isolating single colonies, verifying that the correct subclone is present and then mini-prepping by alkaline lysis.

## References

1. Li RQ, Fan W, Tian G et al (2010) The sequence and de novo assembly of the giant panda genome. Nature **463**:1106–1106
2. Wei F, Zhang J, Zhou S et al (2009) The Physical and Genetic Framework of the Maize B73 Genome. PLoS Genetics **5**:e1000715
3. Documentation relating to the base caller 'phred', DNA sequence assembler 'phrap' and database viewing and manipulation tool 'consed'. http://www.phrap.org/phredphrapconsed.html. Accessed 13 November 2010
4. Documentation relating to the Staden package. http://staden.sourceforge.net/overview.html. Accessed 13 November 2010
5. Bonfield JK, Smith KF, Staden R (1995) A new DNA sequence assembly program. Nucleic Acids Res **23**:4992–4999
6. Staden R, Beal KF, Bonfield JK (2000) The Staden package, 1998. In: Krawetz S, Misener S (eds) Bioinformatics Methods and Protocols: Methods in Molecular Biology. Humana Press, New Jersey
7. Gordon D, Abajian C, Green P (1998) Consed: a graphical tool for sequence finishing. Genome Research **8**:195–202
8. EMBL Nucleotide Sequence Database. http://www.ebi.ac.uk/embl/ Accessed 13 November 2010
9. Summaries of the International Strategy Meetings in Bermuda. http://www.ornl.gov/sci/techresources/Human_Genome/research/bermuda.shtml. Accessed 13 November 2010
10. NCBI High-Throughput Genomic Sequences. http://www.ncbi.nlm.nih.gov/HTGS/. Accessed 13 November 2010
11. Documentation relating to Primer3. http://primer3.sourceforge.net/. Accessed 13 November 2010

12. Rozen S, Skaletsky HJ (2000) Primer3 on the WWW for general users and for biologist programmers. In: Krawetz S, Misener S (eds) Bioinformatics Methods and Protocols: Methods in Molecular Biology. Humana Press, New Jersey
13. McMurray AA, Sulston JE, Quail MA (1998) Short-insert libraries as a method of problem solving in genome sequencing. Genome Research **8**:562–566
14. Quail MA (2001) M13 cloning of mung bean nuclease digested PCR fragments as a means of gap closure within A/T-rich, genome sequencing projects. DNA Sequence **12**:355–359
15. Devine SE, Chissoe SL, Eby Y et al (1997) A transposon-based strategy for sequencing repetitive DNA in eukaryotic genomes. Genome Research 7:551–563
16. Documentation relating to restrictionmapper. http://www.restrictionmapper.org/. Accessed 13 November 2010
17. Documentation relating to dotter. http://sonnhammer.sbc.su.se/Dotter.html. Accessed 13 November 2010
18. Ewing B, Green P (1998) Basecalling of automated sequencer traces using phred. II. Error probabilities. Genome Research **8**:186–194
19. Submissions to the EMBL-EBI database. http://www.ebi.ac.uk/Submissions/. Accessed 13 November 2010
20. Submissions to the Genbank database. http://www.ncbi.nlm.nih.gov/genbank/submit.html. Accessed 13 November 2010
21. Submissions to the DDBJ. http://www.ddbj.nig.ac.jp/submission-e.html. Accessed 13 November 2010
22. International Nucleotide Sequence Database Collaboration Policy. http://www.insdc.org/policy.html. Accessed 13 November 2010
23. Chain PSG, Grafham DV, Fulton RS et al (2009) Genome Project Standards in a New Era of Sequencing. Science **326**:236–237

# Part II

## Targeting Regions of the Genome

# Chapter 5

# Reduced Representation Methods for Subgenomic Enrichment and Next-Generation Sequencing

**Jeffrey M. Good**

## Abstract

Several methods have been developed to enrich DNA for subsets of the genome prior to next-generation sequencing. These front-end enrichment strategies provide powerful and cost-effective tools for researchers interested in collecting large-scale genomic sequence data. In this review, I provide an overview of both general and targeted reduced representation enrichment strategies that are commonly used in tandem with next-generation sequencing. I focus on several key issues that are likely to be important when deciding which enrichment strategy is most appropriate for a given experiment. Overall, these techniques can enable the collection of large-scale genomic data in diverse species, providing a powerful tool for the study of evolutionary biology.

**Key words:** Reduced representation, Sequence capture, Targeted resequencing, Ancient DNA, Sample bar coding

## 1. Introduction

The introduction of high-throughput, massively parallel sequencing technologies (i.e., next-generation sequencing, or NGS) has fundamentally changed the scale at which nucleotide sequence data can be collected. For example, it is now technologically feasible to shotgun-sequence an entire mammalian genome within a few weeks. However, whole-genome sequencing is still sufficiently cost-prohibitive that genome sequencing is not yet commonplace for most organisms. To help circumvent these limitations, several approaches have been developed to enrich DNA for subsets of the genome prior to sequencing. These front-end enrichment strategies allow researchers to fully leverage the high-throughput capacity of NGS technologies to collect genome-wide nucleotide sequence data in an efficient and directed manner.

Virginie Orgogozo and Matthew V. Rockman (eds.), *Molecular Methods for Evolutionary Genetics*, Methods in Molecular Biology, vol. 772, DOI 10.1007/978-1-61779-228-1_5, © Springer Science+Business Media, LLC 2011

Whereas many powerful genetic tools are restricted to well-developed model systems, NGS does not in principle require prior genomic knowledge from the organism to be sequenced. Thus, these emerging technologies offer tremendous potential for the field of evolutionary genetics by enabling large-scale genomic analysis of organisms across the tree of life. Nevertheless, much of the research implementing NGS enrichment strategies has focused on humans and a handful of other model systems. Several good technical reviews have been published recently on these topics (1–5). The purpose of this chapter is to provide a general and non-technical overview of strategies that are commonly employed to construct NGS libraries that are enriched for subsets of the genome. I focus on several of the key issues that are important to consider when designing an enrichment-based NGS experiment to address common evolutionary questions. A related topic, namely, the high-throughput screening of previously identified variable nucleotide positions (single-nucleotide polymorphisms or SNPs), is not discussed here (but see Chapters 10 and 11).

## 2. An Overview of Methods for Reduced-Representation Genomic Enrichment

Several competing NGS technologies have been developed (for technical reviews see (6, 7)), and several more are expected to become commercially available within the near future. For the purposes of this review, I primarily focus on examples that have utilized Roche 454 (8) or Illumina (9) sequencing. These platforms are currently two of the most widely implemented technologies and thus are likely to be readily accessible to individual laboratories interested in collecting NGS data. However, most of the enrichment techniques I discuss here are highly flexible and easily adaptable to other NGS platforms, such as AB SOLiD (10).

NGS technologies typically yield several orders of magnitude more data than traditional Sanger sequencing. However, NGS data tend to involve shorter sequences (e.g., <50–400 bp) that have a much higher error rate. These shortcomings complicate sequence assembly and analysis but can be partially overcome by deep sequencing to assure that each base pair is sampled with high redundancy. Shotgun genome sequencing with Sanger chemistry typically has involved less than tenfold average sequence redundancy (i.e., whole-genome shotgun sequencing coverage) to produce a draft genome assembly. So-called finished genomes require even deeper coverage, sufficient to obtain an estimated error rate of less than 1 in 10,000. If a reference genome has already been constructed, then low coverage NGS data can be used to quickly resequence additional genomes that can be assembled with comparative mapping (9, 11, 12). Considerably higher coverage may be necessary if no reference is available. For example, the recently published panda genome was sequenced and de novo assembled using shotgun Illumina sequencing to approximately 73× redundancy (13). Even at this high coverage, the panda genome assembly does not approach finished sequence quality.

Obtaining many-fold sequencing redundancy across an entire genome remains expensive and analytically demanding for organisms with large and complex genomes. Moreover, researchers are often primarily interested in specific functional regions of the genome (e.g., protein-coding genes) or in obtaining anonymous diagnostic markers dispersed across the genome. Thus, it may be highly desirable to subsample genomic regions for deeper sequencing. Genomic subsampling may be especially relevant to evolutionary studies focused on surveys of population-level variation or comparative contrasts between different species.

Both Illumina and 454 sequencing require constructing sequencing libraries by ligating universal adapter sequences to a fragmented DNA sample. These adapters are used directly in the sequencing process and can be exploited for several useful library manipulations (discussed more below). If the sample DNA was isolated from standard somatic cells or tissue, then an organism's entire genome will be represented in the constructed sequencing library. Even relatively small quantities of genomic DNA can represent many-fold copies of the genome. For example, 100 pg of human DNA would contain approximately 30 haploid copies of the genome. Most methods of genomic enrichment aim to reduce the representation of sequencing libraries to specific regions of the genome so that downstream sequencing efforts are enriched for these regions. Reduced representation (RR) methods have been widely used for several years in genome sciences (14) and predate the development of NGS technologies (see Note 1). However, with the advent of ultrahigh-throughput NGS platforms, RR enrichment has quickly become a powerful tool in genetics and genomics. For simplicity, the numerous RR approaches can be classified into two groups based on if genomic enrichment is general or targeted (Table 1).

### 2.1. General RR Enrichment Methods

Several RR methods leverage general sequence features of genomic DNA as a basis for enrichment. One commonly used method of general RR enrichment has been to anonymously fragment genomic DNA using restriction endonuclease digestion (14–16). RR sequencing libraries can then be created by ligation of NGS adapters to the ends of restriction-digested DNA and thus adjacent to restriction sites. NGS data derived from restriction-digested libraries will be enriched for adjacent *r*estriction-site *a*ssociated *D*NA (RAD). Repeating this process across several individuals should enrich for sequences from the same arbitrary genomic regions because closely related individuals are expected to share most

**Table 1**
**Reduced representation methods for sequencing enriched genomic regions**

| Method | Specificity | No. targets | Example protocols |
|---|---|---|---|
| Enzyme enrichment | General | Medium–large | RAD sequencing (Chapter 9) |
| Transcriptome sequencing | General | Large | RNA-seq (23)[a] |
| Multiplex PCR | Targeted | Small | Direct multiplex sequencing (29) |
| On-array capture | Targeted | Medium–large | Agilent (41), NimbleGen (1) |
| In-solution capture | Targeted | Medium–large | Agilent (1) |
| Molecular inversion probes | Targeted | Small–medium | MIP (1) |
| Primer extension capture | Targeted | Small | PEC (Chapter 8) |

[a] For library normalization, see Chapter 6

restriction sites. With sufficient sequencing depth, genetic variation at nucleotides adjacent to restriction sites (RAD markers) can be accessed across several individuals (see Note 2). Variations on this general method of enrichment have been used to identify SNPs in humans (14) and several agriculturally (15, 17) or ecologically important organisms (18, 19). A protocol for developing RAD markers is presented in Chapter 9.

One powerful feature of RAD sequencing is that researchers can manipulate the degree of genomic reduction (15). The expected density of RAD markers will depend on the frequency of restriction sites in the genome (15, 16). Restriction endonucleases that target relatively rare recognition sequences will produce larger intervals between RAD markers. Higher marker densities can be achieved by targeting common sites or by using a combination of different restriction enzymes. The actual density of restriction sites is only known in species with sequenced genomes, but related species are expected to have similar genomic base compositions and thus have similar restriction site frequencies. The genomic representation of restriction-digested DNA can be further refined with an additional size selection step (15). Electrophoresis of restriction-digested DNA through a gel medium should generate a broad smear of DNA fragments of different lengths. Digested DNA of a given size range can then be excised and used to further select for regions of the genome that share a particular density of restriction sites, and to avoid fragments sizes that are enriched for repetitive elements (15).

Another powerful method of general RR enrichment is the direct sequencing of transcribed portions of the genome. Transcript sequencing has long been used for the identification and annotation of protein-coding genes (20), and to study the relative abundance of transcripts within a given cell or tissue (21, 22). The ultrahigh level of throughput afforded by several NGS technologies now enables the deep sequencing of whole transcriptomes (all of the DNA transcribed within a given cell or tissue), thereby allowing researchers to determine the complete nucleotide sequence and the relative abundance of transcribed genes. One commonly used method, known as RNA-seq (5, 23), involves generating millions of sequence reads (usually with Illumina sequencing) from cDNA derived from reverse transcription of the polyadenylated fraction of total RNA. The NGS reads can then be de novo assembled into consensus transcript sequences (24) or mapped to a reference genome.

The potential for transcriptome sequencing to facilitate evolutionary genetic research is tremendous, yet there are several important experimental considerations. While only a small fraction of the genome is transcribed within a given cell, most tissues express thousands of genes (25). Therefore, tissue transcriptomes still represent millions of genomic base pairs. Because the relative abundance of transcripts between genes can vary by several orders of magnitude (26), highly expressed genes will tend to dominate sequencing coverage of cDNA libraries. If RNA-seq and related approaches are to be used primarily as a RR tool for genomic enrichment and sequencing, and not to directly study relative transcript abundances, then it may be desirable to normalize cDNA or RNA libraries with some form of subtractive screening (27) prior to sequencing (see Chapter 6). Ideally, this will reduce the representation of highly expressed genes within an NGS library and thereby increase the probability that rare transcripts will be detected.

### 2.2. Targeted RR Enrichment Methods

Several approaches have been developed to enrich for specific segments of the genome using targeted oligonucleotide probes (Table 1, Fig. 1). The oldest and most familiar of these is direct PCR, which uses a pair of targeted oligonucleotide primers to amplify a specific genomic region. As with any DNA source, PCR-amplified product can easily be converted into a NGS library. However, it is necessary to generate thousands of individual amplicons to utilize the massively parallel throughput of NGS. In principle, it is possible to combine several amplicons within a single reaction (i.e., multiplex PCR). While considerable progress has been made in streamlining multiplex PCR enrichment for NGS (28–30), multiplex PCR remains challenging to optimize and often loses robustness as the number of amplified regions increases.

Targeted oligonucleotide probes can also be used to create RR libraries by capturing DNA with direct hybridization. The general concept of using hybridization for RR enrichment has long been

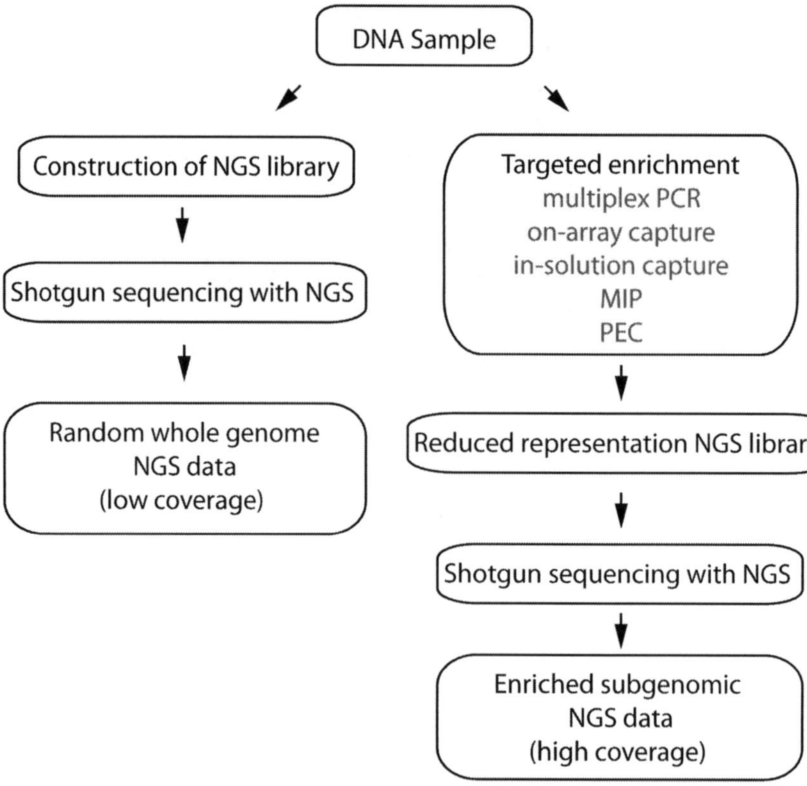


Fig. 1. Experimental overview of generating whole-genome versus target-enriched NGS data.

used in human genetics (31) and has recently been extended to leverage NGS technologies (32–35). Adapter-ligated genomic DNA can be directly hybridized to a collection oligonucleotide probes, commonly referred to as "baits". Targeted genomic regions will anneal to complementary baits, forming a strong double-stranded bond. The bait probes are typically either bound to a solid surface, such as a glass microarray slide, or prelabeled with biotin and immobilized using magnetic beads. The background or nontarget genomic DNA remains in solution and can be removed with rinsing. The captured targeted regions are then eluted, typically using heat or chemical treatment, and the resulting target-enriched NGS library is then prepared for sequencing.

Sequence captures on the order of thousands or millions of bases of bait DNA have become economically tractable with the development of large-scale oligonucleotide synthesis using programmable microarrays (36, 37). Probes synthesized with these arrays can then be used for direct sequence capture (32–34). Two competing commercial platforms are available for target enrichment with on-array hybridization capture. The Agilent SureSelect on-array platform uses 60-bp probes and arrays are currently available with 244,000 or one million (1 M) individual probes. Alternatively, the NimbleGen platform uses 60–90 bp probes isothermally adjusted for base composition and is available in 385,000 or 2.1 M probe platforms. The total number of probes determines the maximum target size. Probes are designed to overlap or tile across a target region and the wider the tiling the larger the maximum target size. Total target sizes commonly range from less than 1 M to more than 25 Mbp. Both platforms have been shown to provide comparable results for a given target size (1). The Agilent platform allows for highly customized designs through a flexible, Web-based application (38), which may be particularly useful to researchers wishing to develop capture experiments in nonmodel organisms.

On-array capture has primarily been used for targeted resequencing in humans (32–34, 39, 40). In these experiments, large quantities of NGS libraries (5–20 μg) are hybridized to targeted arrays using specialized hybridization chambers and an oven. The arrays are then washed with a series of buffers to remove nonhybridized molecules, and returned to the hybridization chamber with fresh water or elution buffer. Captured sequences are eluted into solution by melting off the hybridized strands with a chemical treatment (sodium hydroxide) or by eluting them through heat denaturation (95°C). The eluted target-enriched library can then be prepared for sequencing. Because the amount of target DNA that is recovered is often small (~30–60 pg (32)), it may be necessary to PCR amplify the enriched libraries using primers that target the universal adapter sequences. Captures typical yield very high efficiency with ~50% or greater of identifiable sequences reads matching targeted bases pairs (see Note 3). Highly optimized laboratory protocols for on-array capture have been developed for both the Agilent (41) and NimbleGen (1) platforms.

Targeted enrichment can also be performed with bait probes that are in solution rather than fixed to an array. Programmable microarrays are used to synthesize large pools of oligonucleotides that are cleaved into solution. Commercial in-solution reactions for medium to large-scale captures are available through both NimbleGen and Agilent. Agilent's SureSelect in-solution target enrichment system then converts the cleaved probes into biotinylated RNA baits using in vivo transcription (35). The RNA baits are then hybridized to adapter-ligated genomic DNA in solution and immobilized with streptavidin-coated magnetic beads. Currently, up to 55,000 120 bp baits can be designed per in-solution capture experiment. In-solution capture typically requires less DNA template (0.5–3 μg) and appears to provide similar target enrichment to on-array capture (1). In-solution capture also does not require as much supporting equipment as on-array capture, such as dedicated hybridization stations and ovens, and may be more easily scalable for projects with many individual samples.

Other forms of probe-based enrichment have been developed that are useful for certain applications but may not be as suitable for enrichment of a very large number of targets. One approach, molecular inversion probes (MIP), has been developed to selectively capture specific regions using two targeted oligonucleotides linked with an intervening universal sequence (42). The two linked probes are designed to flank a desired target, which is then copied with DNA polymerase. Circularization fill-in of the target is completed with DNA ligase and noncircularized DNA is digested with an enzymatic treatment. The circularized targets are then enriched with amplification using priming sites within the universal linker sequences. Though highly parallelizable, this technique performs best when targeting a small number of targets that need to be captured in many individual samples (1). Another approach, Primer-Extension-Capture or PEC (43), utilizes short biotinylated probes and a single PCR extension step to capture specific genomic regions (see Chapter 8). The PEC procedure is particularly well suited for enrichment of smaller genomic regions from highly degraded DNA samples, as is commonly retrieved from historical or ancient specimens. For example, PEC has been used to rapidly sequence several complete mitochondrial genomes from ancient bone samples of archaic humans (43–45). Custom baits can also be generated by ligating biotinylated adapters to PCR products (46). This approach works quite well when dealing with smaller targets that can be PCR amplified using one or a few long-range reactions. For example, a recent study generated biotinylated probes from two overlapping PCR products spanning the complete human mtDNA genome (46). The probes were then immobilized on streptavidin-coated magnetic beads and used to capture and sequence 46 complete human mtDNA genomes in parallel.

## 3. Which Enrichment Method Is Most Appropriate for My Experiment?

The first decision to be made when designing a RR enrichment experiment is to determine what biological questions the sequence data will be used to address. For example, studies that are focused on understanding the role of natural selection on protein evolution must employ enrichment strategies that can efficiently target genic sequences (e.g., RNA-seq or hybridization capture). Alternatively, RAD sequencing and other general sequencing approaches may be ideal for addressing population-genetic or evolutionary questions that require large sets of informative but functionally anonymous SNPs. The three most important additional considerations between various RR approaches are (1) whether prior genomic information is required for the experimental design, (2) what kinds of biological samples are to be used, and (3) the cost of enrichment.

### 3.1. Technical Considerations

The availability of genomic resources can have a large influence on which RR approaches will be best suited for a given study. Existing genomic resources, and a high-quality reference genome in particular, greatly facilitate the design, implementation, and data analysis of all RR enrichment methods. However, some approaches are more robust than others to the absence of a reference genome. Specifically, transcriptome sequencing provides a logical and powerful first step to facilitate research in species without developed genomic tools. Deep sequencing of cDNA libraries and de novo assembly of tissue transcriptomes is rapidly emerging as a common genomic tool to facilitate evolutionary and ecological genomic studies (e.g., (47)).

Anonymous enrichment approaches, such as RAD sequencing, also do not require prior genomic knowledge and, therefore, provide a powerful platform for anonymous SNP identification in nonmodel organisms (19). RAD markers are ideal for many evolutionary applications, such as marker-assisted genetic mapping (16) or genomic scans for positive selection (18), which rely on surveying genome-wide sets of diagnostic SNPs. One important consideration is that RAD markers are expected to be random with respect to functional aspects of the genome and, therefore, cannot be assumed to be neutral genetic markers. For organisms with no available reference genome, there is no way to tell if a given SNP reflects a functionally constrained portion of the genome (e.g., a constrained codon site within a protein coding gene). Therefore, some caution should be taken with using RAD markers for population genetic analyses that are sensitive to the influence positive or negative selection.

By definition, all targeted approaches require some a priori genomic information. Genome data are important for three steps of RR enrichment with targeted hybridization. First, both on-array and in-solution bait probes must be designed directly from a genome that is related to the samples that are to be sequenced. Hybridization enrichment can tolerate some level of sequence mismatch between targets and baits. For example, allelic enrichment bias (i.e., preferential capture of the allele matching the reference genome) appears to be minor in capture experiments in human populations where nucleotide variation is low (33). Hybridization capture also appears to work relatively well when applied to closely related organisms separated by relatively low levels of sequence divergence (48). However, it remains to be seen how evolutionarily distant a reference genome can be and still be effectively used as a basis for target enrichment.

Second, hybridization enrichment is most effective when targeting single-copy regions of the genome. Most probe designs utilize some form of repeat masking to avoid probes that would enrich for repetitive or low complexity DNA (41). Repetitive DNA is often overcollapsed into single sets of contiguous sequence in low coverage de novo genome or transcriptome assemblies. Targeted enrichment designs based on incomplete or low coverage draft genome resources will be blind to many issues associated with repetitive DNA.

Third, downstream analysis of NGS data typically relies on the accurate mapping of sequences to a reference genome (32, 39). The accuracy and confidence of resulting consensus sequences depends, in part, on the extent to which a given sequencing read uniquely matches the genome. De novo assembly tools have been developed for NGS data, including those commonly used to assemble transcriptomic data (24), but mapping-based assembly tools are much faster and less computationally demanding (49–52). In the absence of any available reference genomic data, targeted approaches may be facilitated by a two-tiered experimental design. For example, deep sequencing of cDNA from one individual could be used to generate a de novo transcriptome assembly. The assembled transcriptome could then be used to design a target enrichment experiment for downstream use on additional individuals or closely related species. Multicopy genes and regions of low sequence complexity may still be problematic when using this approach. However, it should be possible to identify and exclude many repetitive regions with post hoc analyses. For example, highly repetitive regions should result in unusually high sequence coverage (53) or an excess of nucleotide heterozygosity.

### 3.2. Sample Considerations

Enrichment strategies differ considerably in both the quality and quantity of sample DNAs that are required (Table 2). Careful considerations of these requirements can be particularly important for

**Table 2**
**Experimental and technical requirements of various enrichment methods**

| | | Typical sample requirements | | |
|---|---|---|---|---|
| **Method** | **Genomic info**[a] | **Type** | **Quantity** | **Min. quality** |
| RAD sequencing | No | gDNA | 0.1–1 μg | Medium |
| Transcriptome sequencing | No | RNA | 10 μg[b] | High |
| On-array capture | Yes | gDNA | 5–20 μg | Low, aDNA |
| In-solution capture | Yes | gDNA | 0.5–3 μg | Low[c] |
| Molecular inversion probes | Yes | gDNA | ≥0.2 μg | Medium–high |
| Primer extension capture | Yes | gDNA | Very low, aDNA | Low, aDNA |

[a] Specifies if genomic data are needed to design the enrichment experiment

[b] Typical starting amount of total RNA. The total amount of starting material is flexible and may be quite low (<0.1 μg) but does require high-quality RNA to assure proper synthesis of cDNA

[c] Although effective in-solution capture and enrichment of aDNA has not yet been demonstrated, the quality of DNA required is probably similar between in-solution and on-array capture. Other solution-based methods of targeted enrichment, such as PEC, work exceptionally well on aDNA

evolutionary studies that rely on precious DNA samples of low quantity or quality. Transcriptome sequencing is among the more demanding of RR approaches, requiring high-quality RNA samples for library generation and normalization. By contrast, RAD sequencing can be performed on relative small DNA quantities and does not require high-quality (i.e., high molecular weight) genomic DNA. Hybridization-based enrichments often require large total amounts of sample DNA, ranging from 5 to 20 μg of sequencing library per hybridization experiment for array-based enrichment to ~3 μg for in-solution approaches. These sample requirements are based on the stoichiometric demands of the respective hybridization reactions and the use of lower amounts of DNA is expected to reduce the robustness of the enrichment.

While these high sample demands may be difficult to meet with many commonly used DNA sources, there are a number of techniques that can be employed to achieve the necessary total amount of DNA when working with limited starting templates. Small amounts of genomic DNA can be amplified using multiple displacement enzymes. Whole-genome-amplified DNA has been successfully used for on-array capture (32–34), though this technique may result in DNA samples with biased genome coverage (33). Alternatively, NGS libraries can be prepared from small amounts of sample DNA and then amplified with PCR using primers that target sites within the universal adapters (41, 54). PCR amplification can quickly yield large amounts of sequencing library constructed from small amounts of starting template. In principle, once DNA has been converted to an adapter-ligated sequencing library it can be immortalized through repeated rounds of amplification. In practice, heavily amplified libraries can result in some skew in genome coverage due to amplification bias and provide an additional source of sequencing error. It is, therefore, advisable to keep the total number amplification cycles at a minimum. Library immortalization with PCR has proven to be an especially powerful resource for preserving DNA extracts from rare or precious samples (43, 55), such as ancient DNA (aDNA).

Using amplified Illumina sequencing libraries in targeted hybrid enrichment may result in reduced capture efficiencies relative to unamplified libraries (1). Unamplified Illumina libraries contain forked adapter sequences that are partially noncomplementary. PCR amplification generates double-stranded complementary amplicons, resulting in increased potential for cross hybridization between universal adapter sequences and subsequent capture of nontarget regions (41). Nevertheless, amplified sequencing libraries are commonly used for targeted hybridization enrichment and nonspecific capture can be greatly reduced by introducing blocking probes that match adapter sequences (41).

Another powerful tool is the use of sample indexing to bar-code individual sequencing libraries (56). Sample multiplexing can greatly improve the efficiency of NGS experiments while dramatically reducing the overall cost. Given the broad application and potential of library multiplexing for evolutionary studies, I discuss the construction of indexed NGS libraries in more detail below. With respect to sample requirements, individual bar coding enables several individuals to be combined into a single multiplex hybridization capture, greatly reducing the amount of sequencing library required per individual. A recent on-array targeted capture experiment in humans demonstrated the power of multiplex sample bar coding by capturing 50 indexed sequencing libraries on a single enrichment array (48). For this experiment, approximately 400 ng of each indexed sequencing library was combined into a 20 μg pool and hybridized to a single Agilent SureSelect 1 M capture array. Some loss of enrichment efficiency was observed in this initial experiment (~25% of sequences mapped to targeted bases). However, sequencing coverage across individuals was fairly uniform, and the overall cost and time of the experiment was dramatically reduced relative to nonmultiplexed on-array (or in-solution) enrichment of 50 samples.

Many evolutionary genetic studies must rely on suboptimal sources of DNA. For example, DNA derived from noninvasive sources, such as saliva, hair, or fecal samples, are often degraded and may include environmental contaminants that increase the overall sequence complexity of NGS libraries. Likewise, aDNA is often highly degraded and may include damaging chemical modifications that cause sequencing errors (57). One advantage of many targeted enrichment strategies, and NGS sequencing in general, is that these technologies tend to be fairly robust to variation in DNA template quality. The first step to generating an adapter-ligated sequencing library is to fragment high molecular weight DNA into short fragments (e.g., typically ~200–300 bp for Illumina sequencing) with sample nebulization or sonication. This step is not necessary when using degraded samples with average fragment sizes less than 300 bp. Indeed, NGS libraries can be constructed from very highly fragmented aDNA, where average fragment sizes are less than 50 bp (58, 59). Likewise, on-array capture enrichment approaches appear to work relatively well on aDNA libraries. A recent study used large-scale targeted capture and sequencing of genomic DNA libraries derived from a ~49,000-year-old Neandertal bone (48). Only ~0.2% of the DNA fragments in these libraries came from Neandertals, with the rest largely deriving from bacteria that posthumously colonized the bone. The sequencing library was enriched for ~14,000 genomic positions with two rounds of library amplification and Agilent 1 M on-array capture enrichment. This serial capture experiment resulted in ~5× coverage of targeted positions and a large proportion (~37%) of the total sequencing reads falling with targeted regions. This represents an almost 190,000-fold target enrichment, given the large proportion on background microbial DNA in this library (~99.8%).

### 3.3. Cost of Enrichment and Sequencing

Experimental cost is likely to be a key issue when designing an NGS experiment. For most targeted enrichment strategies, the highest costs are usually associated with the sequencing. The per-base-pair cost of NGS continues to plummet with each new advance in throughput. Nevertheless, for enrichment platforms that allow for flexibility in the total target size, researchers must evaluate the trade-off between total target size and average sequencing coverage per individual. For example, adjusting the tiling density of probes can scale the total target size of an on-array enrichment capture. Very large captures usually show levels of enrichment efficiency similar overall to smaller captures but will require more sequencing per individual to obtain a given average sequencing coverage per target base pair. There are no hard and fast rules for how much sequencing coverage is necessary and the answer depends in part on the desired consensus sequence accuracy and the specific goals of an experiment. A recent on-array study of the human exome targeted 26.6 Mb of protein-coding sequence in 12 individuals (39). Each individual was sequenced to an average coverage of 51×, after filtering out duplicate PCR amplicons generated during library amplification. With this depth of sequencing, more than 99% of targeted bases were sequenced at least once and ~96% of targeted bases were sampled to at least 8× coverage, the minimum coverage required by the authors to resolve heterozygous positions.

In addition to sequencing costs, each procedure requires additional expenses associated with library construction and enrichment. Several protocols have been developed to reduce the costs and time associated with NGS library construction relative to commercially available kits (see below). Enzyme enrichment strategies, such as RAD sequencing, are relatively inexpensive and can be performed using equipment found in most molecular laboratories. Some probe-based approaches, such as PEC or MIP enrichment, require an initial investment in stocks of targeted probes that can then be used on large collections of samples. For certain applications, the initial cost of probe stocks can be further reduced by generating custom baits directly from amplified PCR products (46). On-array and large-scale in-solution capture probes must be purchased for each enrichment experiment. Individual capture arrays are reasonably affordable (starting at ~$500 per array) but also may require additional investment in specialized hybridization chambers and ovens. In-solution capture does not require as much specialized equipment; however, one current limitation for in-solution enrichment is that bait libraries are synthesized in bulk with a minimum scale of several capture experiments per design (e.g., Agilent currently requires a minimum order of ten captures per design). Thus, while on-array capture incurs more initial investment in specialized instrumentation, in-solution capture experiments still require a considerable minimum investment that may not be necessary for smaller experiments or designs that utilize bar coding and sample multiplexing (multiple individuals combined in a single capture, see below). Several after-market derivatives based on the core principles developed by Agilent and NimbleGen are becoming available and should help lower the consumer cost of both on-array and in-solution technologies.

## 4. Construction of Indexed Sequencing Libraries for Multiplexed Enrichment and Sequencing

The high throughput of NGS, when combined with RR enrichment of specific regions of the genome, enables the parallel analysis of multiple individuals. If the primary goal of an experiment is to identify fixed differences between two or more groups then it may be sufficient to analyze pools of samples without maintaining individual sample identity. For example, RAD sequencing has been used for genetic mapping in sticklebacks using bulk segregant analysis (16) and to estimate approximate allele frequencies of SNPs identified from pooled samples of cattle (15). When using bulked analysis for such applications, it is crucial that care is taken to assure that each individual is represented more or less in equal proportions.

Alternatively, individual sequencing libraries can be labeled with a specific index or bar code to allow for parallel sequencing. Once indexed, several sequencing libraries can then be pooled for sequencing and later differentiated with low-level bioinformatic data analysis. Individual sequencing libraries can be differentiated through the addition of a nucleotide index or bar code within one of the two adapter sequences (1, 16, 54, 56). The current Illumina indexing system uses a unique 6-bp (or greater) index embedded within one of adapters. The index is read using a separate sequencing read (i.e., a third 7-bp sequencing read, if using the Illumina paired-end module). Commercial kits are available that include all the necessary reagents for generating indexed Illumina sequencing libraries. However, these kits are expensive, only allow for indexing of relatively few samples, and include several time-intensive steps.

Fortunately, multiple protocols have been developed that greatly streamline the process and reduce the per-library cost (1, 54). For example, a recently published protocol (54) allows for the rapid construction of indexed Illumina sequencing libraries at a fraction of the cost of commercial kits (Fig. 2). This method extends the basic principles of library preparation developed for the Roche 454 sequencing platform to generate indexed Illumina paired-end sequencing libraries. Universal adapters are added to fragmented DNA using blunt-end ligation. Specific bar codes can then be added with PCR amplification using indexed primers. Several of the time intensive steps, such as fragment size selection with gel excision, have been removed or modified from the procedure.

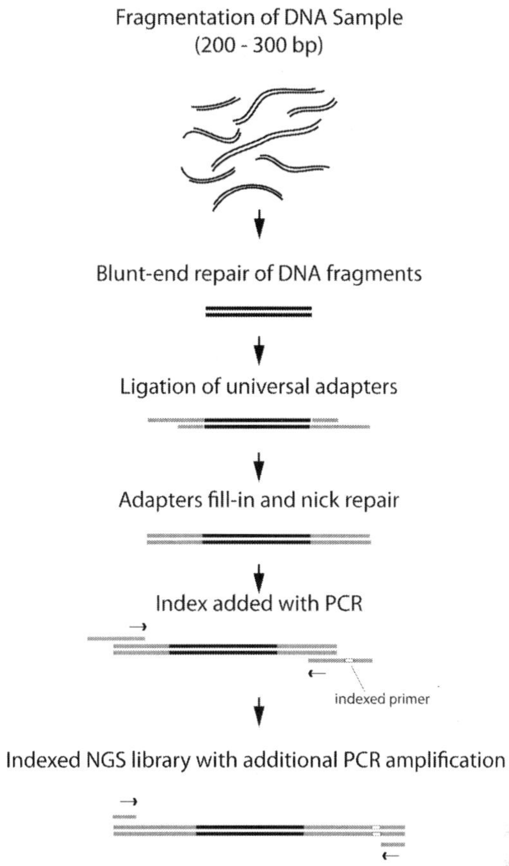


Fig. 2. Construction of indexed NGS libraries. Sample DNA is fragmented (if necessary) and blunt-end repaired. Universal adapters are added with blunt-end ligation and made completely double-stranded with a fill-in reaction. Indices are added with PCR, using one primer that includes a unique bar-code sequence (6 or 7 bp). This reaction also adds the P5 and P7 attachment sites used in Illumina sequencing. If necessary, indexed libraries can be further amplified using universal primers that target the ends of the adapter sequence, thereby preserving the internal sample index. See refs. 48 and 54 for a detailed protocol and a representative experimental application.

The entire protocol can be completed in approximately 3 days using standard equipment found in most molecular laboratories. The approach is highly flexible and can be performed on many samples in parallel using a 96-well plate format. The method is also robust across a broad range of starting quantities of DNA (100 pg–1 μg). As discussed above, highly multiplexed, indexed libraries usually result in some reduction in enrichment efficiency. However, this loss in specificity is likely to be minor when compared to the added time and costs associated with nonmultiplexed capture enrichment of multiple samples. One important consideration when using sample multiplexing in tandem with targeted enrichment is the potential for bar-code misassignment (i.e., incorrectly associating the wrong bar code to a given sequence). One way that this may occur is through recombinant PCR (60). Target-enriched samples may require a bulk PCR amplification step prior to sequencing. During this reaction, it is possible that recombination between samples could result in mosaic sequences. For many applications, low levels of bar-code misassignment are unlikely to be a major problem. However, when designing an experiment it is important to consider the possible impact of low levels of misassigned bar codes. Keeping the number of bulk amplification cycles to a minimum and avoiding large between-individual variation in DNA concentrations of pooled samples should further reduce the frequency and impact of bar-code misassignment.

## 5. Future Prospects

The targeted enrichment approaches reviewed here offer a broad range of options for researchers interested in comparative genomic analysis. As the cost of NGS continues to fall, complete genome sequencing will eventually replace targeted enrichment strategies as the preferred method for generating large-scale sequence data. However, for many studies complete genome sequences are simply unnecessary. Moreover, the computational demands of sequencing and analyzing whole genomes in many species and/or individuals are far from trivial. Evolutionary studies that rely on comparisons between several species or surveys of population-level variation may often be better served by targeted genomic analysis tailored to address specific questions. All of the methods discussed here help facilitate genomic analysis in diverse species and, thus, are likely to provide an important tool to evolutionary biologists for the foreseeable future.

## 6. Notes

1. The term 'reduced representation' has often been used specifically in the context of enzyme enrichment (14, 15). For the purposes of this review, I use 'reduced representation methods' more generally to refer to diverse approaches used to construct NGS libraries that are enriched for subsets of the genome.
2. RAD sequencing is conceptually very similar to the classical molecular technique of characterizing genetic variation by screening for restriction fragment length polymorphisms caused by the disruption of restriction sites (61). However, the

most informative RAD markers will be those where the recognition sequences are invariant across sequenced individuals.

3. Without RR enrichment, targeted base pairs will be sampled with shotgun sequencing according to their frequency in the genome. For example, approximately 0.03% of sequenced base pairs would be expected to overlap a target of one million base pairs in the human genome, assuming a total genome size of ~3 Gb.

## Acknowledgments

I thank Emily Hodges, Frank Albert, Martin Kircher, Adrian Briggs, Hernán Burbano, Gordon Luikart, and Matthias Meyer for many helpful conversations on NGS and targeted enrichment. Research contributing to this review was supported by an NSF international postdoctoral fellowship (OISE-0754461).

### References

1. Mamanova L, Coffey AJ, Scott CE et al (2010) Target-enrichment strategies for next-generation sequencing. Nat Methods 7:111–118
2. Turner EH, Ng SB, Nickerson DA et al (2009) Methods for genomic partitioning. Ann Rev Genomics Hum Genet **10**:263–284
3. Lee H, O'Connor BD, Merriman B et al (2009) Improving the efficiency of genomic loci capture using oligonucleotide arrays for high throughput resequencing. BMC Genomics **10**:646
4. Summerer D (2009) Enabling technologies of genomic-scale sequence enrichment for targeted high-throughput sequencing. Genomics **94**:363–368
5. Wang Z, Gerstein M, Snyder M (2009) RNA-Seq: a revolutionary tool for transcriptomics. Nat Rev Genet **10**:57–63
6. Metzker ML (2010) Sequencing technologies - the next generation. Nat Rev Genet **11**:31–46
7. Shendure J, Ji HL (2008) Next-generation DNA sequencing. Nat Biotechnol **26**:1135–1145
8. Margulies M, Egholm M, Altman WE et al (2005) Genome sequencing in microfabricated high-density picolitre reactors. Nature **437**:376–380
9. Bentley DR, Balasubramanian S, Swerdlow HP et al (2008) Accurate whole human genome sequencing using reversible terminator chemistry. Nature **456**:53–59
10. Valouev A, Ichikawa J, Tonthat T et al (2008) A high-resolution, nucleosome position map of C. elegans reveals a lack of universal sequence-dictated positioning. Genome Res **18**: 1051–1063
11. Wheeler DA, Srinivasan M, Egholm M et al (2008) The complete genome of an individual by massively parallel DNA sequencing. Nature **452**:872–876
12. Wang J, Wang W, Li R et al (2008) The diploid genome sequence of an Asian individual. Nature **456**:60–U61
13. Li RQ, Fan W, Tian G et al (2010) The sequence and de novo assembly of the giant panda genome. Nature **463**:311–317
14. Altshuler D, Pollara VJ, Cowles CR et al (2000) An SNP map of the human genome generated by reduced representation shotgun sequencing. Nature **407**:513–516
15. Van Tassell CP, Smith TP, Matukamalli LK et al (2008) SNP discovery and allele frequency estimation by deep sequencing of reduced representation libraries. Nat Methods **5**:247–252
16. Baird NA, Etter PD, Atwood TS et al (2008) Rapid SNP discovery and genetic mapping using sequenced RAD markers. PLoS ONE 3:e3376
17. Wiedmann RT, Smith TPL, Nonneman DJ (2008) SNP discovery in swine by reduced representation and high throughput pyrosequencing. BMC Genet **9**:81

18. Hohenlohe PA, Bassham S, Etter PD et al (2010) Population genomics of parallel adaptation in threespine stickleback using sequenced RAD tags. PLoS Genet. 6:e1000862
19. Van Bers NEM, Van Oers K, Kerstens HHD et al (2010) Genome-wide SNP detection in the great tit Parus major using high throughput sequencing. Mol Ecol **19**:89–99
20. Adams MD, Kelley JM, Gocayne JD et al (1991) Complementary DNA sequencing: Expressed sequence tags and the human genome project. Science **252**:1651–1656
21. Velculescu VE, Zhang L, Vogelstein B et al (1995) Serial analysis of gene expression. Science **270**:484–487
22. Velculescu VE, Zhang L, Zhou W et al (1997) Characterization of the yeast transcriptome. Cell **88**:243–251
23. Mortazavi A, Williams BA, McCue K et al (2008) Mapping and quantifying mammalian transcriptomes by RNA-Seq. Nat Methods **5**:621–628
24. Zerbino DR, Birney E (2008) Velvet: Algorithms for de novo short read assembly using de Bruijn graphs. Genome Res **18**:821–829
25. Su AI, Cooke MP, Ching KA et al (2002) Large-scale analysis of the human and mouse transcriptomes. Proc Natl Acad Sci USA **99**:4465–4470
26. Montgomery SB, Sammeth M, Gutierrez-Arcelus M et al (2010) Transcriptome genetics using second generation sequencing in a Caucasian population. Nature **464**:773–777
27. Carninci P, Shibata Y, Hayatsu N et al (2000) Normalization and subtraction of cap-trapper-selected cDNAs to prepare full-length cDNA libraries for rapid discovery of new genes. Genome Res **10**:1617–1630
28. Varley KE, Mitra RD (2008) Nested Patch PCR enables highly multiplexed mutation discovery in candidate genes. Genome Res **18**:1844–1850
29. Stiller M, Knapp M, Stenzel U et al (2009) Direct multiplex sequencing (DMPS): a novel method for targeted high-throughput sequencing of ancient and highly degraded DNA. Genome Res **19**:1843–1848
30. Tewhey R, Warner JB, Nakano M et al (2009) Microdroplet-based PCR enrichment for large-scale targeted sequencing. Nat Biotechnol **27**:1025–1031
31. Lovett M, Kere J, Hinton LM (1991) Direct selection: a method for the isolation of cDNAs encoded by large genomic regions. Proc Natl Acad Sci USA **88**:9628–9632
32. Hodges E, Xuan Z, Balija V et al (2007) Genome-wide in situ exon capture for selective resequencing. Nat Genet **39**:1522–1527
33. Albert TJ, Molla MN, Muzny DM et al (2007) Direct selection of human genomic loci by microarray hybridization. Nat Methods **4**:903–905
34. Okou DT, Steinberg KM, Middle C et al (2007) Microarray-based genomic selection for high-throughput resequencing. Nat Methods **4**:907–909
35. Gnirke A, Melnikov A, Maguire J et al (2009) Solution hybrid selection with ultra-long oligonucleotides for massively parallel targeted sequencing. Nat Biotechnol **27**:182–189
36. Cleary MA, Kilian K, Wang Y et al (2004) Production of complex nucleic acid libraries using highly parallel in situ oligonucleotide synthesis. Nat Methods **1**:241–248
37. Hughes TR, Mao M, Jones AR et al (2001) Expression profiling using microarrays fabricated by an ink-jet oligonucleotide synthesizer. Nat Biotechnol **19**:342–347
38. https://earray.chem.agilent.com/earray/
39. Ng SB, Turner EH, Robertson PD et al (2009) Targeted capture and massively parallel sequencing of 12 human exomes. Nature **461**:272–276
40. Ng SB, Buckingham KJ, Lee C et al (2010) Exome sequencing identifies the cause of a mendelian disorder. Nat Genet **42**:30–35
41. Hodges E, Rooks M, Xuan Z et al (2009) Hybrid selection of discrete genomic intervals on custom-designed microarrays for massively parallel sequencing. Nat Protocols **4**:960–974
42. Porreca GJ, Zhang K, Li JB et al (2007) Multiplex amplification of large sets of human exons. Nat Methods **4**:931–936
43. Briggs AW, Good JM, Green RE et al (2009) Targeted retrieval and analysis of five Neandertal mtDNA genomes. Science **325**:318–321
44. Krause J, Fu Q, Good JM et al (2010) The complete mitochondrial DNA genome of an unknown hominin from southern Siberia. Nature **464**:894–897
45. Krause J, Briggs AW, Kircher M et al (2010) A complete mtDNA genome of an early modern human from Kostenki, Russia. Curr Biol **20**:231–236
46. Maricic T, Whitten M, Pääbo S (2010) Multiplexed DNA sequence capture of mitochondrial genomes using PCR products. PLoS ONE **5**:e14004

47. Wolf JBW, Bayer T, Haubold B et al (2010) Nucleotide divergence vs. gene expression differentiation: comparative transcriptome sequencing in natural isolates from the carrion crow and its hybrid zone with the hooded crow. Mol Ecol **19**:162–175
48. Burbano HA, Hodges E, Green RE et al (2010) Targeted investigation of the Neandertal genome by array-based sequence capture. Science **328**:723–725
49. Li H, Durbin R (2009) Fast and accurate short read alignment with Burrows-Wheeler transform. Bioinformatics **25**:1754–1760
50. Li H, Handsaker B, Wysoker A et al (2009) The Sequence Alignment/Map format and SAMtools. Bioinformatics **25**:2078–2079
51. Li H, Ruan J, Durbin R (2008) Mapping short DNA sequencing reads and calling variants using mapping quality scores. Genome Res **18**:1851–1858
52. Langmead B, Trapnell C, Pop M et al (2009) Ultrafast and memory-efficient alignment of short DNA sequences to the human genome. Genome Biology **10**:R25
53. Alkan C, Kidd JM, Marques-Bonet T et al (2009) Personalized copy number and segmental duplication maps using next-generation sequencing. Nat Genet **41**:1061–1067
54. Meyer M, Kircher M (2010) Illumina sequencing library preparation for highly multiplexed target capture and sequencing. Cold Spring Harb Protoc. doi:10.1101/pdb.prot5448
55. Blow MJ, Zhang T, Woyke T et al (2008) Identification of ancient remains through genomic sequencing. Genome Res **18**:1347–1353
56. Meyer M, Stenzel U, Hofreiter M (2008) Parallel tagged sequencing on the 454 platform. Nature Protocols **3**:267–278
57. Briggs AW, Stenzel U, Johnson PLF et al (2007) Patterns of damage in genomic DNA sequences from a Neandertal. Proc Natl Acad Sci USA **104**:14616–14621
58. Green RE, Krause J, Briggs AW et al (2010) A draft sequence of the Neandertal genome. Science **328**:710–722
59. Green RE, Krause J, Ptak SE et al (2006) Analysis of one million base pairs of Neanderthal DNA. Nature **444**:330–336
60. Meyerhans A, Vartanian JP, Wainhobson S (1990) DNA recombination during PCR. Nucleic Acids Res **18**:1687–1691
61. Botstein D, White RL, Skolnick M et al (1980) Construction of a genetic linkage map in man using restriction fragment length polymorphisms. Am J Hum Genet **32**:314–331

# Chapter 6

# Accessing the Transcriptome: How to Normalize mRNA Pools

## Heiko Vogel and Christopher W. Wheat

## Abstract

As advances in next generation sequencing continue to provide increasing access to the genomics revolution for research systems having few or no genomic resources, transcriptome sequencing will only increase in importance as a fast and direct means of accessing the genes themselves. However, constructing a comprehensive cDNA library for deep sequencing is very difficult, as highly abundant transcripts hamper de novo identification of low-expressed genes, and genes expressed only under very specific conditions will remain elusive. The reduction of variance in gene expression levels to within a tenfold range of differences by cDNA normalization provides an important means of allocating sequencing across a greater fraction of genes, directly translating into a more even coverage across genes. Here, we outline two different normalization methods, addressing many of the important issues we think need consideration when going from RNA isolation to the cDNA material required for sequencing. This will provide coding gene information across thousands of genes from any organism, providing rapid insights into topics such as gene family member identification and genetic variation that may be associated with a studied phenotype.

**Key words:** Transcriptome sequencing, cDNA, Normalization

## 1. Introduction

The advent of new sequencing technologies, such as next generation sequencing (NGS) and the upcoming 3rd Generation Sequencing (3GS), has opened the door to the genomics revolution for research systems having few or no genomic resources. This provides an opportunity for researchers studying these systems to develop functional genomic tools and work toward a mechanistic understanding of their phenotypes of interest. The field of NGS and 3GS is rapidly advancing, with changes in the near future likely to continue manifesting as increasing sequence read length, coverage, and accuracy, and a decrease in cost per basepair sequenced.

Yet, in this rapidly advancing field of sequencing innovations, we see an ongoing need for two things well into the coming decade: the normalization of mRNA pools and the ability to assemble the

Virginie Orgogozo and Matthew V. Rockman (eds.), *Molecular Methods for Evolutionary Genetics*,
Methods in Molecular Biology, vol. 772, DOI 10.1007/978-1-61779-228-1_6, © Springer Science+Business Media, LLC 2011

transcriptome and to assess its quality. Much as prices for reliable and fast personal computers have remained somewhat stable around $1,000.00 over the last decade while processing speed has doubled nearly every 2 years (following Moore's law), the cost of a given sequencing run on a NGS machine has begun to stabilize while coverage has actually increased faster than Moore's doubling rule. Thus, while current and coming innovations will certainly lead to dramatic decreases in per-bp sequencing cost, the overall cost of a full sequencing run will likely not change much. We predict that during this time the partitioning and pooling of individual samples will grow in importance. Insightful experimental design will then, as now, provide increasingly cost-effective means of obtaining genomic scale data from ever increasing biological replicates. During this period, transcriptome sequencing will only increase in importance as a fast and direct means of accessing the genes themselves. Transcriptome data are extremely rich, as they can be used for determining mRNA sequences, assessing their relative expression, and characterizing alternative splicing and allele specific expression variation. While today a 454 sequencing run of a normalized mRNA pool may provide full coverage of some genes, and partial coverage of most genes in the genome, tomorrow, researchers will likely be pooling multiple individuals into such runs labeled with barcodes and getting near full length coverage of most genes. This will provide coding gene information across thousands of genes from many individuals, providing rapid insights into topics such as gene family member identification and genetic variation that may be associated with the studied phenotype. Additionally, this transcriptome data will provide the necessary template (backbone) for RNA-seq mapping in the absence of, or in combination with, whole genome sequence. Finally, mRNA sequence information is extremely important for gene prediction and annotation of whole genome sequences, as transcriptome sequencing routinely identifies genes missed by prediction algorithms and standard EST sequencing (via cloning and Sanger sequencing) (1–3).

Gaining access to a large fraction of the transcriptome via transcriptome sequencing necessarily must consider two issues. First, in a typical pool of mRNA isolated from a single tissue, fewer than 20 genes can constitute upward of 50% of the mRNA pool. Normalization, or the reduction of this variance in gene expression levels to within a tenfold range of differences, provides an important means of allocating sequencing across a greater fraction of genes. In terms of sequencing, this also directly translates into a more even coverage across genes. This is critically important for the reassembly of short reads into full-length gene models and the identification of single nucleotide polymorphism variation. Here, it should also be mentioned that over-normalization can result in the random removal of individual transcripts, based on the partial cDNA degradation under nonoptimal conditions. Second, as a rule of thumb estimate roughly 70% of the transcriptome is expressed in any one tissue at any one time (1). Additionally, the total number of genes expressed by tissue and environmental or experimental condition can be highly variable, both qualitatively and quantitatively. With this in mind, obtaining a pool of mRNA for all the genes in the genome becomes a holy grail as literally nearly every combination of tissue by developmental stage by environmental treatment to some extent becomes necessary to approach 100% of the transcriptome. Stated another way, constructing a comprehensive cDNA library for later deep sequencing is very difficult as genes expressed only under very specific conditions will remain elusive.

This chapter is therefore focused on how to accurately and rather inexpensively normalize mRNA pools for the construction of representative cDNA libraries for deep sequencing (*Normalization*). We take the reader through two different normalization methods, from RNA extraction through to the size-selected cDNA that is needed as input for the next generation platform of choice. Chapter 7 in this volume is focused on the steps that come after one has generated a cDNA pool for deep sequencing, normalized or not (*Transcriptome sequencing goals, assembly and assessment*).

## 2. Materials

### 2.1. Total RNA / and mRNA Isolation

1. Phenol-based total RNA isolation: e.g., TriZol (Invitrogen).
2. RNAlater (Ambion).
3. Handheld motorized Biovortexer (BioSpec Products, Bartlesville, OK).
4. 1-Bromo-3-chloro-propane (Sigma).
5. Total RNA isolation from problematic plant and insect material: InviTrap Spin Plant RNA Mini Kit (Invitek, Berlin, Germany).
6. RNeasy MinElute kit (Qiagen).
7. DNase: TURBO DNase (Ambion).
8. Poly(A)Purist kit (Ambion).
9. THE RNA Storage Solution (Ambion).
10. Nanodrop ND-1000 spectrophotometer (Thermo Scientific).
11. Agilent 2100 Bioanalyzer using the RNA Nano (or Pico) chips (Agilent Technologies).
12. 80% Ethanol.
13. Isopropanol.

### 2.2. RNA Isolation from Few Cells

1. PicoPure RNA isolation kit (Arcturus Bioscience, CA).
2. Chemical nuclease inhibitor: NucleoGuard stock solution (AmpTec, Hamburg, Germany).
3. Carrier for the precipitation of low RNA amounts: N-Carrier (AmpTec, Hamburg, Germany).
4. RNeasy MinElute columns (Qiagen).
5. RNaseZap decontamination solution (Ambion).

### 2.3. RNA Amplification

1. ExpressArt mRNA amplification kit (AmpTec, Hamburg, Germany).
2. Primer used for RNA to cDNA conversion: anchored oligo(dT)-T7-promoter primer (Metabion, Germany).
3. Mixture of the AmpTec reverse transcriptase enzyme and the ArrayScript reverse transcriptase (Ambion).
4. SUPERase•In RNase Inhibitor (Ambion).
5. Double-stranded cDNA generation: Superscript II dscDNA synthesis kit (Invitrogen), the ExpressArt mRNA amplification kit (AmpTec, Hamburg, Germany), and a 5′-biotinylated primer (5′-CTCATCTAGAGACCGCATCCCAGCAGTTTT TTTTTTTTTTTTTTTVN-3′) (V = G, C, A).

### 2.4. ds-cDNA Synthesis and Normalization

1. PCR Thermal cycler with heated lid (e.g., ABI 9700, Applied Biosystems).
2. First-strand cDNA synthesis buffer: 5× PowerScript buffer (TaKaRa).
3. SUPERase•In RNase inhibitor (Ambion).
4. Reverse transcriptase: ArrayScript (Ambion) or PowerScript (TaKaRa) or AffinityScript (Agilent Technologies).
5. 20 mM Dithiothreitol (DTT).
6. 10 mM dNTPs (10 mM each dATP, dCTP, dGTP, and dTTP solution).
7. Advantage UltraPure PCR Deoxynucleotide Mix (TaKaRa).
8. 5′ end adapter: 5′-AAGCAGTGGTATCAACGCAGAGTGGC CATTACGGCCGGGGG-3′, 15 μM, HPLC purified.
9. 3′ end Oligonucleotide/Primer: 5′-AAGCAGTGGTATC AACGCAGAGTGGCCGAGGCGGCC$(T)_{20}$VN-3′ 10 μM, HPLC purified (V = G, C, A).
10. For the normalization step and in cases where an out-of-the-box solution is preferred: SMART cDNA library construction kit (TaKaRa) and Trimmer-Direct cDNA normalization kit (Evrogen, Moscow, Russia).
11. 4× Hybridization buffer: 200 mM HEPES (pH 7.5), 2 M NaCl.

12. 2× DNase master buffer: 100 mM Tris–HCl (pH 8.0), 10 mM $MgCl_2$, 2 mM DTT.
13. Duplex-specific nuclease (DSN) enzyme (Evrogen, Moscow, Russia).
14. 50 mM Tris–HCl (pH 8.0).
15. DSN stop solution: 5 mM EDTA.
16. PCR Primer M1: 5′-AAGCAGTGGTATCAACGCAGAGT-3′, 10 μM, HPLC purified.
17. A proofreading PCR enzyme or enzyme mixture (e.g., Advantage 2 Polymerase mix (TaKaRa), Phusion (Finnzymes, Espoo, Finland), AccuPrime (Invitrogen)).

#### 2.5. cDNA Cleanup, Size Fractionation, Concentration, and Enzymatic Digestion

1. DNA Clean & Concentrator-5 (-25) Kit (Zymo Research).
2. Size-Sep 400 spin columns (GE Healthcare).
3. Standard 1% agarose gels (molecular biology grade agarose).
4. GeneRuler DNA ladder mix (Fermentas).
5. Zymoclean Gel DNA Recovery Kit (Zymo Research).
6. pDNR-Lib vector, *Sfi*I-digested (TaKaRa).
7. *Sfi*I enzyme with reaction buffer 4 (20 mM Tris–Acetate, 10 mM magnesium acetate, 50 mM potassium acetate, 1 mM DTT (pH 7.9), and 100 μg/ml BSA (New England Biolabs)).

#### 2.6. Cloning and Plasmid Isolation

1. ELECTROMAX DH5α-E electro-competent cells (Invitrogen).
2. Gene Pulser XCell Electroporation device (Bio-Rad, Hercules, CA).
3. DYT broth: per 1 l: 16 g Tryptone, 10 g yeast extract, 10 g NaCl; pH 7.0, with chloramphenicol (34 μg/ml).
4. 96-Deep-well plates.
5. A 96-well robot plasmid isolation kit (Nexttec, Leverkusen, Germany).
6. A Tecan Evo Freedom 150 robotic platform (Tecan).

#### 2.7. Alternative Method of Normalization

1. Random (N6) primer (can be obtained from Metabion, Germany).
2. A proofreading PCR enzyme (e.g., Phusion (Finnzymes, Espoo, Finland) or AccuPrime (Invitrogen)).
3. 5′Adapter for PCR amplification: AdapA (5′-GACCTTGGC TGTCACTCA).
4. 3′Adapter for PCR amplification: AdapB (5′-TCGCAGTG AGTGACAGGCCA).
5. Reassociation buffer: 0.3 M sodium phosphate, 0.4 M EDTA, 0.04% SDS, pH 6.8.

6. Equilibration buffer A: 10 mM sodium phosphate, 0.1% SDS, pH 6.8, 65°C.
7. 500 μl of batch hydroxyapatite (HAP): DNA Grade M Bio-Gel HTP (Bio-Rad).
8. Hydroxyapatite rehydration buffer: 0.01 M sodium phosphate (pH 7.0), 0.1% SDS.
9. Glass barrel Econo-Column chromatography columns (Bio-Rad).
10. Gradient buffer B: 0.4 M sodium phosphate, 0.1% SDS, pH 6.8.
11. DNA Clean & Concentrator-5 Kit (Zymo Research).

### 2.8. Sanger, NextGen (454 and Illumina) Sequencing

1. Sanger sequencing: ABI 3730 xl automatic DNA sequencer (Applied Biosystems) with BigDye chemistry v3.1.
2. pDNR-Lib forward primer: CGCAGCGAGTCAGTGAGC.
3. pDNR-Lib reverse primer: ACCATGTTCACTTACCTACT.
4. DNA or ds-cDNA shearing: Hydroshear device (Zinsser Analytic GmbH, Frankfurt, Germany) or NEBNext dsDNA Fragmentase (New England Biolabs).
5. NextGen sequencing: Roche 454 FLX with Titanium Chemistry and Illumina GAIIx genomic sequencer with mRNA-SEQ and Sequencing Kits v3.
6. 5′-454 Adapter: CCATCTCATCCCTGCGTGTCTCCGAC TCAG; 3′-454 Adapter: CTGAGACTGCCAAGGCACACAG GGGATAGG (The first four bases of adapter primers A1 and B1 represent phosphorothioate-modified bases as specified by Roche. In addition, primer B1 is 5′ biotinylated).

## 3. Methods

The detailed methods described in this chapter address several important aspects of the processes involved in RNA isolation, normalization, and sample preparation for subsequent NextGen sequencing. It also addresses issues related to very limited starting materials (e.g., few cells), provides two alternative normalization methods and points out critical parts of the protocols necessary for a successful generation of representative cDNA libraries. It should be noted here that the initial steps (RNA and/or poly(A)+ mRNA isolation) are very important as both RNA quality (e.g., impurities) and integrity will affect all subsequent steps and should be done with extra care.

We also provide a method for directionally cloning and Sanger sequencing cDNAs. Doing mass cloning for subsequent Sanger sequencing may introduce biases in the transcriptome data, such as enrichment in shorter cDNA fragments and absence of unclonable DNA (4, 5). Direct sequencing with NGS methods avoids such problems and leads to a much larger amount of sequence data. However, two significant advantages of the Sanger approach still remain (1) the existence of individual clones which can subsequently (and specifically) be fully sequenced and also used for generating expression constructs and (2) the unambiguous sequencing of true 5′- and 3′-ends of individual cDNAs with the directional cloning and sequencing approach. Thus, the sequencing approaches are, to some extent, complementary.

### *3.1. Total RNA and mRNA Isolation, with an Insect Tissue Focus*

1. Immediately submerge material for intended RNA extraction (e.g., whole insects, dissected insect tissue or isolated plant tissues) in liquid nitrogen and store at –80°C or (in case of very small amounts of material) immediately submerge in RNAlater solution and store at –20°C until isolation of RNA.
2. For total RNA isolation, homogenize whole insects and larger tissues to a fine powder by grinding in liquid nitrogen with a mortar and pestle (see Note 1). Wear gloves at all times during the RNA isolation procedures and while handling materials and equipment to prevent contamination by ribonucleases (RNases).
3. Carefully transfer an aliquot (approximately 100 mg) of the ground material with a precooled (in liquid N2) spatula to 1.5-ml Eppendorf tubes with pre-aliquoted TriZol (1 ml) and immediately homogenize and mix with a vortexer.
4. Incubate the samples at room temperature for dissolution of RNA–protein complexes for 5–10 min, add 150 μl of 1-Bromo-3-chloro-propane to the samples, mix well by vortexing for 1 min, and place the samples on ice for 10 min for phase preseparation.
5. Centrifuge samples for final phase separation in a precooled (4°C) centrifuge for 10 min at >10,000 × *g* and carefully transfer the upper aqueous phase to a new 1.5-ml tube containing 600 μl of isopropanol at room temperature (see Note 2). Mix immediately and thoroughly by either tube inversion or vortexing.
6. RNA precipitation can be performed at room temperature or overnight at –20°C. Pellet RNA by spinning in a precooled (4°C) centrifuge for 30 min at >10,000 × *g*. Wash RNA pellets twice with 80% ethanol and air-dry for 10–15 min. Do not dry the RNA pellets too long as this might lead to problems when trying to resuspend the RNA in buffer or water. However, any remaining ethanol might lead to subsequent inhibition of enzymatic steps.

7. Resuspend the dried RNA pellet with 90 μl of RNA Storage Solution, vortex thoroughly, and incubate on a heat block at 50–55°C (do not exceed 65°C) for 10 min or until no RNA pellet is visible. Repeat vortexing and prolong heat incubation if necessary but do not exceed 1 h of incubation at 55°C.
8. In case the starting material for the normalization procedure will be total RNA (see Note 3), an additional DNase treatment prior to a subsequent second (column-based) purification step to eliminate any contaminating DNA is highly recommended. Add 10 μl of DNase buffer and 2 μl of TURBO DNase to the resuspended RNA, incubate on a heat block or hybridization chamber at 37°C for 30 min, and purify the RNA with a column-based RNA clean-up method.
9. Test RNA integrity and quantity by verification on an Agilent 2100 Bioanalyzer using the RNA Nano chips. RNA quantity should be determined photospectrometrically on a Nanodrop ND-1000 spectrophotometer. Alternatively, RNA integrity can be approximated by standard RNA agarose gels and RNA quantity can be measured with fluorescent dyes. However, the combination of the Agilent Bioanalyzer and the Nanodrop is now seen as the standard reference for the analysis of good quality RNA.
10. Poly(A)+ RNA can be fractionated from total RNA by oligo(dT)-cellulose chromatography, using the MicroPoly(A)Purist method (see Note 4). Combine total RNA in RNA Storage Solution with Binding Solution, thoroughly mix, and add oligo(dT)-cellulose. Incubate the slurry at 70°C for 5 min to denature any secondary structures in the RNA and to allow subsequent hybridization between the poly(A) sequences on mRNAs and the poly(T) sequences of the Oligo(dT) Cellulose.
11. Mix the solution for 60–90 min at room temperature with continual rocking on a horizontal (or alternatively an orbital) shaker/rocker. Constant rocking is important to obtain maximum efficiency of poly(A) RNA binding. After hybridization, pellet the oligo(dT)-cellulose by centrifugation at 4,000 × *g* for 4 min at room temperature and carefully remove the supernatant by aspiration.
12. Wash the bound mRNA twice by adding an aliquot of wash buffer I, vortexing the slurry, and transferring the oligo(dT)-cellulose suspension to a spin column. Centrifuge at 4,000 × *g*, discard the flow-through, and repeat the process with a new aliquot of wash buffer I. Repeat the process with two cycles of wash buffer II. These washes remove nonspecifically bound material and ribosomal RNA and should be performed with care.
13. Elute the bound poly(A)+ mRNA by adding 100 μl preheated (70°C) RNA storage solution to the spin column. Vortex the complete column and immediately centrifuge for 2 min at 5,000 × *g*. Repeat the above steps with one additional volume of

preheated RNA storage solution. If necessary, the eluted RNA can be concentrated with standard ethanol precipitation or by using a commercial RNA purification and concentration kit.

### 3.2. RNA Isolation from Few Cells and RNA Amplification

The method described below should be used in cases where the amount of starting material is extremely limited, such that a successful RNA extraction by standard methods will be unlikely. We have used this method with different kinds of tissue/cell materials. However, here we will describe the approach we have taken with plant cell material using a commercially available kit with several modifications and enhancements for producing cDNA ready for NextGen sequencing (6).

Before starting please note the following: Take extra care not to touch anything in use with bare hands. Wear disposable gloves at all stages of the protocol and change them frequently. Use only certified RNase-free pipet tips and plastic ware. We recommend cleaning work surfaces with commercially available RNase decontamination solution prior to starting the reactions. Use only certified RNase-free DNase.

1. Isolate RNA from small amounts of material using the PicoPure RNA isolation kit with the following modifications. To prevent any degradation of the minute amounts of RNA during the isolation procedure and to enhance the binding efficiency of the RNA on the purification columns, the lysis buffer should be supplemented with 1% (v/v) of NucleoGuard stock solution (which will prevent degradation of the minute amounts of RNA during the purification steps) and 2 μl of N-Carrier which is used as a co-precipitant.
2. The isolated RNA should be treated with DNase as mentioned above (Subheading 3.1, step 8) prior to the second purification step to eliminate any contaminating DNA. This DNA elimination step is strongly recommended, as any co-purifying DNA might interfere with downstream reactions and RNA analysis (see Note 5).
3. Perform a second purification step with RNeasy MinElute columns to eliminate contaminating polysaccharides, proteins, and the DNase enzyme. It is very important to remove any traces of wash buffer prior to elution of the purified RNA, as these will negatively affect downstream amplification methods. Elute the RNA from the columns with 12 μl of RNase-free water or buffered TE solution (pH 8.0). Verify RNA integrity and quantity on an Agilent 2100 Bioanalyzer using the RNA Pico chips and applying standard RIN (RNA Integrity) parameters if possible (see Note 6). In case of insect RNA, RIN values cannot be used as the 28S rRNA band contains a cryptic, hidden break, characterized by the dissociation of the 28S rRNA into two equally sized subunits under denaturing conditions.

4. In order to generate the required amounts of ds-cDNA for NextGen sequencing applications, the RNA has to be amplified before reverse transcription and ds-cDNA generation. Linear mRNA amplification can be achieved by using the ExpressArt mRNA amplification kit but with several important modifications. Use approximately 1–4 ng (see Note 7) of total RNA as starting material in two independent reactions per sample to level out any random methodological effects. Convert the RNA to cDNA with an anchored oligo(dT)-T7-promoter primer using a mix of the AmpTec RT enzyme and the ArrayScript reverse transcriptase (or an equivalent enzyme) and SUPERase•In RNase Inhibitor. Generate ds-cDNA with a specific trinucleotide (Box–random–trinucleotide) primer included in the AmpTec kit.
5. Generate amplified RNA according to the manual and purify the resulting RNA after the first amplification round with RNeasy MinElute columns to eliminate any contamination, including the enzymes used in the amplification step. Elute the RNA from the columns with 12 μl of buffered TE solution (pH 8.0). This first round of RNA amplification can be followed by a second and third amplification round if necessary, depending on the amount of input material used at the beginning of the method (see Note 8).
6. Before starting the cDNA synthesis, RNA integrity and quality should be verified on an Agilent 2100 Bioanalyzer using the RNA Nano chips (see Note 9). Measure RNA quantity on a Nanodrop ND-1000 spectrophotometer and specifically control for any impurities (OD 230/260/280). Good quality RNA will have an OD 260/280 ratio of 1.8–2 and an OD 260/230 of 1.8 or greater. Low OD 260/280 and OD 260/230 ratios are clear signs of contaminants that produce peaks in the 230 and/or 280 nm region, such as phenolics, chaotropic salts, and proteins. Therefore, it is important that not only the OD A260/A280 ratio should be above 1.8 or ideally very close to 2.0, but that in addition, the OD A260/A230 ratio should be above 1.8 and ideally very close to or above 2.0. Please keep in mind that the OD 260/280 ratio is considerably influenced by pH, such that the same RNA measured in buffered TE solution (pH 8.0) and water shows different OD 260/280 ratios.
7. For the generation of double-stranded cDNA for NextGen library generation and sequencing, 5–10 μg of DNA-free amplified mRNA should be converted into double-stranded cDNA in two or three different reactions in order to avoid inefficient reverse transcription. Reverse transcription and ds-cDNA generation can be done with any standard cDNA synthesis kit, for example, with the SuperScript II ds-cDNA synthesis kit and the ExpressArt mRNA amplification kit, using

a 5′-biotinylated primer. After cDNA synthesis, pool all reactions and purify cDNA with a commercial column-based purification system (e.g., DNA Clean & Concentrator).

### 3.3. Normalization Using Kamchatka Crab Nuclease

The Kamchatka crab DSN method is a normalization technique to prevent over-representation of the most common transcripts (7, 8). For this method, ds-cDNA is generated and is then subjected to a denaturation–reassociation step. The double-stranded cDNAs that are reformed during the reassociation step are subsequently degraded using DSN enzyme. As highly expressed genes will be reflected by many identical cDNAs, these will have a higher chance of reassociating during the hybridization step. As the DSN enzyme shows a strong preference for cleaving ds-DNA, the majority of the highly abundant, reassociated transcripts will be cleaved and thus eliminated from downstream analysis. Normalized, full-length enriched cDNA libraries can be generated using either a combination of the SMART cDNA library construction kit and the Trimmer-Direct cDNA normalization kit or simply using the Kamchatka crab ds-DNA specific nuclease, which is included in the Trimmer kit. When using the combination of the SMART and the Trimmer kit, we recommend several important modifications and enzyme replacements. The normalization described here results in the reduction of many over-abundant transcripts detected as strong bands in the non-normalized total cDNA, thus drastically reducing the number of repeated gene objects sequenced per sequencing run. Each step of the normalization procedure should be carefully monitored to avoid the generation of artifacts and overcycling. The resulting normalized cDNAs can be used as a template for both Sanger and NextGen sequencing.

These instructions assume the use of either the Kamchatka crab nuclease or the use of parts of the commercially available kits mentioned in Subheading 2. In case the kit is not used, there is a requirement to order primers separately and to generate some of the buffers before starting the procedure.

The procedure described here is optimized to convert 100–3,000 ng of total RNA or up to 500 ng of poly(A)+ RNA into first strand cDNA. However, as little as 20 ng of total RNA can be successfully used in cases where RNA material is limited. It is not advised to use more RNA than we suggest as this will lead to either incomplete conversion of the RNA to cDNA or sometimes even to inhibition of the complete reaction.

The quality of the starting RNA material (whether total RNA or poly(A)+ RNA) is of utmost importance and should therefore be carefully monitored, both quantitatively (by, e.g., Nanodrop or specific fluorescent dye methods like RiboGreen) and qualitatively (e.g., with the Agilent Bioanalyzer). Wear gloves at all times during the first-strand cDNA synthesis and PCR amplification procedures and while handling materials and equipment to prevent contamination by ribonucleases.

The first step, described below, is to perform reverse transcription with a mixture of several reverse transcription enzymes (ArrayScript, Ambion; AffinityScript, Agilent Technologies; PrimeScript, TaKaRa).

1. Use a thermal cycler with a heated lid. Prepare the first-strand cDNA synthesis reaction in a microcentrifuge tube (RNase-free 0.2-ml thin-walled PCR tubes). Mix and spin each component (except the enzymes) in a microcentrifuge before use to avoid biased drawing from a formed gradient. Add the following components in order:

   100 ng to 3 μg of total RNA or 20–500 ng of poly(A)+ mRNA

   RNase-free water to total volume 3 μl

   1 μl of 5′ end adapter

   1 μl 3′ end Oligonucleotide/Primer.

2. Mix well by gentle vortexing and incubate the reaction tube at 72°C for 2 min. Place the tubes on ice immediately and cool the reaction for ~2 min to allow the primer to anneal to the RNA.

3. After the reaction has cooled to room temperature, add the following components to each reaction tube, in order, for a final reaction volume of 10 μl:

   2 μl of 5× PowerScript RT Buffer

   1 μl of 20 mM DTT

   1 μl of 10 mM dNTPs

   *Optional*: 0.2 μl of SUPERase•In Ribonuclease Inhibitor (20 U/μl)

   1 μl Reverse transcriptase enzyme mixture: equal units of each of the RT enzymes described above (see Note 10).

   Note that to prevent heat inactivation, the reverse transcriptase enzymes and RNase Inhibitor must be added after the annealing reaction has cooled to room temperature.

   The addition of the Ribonuclease Inhibitor is optional but is recommended for low amounts of starting RNA and for RNA isolated from tissues with high intrinsic RNase activity (e.g., mammalian pancreas and spleen).

   Mix the contents by gentle pipetting and briefly spin tubes in a microcentrifuge to collect contents at the bottom of the tube.

4. Incubate the reaction tubes in a temperature-controlled thermal block (e.g., thermal cycler with a heated lid) for 1 h at 42°C and 90 min at 50°C (see Note 11). Place the tubes on ice to terminate first-strand synthesis and for subsequent ds-cDNA generation by PCR amplification. Reaction products should stay on ice if proceeding directly to the ds-cDNA synthesis step, or be stored at –20°C until needed.

5. Next, generate and amplify double-stranded cDNA using a PCR-based approach. Prepare a PCR master mix for all

reaction tubes of the previous step by combining the following reagents in the order shown (volumes per reaction):

39 μl RNase-free water

5 μl 10× PCR buffer (e.g., Advantage 2)

1 μl 10 mM dNTPs

2 μl PCR Primer M1

1 μl Polymerase enzyme (e.g., Advantage 2 Polymerase Mix)

Mix well by vortexing and aliquot 48 μl of the PCR master mix in a thin-walled 0.2-ml PCR reaction tube with 2 μl of the first-strand cDNA synthesis step (Subheading 3.3, step 4). Place the tube(s) in a thermal cycler and run the following program:

95°C for 1 min; (95°C for 7 s, 66°C for 10 s, 72°C for 6 min 30 s) × *n* cycles.

Use *n* = 13 for total RNA (0.5–2 μg) and *n* = 15 for poly(A)+ RNA (0.1–0.5 μg).

After cycling analyze 6 μl of each PCR reaction on agarose gels and check for correct cycling parameters by estimating product concentration and size distribution in order to avoid overcycling (Fig. 1, lanes A-15 and B-15). The non-normalized cDNA should appear as a broad smear on agarose gels, ranging (for most species and tissues) from 200 bp to >3 kb, often with several distinct, strong bands (see Fig. 1, lanes A-11 and B-11) reflecting abundant transcripts.

Overcycling by using too many PCR cycles will lead to a high molecular weight "smear" on agarose gels (see Fig. 1, A-15, B-15) which should be avoided as this leads to the generation of cDNA artifacts. However, undercycling (too little cDNA

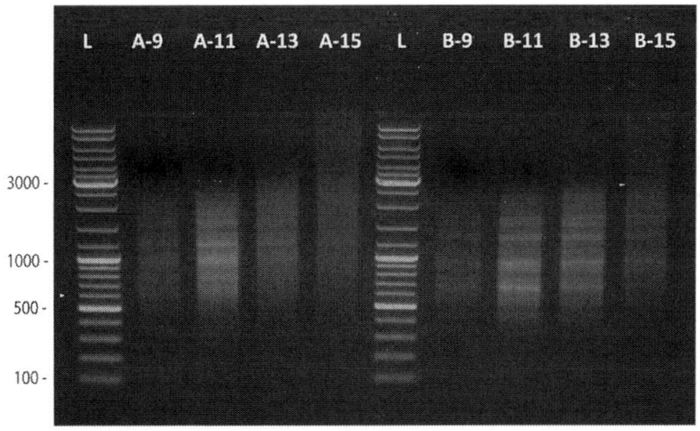


Fig. 1. Comparison of cycling condition parameters for non-normalized cDNAs. Examples of correct cycling conditions and overcycling of non-normalized complex ds-cDNAs from two different tissues (A: insect midgut; B: plant ovule; L: DNA size marker). Numbers after letters indicate the number of PCR cycles used. The cycling parameters depicted here clearly show undercycling (too little cDNA produced, A-9 and B-9), optimal cycling (good amount of cDNA but no production of PCR artifacts, A-11 and B-11), and overcycling (artifact production seen as a high-molecular smear, A-13, A-15, and B-15).

material produced) can easily be corrected by placing the tubes back in the thermal cycler for additional PCR cycles.

Purify and concentrate the amplified cDNA with a commercial PCR purification kit (e.g., DNA Clean & Concentrator) and use approximately 800–1,500 ng for the subsequent normalization step.

6. Thaw the 4× hybridization buffer and equilibrate to room temperature for 20 min. Add the following material to a 0.2-ml PCR tube:

   Up to 13.5 μl of the ds-cDNA prepared above (about 800–1,500 ng)

   4.5 μl 4× Hybridization buffer

   RNase-free water to a final volume of 18 μl

   Mix the contents by gentle vortexing, aliquot 6 μl of the reaction mixture into each of three PCR tubes (control, high nuclease (HN), and low nuclease (LN)), and incubate in a thermal cycler at 98°C for 2 min (for strand dissociation) followed by a 5-h incubation at 68°C (slow reassociation of the single-stranded cDNAs).

7. Preheat the DSN master buffer at 68°C for at least 10 min. Add 7 μl of the preheated buffer to each tube and incubate all tubes at 68°C for 10 min in the thermal cycler. Do not remove the tubes from the thermal cycler except for the time necessary to add the buffer. Prolonged exposure to room temperature will lead to reannealing of ss-cDNAs to form ds-cDNAs and potentially also to subsequent nonspecific digestion of ss-DNA secondary structures, thus decreasing normalization efficiency.

   Carefully add 1 μl of the Nuclease storage buffer only (control tubes), high nuclease (1:1 parts by volume nuclease to storage buffer ratio; HN), and low nuclease (1:3 parts by volume nuclease to storage buffer ratio; LN) to the three tubes, respectively. Incubate the tubes in a thermal cycler at 68°C for 20 min, stop the nuclease reaction by adding 14 μl of DSN stop solution, and place the tubes on ice. Add 12 μl of sterile water to each tube and keep on ice.

8. Amplify the resulting control and normalized cDNAs by adding the following to 1.5 μl of the diluted cDNA prepared above:

   40.5 μl RNase-free water

   5 μl 10× PCR buffer (e.g., Advantage 2)

   1 μl 10 mM dNTPs

   1.5 μl PCR primer M1

   1 μl PCR Polymerase (e.g., Advantage 2)

   Generate a cycling series for the nuclease (LN and HN) and control tubes, using an initial seven cycles. Keep the LN and HN tubes on ice and proceed with the control tube for a total of 9,

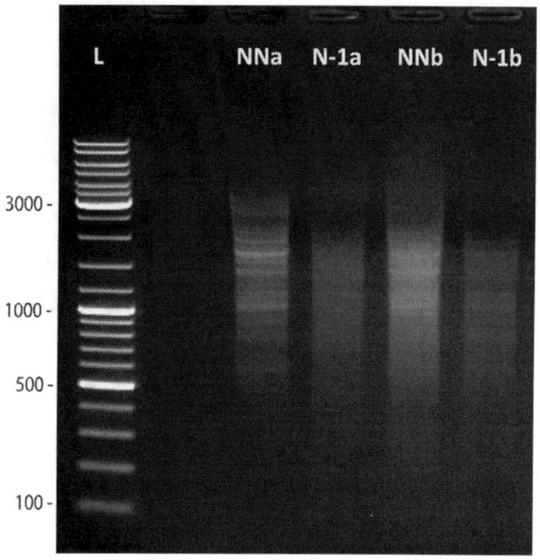


Fig. 2. Example of successful normalization. Modest (N-1a) and incomplete (N-1b) normalization with the Kamchatka crab nuclease method, each compared to non-normalized starting ds-cDNA.

11, and 13 cycles, each time taking a 12-μl aliquot from the PCR tube for subsequent analysis on an agarose gel. The normalization procedure and the number of PCR cycles used to amplify the ss-cDNAs should be carefully monitored to avoid the generation of artifacts and overcycling (Figs. 1 and 2; see Note 12).

9. Based on the optimal number of cycles for the control to reach the plateau but avoiding overcycling ($N$), determine the number of PCR cycles required for the LN and HN samples, which is given in the Trimmer-Direct manual as $N-7$ (+9), such that in case the optimal number of cycles is 8, one would subject this sample to $8-7$ (+9) = 10 additional cycles. Subject the LN and HN tubes to the additional cycles determined and load 8 μl of each PCR product alongside with the control PCR with optimal cycle number.

   It is important to determine the success of the normalization procedure by checking for the disappearance of (most of) the pronounced bands visible in the background smear of the cDNA, which represents highly abundant transcripts. This is done by comparing the "before normalization" condition with the normalized samples. In Fig. 2, we have depicted two different outcomes of such a comparison between non-normalized (NNa, NNb) and normalized (N1a, N1b) samples. In the case of successful normalizations, no distinct banding patterns are visible (N1a), whereas in incomplete normalization reactions all (or parts) of the banding patterns are still visible (N1b).

   In cases where the samples are not sufficiently normalized, the amount of nuclease and/or the incubation time should be increased. However, in some cases the normalized cDNAs

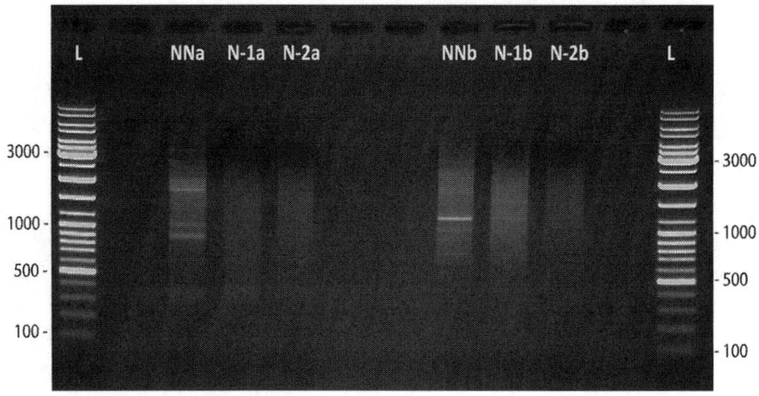


Fig. 3. Comparison of successful normalizations with over-normalization. Example of correct conditions for normalization with the Kamchatka crab nuclease where NN represents the non-normalized cDNA material and N-1 and N-2 represent two different levels (i.e., amounts of nuclease) of normalization. A moderate normalization is represented by sample N1a, where a moderately strong band around 350 bp is still visible, which is almost gone in N-2a (successful complete normalization). In contrast, in N-1b several moderately strong bands are still visible which completely disappear in N-2b. However, please note that in N-2b the smear is much fainter and the cDNA size distribution is shifted toward the lower molecular weight.

appears as a smear shifted toward lower size (see Fig. 3) or an overall much lower concentration. This is very likely due to excessive nuclease treatment, resulting in partial cDNA degradation. Avoid this excessive nuclease treatment as this will lead to subsequent losses of sequence information on the degraded cDNAs.

10. The resulting full-length-enriched, optimally normalized cDNAs can be linearly amplified (starting from the ss-cDNAs obtained in step 9) to the amounts required by the different sequencing technologies (e.g., usually 5–10 μg ds-cDNA for the 454 FLX).

    We suggest digesting the ds-cDNA with *Sfi*I enzyme to remove most of the adaptor sequences for NextGen sequencing (see Note 13), and subsequently column-purifying and concentrating the material. Measure DNA quantity on a Nanodrop ND-1000 spectrophotometer.

### 3.4. Alternative Method of Normalization Using Hydroxyapatite Columns

This normalization technique utilizes renaturation kinetics of complementary DNA strands and differential fractionation of single-stranded DNA vs. double-stranded DNA and is based on hydroxyapatite column chromatography. Here, we describe the technique essentially as developed by Soares et al. (9), with modifications by Bonaldo et al. (10), and adaptation of the technique to the FPLC system by Lo et al. (11).

This method has an advantage in cases where there is a requirement for the use of random priming or a combination of random and Poly(A)+ priming. This can be an absolute requirement for prokaryotic RNA material or optional when the starting RNA material is partially (or strongly) degraded. Furthermore, when used in combination with a random priming method for cDNA generation this approach can minimize 3′ end bias of cDNA generation and optimize potential representation of the complete 5′ end of long cDNAs. For this purpose, the starting material for eukaryotes needs to be poly(A)+ mRNA as, when starting with total RNA, massive amounts of nonprotein coding RNAs would be reverse transcribed. A potential additional benefit is the removal of the requirement for subsequent concatamerization and shearing, depending on the NextGen sequencing platform used.

After ds-cDNA generation with a random (e.g., N6) primer, normalization can be carried out by one cycle of denaturation followed by a reassociation step of the cDNAs, resulting in a mixture of double- and single-stranded cDNAs. Reassociated ds-cDNA is separated from the remaining ss-cDNA by passing the mixture over a hydroxyapatite column, which selectively binds double-stranded DNA. After hydroxyapatite chromatography, the ss-cDNA is amplified by 9–12 PCR cycles using a proofreading enzyme. Our protocol for the denaturation and reassociation of cDNA fragments in solution principally follows established methods, with some minor modifications.

1. Isolate poly(A)+ RNA (1 μg) from total RNA by oligo(dT)-cellulose chromatography as described above (Subheading 3.1). Perform the first-strand cDNA synthesis by using a mixture of random hexanucleotides (300 μg/ml) and a modified MMLV reverse transcriptase or a mixture of different enzymes (see Subheading 2 for enzyme choices).
2. Carry out second-strand cDNA synthesis by primer-extension PCR using a proofreading/Taq polymerase enzyme mix (see Subheading 3.3). Two primers, AdapA (5′-) and AdapB (complementary strand 5′-3′) should be annealed at equal molar ratio and used as adaptors to ligate to the blunt-ended ds-cDNA. Add 2 μl of 10 μM adapter (mixture of two adapter oligos 10 μM each, see above), 2 μl of 10× ligation buffer (provided with the ligase), and 1 μl (1–5 U) of T4 DNA ligase to the cDNA solution for a final volume of 20 μl. Leave the reaction at 18°C overnight. Subject the ligated product to a PCR-based method of subsequent amplification using AdapA and AdapB primers with 9–12 PCR cycles (denaturation at 94°C, 10 s; annealing at 60°C, 15 s; extension at 72°C, 6 min) using a proofreading enzyme mix. The number of PCR cycles should be chosen such that the required amount of ds-cDNA will be obtained but without any overcycling artifacts being produced in the PCR amplification process (see Fig. 1).
3. Perform the reassociation reactions in a 50-μl reaction mixture containing 0.3 M sodium phosphate (pH 7.0), 0.4 mM EDTA, 0.04% SDS, and 4 μg of amplified cDNA. Heat-denature the reaction mixture in a thermal cycler for 5 min at 100°C and then immediately cool to and maintain the tube(s) at 65°C. Allow the DNA molecules to reassociate for 24 h.

4. Inhibit the reassociation by chilling the reaction tube on wet ice and further dilute the mixture to 1.0 ml in column equilibration buffer A at 65°C.
5. For rehydration suspend hydroxyapatite at a 1:10 ratio in 0.01 M sodium phosphate (pH 7.0) containing 0.1% SDS and gently swirl the solution to obtain a slurry (see Note 14). Let the hydroxyapatite/buffer slurry settle for 10–20 min and carefully decant the buffer to get rid of any fragmented floating crystals and the cloudy upper level at the top of the settled bed. Repeat the mixing and decanting step twice by adding an equal volume of starting buffer to the bed, mix by gentle swirling and perform the decanting step as described above. Resuspend the rehydrated hydroxyapatite material in the starting buffer and pour the slurry onto a column. Pack the washed slurry to 1.0-ml bed volume in waterjacketed 1-cm column using the FPLC system and run at flow rates of 8–10 ml/h.
6. Apply the diluted reassociated DNA sample mixture of ss- and ds-cDNA from step 4 to the rehydrated, pre-equilibrated hydroxyapatite jacketed column maintained at 65°C.
7. Wash with 3 CV (column volumes) of buffer A, then elute with a continuous gradient from 0 to 100% Buffer B (65°C) on the FPLC over 10 CV, followed by 4 CV of Buffer B to wash the column.
8. Calibrate the elution profiles of single-stranded and double-stranded DNA using a step gradient of 0.05–0.4 M sodium phosphate (pH 7.0, containing 0.1% SDS) with 0.02 M increments in the concentration of the phosphate buffer. ss-DNA elutes at ~120 mM sodium phosphate and dsDNA at ~300 mM sodium phosphate under these conditions. Desalt and concentrate the resulting single-stranded cDNA fraction by using a column-based commercial kit. The purified ss-cDNA prepared by this method is used for subsequent amplification and generation of ds-cDNA by a PCR-based method with 9–12 PCR cycles using a proofreading enzyme mix and primers described in Subheading 2 (see also Subheading 3.3 for optimizing cycling conditions and avoiding overcycling).

### 3.5. Preparation of Size-Fractionated, Directionally Cloned cDNA Libraries for Sanger Sequencing

Directionally cloning cDNAs into a vector with subsequent directional Sanger sequencing (e.g., 5′-ends) allows for the potential capture of the true 5′ end of transcripts. Thus, the cloned cDNAs may serve as both a resource for full-length sequencing of individual cDNAs as well as a complementary approach to NextGen sequencing methods where sometimes the true 5′ end of cDNAs is questionable. Although generally being reliable and providing a good representation of all possible cDNAs, there are cases where cDNAs are unclonable. Thus, the (additional) direct sequencing of cDNAs by NextGen methods without prior cloning will likely provide a more complete/unbiased representation of the transcriptome.

For cloning and subsequent Sanger sequencing, the very small (and likely incomplete, prematurely terminated) cDNAs should be removed by size exclusion chromatography. The resulting larger cDNAs are separated on agarose gels and three different size ranges are eluted from a preparative agarose gel. It is important to confirm the size ranges by analyzing an aliquot of the size-fractionated cDNA by gel or capillary electrophoresis. This size fractionation before cloning is important to minimize the size-bias in cloning (see Note 15) mentioned in the introduction of the methods chapter.

1. Perform cDNA size fractionation with SizeSep 400 spun columns that will result in a cutoff at ~200 bp. Digest the full-length enriched cDNAs with *Sfi*I to remove parts of the adapters used for normalization and to allow directional cloning.
2. Load digested cDNA on a standard agarose gel and excise three different size fractions (200–900; 900–1,800; and 1,800–8,000 bp) from the gel with a clean scalpel. Dissolve the agarose gel blocks at 50°C in agarose melting buffer and isolate and concentrate the ds-cDNA by using a column-based purification method. Measure both the concentration and quality of the purified cDNA on a Nanodrop-1000 photospectrometer.
3. The purified, concentrated cDNA can be ligated to the *Sfi*I-digested pDNR-Lib plasmid vector with T4 DNA ligase. Transform an aliquot of the ligation reactions into *E. coli* ELECTROMAX DH5α-E electro-competent cells with a Gene Pulser XCell, streak out onto selective (chloramphenicol) agarose plates, and estimate colony-forming units (cfu). Based on the cfu calculations prepare large agarose plates for clone-picking with no more than 20 colonies per square cm.
4. If performing higher-throughput sequencing, pick bacterial colonies grown on square agar plates with a clone-picking robot (QPixII) and grow bacterial cells to confluency overnight in flat-bottom 96-well square block plates with a volume of 0.7 ml DYT-chloramphenicol medium per well. Plasmid minipreparation from bacterial colonies can be performed either manually or by using the 96-well robot plasmid isolation kit (Nexttec) on a robotic platform (Tecan).
5. Carry out single-pass sequencing of the 5′ termini of the cloned cDNA libraries on an ABI 3730 xl automatic DNA sequencer with pDNR-lib forward primer. Vector clipping, quality trimming, and sequence assembly can be done with free software programs such as the STADEN package or with commercial software solutions (e.g., Lasergene software package (DNAStar Inc.)).

### 3.6. Preparation of Size-Fractionated, Sheared cDNAs for NextGen Sequencing

The transcripts of cells are not an ideal starting material for NextGen sequencing methods. This is basically due to two factors: the length of the starting material and the read length of the most prominent NextGen sequencing methods. In comparison to genomic DNA (which usually is high-molecular weight with >100 kb after isolation) as starting material for NextGen sequencing, cDNAs have a very different size distribution. In general, cDNAs can cover sizes (dependent on the species and/or tissue material) ranging from 150 bp up to 10 kb and larger. For efficient PCR amplification and subsequent sequencing, the size range has to be minimized, typically by random shearing. While this is not a problem with high-molecular weight genomic DNA, cDNAs can be often too small to be efficiently sheared. Even if the random shearing process itself is optimized, the resulting fragments would be too small for the newer generation of the longer read technologies (e.g., 454 FLX with Titanium chemistry) and the very small cDNAs would be altogether omitted in the subsequent size-fractionation step. The shearing can be done using different methods, including the standard nebulization method, or by using shearing devices such as the Hydroshear, Bioruptor, or Covaris. The Hydroshear is based on hydrodynamic forces, the Bioruptor uses sonication, and the Covaris uses Adaptive Focused Acoustics for DNA (or RNA) shearing. Based on our experience, we would recommend the use of the shearing devices over the nebulization method for the final step of fragment generation, as those will result in a much more compact size range and a higher proportion of fragment recovery, which can be critical with limited amounts of starting material. Alternatively, an enzymatic method can be used, avoiding the requirement for expensive equipment. In our hands the Fragmentase enzyme mixture from NEB has proven to be reliable for most samples, generating the required fragment sizes for both the 454 FLX and Illumina/SOLID/Helicos sequencing. Please note that the size fraction eluted from the preparative agarose gel largely depends on both the smallest full-length cDNAs known for the species of interest as well as the method and chemistry used for NextGen sequencing.

One possible solution to the problem of the small cDNA sizes is the concatamerization (coligation) of smaller cDNAs before shearing and size fractionation. However, this concatamerization step poses some problems in downstream bioinformatics analysis. More specifically, any adapters used for cDNA generation and normalization have to be identified not only at the ends of the reads but also anywhere in the middle of reads. Not all adapters can be identified by perfect matches as one has to take many kinds of sequencing or basecalling errors into account, leading to artificially "mutated" versions of the adapter sequences.

None of the problems discussed above should (at least theoretically) occur for random-primed samples, as the resulting cDNAs are usually in the correct size ranges for most direct

NextGen sequencing methods without the need of concatamerization and/or fragmentation. However, on the other hand, the resulting cDNA fragments can be too small for the ultra-long read technologies (1,000 bp 454 technology and 3rd generation sequencers).

## 4. Notes

1. Alternatively, small amounts of tissue material can also be homogenized directly in TriZol with a motorized handheld pestle. However, care has to be taken such that the obtained level of homogenization is sufficient to extract RNA from hard-to-homogenize tissues. Specifically, the direct cell lysis and homogenization of some insect tissues such as head capsules, and some fungal spores and unicellular algae, can be close to impossible, thus requiring prolonged grinding in liquid nitrogen.
2. Extra care should be taken to avoid the transfer of interface and lower phase in order to reduce the risk of DNA and protein contamination in the RNA preparation. In some cases (e.g., fat body tissue of insects) phase separation is not as clean as required. In these cases a transfer of the upper aqueous phase to a new tube and a second wash step with 1-bromo-3-chloropropane is strongly advised.
3. Poly(A)+ RNA isolation is recommended in cases where the starting material (e.g., total RNA) is not limited, allowing the isolation of sufficient amounts of poly(A)+ RNA for cDNA synthesis. However, poly(A)+ RNA isolation can also often help to overcome problems with co-purified contaminants in total RNA isolations which can affect downstream enzymatic reactions, such as PCR amplification steps. Poly(A)+ RNA isolation is an absolute requirement in case one would like to use random priming for cDNA synthesis.
4. Any method based on either the oligo(dT)-cellulose or magnetic beads can be used. In our hands the oligo(dT)-cellulose-based method was very robust and performed well with both plant and insect tissue and cell material. However, oligo(dT)-cellulose-based methods are sensitive to large amounts of salts in the total RNA solution used for Poly(A)+ RNA fractionation. In case the RNA was extracted with an organic extraction method (i.e., without a second purification step), make sure to wash the pellet thoroughly after precipitation or perform a second precipitation.
5. Please be aware that in some cases the DNase incubation step might have a negative impact on RNA integrity and should be omitted in these cases. Whether there is a negative effect of the

DNase treatment step on RNA integrity and/or quantity can unfortunately only be found out by testing.

6. We strongly recommend the analysis of the RNA quality by using the Bioanalyzer (or equivalent) with the RNA Pico chips. Only the Pico chips will have the required sensitivity for the low amounts of total RNA extracted with the above method. Do not try any gel-based RNA analysis methods, as they are by far too insensitive and one would lose valuable sample material. In case access to a Bioanalyzer is not available, proceed with the RNA amplification steps and analyze the amplified RNA.
7. It is possible to start with even lower amounts of total RNA. However, best results will be obtained in cases where the amount of starting material exceeds 1 ng of total RNA as it will be possible in these cases to avoid more than two rounds of RNA amplification.
8. The second round of amplification is usually necessary when starting with total RNA in the picogram or low nanogram range. However, a third round of RNA amplification should only be performed in cases where the second amplification did not lead to sufficient amounts of amplified RNA as additional rounds of amplification may lead to a representation bias and artifacts.
9. The amplified RNA looks very different from total or poly(A)+ mRNA on the Bioanalyzer chips or on agarose gels. The general appearance is a smear, reflecting an overall smaller size range distribution. Do not be alarmed by this as it is typical for any RNA amplification procedure. However, the size range distribution is also dependent on the integrity and quality (e.g., purity) of the starting RNA material.
10. The choice of the reverse transcriptase is of utmost importance. The fraction of incomplete (prematurely terminated) cDNAs generated with a range of commercial reverse transcriptases varies greatly. Any incomplete cDNA (mostly 5′ ends) will lead to an incomplete representation of the full-length cDNAs in the downstream read assembly. Based on our own experience, there is a range of enzymes that work well with different kinds of starting materials and amounts of RNA, while others perform rather poorly. One of the options we have used is a mixture of different reverse transcriptases, which has worked well in our hands.
11. The prolonged, multitemperature incubation allows for efficient reverse transcription at different optimal temperatures of the enzymes used here. Some reverse transcriptases are able to perform extremely well at elevated temperatures, which can also lead to a better resolution of RNA secondary structures and thus to successful complete reverse transcription of even long mRNAs. Thus, for the enzyme mixture used here, for RNAs containing secondary structure and other challenging

targets, a synthesis temperature of more than 42°C (e.g., up to 55°C) may be used without loss of performance.

12. The right choice of the optimal number of PCR cycles ensures that the ds-cDNA will remain in the exponential phase of amplification, thus avoiding overcycling. If in doubt, always chose one or two fewer cycles as this will only lead to lower amounts of ds-cDNA material but not to the generation of artifacts.
13. The digestion with *Sfi*I and thus removal of large parts (approximately 30 bp) of the adapters used for the normalization procedure is a very important step as the adapters are long. This step is important irrespective of the sequencing method, as non-cDNA sequence (in this case adapter sequence) will affect the efficiency of the subsequent NextGen sequencing.
14. Hydroxyapatite column material (e.g., Bio-Rad Bio-Gel HTP), when supplied in a dry powder form, has a small particle size that can significantly increase the binding capacity and may enhance its selectivity for ds-cDNA molecules. When calculating the amount of hydroxyapatite powder one has to consider that the hydrated hydroxyapatite occupies approximately 2–3 ml per dry gram. All buffers should be degassed in an ultrasound bath or in a vacuum manifold prior to the addition of the dry hydroxyapatite. Do not use magnetic stir bars or stirring rods, as these will likely damage the hydroxyapatite crystals, leading to greatly reduced binding capacity and/or incomplete separation of ss- and ds-cDNA.
15. The size-fractionated, size-dependent cloning has significant advantages over simple total cDNA cloning. The efficiency of the ligation step can be very different in cases where there is an enrichment of large fragments, as is the case for full-length enriched cDNAs. Thus, performing individual ligation and transformation steps with the different size-fractions leads to a better representation of specifically the larger cDNAs.

## Acknowledgments

Support for this work comes from the Max Planck Society and Finnish Academy Grant 131155.

### References

1. Weber APM, Weber KL,Carr K et al (2007) Sampling the *Arabidopsis* transcriptome with massively parallel pyrosequencing. Plant Physiology **144**:32–42
2. Shendure J, Hanlee J (2008) Next-generation DNA sequencing. Nature Biotechnology **26**: 1135–1145
3. Schuster SC (2008) Next-generation sequencing transforms today's biology. Nature Methods **5**:16–18
4. Carninci P, Shibata Y, Hayatsu N et al (2001) Balanced-size and long-size cloning of full-length, cap-trapped cDNAs into vectors of the novel lambda-FLC family allows enhanced

gene discovery rate and functional analysis. Genomics 77:79–90
5. Kieleczawa J (2005) DNA sequencing: optimizing the process and analysis. Jones and Bartlett, Sudbury MA
6. Sharbel TF, Voigt ML, Corall JM et al (2010) Apomictic and sexual ovules of Boechera display heterochronic global gene expression patterns. Plant Cell **22**:655–671
7. Zhulidov PA, Bogdanova EA, Shcheglov AS et al (2004) Simple cDNA normalization using Kamchatka crab duplex-specific nuclease. Nucleic Acids Res **32**:e37
8. Shcheglov A, Zhulidov P, Bogdanova E et al (2007) Normalization of cDNA libraries. In: Buzdin A, Lukyanov S (eds) Nucleic acids hybridization: modern applications. Springer
9. Soares B, Bonaldo MF, Jelene P et al (1994) Construction and characterization of a normalized cDNA library. Proc Nat Acad Sci USA **91**:9228–9232
10. Bonaldo MF, Lennon G, Soares MB (1996) Normalization and subtraction: two approaches to facilitate gene discovery. Genome Res **6**:791–806
11. Lo L, Zhang Z, Hong N et al (2008) 3640 Unique EST clusters from the medaka testis and their potential use for identifying conserved testicular gene expression in fish and mammals. PLoS ONE **3**:e3915

# Chapter 7

# Transcriptome Sequencing Goals, Assembly, and Assessment


## Christopher W. Wheat and Heiko Vogel



## Abstract

Transcriptome sequencing provides quick, direct access to the mRNA. With this information, one can design primers for PCR of thousands of different genes, SNP markers, probes for microarrays and qPCR, or just use the sequence data itself in comparative studies. Transcriptome sequencing, while getting cheaper, is still an expensive endeavor, with an examination of data quality and its assembly infrequently performed in depth. Here, we outline many of the important issues we think need consideration when starting a transcriptome sequencing project. We also walk the reader through a detailed analysis of an example transcriptome dataset, highlighting the importance of both within-dataset analysis and comparative inferences. Our hope is that with greater attention focused upon assessing assembly performance, advances in transcriptome assembly will increase as prices continue to drop and new technologies, such as Illumina sequencing, start to be used.



**Key words:** Next generation sequencing, cDNA, Transcriptome, Assembly


## 1. Introduction

The first goal of this section is to present some of the issues we think are important to consider when planning a transcriptome sequencing project using next generation techniques. Our second goal is to present what we think are currently the best methods for assembling transcriptome sequences and importantly, why and how to assess a given transcriptome assembly in the absence of whole genome sequence.

Making an informed and insightful choice of experimental design and execution using next generation technologies is challenging. Unlike many research endeavors, next generation sequencing project can cost more than $10,000 and result in near


Virginie Orgogozo and Matthew V. Rockman (eds.), *Molecular Methods for Evolutionary Genetics*,
Methods in Molecular Biology, vol. 772, DOI 10.1007/978-1-61779-228-1_7, © Springer Science+Business Media, LLC 2011

complete failure. We have both unfortunately heard many such horror stories that in several cases were very much avoidable. RNA quality and its ability to make quality cDNA should certainly be verified in-house before being sent to a core facility for sequencing. Private "for profit" companies may demand payment regardless of whether the sample is of usable quality, or from the intended material. Examples of such mishaps range from full sequencing runs of low quality RNA that yielded no usable data to the case of a plant lab that was returned mouse data – after nearly a year of finger pointing, no usable data has been generated despite the bills having already been paid. University core facilities are not necessarily better, as some researchers have been on waiting lists for nearly a year, with each month bringing promises that their run is next in line. Such turnaround times can cripple research progress, for principal investigators and PhD students alike. Thus, our first goal in this section is to prepare the uninitiated for wading into this complex landscape.

An increasing number of research labs are sequencing the transcriptome of their research species. For most of these species, this sequencing is the first genomic dataset ever generated as no whole genome sequence exists. Moreover, the closest species for which whole genomic sequence exists is usually quite divergent, and sometimes over 100 million years divergent. Under such circumstances, these research labs face the difficulty of assessing the performance of their transcriptome sequencing project in the absence of a genomic reference sequence for their species.

Assessing assembly performance is important for several reasons. Quite simply, one needs to have the best possible assembly in order to increase the speed, accuracy, and ultimately success of downstream projects. To visualize this problem, consider the following. There exists a continuum of data structures, with on one end all of the single reads from the shotgun sequencing of the sheared transcriptome. From a single current 454 sequencing run, there are roughly a million of these, each approximately 400 bp in length. At the other end of the continuum, there are ~20,000 contigs that represent the full-length sequences of all of the mRNAs in the sample (i.e., all of the shotgun reads have been used and assembled into these contigs, assuming the sample has about 20,000 unique mRNA transcripts). Consider how research would progress working only with the full set of unassembled single reads. Annotating this would be problematic as the reads are short and without assembly, individual errors in each read do not have a chance of being swamped out by other sequencing reads for an accurate consensus sequence (this is where the high accuracy of next generation sequencing derives from). Blasting a gene of interest (using the known sequence from another species) against this data will require a fair bit of computing power and the result will only be all of the reads matching your gene of interest, which could be hundreds. Designing PCR primers for this gene will require looking at the alignment of these individual reads across the gene and accounting for genetic variation in the sample. Identifying SNP variation would require looking at multiple independent reads for each gene region, etc. Multiply this across even 50 genes, and this becomes a prohibitive time sink. At the other end of the spectrum, there is a single full-length sequence per gene, which is highly accurate as its assembly has been able to take advantage of overlapping sequencing reads. Telling your assembly program to code polymorphism into the consensus sequence, when such information comes from frequent and high quality sequencing reads, also provides information regarding SNP variation in your sample, important for primer design for PCR and probe design in microarray analysis, as well as in identifying SNPs themselves. Thus, getting as close as we can to a full assembly is the goal, as this decreases the time spent in avoidable bioinformatics tasks and therefore accelerates data interpretation and advances in biological research.

A transcriptome assembly is affected by the number and quality of the reads, the software used to assemble it, and the parameters chosen within the software. To get at these issues, the sequencing quality first needs to be checked. Second, the extent of transcriptome coverage needs to be quantified. This is important both for the individual lab and the community as a whole, since advances in methodology need to be assessed and published. There is a significant range of performance differences among currently existing software packages and without these assessments, knowing where your assembly exists along the range of bad to good assemblies is impossible. Packages differ in terms of what types of next generation sequencing data they can accept, how quickly and efficiently they run it, and how well they assemble the data into contigs. Finally, they also differ in their end goal performance for operations such as calling SNPs. While we will not be covering SNP issues, such end-user goals need to be considered early on during experimental design. Our second goal for this chapter is therefore to provide the user a guide for assembling and assessing a transcriptome in the absence of a genomic reference.

In this chapter, we are primarily going to focus on the Roche 454 technology for transcriptome sequencing. This is for the simple reason that this method gives the longest read lengths of any of the currently available next generation methods. For example, the current version of the Roche 454 technology, using the Genome Sequencer FLX Instrument with GS FLX Titanium chemistry returns a reported 1.2 million reads averaging approximately 400 bp each and is expected to reach over 800 bp by the end of 2010. This is in comparison to the second longest read method by Illumina, which has flow cell runs currently generating 180–200 million reads which can reach lengths up to 100 bps. The increased read lengths of 454 are a significant advantage for de novo assembly, but it should be noted that the paired end sequencing provided by Illumina coupled with its nearly 200-fold higher coverage is likely to result in similar and potentially better assembly success with bioinformatics advances (1).

As a final point of discussion, we wish to provide the beginning researcher with a powerful approach to ensure that they are quickly able to attain the research goals of their project. We strongly recommend that researchers decide upon and test the assembly pipeline they are planning to use. Doing this before or even in parallel to the actual lab sequencing project, while waiting for the data to return from a core facility, should facilitate and accelerate future data analysis. First, obtain a dataset that is as similar to the expected as possible, in terms of format (e.g., 454 or Illumina), material sequenced (normalized or unnormalized, transcriptome size, etc.), and size (both read length and number of reads). The short read archive of NCBI provides such datasets for downloading (http://www.ncbi.nlm.nih.gov/sra). Be aware that you may need to trim out adapter sequences prior to assembly. Second, upload and run that dataset through your assembly program. Determine how long it takes to run, whether your computer crashes or slows to a snail's pace, etc. Third, assess the assembly results. How long are the assembled contigs? Could they be longer? Compare across different setting of your software package, and across different packages. Follow the instructions below for assessing assembly performance. Fourth, can you view your data in a way that is intuitive? Do you like the software you have committed to using? Fifth, assess your desired end goal performance. How the SNPs are being called? Are you able to decide upon frequency thresholds both at the candidate SNP location and in neighboring regions? This latter filtering step is important. For example, consider three polymorphic sites located within 5 bp. These may not be SNP variation but rather an alternatively spliced codon that your assembler simply cannot detect. Working through these steps ahead of time will prepare you for the coming data, essentially identifying the holes, bottlenecks, and flow rate through your proposed pipeline before your real data are ready to be poured into it.

## 2. Materials

1. A list of the companies and technologies available, and their latest statistics.
2. Sufficient technical understanding.
3. Places to do the work and their costs.
4. Contact information for people with experience: Names of people who have used specific methods, core facilities, or companies.

5. A clear end goal and/or biological question.
6. Bioinformatics: A list of the software available and their functions; computer requirements of these packages for handling data of your expected type and size; and assistance from collaborators or a core facility.

## 3. Methods

### 3.1. Taking the First Steps

1. Between the time you are writing your grant and when you are getting ready to implement your grant scheme, you should be sure to update Subheading 2, item 1 given the 6–12 month rate of technological advancement in this field. Getting this information will require speaking with company representatives as well as your local genomics core facility representative. The latter is more likely to provide you with the down to earth details of how things are working day to day in that core facility, rather than an idealized version generally provided by company representatives. These can be quite different, in both positive and negative directions. We also strongly suggest finding someone with actual experience so you can directly hear what has worked well, easily, robustly, etc. vs. what one reads in published journals or pamphlets. A commonly asked question is how can I tell if my sample really is next in line at the core facility? One way to cut through to the truth is ask for the contact information of those whose samples were just finished. They will likely have much insight to share with you, and it will keep the core facility focused in discussions with you.
2. Developing a technological understanding of the sequencing methods is very important. These methods have fundamental differences in the way they sequence DNA, which results in important tradeoffs in sequencing read length, number of sequencing reads, their error rates and types, and their ability to partition runs efficiently and cheaply. Importantly, these issues may change in the near future.

### 3.2. References and Contact Information from People with Experience

1. We have gathered quite a bit of valuable insights from conversations with people using these methods. In addition, much has been gained by talking with people who have used specific core facilities or companies. Most of our conversations have happened at conferences or workshops focused on next generation sequencing. We recommend any of the workshops being funded by the European Science Foundation, and core facilities themselves. Many medical schools also organize similar symposia. An excellent and savvy genomics community working on a wide range of taxa attends the Society for

Molecular Biology and Evolution (http://www.smbe.org/) and the UK Population Group (http://www.populationgeneticsgroup.org/) meetings. Such interactions are very important in order to make informed decisions regarding experimental design and which core facilities to chose. Importantly, this landscape is constantly shifting with, for example, core facility turn around time changing quite dramatically within a 6-month period (and not always for the best).

2. We highly recommend taking additional steps after finding what appears to be a suitable core facility or company. Getting contact information from actual people who have used these facilities recently is a valuable resource, and if they got good service, more than likely they will be more than happy to provide a short account of their experience. These people can also provide price estimates for comparisons with quotes from company representatives.

### *3.3. A Clear Goal and/or Biological Question*

1. We assume that many of the people reading this chapter are interested in finding the genetic basis of the phenotypic variation they study. However, some researchers may only be interested in obtaining SNPs or microsatellites for use in molecular ecological studies of population dynamics. Sequencing normalized cDNA in a full 454 run will certainly provide these resources, but full-length coverage or broad coverage of the transcriptome is perhaps not as important in such cases. Rather, half a sequencing plate of 454 may be more than sufficient to generate the needed data, with shearing and normalization potentially not necessary (as most microsatellites found in the transcriptome are located in UTR regions, e.g., (2)).
2. When trying to develop molecular insights into phenotypes of interest, some assumption of the genetic architecture underlying this phenotype should be made. Studies targeting protein-coding sequence evolution require different approaches to next generation transcriptome sequencing and assembly than do studies targeting changes in gene expression. There has been some discussion in the literature regarding the genetic basis of morphological variation, with different camps emphasizing coding or expression variation. While there are clearly empirical examples of both and little conclusive data sufficient for generalities (3), what is clear is the need for researchers to decide early on whether they are interested in gaining genomic insights into coding or expression variation. Such a decision needs to be made, for obtaining good data for both questions currently requires considerable sequencing effort (discussed below).
3. If one wants to assess relative expression differences among individuals with good biological replication, we highly recommend

using microarrays since RNAseq is still very expensive. One can design a very high quality microarray from transcriptome sequencing data by designing the microarray probes based on the assembly. Transcriptome sequencing for this purpose should sequence a normalized transcriptome, which will generate partial sequences typically covering between 50 and potentially over 70% of unique genes in the transcriptome (e.g., (4, 5)). However, if one wants to compare coding sequences between samples (e.g., populations or species), very deep sequencing will be required in order to get sufficient sequencing reads across enough genes for analysis. Indeed, typical sequencing runs obtained from a normalized pool of mRNA rarely produces full-length sequence for more than 1,000 genes. For example, recent transcriptome sequencing of normalized mRNA pools from two closely related fish species, ½ each on a full GS FLX 454 run, found 13,106 pairs of putative orthologs from the assembled contig ESTs (6). These had a mean shared coverage length of 264 bp (range from 153 to 767 bp). Of these, only 1,721 matched the open reading frames of known proteins making inference of biological function challenging. However, with the dramatic increases in sequencing coverage and length, shared coverage is likely to dramatically improve.

4. A final question for consideration is how much variation in the genetic mechanism among individuals and populations is there likely to be for your given phenotype of interest. As our genetic understanding of phenotypes of interest continues to grow, we are faced with an increasing body of evidence indicating that what may appear to be a single phenotype at the morphological level may indeed have several different genetic origins both among and within populations. This is true for clear morphological phenotypes such as coat color variation in mice (7) as well as metabolic phenotypes in fish (8). Failure to consider such a possibility in experimental design can lead to the pooling of homogeneous phenotypes that have heterogeneous genetic architecture, or great confusion when trying to extend lab observations across independent wild populations.

### 3.4. Assembly

1. Filtering and trimming. Prior to assembly, the raw sequencing output needs to be cleaned in order to remove the sequences of adapter oligos that were added prior to sequencing. In many cases, these may have been sequenced and they could provide spurious alignment similarities. Following this, research into sources of error in 454 sequencing data recommend simply trimming reads that are larger or smaller than a given range around the mean (9). For example, if the mean is 400 bp, it may be wise to remove reads that are shorter than 200 bp in

length, as these may contain a larger number of errors than expected. For sequences much longer than 500 bp, these extra reads may or may not be accurate. Along with this trimming or independent of it, one needs to consider how to handle low complexity regions and low quality sites. Most methods will allow for the former to be masked and the quality information of the latter to be considered during assembly. A simple example unique to transcriptome sequencing are poly-A tails, which of course should be masked or removed from sequences prior to assembly. Varying the number of homopolymer As may be needed to optimize masking of poly-A tails vs. real poly-A runs within genes.

2. Parameter settings for assembly will need to be determined empirically, but generally the default setting of many methods work relatively well. While many people first use the software package included with the Roche 454 machine, called Newbler, we have not had good success with this software and recommend as a first start Mira3 (10), especially because it is freeware. Our own experience and that of some others have found several of the expensive commercial software programs to be prohibitively RAM intensive. Due to extreme amount of variation among software programs, data sets, and local computer configurations, a comparison of assembly programs is beyond the scope of this chapter. We recognize this as a current gaping hole in transcriptome sequencing literature.

#### 3.5. Assessing the Assembly Against Itself

1. Within-dataset assessment can take advantage of the general output of most assemblies, using the number of reads per assembled contig, the length of these contigs, and the average number of reads per bp along a contig, which will be referred to as average depth per contig. First, we want to assess the distribution of contig lengths and how many reads have been used to make these (Fig. 1). These graphs provide a first assessment of contig assembly, allowing one to see the how many contigs of a given size have been formed, as well as how many reads have been used for these assemblies. Log scale axes aid in visualizing the distribution of contigs, and to be consistent across figures, when appropriate, all axes use log scale.
2. Contig length plotted against the total number of reads per contig (Fig. 2a) shows the expected trend of increasing contig length as more reads are used to assemble each contig. This is what we would generally expect from a good assembly. However, such a graph can be misleading due to the high density of points being hidden at different values.
3. The distribution of these reads across the contig are also important, as stretches of contig that are <4 bp deep cannot provide reliable information regarding SNPs. For any given site that is

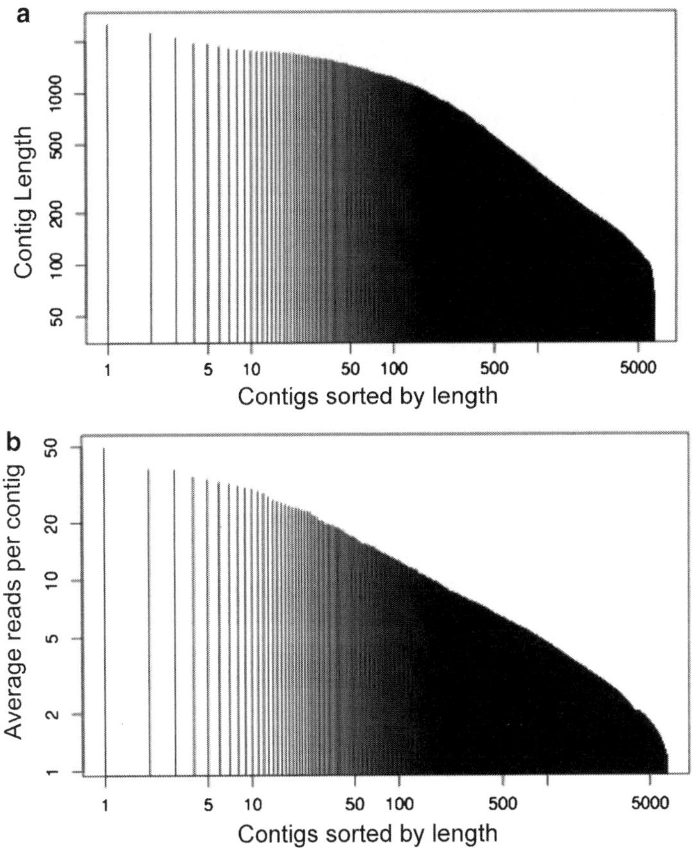


Fig. 1. Distributions of assembled contig lengths (**a**) and the average number of reads per assembled contig (**b**). Each contig is represented by a single thin line. Note that all axes are in $\log_{10}$ scale, with the *x*-axis showing the distribution of contigs ($n = 6{,}530$).

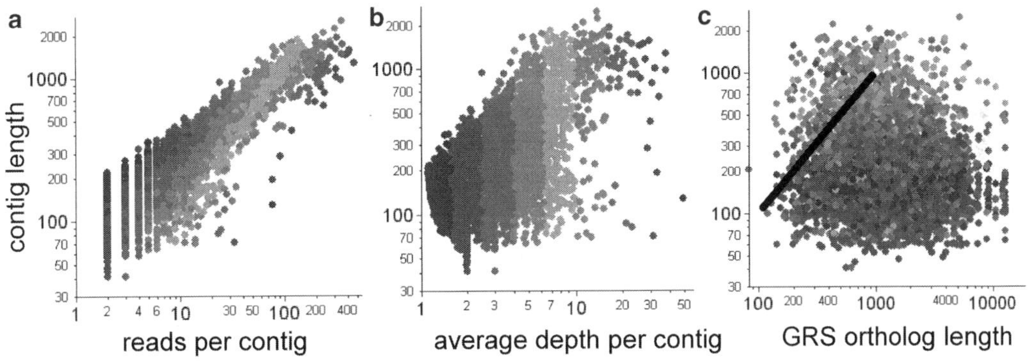


Fig. 2. Plots of contig length against the number of reads per contig (**a**), average number of reads per bp per contig (i.e., depth per contig) (**b**), and the length of the gene for which the contig was assembled, inferred via blast alignment with a genomic reference species' (GRS) orthologous gene (**c**). Each contig is *shaded* according to its average number of reads, as shown on the *x*-axis in (**b**). A linear fit with slope 1 is shown in (**c**), between 100 and 1,000 bp. Note all axes are in $\log_{10}$ scale.

polymorphic, the two reads for each alternative nucleotide establish them as real rather than error. While quality score could be used instead, lowering the requirement to two reads, the four read minimum is robust to assumptions of many quality score calling algorithms. We need to therefore assess the distribution of reads along the contig at different contig lengths. We can gain insight into this by looking at how contig length changes as average depth per contig increases (Fig. 2b). A strong relationship between contig length and the average depth per contig are observed. There appears to be a plateau around a depth of 10, between contig lengths 1–2 kb, suggesting a target of 10× coverage for good assembly (4). Notice also that for many they are short and have few reads (i.e., those located in the lower left of the graph). These contigs suggest that greater sequencing depth and read length are required to increase the contig assembly length, or that bioinformatics assembly problems exist, or some degree of both. Teasing apart these effects is important, and we can only do this via a comparative analysis in the next section.

4. Troubling are contigs that do not follow the positive relationship of increasing contig length with average depth. These are reads that fail to assembly together as very long contigs regardless of the number of reads incorporated (the lower center portion of Fig. 2b). A very good biological reason may account for this, as short genes will naturally form short contigs regardless of how many reads are assembled into a given contig. This may also be due to biases in the shearing of the transcriptome, resulting in many reads of unsheared genes that are only able to come from their terminal ends. Such a 5′ and 3′ biases in read distributions was detected in a comparison of the plant *Arabidopsis thaliana* transcriptome sequencing with its whole genome scaffold (5). Thus, this region is potentially telling us quite a bit about both technical and biological effects. To separate these effects we need to know the expected lengths of the genes that the contigs represent, and this requires the comparative approach detailed in the next section.

### 3.6. Assessing the Assembly Against a Genomic Reference Species

In this section, we consider how to assess transcriptome assemblies in the absence of genomic data for the studied, or focal species (e.g., EST libraries, whole genome sequence and predicted gene sets). For any focal species, there is a genomic reference species (GRS) that can be used for comparative analysis. Here, we refer to a GRS as being a species that has a predicted set of genes from its sequenced genome. These genes provide a good first approximation to a full gene set and they can be used in comparative analyses with the focal species. Focal species naturally vary in how close evolutionarily they are to their nearest GRS.

1. While there are many insights that can be gained from assessing an assembly by comparing it to itself (e.g., Subheading 3.5), comparative analyses are needed to gain important insights and disentangle technical from biological effects as best we can (e.g. Subheading 3.5, steps 3 and 4). The first thing we wish to know is whether our assembled contigs are in fact the mRNA of genes from the target species. Many research groups address this question by blasting their contigs against reference gene databases (ideally protein databases), obtaining estimates of the number of unique genes (unigenes) hit and functional-group membership percentages (e.g., Blast2GO annotations), and assessing the taxonomic relatedness of their hit species to their focal species. This approach provides us an estimate of number of unigenes in the transcriptome assembled database, as there may be many contigs for the same gene. However, researchers need to keep in mind that the databases they compare against can influence their findings. Thus, it is important to compare against both large databases and predicted gene sets from single species (e.g., (4)). Additionally, there are likely to be many genes unique to a given taxon that are not expected to be identified in other species. For example, across the 12 genomes of *Drosophila* (11), spanning approximately 60 million years of divergence (12), 77% of *D. melanogaster* genes are found across the 11 other genomes.
2. Estimates of the number of unigenes can be compared to the expected number of genes for a GRS. This provides some insight into what percentage of the transcriptome was likely "touched." We say "touched" rather than sequenced to emphasize the point that the vast majority of contigs do not represent full-length mRNA, but rather partial fragments. In fact, many contigs will be for separate portions of the same gene and this must be accounted for when estimating the number of unigenes hit in blast database searches. These contigs coming from different parts of the same gene may not have their best blast hit to the same unigene in a given database. In such cases, a single gene in the transcriptome sequenced species could result in three independent contigs which in turn blast to three different genes in a protein database (or the same gene but from different species). This will inflate the number of unique genes identified in a protein database unless care is taken to remove this level of spurious inflation. One way around this is to blast all the assembled contigs and singletons against the predicted gene set of a single GRS, with the number of the predicted genes hit being an estimate of the number of unigenes the contigs represent (e.g., (4)). This of course will still miss many unique genes in the focal species, as these will not find blast hits in comparisons, but it does provide what may be a good lower bound on an estimate of unigenes touched.

3. An important issue to keep in mind when blasting the focal species assembly against the predicted gene set of a GRS is the potential gene family dynamics in both species. One can at least eliminate this effect in the GRS dataset by performing a reciprocal best blast of the GRS predicted genes against itself, thereby identifying the gene sets which share more than 90% amino acid identity, then taking only the longest of these members. This 90% cutoff GRS predicted gene dataset will then only provide a single gene for gene families in the focal species to blast against and this provides a rather robust lower estimate of the number of focal species unigenes.

4. Here, we wish to argue that several additional steps can be easily taken and are needed for insightful transcriptome assessment and assembly advances. Up until now in this chapter, we have only begun to address perhaps the most fundamental question in assessing an assembly: How well have our contigs been assembled? While Fig. 2a indicates a good assembly performance, even a preliminary comparative analysis shows a very different picture and indicates a poor assembly. We can use a comparative approach to get at something we really need to know, that is, the length of the gene each contig represents. Recall that the assembly programs are taking all of the shotgun short sequence reads from the fragmented cDNA library and trying to piece it all back together. We ultimately wish to know how well they have done their job. The best and most common way to do this is to compare contigs to their genes from the focal species, but we need genomic sequence for this (or an extensive Sanger sequence EST library collection). However, in the absence of such resources, we advocate comparing contigs to the predicted gene sets of the nearest GRS. With this data one can then compare the assembled contig length to the expected length of that gene. Graphing this relationship shows how the vast majority of our contigs are much shorter than their expected length, as most contigs fall well below a linear fit indicated for the range of 100–1,000 bp (Fig. 2c).

5. The poor relationship between contig length and expected length in Fig. 2c hints at poor assembly performance, but is that the whole picture? Again, knowing the contig length is really only insightful when compared to the expected length of the corresponding mRNA. By dividing a given contig's length by the length of its inferred ortholog from the GRS, we obtain a ratio representing a contig's percent-coverage of at least the coding region of a given mRNA. We call this an ortholog length ratio. For contigs that contain nearly all their mRNA's coding region, the aligned contig length will be nearly equal to that of the ortholog identified from the GRS, and thus the ortholog length ratio will be near 1. For those that contain

smaller fragments of the coding region, their ortholog length ratio will be much less than 1. Thus, we can use our inferred orthologous genes from blast searches to gain considerable assembly insight. A ratio >1 most likely indicates the untranslated region (UTR) in the contig assembly.

6. Blast results return quite a bit of important information that can be used for assessment purposes. One can use the length of the aligned region to generate a more exact ortholog length ratio. Keep in mind though, this will only be informative for those orthologs that can blast well for their whole length (genes with low functional constraint that diverge quickly may not work as well). Instead of using the total length of a contig as mentioned above, which may include untranslated sequence before and after the coding region (i.e., 5′ and 3′ UTR regions) and chimerical sequence (i.e., incorrectly joined reads from what are separate genes), we can construct a ratio using the aligned contig length indicated by the blast table results (i.e., query length). Plotting this new ortholog length ratio against the average depth per contig provides perhaps one of the most important insights we can obtain into the assembly, that is, the relationship between full-length assembly and average depth (Fig. 3). Figure 3 displays six different panels, which all graph the ortholog length ratio using query length against average depth, with each panel presenting a different range of expected gene sizes. Graphing all of these in one figure hides the high density of low ortholog length ratios for very large genes. Instead, here we have in each panel 1,000 contigs, with the last panel containing 1,530 (Fig. 3). Perhaps a hundred genes have near full-length coverage, being located in the region of an ortholog length ratio of 1. These also have an average depth near 10, suggesting that such coverage is necessary for full-length assembly. Notice how full length coverage is dramatically decreased for increasingly longer genes, reaching a minimum in the longest gene set in the lower right panel.

7. Are these short contigs the result of poor assembly performance? Ascribing these results to poor assembly performance assumes that the necessary sequences have been generated and the software just cannot put them back together again. To address this question we need to know how many of our contigs are for the same gene. Understanding this tells us about how much sequence we have that covers the genes, and how well that was assembled in single or multiple contigs. By summing the length of the contigs that blast to the same orthologous gene, we can plot this against the length of the orthologous gene (Fig. 4). Looking at this figure we can see a sloping tail to the lower right, since contigs cover a decreasing percentage of a given gene as it increases in length. Points that sum near

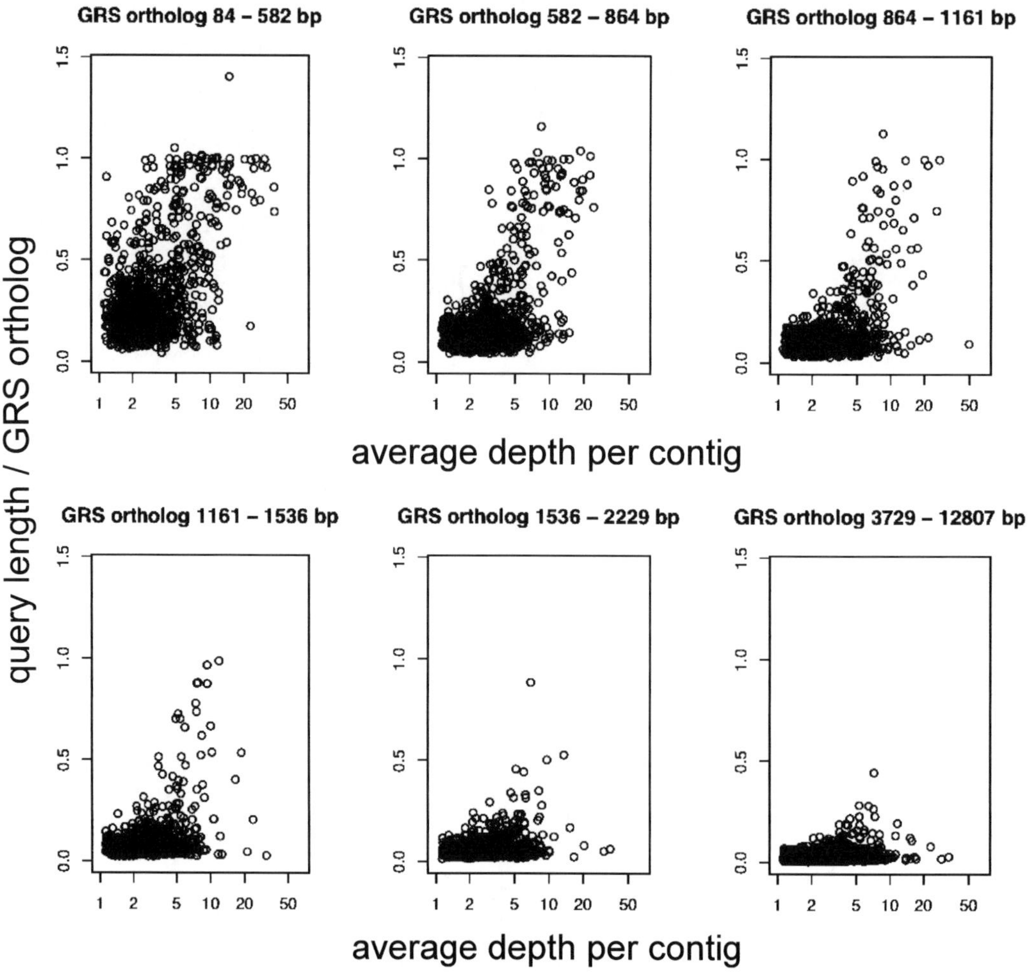


Fig. 3. Expected length of contigs plotted against the average number of reads per bp per contig. The *y*-axis is the contig blast result alignment length divided by the length of its inferred genomic reference sequence (GRS) ortholog (in DNA bp). Each of the six panels is for a different length range of the GRS ortholog. Note that the *x*-axis is in $\log_{10}$ scale.

100% are for genes across a range of coverage depth. Thus, we are getting good sequencing coverage from across a range of gene sizes. Notice also the gray shading of the points, which indicate the number of contigs covering a given ortholog. The vast majority of points indicate that many orthologs are covered by a very small number of contigs, which in turn cover only a small fraction of genes ranging from 600 to 2,000 bp in size. This observation suggests that great sequencing coverage would help provide the data needed to assemble these contigs since there does not appear to be enough reads across genes for their assembly. Had the density of points been higher on the *y*-axis, and composed of many contigs, this would suggest sufficient sequencing coverage that was assembled poorly.

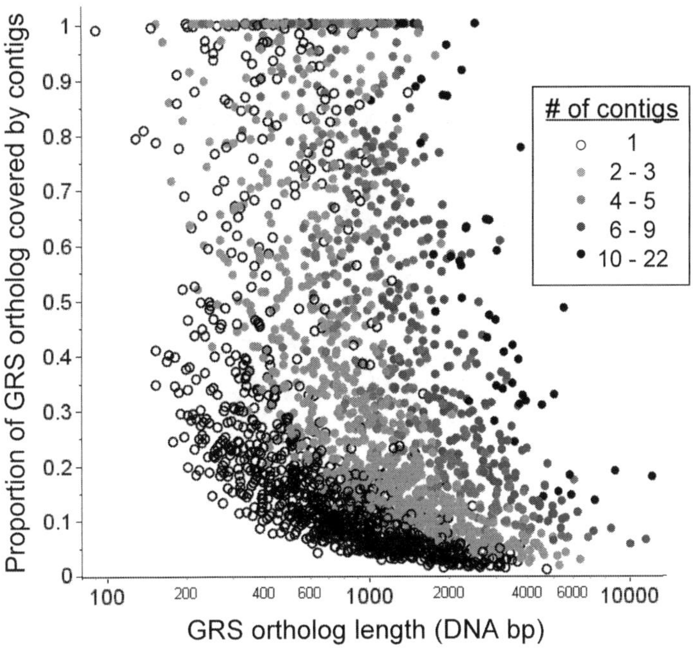


Fig. 4. Proportion of each gene covered by contigs plotted against gene length. Each point represents the sum of contig alignment length for its genomic reference species' (GRS) ortholog, with its shade indicating how many contigs were included in that sum ($\log_{10}$ scale).

8. Readers will be correct in assuming that with longer read lengths, assembly performance will dramatically increase. Nevertheless, assessing assembly performance will continue to be necessary for all of the reasons stated earlier. This is all the more true as users shift toward using the much higher sequencing coverage provided by other platforms such as Illumina. Currently, these reads are only 100 bp in length, which is therefore directly comparable to the average sequencing length presented in this chapter. Recent work suggests that such sequencing can be used for excellent transcriptome assembly, when coupled with an accurate assembly program.

## Acknowledgments

The authors would like to thank many of our colleagues over the past couple of years who have shared their experiences with us. CWW would additionally like to thank W. Stephan, R. Butlin, E. Randi, and D. Tautz for invitations to speak at, and learn from, various Next Generation Sequencing workshops over the past year. CWW would also like to thank Jim Marden for his initial experience with 454 sequencing, as it was he who decided that 454 sequencing could be used for the transcriptome. Support for this work comes from the Max Planck Gesellschaft and Finnish Academy Grant 131155.

## References


1. Birol I, Jackman S, Nielsen C et al (2009) De novo transcriptome assembly with ABySS. Bioinformatics **25**:2872–2877
2. Wheat CW (2010) Rapidly developing functional genomics in ecological model systems via 454 transcriptome sequencing. Genetica **138**:433–51
3. Wray GA (2007) The evolutionary significance of cis-regulatory mutations. Nat Rev Genet **8**:206–216
4. Vera JC, Wheat C, Fescemyer HW et al (2008) Rapid transcriptome characterization for a nonmodel organism using 454 pyrosequencing. Mol Ecol **17**:1636–1647
5. Weber APM, Weber KL, Carr K et al (2007) Sampling the *Arabidopsis* transcriptome with massively parallel pyrosequencing. Plant Physiology **144**:32–42
6. Elmer K, Fan S, Gunter H et al (2010) Rapid evolution and selection inferred from the transcriptomes of sympatric crater lake cichlid fishes. Mol Ecol **19**:197–211
7. Steiner C, Rompler H, Boettger L et al (2008) The genetic basis of phenotypic convergence in beach mice: similar pigment patterns but different genes. Mol Biol Evol **26**:35–45
8. Oleksiak M, Roach J, Crawford D (2004) Natural variation in cardiac metabolism and gene expression in *Fundulus heteroclitus.* Nature Genetics **37**:67–72
9. Huse SM, Huber JA, Morrison HG et al (2007) Accuracy and quality of massively-parallel DNA pyrosequencing. Genome Biology **8**:R143
10. Chevreux B, Pfisterer T, Drescher B et al (2004) Using the miraEST assembler for reliable and automated mRNA transcript assembly and SNP detection in sequenced ESTs. Genome Res **14**:1147–1159
11. Drosophila 12 Genomes Consortium (2007) Evolution of genes and genomes on the Drosophila phylogeny. Nature **450**:203–218
12. Tamura K, Subramanian S, Kumar S (2004) Temporal patterns of fruit fly (*Drosophila*) evolution revealed by mutation clocks. Mol Biol Evol **21**:36–44

# Chapter 8

# Rapid Retrieval of DNA Target Sequences by Primer Extension Capture

Adrian W. Briggs

## Abstract

There is a widespread need for methods to enrich DNA samples for sequences of interest prior to high-throughput sequencing and to reduce the costs associated with a shotgun approach. While useful for targeting megabase-sized regions in a few samples, hybridization capture approaches such as those using microarrays currently involve bulky handling steps, long incubation times, and high per-sample costs. In contrast, the primer extension capture (PEC) method allows direct selection of small genomic regions from DNA sources within 2 h, with low costs for use with parallel samples. PEC promises useful applications in studies such as ancient DNA or forensic sequencing, taxonomic surveying of metagenomic samples, or genomic mapping of repetitive elements.

**Key words:** Capture, Enrichment, Targeted resequencing, Ancient DNA, aDNA, Forensics, Taxonomic barcoding, Metagenomics

## 1. Introduction

Recent advances in sequencing technology have drastically reduced costs of whole-genome sequencing. However, many studies require data only from specific genomic regions of interest. Targeted retrieval of these regions is therefore often economically preferable to a shotgun sequencing approach. This is particularly the case for degraded DNA sources such as forensic samples or ancient remains, since the vast majority of DNA in such degraded samples may represent DNA contamination from microbes that have colonized the dead tissue. Unfortunately, traditional PCR is poorly suited to sequence recovery from degraded samples as it is wasteful of extract and unable to target molecules too short to accommodate both PCR primers (1). Primer extension capture (PEC, Fig. 1) is a

Virginie Orgogozo and Matthew V. Rockman (eds.), *Molecular Methods for Evolutionary Genetics*,
Methods in Molecular Biology, vol. 772, DOI 10.1007/978-1-61779-228-1_8, © Springer Science+Business Media, LLC 2011

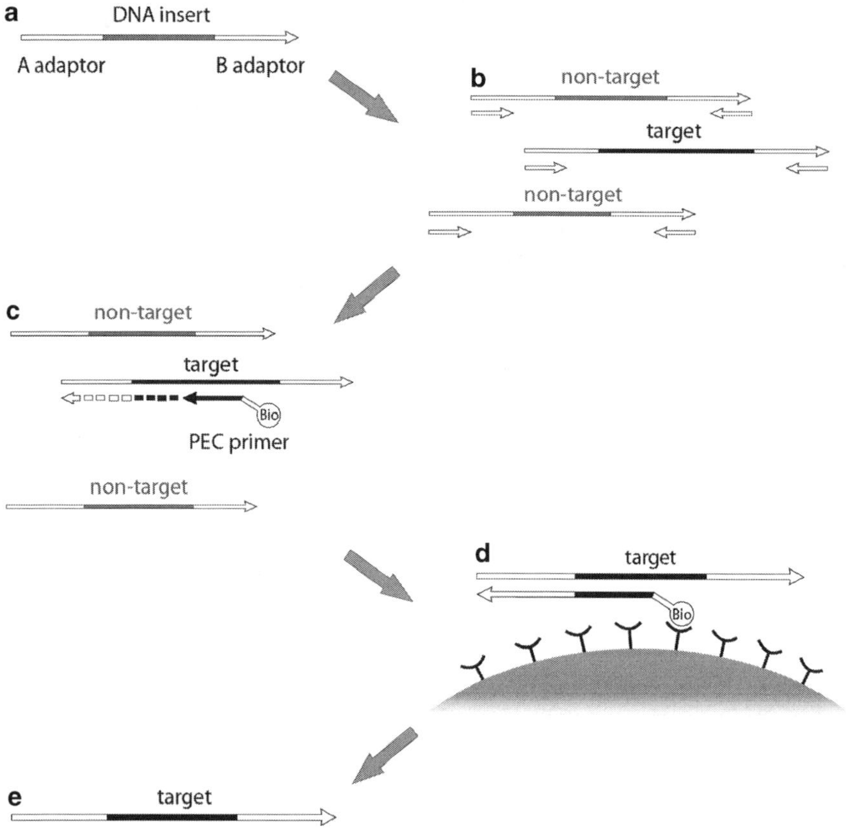


Fig. 1. Principles of primer extension capture. (**a**) A DNA extract is first converted into to a DNA library by attachment of adaptors to the ends of all DNA fragments. (**b**) Before capture, the whole library is PCR amplified for 14 cycles using primers complementary to the adaptors; this produces many copies of each original fragment, including target and nontarget sequences, and immortalizes the sample while improving later capture efficiency. (**c**) The amplified library is then subjected to single primer extension using biotinylated primers (PEC primers) specific for desired target sequences. (**d**) Biotinylated extension products and their attached target templates are captured on streptavidin-coated magnetic beads, and nontargets are washed away. (**e**) The captured and washed target fragments are eluted from the beads, allowing high-throughput sequencing. The primer extension products carry only a single sequencing adaptor and thus do not get sequenced.

method of targeted sequence retrieval that is ideally suited to capturing short target sequences from a highly complex DNA background (1). In contrast to PCR, which works on raw DNA extract, PEC uses a DNA sequencing library as template. A sequencing library is a DNA extract that has had universal adaptor sequences ligated to the ends of all DNA fragments in the extract. The adaptor sequences are required for the high-throughput sequencing process (2, 3). Briefly, one or several biotinylated oligonucleotide primers are mixed with a DNA library containing rare target inserts in a large background of nontargets. Each primer anneals specifically to its targets and extends along the templates in the presence of free nucleotides and a DNA polymerase. Primer-target duplexes are then captured on streptavidin-coated magnetic beads, allowing noncaptured library molecules to be stringently removed by washing. Products are then eluted and sequenced. Importantly, the original library fragments are sequenced and not the primer extension products, as the extension products will not carry both adaptors (Fig. 1) and cannot therefore undergo sequencing.

The PEC procedure has been shown to allow access to many short ancient DNA fragments that are not amenable to traditional PCR (4). In doing so PEC also reduces the problems of present-day DNA contamination (4), which is in general not as degraded as the ancient DNA. In comparison to hybridization capture approaches (5, 6), which also enrich complex adaptor-ligated DNA libraries for targeted sequences, the PEC procedure is substantially quicker, taking a few hours as opposed to several days. PEC can be performed with multiple parallel samples (see Note 1), involves low reagent costs for limited numbers of targets, and can be made extremely specific with careful primer design. In addition, PEC requires only part of a target sequence to be known, unlike hybridization capture approaches, potentially leading to two useful applications of PEC (a) mapping all genomic sites of a multicopy element such as a transposon, by capture of inserts containing the element and sequencing into the flanking sequence; (b) measuring taxonomic diversity in metagenomic samples, by capturing inserts at conserved loci and sequencing outward into phylogenetically informative flanking regions. It should be noted that PEC is less well suited to capture large genomic regions (over a few kb in length – see Note 2).

The template for PEC is an adaptor-ligated DNA library (see Fig. 1a) of the sort used for high-throughput sequencing by platforms such as Illumina/Solexa or Roche/454. For applications involving high quality modern DNA, any of the current sequencing library preparation protocols will suffice. To generate such a library from ancient bone material, I recommend the DNA extraction protocol of Rohland and Hofreiter (7), and the library preparation procedure of Maricic and Pääbo (8), using the relevant adaptor sequences. If the DNA sample is highly damaged, I also recommend including the uracil–DNA–glycosylase/endonuclease VIII DNA repair step described by Briggs et al. (9). A typical ancient DNA experiment involves the following: ~200 mg of bone powder used to produce 100 μl of DNA extract; ~20 μl of this DNA extract used to prepare ~50 μl of DNA library. After the library is prepared it should be quantified. If the amount is too low for fluorescent-based quantification, as is common, a semiquantitative qPCR is recommended. The general procedure for this is described in (10). Once the library has been generated, it should first be universally amplified in order to immortalize the sample and increase capture success. The amplified library can then be used as template in the PEC procedure, generating products enriched for target sequences, which can then directly enter the high-throughput sequencing process.

## 2. Materials

### 2.1. Library Amplification

1. AmpliTaq Gold DNA Polymerase (Applied Biosystems, Foster City, CA).
2. 10× GeneAmp PCR Buffer II (Applied Biosystems).
3. 25 mM $MgCl_2$.
4. dNTP mix (25 mM each of dATP, dTTP, dCTP, and dGTP).
5. 10 mg/ml bovine serum albumin (BSA).
6. Molecular biology-grade water.
7. Adaptor-specific PCR primer pair.
8. Adaptor-ligated DNA library.
9. QIAquick PCR purification kit (Qiagen).

### 2.2. Primer Extension

1. AmpliTaq Gold DNA Polymerase (Applied Biosystems).
2. 10× GeneAmp PCR Buffer II (Applied Biosystems).
3. 25 mM $MgCl_2$.
4. dNTP mix (25 mM each of dATP, dTTP, dCTP, and dGTP).
5. 10 mg/ml BSA.
6. Molecular biology-grade water.
7. Amplified adaptor-ligated DNA library.
8. Biotinylated target primers.
9. MinElute PCR purification kit (Qiagen).

### 2.3. Bead Capture and Isolation

1. M-270 streptavidin Dynabeads (Invitrogen, Carlsbad, CA).
2. 2× Binding and Wash (BW) buffer: 2 M NaCl, 10 mM Tris–Cl, 1 mM EDTA pH 8.0, 0.2% Tween-20.
3. 1× Binding and Wash (BW) buffer: One part 2× BW buffer to one part water.
4. Hot Wash (HW) buffer: 2.5 mM $MgCl_2$, 10× GeneAmp PCR Buffer II (Applied Biosystems), 0.1% Tween-20.
5. EB buffer (supplied with MinElute PCR Purification kit): 10 mM Tris–HCl, pH 8.5.
6. Magnetic Particle Collector (MPC) (Invitrogen).

## 3. Methods

### 3.1. Library Amplification

Before target capture, PCR amplification of the entire library should be performed using primers complementary to the library adaptors (see Note 3). This step is especially necessary when using precious but heavily degraded DNA samples since DNA amounts will be so low that each individual DNA molecule is valuable. Performing capture with many copies of each original fragment maximizes the chance to capture at least one copy of each fragment, and thus recover all of the sequence information available in a sample. However, if the initial library has a concentration greater than 20 ng/μl the amplification step is unnecessary and can be omitted. In this case, proceed directly to the primer extension step.

1. Prepare a PCR reaction mix to a total volume of 100 μl, containing 10 μl of 10× GeneAmp PCR Buffer II, 10 μl of 25 mM $MgCl_2$, 2 μl of 10 mg/ml BSA, 1 μl dNTP mix (25 mM each dNTP), 3 μl each of the forward and reverse adaptor primers (10 μM each primer), 1 μl of 5 U/μl AmpliTaq Gold DNA polymerase, 25 μl of adaptor-ligated DNA library, and 45 μl molecular biology-grade water. The PEC procedure will work for libraries of any DNA concentration, but each library should be used undiluted to maximize sequence complexity of the results.
2. Place the PCR tube in a thermocycler, followed by a denaturation step of 95°C for 12 min, followed by 14 cycles of 95°C for 30 s, 60°C (or the suitable annealing temperature for the primers if different) for 1 min, 72°C for 1 min. Finish the process with 5 min at 70°C and hold at 10°C until ready for purification.
3. After PCR amplification is complete, follow it with purification of the PCR product using a Qiagen QIAquick spin column according to manufacturer's instructions. I recommend to use a microcentrifuge as opposed to a vacuum pump to minimize the retention of PCR primers (see Note 4). Elute DNA from the column with 50 μl of EB Buffer supplied with the kit. It is recommended here to perform qPCR quantification of the amplified library together with an aliquot of the nonamplified library to ensure that pre-amplification worked properly.

### 3.2. PEC Primer Design

PEC primer oligonucleotides consist of a 5′ biotin residue, followed by a 12-base spacer sequence (I use the sequence 5′-CAAGGACATCCG-3′), followed by the target complementary sequence. The 12-base spacer sequence helps to avoid steric hindrance during streptavidin bead capture. I recommend to design the primer target sequence with the program Primer3 (11), using an optimal annealing temperature of 60°C and length range of 16–25 nt (these calculations should not include the 12-base spacer sequence). Make sure that the PEC primers do not have high 3′ complementarity (seven bases or more) to any part of the library adaptors, as this could lead to increased nonspecific capture. I recommend ordering the primers HPLC purified, although desalted primers may also work. I use oligonucleotides from Sigma-Aldrich (St Louis, MO) (see Note 5).

### 3.3. Primer Extension

1. For the Primer Extension reaction, prepare a PCR master mix to a total volume of 50 μl, containing 5 μl of 10× GeneAmp PCR Buffer II, 5 μl of 25 mM $MgCl_2$, 1 μl of 10 mg/ml BSA, 0.5 μl of dNTP mix (25 mM each), 5 μl of 1 μM biotinylated target primer, 0.5 μl of 5 U/μl AmpliTaq Gold DNA polymerase, 10 μl of adaptor-ligated library, and 23 μl of PCR-grade water (see Note 6).
2. Place PCR tube in the thermocycler and perform a single primer extension reaction consisting of 95°C for 12 min, 60°C (or PEC primer annealing temperature) for 1 min, and 72°C for 5 min, then holding at 72°C until the next step.
3. The PCR tube must be kept in the thermocycler at 72°C after primer extension to avoid nonspecific primer annealing and capture. While still in the thermocycler, directly pipette 150 μl PBI or PB buffer (Qiagen) into the reaction tube, mix by pipetting briefly up and down, close the lids and then remove the tubes from the thermocycler.
4. Transfer the mixture to a Qiagen MinElute PCR purification spin column for purification according to manufacturer's instructions. Elute DNA from the column with 30 μl of EB Buffer supplied with the MinElute kit.

### 3.4. Bead Capture and Isolation

*Bead washing*. Streptavidin-coated magnetic beads are used to bind to and isolate the biotinylated PEC primers and any target templates they are annealed to. A critical part of the PEC procedure is handling during the bead washing steps. For all bead washing steps in the PEC procedure, a single wash step consists of the following: (a) add the relevant buffer to the tube while it is still in the magnetic particle collector (MPC); (b) remove the tube from the MPC and resuspend the beads by vortexing at medium speed for 2 s, then repeat the vortexing with the tube upside-down (see Note 7); (c) spin down the tube contents for ~1 s on a table-top centrifuge; (d) return tube to the MPC and remove the supernatant once the beads have collected at the side of the tube.

1. Resuspend a stock solution of M-270 streptavidin beads by vortexing for several seconds in the bottle, and transfer 25 μl of bead suspension to a 1.5-ml tube. Use a MPC to collect beads at the tube wall and remove the supernatant. Wash the beads twice with 500 μl of 2× BW buffer (see Note 8). After the two 500 μl washes, resuspend the beads in 25 μl 2× BW buffer. Note that when performing capture of multiple samples, this prewash step can be performed in a single tube for up to 300 μl stock beads (12 samples); increase the final 2× BW resuspension volume accordingly.
2. Add 25 μl of the purified primer extension DNA products to 25 μl of the washed bead suspension, and save the remaining

5 µl DNA for later quantification. Mix by stirring with a pipette tip while pipetting up and down a few times, then place on a tube rotator and rotate at roughly 10–20 rpm for 15 min at room temperature.

3. Transfer the suspension to a fresh 1.5-ml tube to avoid carry-over of nontarget library fragments that may have adhered to the tube wall. Pellet the supernatant using the MPC and discard the supernatant.
4. Wash the pellet at least five times with 500 µl of 1× BW buffer to remove as many nontarget DNA fragments as possible. Following the final wash supernatant removal, spin down the tube on a table-top centrifuge for 4 s, then return it to the MPC and remove the last traces of supernatant.
5. Add 500 µl 1× HW buffer. Shake the tube for 2 min at 65°C (or 5°C above the PEC primer annealing temperature), 1,000 rpm, on a thermal block shaker. Return to MPC and remove all traces of supernatant.
6. Resuspend the beads in 30 µl EB buffer by flicking a few times then spinning down briefly on a bench-top centrifuge, and transfer the mixture to a fresh 1.5-ml tube. Incubate on a thermocycler at 95°C for 3 min. Remove the tube, flick to mix, spin it down briefly, and return it to the MPC. Transfer the supernatant to a fresh tube, taking care not to transfer any beads. The supernatant contains the captured DNA fragments.

### 3.5. Product Amplification and Sequencing

1. After capture, products are likely to be present in very low copy number. Product amplification is therefore necessary. Prepare a 100-µl PCR mix, containing 10 µl 10× GeneAmp PCR Buffer II, 10 µl of 25 mM $MgCl_2$, 2 µl of 10 mg/ml BSA, 1 µl dNTP mix (25 mM each), 3 µl of each 10 µM adaptor primer, 1 µl of 5 U/µl AmpliTaq Gold DNA polymerase, 25 µl of captured, washed, and eluted DNA, and 45 µl molecular biology-grade water.
2. Place the PCR tube in a thermocycler, followed by a denaturation step of 95°C for 12 min, followed by 14 cycles of 95°C for 30 s, 60°C (or the suitable annealing temperature for the primers if different) for 1 min, 72°C for 1 min. Finish the process with 5 min at 70°C and hold at 10°C until ready for purification.
3. After PCR amplification of the captured product is complete, follow it with purification using a Qiagen MinElute spin column according to manufacturer's instructions. Elute DNA from the column with 50 µl of TE Buffer. The product can now be entered directly into the relevant sequencing process. Alternatively, the product can be used for a second round of capture starting again with the primer extension step, Subheading 3.3 (see Note 9).

## 4. Notes

1. It is possible to perform PEC on pooled samples of multiple individuals, if the adaptors of those samples are modified to contain sample-specific barcodes that can be read during sequencing. An effective barcoding protocol for Illumina sequencing is described by Meyer and Kircher (12).
2. It should be noted that while PEC is excellent for rapid capture of short target regions, and has been used to retrieve complete mitochondrial genomes from Neanderthals and an ancient modern human (1, 4), it is not ideally suited for targeting even larger continuous regions from fragmented DNA sources, due to limits on primer multiplexity and cost. For most applications requiring capture of several kilobases and above, I recommend another hybridization capture method (5, 6). On the other hand, PEC can be used effectively to capture long (several kb) DNA molecules based only on short known parts of the sequences, as has been previously described in a similar method (13).
3. Some sequencing library preparation protocols (e.g., the Illumina standard genomic library) already involve a bulk library amplification step. Although I recommend the PCR conditions described here for amplification of the primary DNA library, the conditions used in other protocols will also produce amplified template that is suitable for use as template for PEC, starting at the primer extension step, Subheading 3.3. Take care that the template amount does not exceed 100 ng, as discussed in Note 6.
4. It is crucial for all the Qiagen spin column purifications to use the Qiagen binding buffer PB or PBI. I find that using an alternative binding buffer such as Qiagen PM increases later nonspecific binding of background DNA to the beads by over tenfold, reducing the target enrichment factor by a corresponding factor.
5. PEC primers can be used in multiplex, with up to 150 PEC primers in the same reaction. For use of primers in multiplex, make up a mix containing 1 μM each primer, and add 5 μl of this mix to the 50 μl primer extension reaction. The concentration of each primer therefore is the same (0.1 μM final concentration) whether one primer or many are used.
6. Too much template DNA in the primer extension step reduces capture efficiency by interfering with primer extension. If the 14-cycle amplified template library contains more than 10 ng/μl amplified DNA, as measured by qPCR (10) or picogreen fluorescence measurement (14), the template should be

diluted so that not more than 100 ng of template are added to the primer extension reaction.

7. Many protocols recommend that streptavidin beads should not be vortexed while carrying biotinylated capture products. However, I find that shaking or flicking tubes to mix beads and wash buffer produces foam, which interferes with supernatant removal. Vortexing for a few seconds at medium speed produces far less foam, and does not seem to affect the binding of biotinylated products to the beads.

8. The Tween-20 is a crucial component of the binding and wash buffer. Omitting Tween results in a huge (over a 1,000-fold) increase of nonspecific DNA carryover by the beads. In addition, the Tween makes the beads far easier to handle by causing them to more reliably remain on the side of the tube while in the MPC as supernatant is removed.

9. Performing PEC with a single target primer will typically increase the proportion of target sequences in the products versus the starting library by 1,000- to 10,000-fold. This enrichment fold is slightly reduced as more primers are used in multiplex, with a target enrichment of 100- to 1,000-fold expected when 100 primers are used in one reaction. For higher enrichment, a second round of PEC can be carried out on the amplified products of the first enrichment step, using the same PEC primers. For a second-step primer extension reaction, I recommend reducing the magnesium chloride concentration by half, and increasing the primer annealing temperature by 5°C. This increases the specificity of capture to further improve the proportion of target sequences in the final products.

## Acknowledgments

I thank Matthias Meyer for laboratory advice, Svante Pääbo for support and supervision, and the whole Neanderthal genome group for discussions. This work was supported by the Max Planck Society.

### References

1. Briggs AW, Good JM, Green RE et al (2009) Targeted retrieval and analysis of five Neandertal mtDNA genomes. Science **325**:318–321
2. Bentley DR (2006) Whole-genome re-sequencing. Curr Opin Genet Dev **16**:545–552
3. Margulies M, Egholm M, Altman WE et al (2005) Genome sequencing in microfabricated high-density picolitre reactors. Nature **437**:376–380
4. Krause J, Briggs AW, Kircher M et al (2010) A complete mtDNA genome of an early modern human from Kostenki, Russia. Curr Biol **20**:231–236
5. Gnirke A, Melnikov A, Maguire J et al (2009) Solution hybrid selection with ultra-long oligonucleotides for massively parallel targeted sequencing. Nat Biotechnol **27**:182–189

6. Hodges E, Xuan Z, Balija V et al (2007) Genome-wide in situ exon capture for selective resequencing. Nat Genet **39**:1522–1527
7. Rohland N, Hofreiter M (2007) Ancient DNA extraction from bones and teeth. Nat Protoc **2**:1756–1762
8. Maricic T, Pääbo S (2009) Optimization of 454 sequencing library preparation from small amounts of DNA permits sequence determination of both DNA strands. Biotechniques **46**:51–57
9. Briggs AW, Stenzel U, Meyer M et al (2010) Removal of deaminated cytosines and detection of in vivo methylation in ancient DNA. Nucleic Acids Res **38**:e87
10. Meyer M, Briggs AW, Maricic T et al (2008) From micrograms to picograms: quantitative PCR reduces the material demands of high-throughput sequencing. Nucleic Acids Res **36**:e5
11. Rozen S, Skaletsky H (2000) Primer3 on the WWW for general users and for biologist programmers. Methods Mol Biol **132**:365–386
12. Meyer M, Kircher M (2010) Illumina sequencing library preparation for highly multiplexed target capture and sequencing Cold Spring Harb Protoc doi:10.1101/pdb.prot5448
13. Dapprich J, Ferriola D, Magira EE et al (2008) SNP-specific extraction of haplotype-resolved targeted genomic regions. Nucleic Acids Res **36**:e94
14. Meyer M, Stenzel U, Hofreiter M (2008) Parallel tagged sequencing on the 454 platform. Nat Protoc **3**:267–278

# Part III

## Measuring Genetic Diversity

# Chapter 9

## SNP Discovery and Genotyping for Evolutionary Genetics Using RAD Sequencing

**Paul D. Etter, Susan Bassham, Paul A. Hohenlohe, Eric A. Johnson, and William A. Cresko**

### Abstract

Next-generation sequencing technologies are revolutionizing the field of evolutionary biology, opening the possibility for genetic analysis at scales not previously possible. Research in population genetics, quantitative trait mapping, comparative genomics, and phylogeography that was unthinkable even a few years ago is now possible. More importantly, these next-generation sequencing studies can be performed in organisms for which few genomic resources presently exist. To speed this revolution in evolutionary genetics, we have developed *R*estriction site *A*ssociated *D*NA (RAD) genotyping, a method that uses Illumina next-generation sequencing to simultaneously discover and score tens to hundreds of thousands of single-nucleotide polymorphism (SNP) markers in hundreds of individuals for minimal investment of resources. In this chapter, we describe the core RAD-seq protocol, which can be modified to suit a diversity of evolutionary genetic questions. In addition, we discuss bioinformatic considerations that arise from unique aspects of next-generation sequencing data as compared to traditional marker-based approaches, and we outline some general analytical approaches for RAD-seq and similar data. Despite considerable progress, the development of analytical tools remains in its infancy, and further work is needed to fully quantify sampling variance and biases in these data types.

**Key words:** Genetic mapping, Population genetics, Genomics, Evolution, Genotyping, Single-Nucleotide Polymorphisms, Next-generation sequencing, RAD-seq

## 1. Introduction

Next-generation sequencing (NGS) technologies open the possibility of gathering genomic information across multiple individuals at a genome-wide scale, both in mapping crosses and natural populations (1, 2). This breakthrough technology is revolutionizing the biomedical sciences (3–5) and is becoming increasingly important for evolutionary genetics (6). The rapidly decreasing

Virginie Orgogozo and Matthew V. Rockman (eds.), *Molecular Methods for Evolutionary Genetics*,
Methods in Molecular Biology, vol. 772, DOI 10.1007/978-1-61779-228-1_9, © Springer Science+Business Media, LLC 2011

cost of NGS makes it feasible for most laboratories to address genome-wide evolutionary questions using hundreds of individuals, even in organisms for which few genomic resources presently exist (7, 8). This innovation has already led to studies in QTL mapping (9), population genomics (10), and phylogeography (11, 12) that were not possible even a few years ago.

Current NGS technology theoretically allows perfect genetic information – the entire genome sequence of an individual – to be collected (2). With rapidly decreasing sequencing costs, it may soon be feasible to completely sequence genomes from the large sample of individuals necessary for many population genomic or genome-wide association studies in organisms other than humans (6). However, genome resequencing is still prohibitively expensive for most evolutionary studies. Fortunately, for many purposes, gathering complete genomic sequence data is an unnecessary waste of resources. For example, because linkage blocks are often quite large in a quantitative trait locus (QTL) mapping cross, progeny can be adequately typed with genetic markers of sufficient density (9). Similarly, many other evolutionary genetic studies require large numbers of genetics markers, but not necessarily complete coverage of the genome (6, 10, 11).

An alternative approach to whole genome resequencing is to use NGS to gather data on dense panels of genomic markers spread evenly throughout the genome. The large number of short reads, provided by platforms such as Illumina, are ideal for this application (7). A methodological difficulty is focusing these large numbers of repeated reads on the same genomic regions to maximize the probability that most individuals in a study will be assayed at orthologous regions. We developed a procedure called *R*estriction site *A*ssociated *D*NA sequencing (RAD-seq) that accomplishes this goal of genome subsampling (9). By focusing the sequencing on the same subset of genomic regions across multiple individuals, RAD-seq technology allows single-nucleotide polymorphisms (SNPs) to be identified and typed for tens or hundreds of thousands of markers spread evenly throughout the genome, even in organisms for which few genomic resources presently exist. Therefore, RAD-seq provides a flexible, inexpensive platform for the simultaneous discovery of tens of thousands of genetic markers in model and nonmodel organisms alike.

In this chapter, we describe the basic protocols for generating RAD markers specifically for sequencing using the Illumina platform. Although we provide details for Illumina sequencing, these protocols can be modified for other sequencing platforms. We also provide a general framework for the analysis of RAD-seq data and discuss several primary bioinformatic considerations that arise from unique aspects of next-generation sequencing data as compared to traditional marker-based approaches. These include inferring marker loci and genotypes *de novo* from RAD tag sequences for an organism with no sequenced genome, distinguishing SNPs from error, inferring heterozygosity in the face of sampling variance, and tracking these sources of uncertainty through further analyses. New bioinformatic advances will certainly be made in this area. We, therefore, present these analytical approaches less as a set of concrete protocols, and more as a conceptual framework with a focus on potential sources of error and bias in next-generation genotyping data produced via protocols such as RAD-seq.

## 2. Materials

### *2.1. DNA Extraction, RNase A Treatment, and Restriction Endonuclease Digestion*

1. DNeasy Blood & Tissue Kit (Qiagen) (see Note 1).
2. RNaseA (Qiagen).
3. High-quality genomic DNA from 2.1: 25 ng/μl (see Note 2).
4. Restriction enzyme (NEB; see Note 3).

### *2.2. P1 Adapter Ligation, Purification and DNA Shearing*

1. NEB Buffer 2.
2. rATP (Promega): 100 mM.
3. P1 Adapter: 100 nM stocks in 1× Annealing Buffer (AB). Prepare 100 μM stocks for each single-stranded oligonucleotide in 1× Elution Buffer (EB: 10 mM Tris–Cl, pH 8.5). Combine complementary adapter oligos at 10 μM each in 1× AB (10× AB: 500 mM NaCl, 100 mM Tris–Cl, pH 7.5–8.0). Place in a beaker of water just off boil and cool slowly to room temperature to anneal. Alternatively, use a boil and gradual cool program in a PCR machine. Dilute to 100 nM concentration in 1× AB (see Notes 4 and 5).
4. Concentrated T4 DNA Ligase (NEB): 2,000,000 U/ml.
5. QIAquick or MinElute PCR Purification Kit (Qiagen).
6. Bioruptor, nebulizer, or Branson sonicator 450.

### *2.3. Size Selection/ Agarose Gel Extraction*

1. Agarose.
2. 5× TBE: 0.45 M Tris–Borate, 0.01 M EDTA, pH 8.3.
3. 6× Orange Loading Dye Solution (Fermentas).
4. GeneRuler 100 bp DNA Ladder Plus (Fermentas).
5. Razor blades.
6. MinElute Gel Purification Kit (Qiagen).

### *2.4. End Repair and 3′-dA Overhang Addition*

1. Quick Blunting Kit (NEB).
2. NEB Buffer 2.
3. dATP (Fermentas): 10 mM.
4. Klenow Fragment (3′–5′ exo$^-$, NEB): 5,000 U/ml.

***2.5. P2 Adapter Ligation and RAD Tag Amplification/ Enrichment***

1. NEB Buffer 2.
2. rATP: 100 mM.
3. P2 Adapter: 10 μM stock in 1× AB prepared as P1 adapter described above (see Notes 4 and 5).
4. Concentrated T4 DNA Ligase.
5. Phusion High-Fidelity PCR Master Mix with HF Buffer (NEB).
6. RAD amplification primer mix: 10 μM. Prepare 100 μM stocks for each oligonucleotide in 1× EB. Mix together at 10 μM (see Note 6).

## 3. Methods

The protocol described below, outlined in Fig. 1, prepares RAD tag libraries for high-throughput Illumina sequencing (see Note 7). In short, genomic DNA is digested with a restriction enzyme and an adapter (P1) is ligated to the fragments' compatible ends (Fig. 1a). This adapter contains forward amplification and Illumina sequencing priming sites, as well as a nucleotide barcode 4 or 5 bp long for sample identification. To reduce erroneous sample assignment due to sequencing error, all barcode differ by at least three nucleotides (see Note 8). The adapter-ligated fragments are subsequently pooled, randomly sheared, and a specific size fraction is selected following electrophoresis (Fig. 1b). DNA is then ligated to a second adapter (P2), a Y adapter (13) that has divergent ends whose two strands are complementary for only part of their length (Fig. 1c). The reverse amplification primer is unable to bind to P2 unless the complementary sequence is filled in during the first round of forward elongation originating from the P1 amplification primer. The structure of this adapter ensures that only P1 adapter-ligated RAD tags will be amplified during the final PCR amplification step (Fig. 1d). The protocol for mapping of the lateral plate locus in threespine stickleback using *EcoRI* RAD markers reported in Baird et al. (9) is described here in detail as an example of the multiplexing

Fig. 1. RAD tag library generation. (**a**) Genomic DNA is digested with a restriction enzyme and a barcoded P1 adapter is ligated to the fragments. The P1 adapter contains a forward amplification primer site, an Illumina sequencing primer site, and a barcode (*shaded boxes* represent P1 adapters with different barcodes). (**b**) Adapter-ligated fragments are combined (if multiplexing), sheared, and (**c**) ligated to a second adapter (P2, *white boxes*). The P2 adapter is a divergent "Y" adapter, containing the reverse complement of the P2 reverse amplification primer site, preventing amplification of genomic fragments lacking a P1 adapter. (**d**) RAD tags, which have a P1 adapter, are selectively and robustly enriched by PCR amplification (reproduced from ref. 9).

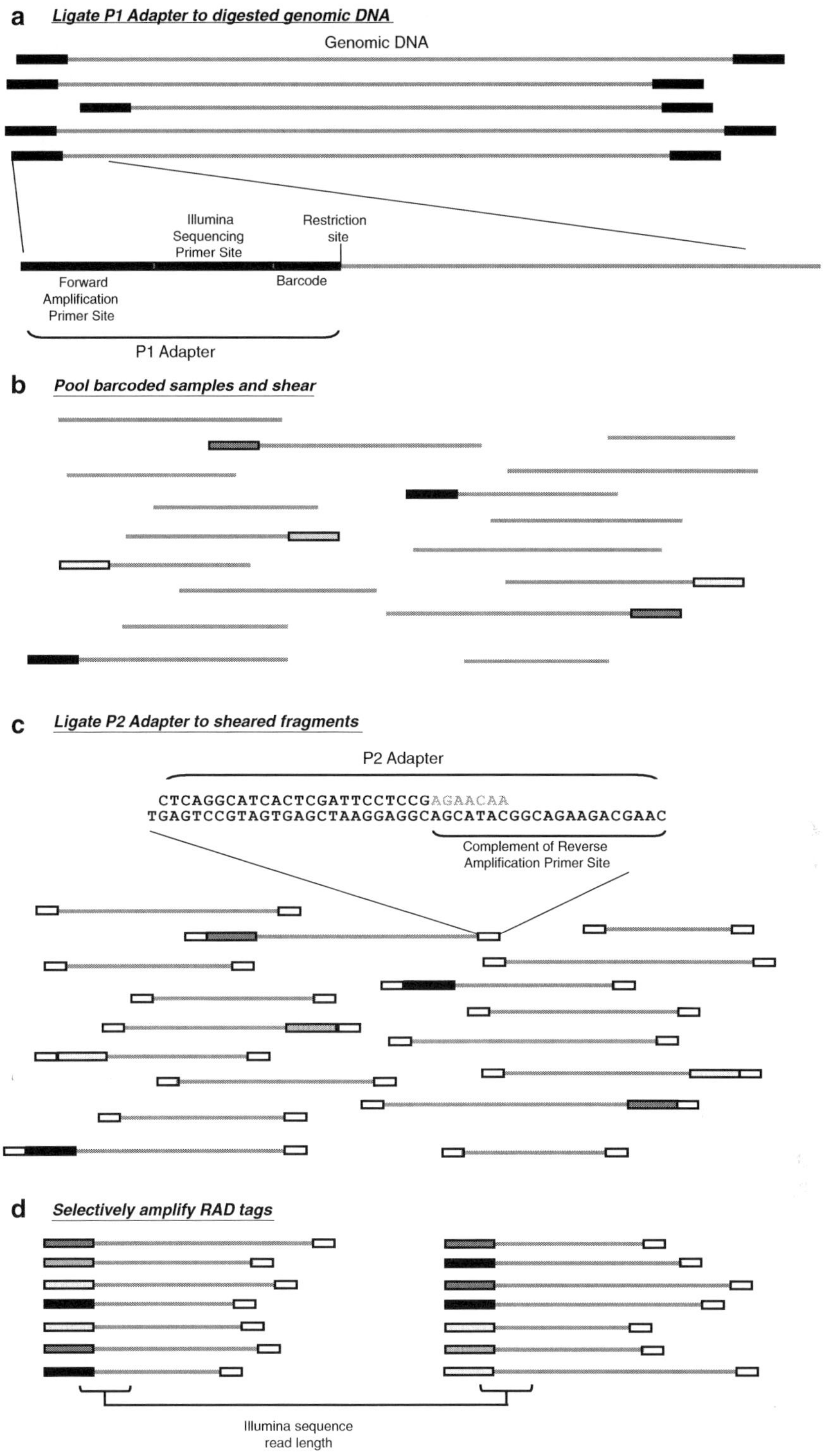
a
Ligate P1 Adapter to digested genomic DNA
Genomic DNA
Illumina Sequencing Primer Site
Restriction site
Forward Amplification Primer Site
Barcode
P1 Adapter
b
Pool barcoded samples and shear
c
Ligate P2 Adapter to sheared fragments
P2 Adapter
CTCAGGCATCACTCGATTCCTCCGAGAACAA
TGAGTCCGTAGTGAGCTAAGGAGGCAGCATACGGCAGAAGACGAAC
Complement of Reverse Amplification Primer Site
d
Selectively amplify RAD tags
Illumina sequence read length

approach. For bulk-segregant analysis, on the contrary, samples of like phenotypes can be pooled prior to digestion and treated as a single sample labeled with a single barcode.

### 3.1. DNA Extraction, RNase A Treatment, and Restriction Endonuclease Digestion

1. We recommend extracting genomic DNA samples using the DNeasy Blood & Tissue Kit (Qiagen) or a similar product that produces very pure, high molecular weight, RNA-free DNA. Follow the manufacturer's instructions for extraction from your tissue type. Be sure to treat samples with RNase A following the manufacturer's instructions to remove residual RNA. The optimal concentration after elution into buffer EB is 25 ng/μl or greater (see Notes 1 and 2).
2. Digest 1 μg of genomic DNA for each sample with the appropriate restriction enzyme in a 50 μl reaction volume, following the manufacturer's instructions. For example, for *EcoRI* digestion, combine in a microcentrifuge tube the following: 5.0 μl 10× NEB Buffer 2, 0.5 μl *Eco*RI, DNA, and $H_2O$ to 50.0 μl (see Notes 9 and 10).
3. Heat-inactivate the restriction enzyme following manufacturer's instructions. If the enzyme cannot be heat-inactivated, purify with a QIAquick column following the manufacturer's instructions prior to ligation. QIAquick purification should work equally well, although conceivably the representation of fragments from distantly separated sites could be reduced when using an infrequent cutter. Allow reaction to cool to ambient temperature before proceeding to ligation reaction or cleanup (see Note 4).

### 3.2. P1 Adapter Ligation

1. Ligate barcoded, restriction site overhang-specific P1 adapters onto complementary compatible ends on the genomic DNA created in the previous step (see Note 11). If you are barcoding only a few individuals or samples, choose barcodes whose sequences differ as much as possible from one another to avoid causing the Genome Analyzer software to lose cluster registry, as it is prone to do when it encounters a nonrandom assortment of nucleotides (see Note 12).
2. To each inactivated digest, add the following: 1.0 μl 10× NEB Buffer 2, 5.0 μl Barcoded P1 Adapter (100 nM), 0.6 μl rATP (100 mM), 0.5 μl concentrated T4 DNA Ligase (2,000,000 U/ml), 2.9 μl $H_2O$; 60.0 μl total volume (see Note 13). Be sure to add P1 adapters to the reaction before the ligase to avoid religation of the genomic DNA. Incubate the reaction at room temperature for 30 min to overnight. Reduce the amount of P1 used in the ligation reaction if starting with less than 1 μg genomic DNA or if cutting with an enzyme that cuts less frequently than *Eco*RI (e.g., we used 2.5 μl of adapter when using *Sbf*I in stickleback, which has close to 23,000 *Sbf*I restriction

sites in its 460 Mb reference genome). It is critical to optimize the amount of P1 adapter added when a given restriction enzyme is used for the first time in an organism (see Note 14).

3. Heat-inactivate T4 DNA Ligase for 10 min at 65°C. Allow reaction to cool slowly to ambient temperature before shearing.

### 3.3. Sample Multiplexing (see Note 15) and DNA Shearing

1. Combine barcoded samples at an equal or otherwise desired ratio. Use a 100–300 μl aliquot containing 1–2 μg DNA total to complete the protocol and freeze the rest at −20°C in case you need to optimize shearing in the next step. In Baird et al. (9), DNA from $F_2$ stickleback progeny that shared a phenotype was pooled and each pool was uniquely barcoded for *Sbf*I bulk-segregant analysis. These samples were then combined at equal volumes with barcoded samples from each parent to create one library. In a second experiment, *Eco*RI-based libraries were made by pooling DNA samples from $F_2$ fish after they were barcoded individually by P1 ligation (see Note 12).
2. Shear DNA samples to an average size of 500 bp to create a pool of P1-ligated molecules with random, variable ends. This step requires some optimization for different DNA concentrations and for each type of restriction endonuclease. The following protocol has been optimized to shear stickleback DNA digested with either *Eco*RI or *Sbf*I using the Bioruptor and is a good starting point for any study (see Note 16). The goal is to create sheared product that is predominantly smaller than 1 kb in size (see Fig. 1).
3. Dilute ligation reaction to 100 μl in water (or take 100–300 μl aliquot from multiplexed samples) and shear in the Bioruptor 10 times for 30 s on high following manufacturer's instructions. Make sure that the tank water in the Bioruptor is cold (4°C) before starting. All other positions in the Bioruptor holder not filled by your sample/s should be filled with balance tubes containing an equal volume of water.
4. Clean up the sheared DNA using a MinElute column following manufacturer's instructions. This purification is performed to remove the ligase and restriction enzyme, and to concentrate the DNA so that the entire sample can be loaded in a single lane on an agarose gel. Elute in 20 μl EB.

### 3.4. Size Selection/ Agarose Gel Extraction and End Repair

1. This step in the protocol removes free unligated or concatemerized P1 adapters and restricts the size range of tags to those that can be sequenced efficiently on an Illumina Genome Analyzer flow cell. Run the entire sheared sample in 1× Orange Loading Dye on a 1.25% agarose, 0.5× TBE gel for 45 min at 100 V, next to 2.0 μl GeneRuler 100 bp DNA Ladder Plus for size reference; run the ladder in lanes flanking the samples until the 300 and 500 bp ladder bands are sufficiently resolved from 200 to 600 bp bands (see Fig. 2; Note 17).

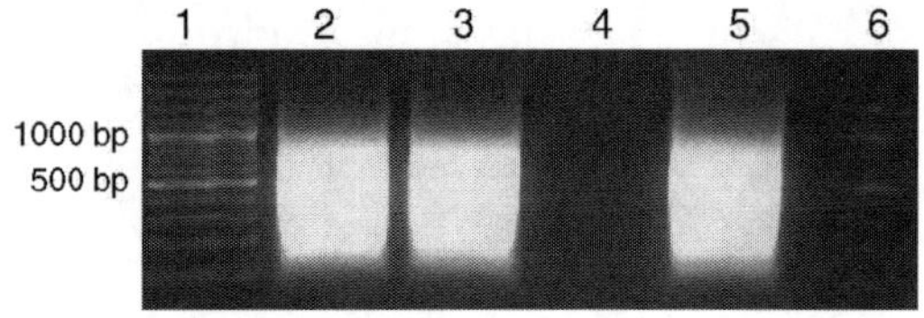


Fig. 2. Three barcoded and multiplexed RAD tag libraries. Lanes 2, 3, and 5 each contain two DNA samples that were restriction digested, ligated to barcoded P1 adapters, combined, sheared, purified, and then loaded on an agarose gel. 2 – parental DNA samples cut with *Sbf*I. 3 – $F_2$ pools cut with *Sbf*I. 4 – blank. 5 – parental DNA samples cut with *EcoR*I. Libraries contain 2 μg total combined genomic DNA each. 1 and 6 – 2.0 μl GeneRuler 100-bp DNA Ladder Plus.

2. Being careful to exclude any free P1 adapters and P1 dimers running at ~130 bp and below, use a fresh razor blade to cut a slice of the gel spanning 300–500 bp (see Note 18). Extract DNA using MinElute Gel Purification Kit following manufacturer's instructions with the following modification: to improve representation of AT-rich sequences, melt agarose gel slices in the supplied buffer at room temperature (18–22°C) with agitation until dissolved (usually less than 30 min) (14). Elute in 20 μl EB into a microcentrifuge tube containing 2.5 μl 10× Blunting Buffer from the Quick Blunting Kit used in the following step (see Note 19).
3. The Quick Blunting Kit protocol converts 5′ or 3′ overhangs, created by shearing, into phosphorylated blunt ends using T4 DNA Polymerase and T4 Polynucleotide Kinase.
4. To the eluate from the previous step, add 2.5 μl dNTP mix (1 mM) and 1.0 μl Blunt Enzyme Mix. Incubate at RT for 30 min.
5. Purify with a QIAquick column. Elute in 43 μl EB into a microcentrifuge tube containing 5.0 μl 10× NEB Buffer 2.

### *3.5. 3′-dA Overhang Addition and P2 Adapter Ligation*

1. This step in the protocol adds an "A" base to the 3′ ends of the blunt phosphorylated DNA fragments, using the polymerase activity of Klenow Fragment (3′–5′ exo$^-$). This prepares the DNA fragments for ligation to the P2 adapter, which possesses a single "T" base overhang at the 3′ end of its bottom strand.
2. To the eluate from the previous step, add: 1.0 μl dATP (10 mM), 3.0 μl Klenow (exo$^-$). Incubate at 37°C for 30 min. Allow the reaction to cool to ambient temperature.
3. Purify with a QIAquick column. Elute in 45 μl EB into a microcentrifuge tube containing 5.0 μl 10× NEB Buffer 2.
4. This step in the protocol ligates the P2 adapter, a "Y" adapter with divergent ends that contains a 3′ dT overhang, onto the ends of DNA fragments with 3′ dA overhangs to create RAD-seq library template ready for amplification.

5. To the eluate from previous step, add: 1.0 μl P2 Adapter (10 μM), 0.5 μl rATP (100 mM), 0.5 μl concentrated T4 DNA Ligase. Incubate the reaction at room temperature for 30 min to overnight.
6. Purify with a QIAquick column. Elute in 50 μl EB and quantify (see Note 18).

### *3.6. RAD Tag Amplification/Enrichment*

1. In this step high-fidelity PCR amplification is performed on P1 and P2 adapter-ligated DNA fragments, enriching for RAD tags that contain both adaptors, and preparing them to be hybridized to an Illumina Genome Analyzer flow cell (see Fig. 1).
2. Perform a test amplification to determine library quality. In a thin-walled PCR tube, combine: 10.5 μl $H_2O$, 12.5 μl Phusion High-Fidelity Master Mix, 1.0 μl RAD amplification primer mix (10 μM), 1.0 μl RAD library template (or a quantified amount; see Note 20). Perform 18 cycles of amplification in a thermal cycler: 30 s 98°C, 18× (10 s 98°C, 30 s 65°C, 30 s 72°C), 5 min 72°C, hold 4°C. Run 5.0 μl PCR product in 1× Orange Loading Dye out on 1.0% agarose gel next to 1.0 μl RAD library template and 2.0 μl GeneRuler 100 bp DNA Ladder Plus (Fig. 3).
3. If the amplified product is at least twice as bright as the template, perform a larger volume amplification (typically 50–100 μl) but with fewer cycles (12–14, to minimize bias), to create enough to retrieve a large amount of the RAD tag library from a final gel extraction (see Note 21). If amplification looks poor, use more library template in a second test PCR reaction. Figure 3 shows three libraries used in Baird et al. (9) that amplified well, which is apparent when comparing the amplified product to the amount of template loaded in the lane to the right of each sample. Template should appear dim, yet visible on the gel. Purify the large volume reaction with a MinElute column. Elute in 20 μl EB.

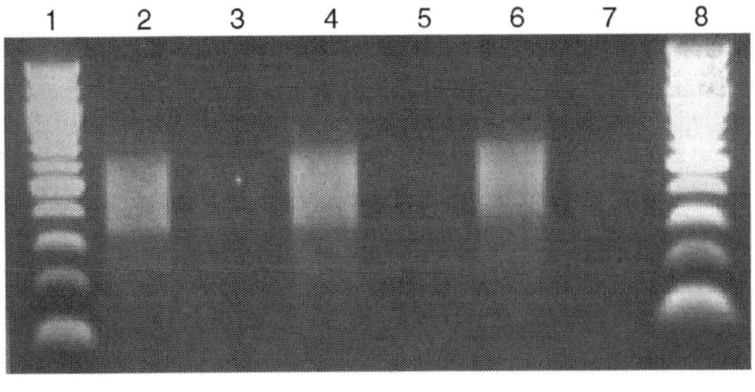


Fig. 3. Test amplification PCR product from the three libraries shown in Fig. 2. Lanes 2, 4, and 6 contain 5.0 μl amplified PCR product. 2 – parental *SbfI* library. 4 – $F_2$ *SbfI* library. 6 – parental *EcoRI* library. Lanes 3, 5, and 7 contain 1.0 μl template used for amplification in the lane to the left. Template was loaded at 5× the amount used in the equivalent volume loaded for amplified reactions. 1 and 8 – 2.0 μl GeneRuler 100-bp DNA Ladder Plus. Libraries are 300–600 bp in size.

4. The following purification step is performed to eliminate any artifactual bands that may appear due to an improper ratio of P1 adapter to restriction-site compatible ends (see Note 14). Load the entire sample in 1× Orange Loading Dye on a 1.25% agarose, 0.5× TBE gel and run for 45 min at 100 V, next to 2.0 μl GeneRuler 100 bp DNA Ladder Plus for size reference (Fig. 4). Being careful to exclude any free adapters or P1 dimers running at ~130 bp and below, use a fresh razor blade to cut a slice of the gel spanning ~350–550 bp. Extract DNA using MinElute Gel Purification Kit following manufacturer's instructions, but melt agarose gel slices in the supplied buffer at room temperature. Elute in 20 μl EB (see Note 22).
5. Quantify the DNA using a fluorometer to accurately measure the concentration. Concentrations will range from 1 to 20 ng/μl. Determine the molar concentration of the library by examining the gel image and estimating the median size of the library smear, which should be around 450 bp. Multiply this size by 650 (the average molecular mass of a base-pair) to get the molecular weight of the library. Use this number to calculate the molar concentration of the library (see Note 23).
6. Sequence libraries on Illumina Genome Analyzer following manufacturer's instructions (see Note 24).

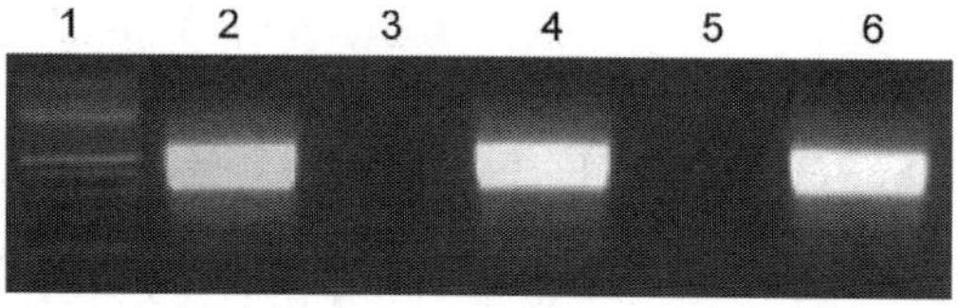


Fig. 4. PCR product from the three libraries shown in Figs. 2 and 3 after the final large volume amplification and purification. Lanes 2, 4, and 6 each contain 20 μl purified PCR product from 100 μl amplifications. 2 – parental *SbfI* library. 4 – $F_2$ *SbfI* library. 6 – parental *EcoRI* library. 1 – 2.0 μl GeneRuler 100-bp DNA Ladder Plus. Lanes 3, 5, and 7 are blank. Libraries are 300–600 bp in size.

Fig. 5. Schematic diagram of population genomic data analysis using RAD sequencing. (**a**) Following Illumina sequencing of barcoded fragments, sequence reads (*thin lines*) are aligned to a reference genome sequence (*thick line*). Depth of coverage varies across tags. Reads that do not align to the genome, or align in multiple locations, are discarded. (**b**) Sample of reads at a single RAD site. The recognition site for the enzyme *SbfI* is indicated along the reference genome sequence (*top*), and sequence reads typically proceed in both directions from this point, at which they overlap. At each nucleotide site, reads showing each of the four possible nucleotides can be tallied (*solid box*). (**c**) Nucleotide counts at each site for each individual are used in a maximum likelihood framework to assign the diploid genotype at the site. In this example, G/T heterozygote is the most likely genotype; the method provides the log-likelihood for this genotype, a maximum-likelihood estimate for the sequencing error rate ε, and a likelihood ratio test statistic comparing G/T to the second-most-likely genotype, G/G homozygote. (**d**) Each individual now has a diploid genotype at each nucleotide site sequenced, and single-nucleotide polymorphisms (SNPs) can be identified across populations. Note, however, that haplotype phase is still unknown across RAD tags. (**e**) SNPs (*ovals*) are distributed across the genome (*thick line*), and population genetic measures (e.g., $F_{ST}$) are calculated for each SNP. (**f**) A kernel smoothing average across multiple nucleotide positions is used to produce genome-wide distributions of population genetic measures.

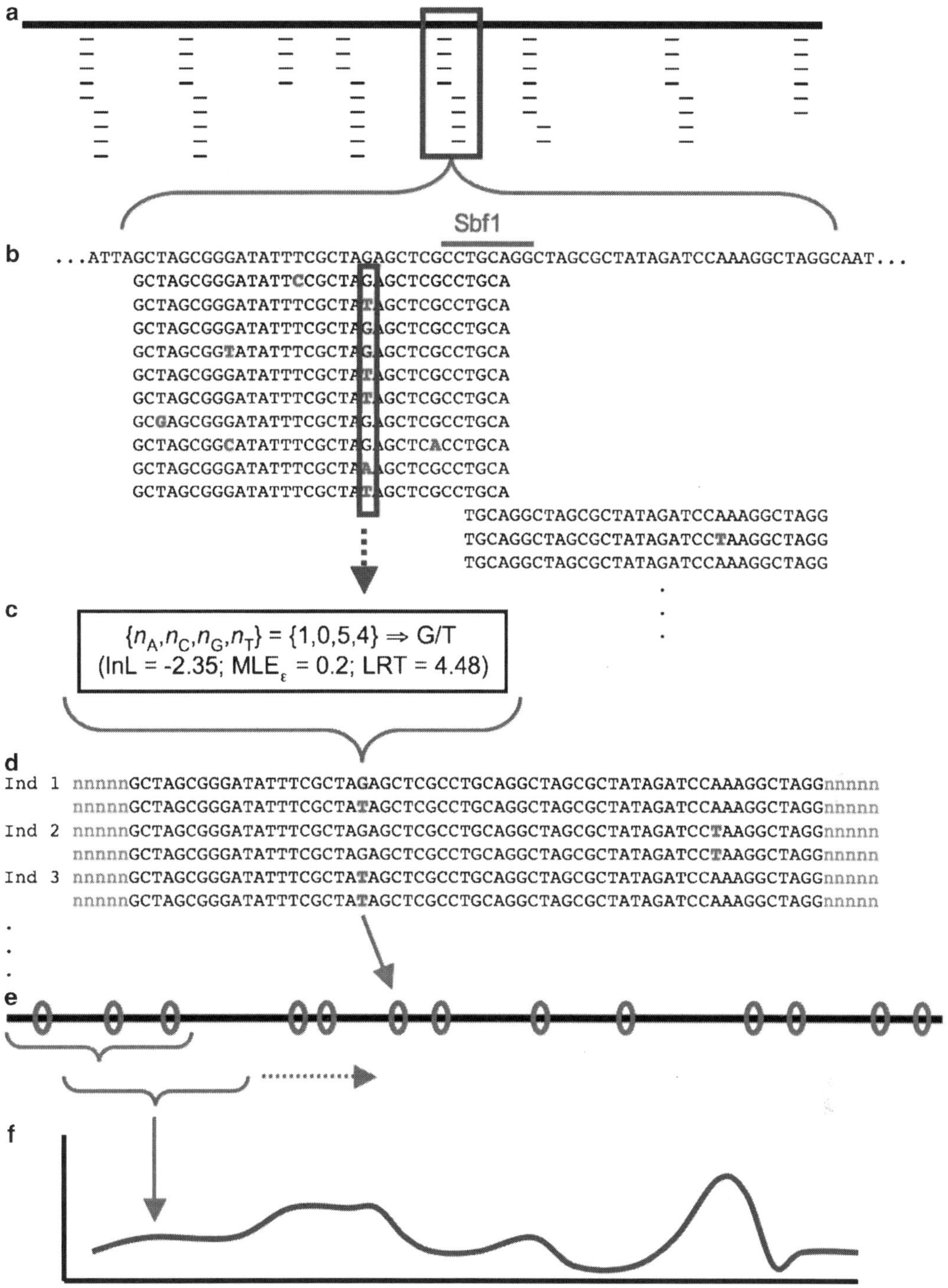


**3.7. Alignment Against a Reference Genome and De Novo Assembly**

A significant consideration for the analysis of RAD sequencing data is whether the organism of interest has a reference genome. If it does, then RAD sequences can be aligned against the genome directly, and SNPs can be called as depicted in Fig. 5 and described below.

However, because the length of reads is still relatively short on most NGS platforms, at least some of the reads will fall in repetitive regions that are similar across several parts of the genome, which will be evidenced by potential assignment with equal probability to these locations. These reads can be removed from the analysis. Alternatively, paired-end sequencing can be performed to help infer the correct location of each read in the genome.

When a reference genome does not exist RAD genotyping can still be performed by assembling reads with respect to one another. For genomic regions that are unique, this assembly works as well as aligning against the genome. The aligned stack of reads can be analyzed to determine SNPs and genotypes that can be used in a genetic map or population genomic analysis. Repetitive regions are problematic as above, but the additional information provided by aligning to multiple genomic regions in the reference genome is absent, making the identification of these repetitive regions even more difficult. Stacks of reads may be abnormally deep because the focal RAD site was by chance sampled significantly more than average, or because paralogous regions with similar sequences were erroneously assembled together. For stacks that fall outside the range of the expected number of reads, the data can simply be expunged from the analysis. More problematic is a situation where two or a small number of paralogous regions are assembled, and the total number of reads is large, but not significantly so, because of sampling variation across all RAD loci.

In situations where paralogous regions are mistakenly assembled, one of several things can be done. First, the length of the reads can be increased, or fragments can be paired-end sequenced, with the hope of obtaining unique information that can be used to tell paralagous regions apart. These solutions increase the cost of the sequencing to an extent that may not be justified by the increase in information. If data are being collected from individuals in a population or mapping cross, tests of Hardy Weinberg Equilibrium (HWE) may allow identification of problematic, incorrectly identified "genotypes" that are really paralogous regions. For example when two monomorphic, paralogous regions are fixed for alternative nucleotides and then mistakenly assembled as a single locus, a SNP will be inferred but no homozygotes will be identified. Lastly, a network-based approach can be employed with the expectation that true SNPs should be at significant frequency and surrounded in sequence space by a constellation of low frequency sequencing errors. In most populations SNPs will be binary, and therefore, the network will consist of two high frequency alleles at the center of the constellation. In situations where paralogous regions are incorrectly assembled, the network will have the easily identifiable topology of three or more high frequency alleles each surrounding by low frequency errors. All of these solutions are imperfect, and extracting information from *de novo* RAD tags and other NGS data will be a significant area of research in the near future.

### 3.8. Inferring Genotypes in the Face of Sequencing Error and Sampling Variance

Another challenge of next-generation sequencing data for bioinformatic analyses is the introduction of sequencing error into many of the reads. Although the sequencing error rate is quite low, in the order of 0.1–1.0% per nucleotide, it still becomes a significant source of inferential confusion when millions of reads are considered simultaneously. Unfortunately, sequencing error compounds the problems of assembling similar paralogous regions, outlined in the previous section, by increasing the probability of misassembly. Error rates can vary across samples, RAD sites, and positions in the reads for each site. In addition, the sampling process of a heterogeneous library inherent in NGS introduces sampling variation in the number of reads observed across RAD sites as well as between alleles at a single site. These issues could be overcome by greatly increasing total sequencing depth, but of course this approach will also increase the cost of a study. A better approach to differentiating true SNPs from sequencing error is a statistical framework that accounts for the uncertainty in genotyping. Undoubtedly significant progress will be made in this area in the near future; here we present one approach as an example of a straightforward, flexible statistical model.

The following maximum-likelihood framework is based upon Hohenlohe et al. (10), designed for genotyping diploid individuals sampled from a population. The expectation is that errors should be differentiated from heterozygous SNPs by the frequency of nucleotides, with errors being represented at low frequency while alleles at heterozygous sites in an individual will be present in near equal frequencies in the total number of reads. Modifications to this approach would be required in other cases, such as haploid organisms, recombinant inbred lines, backcross mapping crosses, or single barcodes representing pools of individuals.

For a given site in an individual, let $n$ be the total number of reads at that site, where $n = n_1 + n_2 + n_3 + n_4$, and $n_i$ is the read count for each possible nucleotide at the site (disregarding ambiguous reads). For a diploid individual, there are ten possible genotypes (four homozygous and six (unordered) heterozygous genotypes). A multinomial sampling distribution gives the probability of observing a set of read counts $(n_1, n_2, n_3, n_4)$ given a particular genotype, which translates into the likelihood for that genotype. For example, the likelihoods of a homozygote (genotype 1,1) or a heterozygote (1,2) are, respectively:

$$L(1,1) = P(n_1, n_2, n_3, n_4 \mid 1,1) = \frac{n!}{n_1!n_2!n_3!n_4!}\left(1 - \frac{3\mathbf{e}}{4}\right)^{n_1}\left(\frac{\mathbf{e}}{4}\right)^{n_2+n_3+n_4} \quad (1a)$$

and

$$L(1,2) = P(n_1, n_2, n_3, n_4 \mid 1,2) = \frac{n!}{n_1!n_2!n_3!n_4!}\left(0.5 - \frac{\mathbf{e}}{4}\right)^{n_1+n_2}\left(\frac{\mathbf{e}}{4}\right)^{n_3+n_4} \quad (1b)$$

where ε is the sequencing error rate. If we let $n_1$ be the count of the most observed nucleotide, and $n_2$ be the count of the second-most observed nucleotide, then the two equations in (1) give the likelihood of the two most likely hypotheses out of the ten possible genotypes. From here, one approach is to assign a diploid genotype to each site based on a likelihood ratio test between these two most likely hypotheses with one degree of freedom. For example, if this test is significant at the $\alpha = 0.05$ level, the most likely genotype at the site is assigned; otherwise the genotype is left unassigned for that individual. In effect this criterion removes data for which there are too few sequence reads to determine a genotype, instead of establishing a constant threshold for sequencing coverage (10). An alternative approach is to carry the uncertainty in genotyping through all subsequent analyses. This can be done by incorporating the likelihoods of each genotype in a Bayesian framework in subsequent calculation of population genetic measures, such as allele frequency, or by using genotype likelihoods in systematic resampling of the data. In either case, information on linkage disequilibrium and genotypes at neighboring loci could also be used to update the posterior probabilities of genotypes at each site.

A central parameter in the model above is the sequencing error rate $\varepsilon$. One option for this parameter is to assume that it is constant across all sites (15), and either estimate it from the data by maximum likelihood or calculate it from sequencing of a control sample in the sequencing run. However, there is empirical evidence that sequencing error varies among sites, and alternatively $\varepsilon$ can be estimated independently from the data at each site. Maximum likelihood estimates of $\varepsilon$ are calculated directly at each site by differentiation of equations (9.1). This technique has been applied successfully to RAD-seq data (10). More sophisticated models could be applied here as well, for instance assuming a probability distribution from which $\varepsilon$ is drawn independently for each site. This probability distribution could be iteratively updated by the data, and it could also be allowed to vary by nucleotide position along each sequence read or even by cluster position on the Illumina flow cell. Further empirical work is needed to assess alternative models of sequencing error.

### 3.9. Future Directions and Alternative Strategies

The analytical method described in the previous section accounts for sequencing error and the random sampling variance inherent in NGS data. However, it does not account for any systematic biases in, for instance, the frequency of sequence reads for alternative alleles at a heterozygous site. For example, biased representation could occur because PCR amplification occurs more readily on one allele or barcode. Barcoding and calling genotypes separately in each individual alleviates some of this bias. In addition, sampling variation among sites and alleles that occurs early in the process can be propagated and amplified in the RAD-seq protocol. Optimizing the protocol to minimize the number of PCR cycles required is an important component of dealing with this issue. However, to date no analytical theory or tools have been developed to handle these sources of variation, and numerical simulations and empirical studies are needed to quantify them. Most simply, individuals of known sequence could be repeatedly genotyped by RAD-seq, using replicate libraries and barcodes, to estimate and partition the resulting variance in observed read frequencies.

Some evolutionary genetic applications will dictate alternative experimental designs, including sequencing of pools of individuals to produce point estimates (with error) of allele frequencies (15). Two examples are pools of individuals from natural populations for phylogeography (11), or groups of individuals of different phenotypic classes in a quantitative trait locus (QTL) mapping cross (9). These approaches lose information about individual genotypes, but because of the volume of data produced by NGS, techniques or analyses that lose some information remain highly effective. For instance, Emerson et al. (11) estimated the fine-scale phylogeographic relationships among populations of the pitcher plant mosquito *Wyeomia smithii* that originated postglacially along the eastern seaboard of USA. Because of the small amount of DNA in each mosquito, six individuals from each population were pooled and genotyped with barcoded adaptors. Rather than directly estimating allele frequencies, which could not be done with high confidence, the analysis focused only on those SNPs for which a statistical model indicated that allele frequency differed significantly between populations. This produced a set of nucleotides that were variable among, and fixed (or nearly so) within, populations. These data were used in subsequent standard phylogenetic analyses. The majority of the potentially informative SNPs were removed from the study, but because such a large number of RAD sites were identified and typed, the remaining 3,741 sites resulted in a beautifully resolved phylogeny, with high branch support and congruity to previous biogeographic hypotheses for this species.

### 3.10. Summary

Ever since the integration of Mendel's laws with evolutionary theory during the Modern Synthesis of the 1930s, biologists have dreamed of a day when perfect genetic knowledge would be available for almost any organism. Nearly a century later, NGS technologies are fulfilling that promise and opening the possibility for genetic analyses that have heretofore been impossible. Perhaps the most critical aspect of these breakthroughs is the unshackling of genetic analyses from traditional model organisms, allowing genomic studies to be performed in organisms for which few genomic resources presently exist. We presented one application of NGS, RAD genotyping, a focused reduced-representation methodology that uses Illumina next-generation sequencing to simultaneously discover and score tens to hundreds of thousands markers in a very cost-efficient manner. The core RAD-seq protocol can be performed in nearly any evolutionary genetic laboratory. Undoubtedly numerous modifications of the core RAD molecular protocols can be made to suit a variety of additional research problems. Despite the ease of use of RAD and other NGS protocols, a significant challenge facing biologists is developing the appropriate analytical and bioinformatic tools for these data. Although we outline some general analytical approaches for RAD-seq, we fully anticipate that the development of bioinformatic tools for RAD and similar data will be a rich area of research for many years.

## 4. Notes

1. Clean, intact, high-quality DNA is required for optimal restriction endonuclease digestion and is important for the overall success of the protocol. We have found that lower quality DNA can be used, but the starting amount will likely need to be increased because a large number of DNA fragments that have a correctly ligated P1 adapter may not end up in the proper size range when the starting DNA is partially degraded. When working with heavily degraded DNA samples is the only option, we have found that parameters of the protocol can be optimized (such as using more input DNA to start with and shearing less) to create usable libraries. These libraries often do not amplify as well as ones made with intact, high molecular weight genomic DNA. The "Best Practices" sections of the most recent Illumina Sample Prep Guides are a good resource for quantification, handling, and temperature considerations.
2. We recommend using a fluorescence-based method for DNA quantification to get the most accurate concentration readings. Since they bind specifically to double-stranded DNA, the dyes used in fluorometric assays are not as affected by RNA, free nucleotides, or other contaminants commonly found in DNA preparations (which can lead to inaccurate concentration predictions when using absorbance). If using another form of DNA quantification, such as UV spectrometer 260/280

absorbance readings, be sure to confirm the concentration by comparing a known calibration sample or running the sample on an agarose gel and comparing to a known quantity of DNA or ladder. We recommend checking the integrity of samples on a gel prior to embarking on this protocol regardless of the quantification method. Genomic DNA should consist of a fairly tight high-molecular-weight band without any visible degradation products or smears.

3. The choice of the particular restriction enzyme to use for a study is based upon several parameters such as the desired frequency of RAD sites throughout the genome, GC content, the depth of coverage necessary, and size of the genome. For example, an average restriction endonuclease with an 8-bp recognition sequence will produce 1 tag every 64 kb in an organism with equal and random frequency of cut sites. Of course, the latter part of the previous sentence is hardly ever true, so the predicted and actual number of restriction sites in a genome can be quite different. For example, the number of SbfI sites (CCTGCAGG) in the stickleback genome (predicted from genome length and assuming equal distribution of each nucleotide) is 7,069, whereas we have identified 22,829 sites found at an average distance of 20.2 kb between sites. Yet *SgrD*I (CGTCGACG), with the same nucleotides as *Sbf*I, but in a different order, has 2892 sites found at an average distance of 160.2 kb between sites, nearly an eight-fold difference. In addition, the depth of coverage for calling a genotype in an outbred sample is quite a bit higher than what is necessary for an isogenic, recombinant inbred line. In general, RAD-seq experimental design is a challenge of optimizing the number of individuals, markers, and coverage given a fixed sequencing effort due to budgetary constraints.

4. The P1 and P2 adapters are modified Solexa© adapters (2006 Illumina, Inc., all rights reserved). The presence of some salt is necessary for the double-stranded adapters used in this protocol to hybridize and remain stable at ambient temperatures and above. At a 1 mM salt concentration, the P1 adapter, which has 64 bases of complementary double-stranded sequence (assuming a 5-bp barcode), has a $T_m$ of approximately 41°C (depending on barcode composition). P2, which has only 24 complementary bases, has a $T_m$ of only 27°C at the same salt concentration. At 50 mM salt the $T_m$s increase significantly to ~69° and 56°, respectively. Care should be taken to allow reagents to cool to ambient temperature before double-stranded adapters are ligated to digested fragments so as not to denature them. In addition, heating short AT rich RAD fragments may result in their denaturation. Since single-stranded RAD fragments will not ligate to the double-stranded adapter overhangs, these RAD tags may be underrepresented in the final library. The P2 adapter used in Hohenlohe et al. (10) is longer than the adapter we used for our first forays

into RAD sequencing. The new, longer P2 adapter has a higher $T_m$ closer to that of the P1 adapters and the added benefit of being paired-end compatible. Thus, the salt concentration in the P2 ligation becomes less important. However, the longer P2 doesn't get effectively eliminated with a column cleanup, necessitating a gel extraction after amplification no matter how well P1 adapter titration has gone (see Note 14).

5. Below are example barcoded *EcoR*I P1 and P2 adapter sequences. "P" denotes a phosphate group, "x" refers to barcode nucleotides, and an asterisk denotes a phosphorothioate bond in the P2 adapter that is introduced to confer nuclease resistance to the double-stranded oligo (14). Phosphorothioate bonds should be added to any 3′ overhangs on P1 adapters (e.g., *Sbf*I adapters).

   P1 top: 5′-AATGATACGGCGACCACCGAGATCTACACTCTTTCCCTACACGACGCTCTTCCGATCTxxxxx-3′

   AATTxxxxxAGATCGGAAGAGCGTCGTGTAGGGAAAGAGTGTAGATCTCGGTGGTCGCCGTATCATT-3′

   P2 top: 5′-P-CTCAGGCATCACTCGATTCCTCCGAGAACAA-3′

   P2 bot: 5′-CAAGCAGAAGACGGCATACGACGGAGGAATCGAGTGATGCCTGAG*T-3′

6. RAD amplification primers are Modified Solexa Amplification primers (2006 Illumina, Inc., all rights reserved).

   P1-forward primer: 5′-AATGATACGGCGACCACCG*A-3′

   P2-reverse primer: 5′-CAAGCAGAAGACGGCATACG*A-3′

7. This protocol has been modified from that used in Baird et al. (9) and now incorporates critical improvements made since publication, including ones adopted from Quail et al. (14) and Illumina library preparation protocols. Although we recommend following the protocol as described, other companies may offer superior (or cheaper) versions of reagents that come at different enzyme concentrations or activities, which should work just as well. Using them may require additional optimization, including different incubation times or reaction volumes for efficient RAD-seq library preparation. Many other brands of DNA cleanup and gel extraction columns could instead be used also, but an important consideration is the minimum required elution volume. We have successfully substituted Zymo's DNA Clean and Concentrator for Qiagen's MinElute kit and 10 Weiss units/μl Epicentre T4 ligase instead of NEB's 2000 cohesive end units/μl ligase.

8. Three-mismatch barcodes are optimal because although a significant number of reads will have a sequencing error in the barcode, it is very unlikely that a single read will have two errors in the same 5-bp sequence. Therefore, most of the reads that

have an error in the barcode can still be assigned to the correct sample when the adapters are designed to have three mismatches, whereas with only two mismatches a read with a sequencing error in the barcode may have come from one of two samples.

9. "$H_2O$" in this text refers to water that has a resistivity of 18.2 MΩ-cm and total organic content of less than five parts per billion.

10. Set up larger reactions if necessitated by dilute DNA and then concentrate the samples with a column before proceeding to ligation. This will cut down on throughput of the protocol, of course.

11. In general, when making master mixes, using multichannel pipettes and working with samples in 96- or 384-well plates will speed up the restriction digest and P1 ligation steps when multiplexing multiple barcoded individuals.

12. In Baird et al. (9) DNA samples from 96 recombinant $F_2$ individuals were uniquely barcoded, which allowed us to track RAD markers and associate them with differing phenotypes. For example, $F_2$ individuals used in the mapping analysis included 60 possessing a complete compliment of lateral plate armor and 31 with a reduced number of plates. Up to 60 uniquely barcoded samples were pooled in a single library, and all samples were sequenced in two sequencing lanes. Sequences from each individual fish were sorted out in silico by barcode, allowing the genetic mapping of variation in the lateral plates as well as variation in another skeletal trait, the pelvic structure. For the bulk-segregant analysis, DNA from $F_2$ individuals was pooled by phenotype prior to digestion with *Sbf*I. Each digested pool was labeled with a unique barcode and then combined into a single library. In both cases, the parental samples were uniquely barcoded and combined into single libraries that were sequenced along with the $F_2$ libraries.

13. NEB Buffer 2 is used in the ligation reactions instead of ligase buffer because the salt it contains (50 mM NaCl) ensures the double-stranded adapters remain annealed during the reactions (see Note 4). T4 DNA Ligase is active in all 4 NEB Buffers if supplemented with 1 mM rATP, but doesn't work at maximum efficiency in NEB 3 because of the high levels of salt in that buffer. The presence of some salt is necessary for the double-stranded adapters to remain stable at ambient temperature during the ligation, but too much may cause a problem. Be aware of the amount of salt put into the ligation reactions and adjust the concentration of the adapters accordingly (for instance, if working with a frequent cutter, use lower volumes of P1 at 1 μM instead of higher volumes at 100 nM to cut down on salt added to the reaction). If the restriction buffer used for digestion does not contain 50 mM potassium or sodium ions, or if

the restriction endonuclease cannot be heat-inactivated, purify the reaction in a column prior to P1 ligation and add 6.0 μl NEB Buffer 2. This will negate the benefits of multiplexing somewhat but may be useful in certain RAD library applications involving one or only a few individuals.

14. *EcoRI* has been shown to work robustly in multiple organisms in our labs. Restriction enzymes that cut less frequently create fewer RAD tags and, thus, require more input DNA and less P1 adapter to keep the molar ratio approximately equal. Libraries produced with less frequent cutters are more difficult to amplify in general and protocol parameters may take some optimization for favorable results. It is critical to perform preliminary studies to optimize the appropriate amount of P1 adapter for a given restriction enzyme that is used for the first time in an organism, unless the actual number of sites is known (i.e., if a genome sequence is available). A range of P1 adapter to DNA ratios can be used in a preliminary study, and the efficiency of ligation can then be assayed via gel visualization. Alternatively, a more precise estimate of the quantity of correctly adapted fragments in each P1-DNA ratio can be determined after ligation of both adaptors via a qPCR reaction using primers designed to the P1 and P2 adapters. Over the correct range of adapter-DNA ratios, the amount of ligated DNA should increase and then asymptote. The inflexion point of this relationship is the ideal ratio of P1 adapter to DNA. If the ratio of P1 adapter overhangs to available genomic compatible ends is too low, you can get insufficient amplification and/or biased representation of some RAD tags. However, if the ratio of P1 to genomic overhangs is too high, a contaminant band that runs around 130 bp will appear after the final PCR reaction. If this contaminant overwhelms the amplification reaction it can lead to significant adapter sequence reads in the final sequencing output (even after gel extraction following the final PCR). This phenomenon is completely dependent upon the number of actual cut sites present in that genome and the corresponding amount of P1 adapter used. Our *SbfI* study in stickleback used 2.5 μl P1 per microgram starting material and performed very well for library construction (see Figs. 3 and 4; lanes 2 and 4); however, this is likely due to the fact that there are actually more *SbfI* sites than expected by chance (see Note 3). Therefore, it may be preferable to start with less P1 when working on genomes with closer to the expected number of sites. In addition, the prescribed amounts of P1 adapters used in this protocol were optimized for the studies published in Baird et al. (9), using adapters lacking phosphorothioate bonds. In our hands, RAD-seq libraries created using adapters that have the phosphorothioate modifications amplify better and appear much less prone to adapter contamination. Though we have not optimized the maximum amount to use for these new adapters, P1 concentrations in the ligation reactions can be increased.

15. This step allows multiple individually barcoded samples to be combined and processed as well as to cut down on cost, work time, and differences in amplification efficiency that may arise between different library preparations when processing many samples at once.

16. Although we have optimized our protocol for shearing via sonication, other forms of shearing should work (the "Alternate Fragmentation Methods" sections of the Illumina Sample Prep Guides are a good resource for important considerations when choosing a shearing method).

17. We have found that it is unwise to run more than one library sample on the same agarose gel, as is shown in the figures (unless they will be combined and sequenced in the same lane on the flow cell) since it can lead to contamination between samples. This is especially important when dealing with samples following PCR amplification. We also recommend using aerosol-resistant filter tips for all amplification and downstream steps in the protocol to avoid library contamination.

18. A wider size range can be isolated (Subheading 3.4, step 2) to have more RAD fragments to carry through the protocol if low template amounts are evident after the P2 ligation (see Note 2).

19. Use MinElute columns and not QIAquick columns, which require a larger elution volume.

20. The optimal amount of template is dependent on the restriction enzyme used and its occurrence throughout the particular genome. It is difficult to be confident of the true concentration of amplified RAD tag molecules in your final sample, which have both P1 and P2 sequences, and are, therefore, able to bind the adapter oligonucleotides present on the Illumina flow cell. Poorly amplified libraries will contain a greater number of background sheared genomic DNA fragments with only P2 adapters attached, which cannot bind to the flow cell. A more precise estimate of fragments that have correctly ligated both P1 and P2 adaptors, and can therefore form clusters on the flow cell, can be ascertained by using qPCR with primers that are specific to the amplification priming sites on each adaptor.

21. Libraries that amplify robustly, such as those shown in Fig. 3, can be amplified with only 14 or fewer cycles of amplification to avoid skewing the representation of the library (14). The goal is to use as few PCR cycles as possible to obtain robustly amplified libraries without amplification bias.

22. For long-term storage of DNA samples, Illumina recommends a concentration of 10 nM and adding Tween-20 to the sample to a final concentration of 0.1%. This helps to prevent adsorption of the template to plastic tubes upon repeated freeze–thaw cycles, which would decrease the effective DNA concentration and, therefore, the number of sequencing clusters the library will produce.

23. For example, a measured DNA concentration of 10 ng/μl expressed in grams per liter is 0.01 g/l. 650 g/mol/bp × 400 bp = 292,500 g/mol = 0.0002925 g/nmol. To calculate the nanomolarity, divide 0.01 g/l by 0.0002925 g/nmol to get 34.2 nmol/l or 34.2 nM.
24. We recommend that you validate your first one or two RAD-seq libraries by cloning 1.0 μl of the gel-purified library into a blunt-end compatible sequencing vector. Sequence individual clones by conventional Sanger sequencing. Confirm that insert sequences contain the correct barcodes and restriction cut site overhang and are from the genomic source DNA.

## Acknowledgments

The authors thank the University of Oregon researchers who, over the past 3 years, have helped troubleshoot many preliminary versions of this protocol. This work was funded by grants from the National Institutes of Health (1R24GM079486-01A1 and Ruth L. Kirschstein National Research Service Award F32 GM078949) and the National Science Foundation (IOS-0642264 and DEB-0919090).

### References

1. Mardis ER (2008) The impact of next-generation sequencing technology on genetics. Trends Genet **24**:133–141
2. Shendure J, Ji H (2008) Next-generation DNA sequencing. Nat Biotech **26**:1135–1145
3. Asmann YW, Wallace MB, Thompson EA (2008) Transcriptome profiling using next-generation sequencing. Gastroenterology **135**:1466–1468
4. Marguerat S, Wilhelm BT, Bahler J (2008) Next-generation sequencing: applications beyond genomes. Biochem Soc Trans **36**: 1091–1096
5. Mortazavi A, Williams BA, McCue K et al (2008) Mapping and quantifying mammalian transcriptomes by RNA-Seq. Nat Methods **5**:621–628
6. Rokas A, Abbot P (2009) Harnessing genomics for evolutionary insights. Trends Ecol Evol **24**:192–200
7. Mardis ER (2008) Next-generation DNA sequencing methods. Annu Rev Genomics Hum Genet **9**:387–402
8. Van Tassell CP, Smith TP, Matukumalli LK et al (2008) SNP discovery and allele frequency estimation by deep sequencing of reduced representation libraries. Nat Methods **5**:247–252
9. Baird NA, Etter PD, Atwood TS et al (2008) Rapid SNP discovery and genetic mapping using sequenced RAD markers. PLoS ONE **3**:e3376
10. Hohenlohe P, Bassham S, Stiffler N et al (2010) Population genomics of parallel adaptation in threespine stickleback using sequenced RAD tags. PLoS Genet **6**:e1000862
11. Emerson KJ, Merz CR, Catchen JM et al (2010) Resolving post-glacial phylogeography using high throughput sequencing. Proc Natl Acad Sci USA **107**:16196–200
12. Gompert Z, Lucas LK, Fordyce JA et al (2010) Secondary contact between *Lycaeides idas* and *L. melissa* in the Rocky Mountains: extensive admixture and a patchy hybrid zone. Mol Ecol **19**:3171–3192
13. Coyne KJ, Burkholder JM, Feldman RA et al (2004) Modified serial analysis of gene expression method for construction of gene expression profiles of microbial eukaryotic species. Appl Environ Microbiol **70**:5298–5304
14. Quail MA, Kozarewa I, Smith F et al (2008) A large genome center's improvements to the Illumina sequencing system. Nat Methods **5**:1005–1010
15. Lynch M (2009) Estimation of allele frequencies from high-coverage genome-sequencing projects. Genetics **18**:295–301

# Chapter 10

# DNA Microarray-Based Mutation Discovery and Genotyping

**David Gresham**


## Abstract

DNA microarrays provide an efficient means of identifying single-nucleotide polymorphisms (SNPs) in DNA samples and characterizing their frequencies in individual and mixed samples. We have studied the parameters that determine the sensitivity of DNA probes to SNPs and found that the melting temperature ($T_m$) of the probe is the primary determinant of probe sensitivity. An isothermal-melting temperature DNA microarray design, in which the $T_m$ of all probes is tightly distributed, can be implemented by varying the length of DNA probes within a single DNA microarray. I describe guidelines for designing isothermal-melting temperature DNA microarrays and protocols for labeling and hybridizing DNA samples to DNA microarrays for SNP discovery, genotyping, and quantitative determination of allele frequencies in mixed samples.


**Key words:** DNA microarray, Single-nucleotide polymorphisms, Isothermal melting temperature, SNPscanner, Bulk segregant mapping

## 1. Introduction

The original motivation for the development of DNA microarrays was the detection of genome sequence variation (1, 2). Although myriad applications of DNA microarrays were subsequently developed, including the analysis of mRNA expression levels (3), protein–DNA interactions (4), and genome amplifications and deletions (5, 6), the discovery and analysis of single-nucleotide polymorphism (SNP) variation using microarrays has remained a mainstay of modern molecular genetics.

All DNA microarray methods for detecting sequence differences rely on the chemistry of DNA duplex formation. Under appropriate reaction conditions, duplexes that are perfectly complementary in their DNA sequence are strongly favored over duplexes that contain one or more mismatched bases. In a typical

Virginie Orgogozo and Matthew V. Rockman (eds.), *Molecular Methods for Evolutionary Genetics*,
Methods in Molecular Biology, vol. 772, DOI 10.1007/978-1-61779-228-1_10, © Springer Science+Business Media, LLC 2011

experiment, the efficiency of duplex formation is measured by labeling a DNA sample with a fluorophore and quantifying the fluorescent signal at thousands to millions of probes following a hybridization reaction. Sample DNA fragments that are perfectly complementary to the probe sequence will exhibit maximal fluorescent signals, whereas the presence of even a single base difference that reduces complementarity results in diminished signals.

For the purpose of DNA sequence comparison, it is necessary to maximize the difference in efficiency of matched and mismatched duplex formation. Although several factors determine the efficiency of these reactions, two factors dominate. The first is the position of the mismatched base within the probe. Empirical studies have shown that mutations corresponding to mismatches in the central portion of the probe have the greatest impact on hybridization efficiency (7, 8). The second is the relationship between the predicted probe melting temperature ($T_m$) and the temperature at which the hybridization reaction is performed (9). The $T_m$ of a probe is defined as the temperature at which 50% of the DNA molecules are in a duplex state. Previously, we performed a systematic study of the relationship between probe $T_m$ and the discriminatory power of a probe sequence. We found that a probe melting temperature 2–5°C lower than the temperature at which hybridization is performed maximizes the sensitivity of duplex formation to single-base mismatches (9).

Here, I describe guidelines for designing DNA microarrays that employ these two simple principles. The manufacture of DNA microarrays corresponding to these designs is best realized using commercial manufacturers such as Agilent, Nimbelgen (Roche), or Affymetrix. These designs are well suited to SNP discovery on a genome scale (7) or targeted SNP genotyping of either individuals or pools of millions of individuals (10). I provide methodological details on preparation of samples and DNA hybridization experiments. The detailed steps are specific to the Agilent system, but should be readily adapted to other two-color hybridization platforms. In addition, I provide guidelines for analysis of hybridization data.

## 2. Materials

### 2.1. DNA Preparation and Labeling

1. High-quality genomic DNA is purified using Genomic Tip 100/G (Qiagen).
2. A sonicator is required for fragmenting DNA. Alternative means of random fragmentation are also possible, such as nebulization.
3. A Qubit Fluorometer (Invitrogen) provides the most accurate means of determining DNA concentration.

4. Quant-iT dsDNA Assay Kit, Broad Range (Invitrogen).
5. DNA Clean and Concentrator-5 columns (Zymo Research).
6. BioPrime Array CGH Genomic Labeling System (Invitrogen) contains all the components for labeling DNA except the cyanine-labeled nucleotides. These components include random primers (hexamers), a mix of nucleotides and the Klenow enzyme.
7. Cyanine-5 and cyanine-3 labeled dUTP (suppliers include Perkin Elmer and GE Healthcare).
8. 3 M sodium acetate, pH 5.2.
9. 100% ethanol.

### 2.2. DNA Hybridization and Washing

1. 2× Hi-RPM Hybridization Buffer, 25 ml (Agilent).
2. 10× GE Blocking Agent (lyophilized pellet) (Agilent).
3. Hybridization gasket slide (Agilent). Note that Agilent DNA microarrays come in a variety of formats ranging from 1 array/slide to 8 arrays/slide. It is important to purchase the appropriate corresponding hybridization gasket slide.
4. Express Plus 0.22-µm Stericup and Steritop filter (Millipore).
5. Wash A: 700 ml water, 300 ml 20× SSPE, and 0.25 ml 20% *N*-lauroylsarcosine. Filter Wash A using a Stericup 0.22-µm filter into a 1 liter bottle.
6. Wash B: 997 ml water, 3 ml 20× SSPE, and 0.25 ml 20% *N*-lauroylsarcosine. Filter Wash A using a Stericup 0.22-µm filter into a 1 liter bottle.
7. Acetonitrile. Acetonitrile is mildly toxic and should be handled with care.
8. Hybridization chambers and tweezers (Agilent) (see Note 1).
9. Four wash chambers and one rack. I use a 20-slide unit staining dish and slide rack from Electron Microscopy Sciences.
10. Four magnetic stir plates and mini stir bars.

## 3. Methods

### 3.1. Microarray Probe Design

Depending on whether one seeks to identify unknown SNPs by hybridizing to probes of known sequence or to genotype known SNPs in individual or mixed samples, two distinct microarray designs are required. In both cases, a reference genome sequence is required, and for genotyping microarrays the alternate allele for each SNP must be known. For SNP identification, probes are designed to overlap in a tiled manner. For genotyping, it is necessary to design probes in which the known SNP lies within the central region of the probe. For both applications, an isothermal-melting probe design should be employed to maximize the potential for SNP identification or the discriminatory power of an allele-specific probe. I provide algorithmic guidelines, and examples in the notes, for simple computer code that must be written to generate either of these two microarray designs.

#### 3.1.1. Isothermal Probe Design

1. The $T_m$ (in °C) for a given DNA sequence is calculated using the relationship $T_m = \Delta H° \times 1{,}000/(\Delta S° + R \times \ln(C_T/x)) - 273.15$ where the $R = 1.9872$ cal/Kmol is the gas constant, $x = 4$ for nonself-complementary duplexes, and a total strand concentration ($C_T$) of $0.6 \times 10^{-12}$ M is appropriate.
2. To calculate the $T_m$ of a probe, it is necessary to determine the total enthalpy ($\Delta H°$) and entropy ($\Delta S°$) of the DNA sequence using the nearest neighbor parameters (Table 1). These parameters are determined for a salt concentration of 1 M NaCl, but they also provide suitable estimations for lower salt concentrations.
3. A target probe $T_m$ should be selected. We have found that a $T_m$ of 60°C results in probes of a median length of 25 bases and is a suitable target $T_m$ for isothermal probe design.
4. Following completion of microarray probe design, each probe should be tested for uniqueness in the genome using a program such as BLAT. Nonunique probes should be excluded from the design. In addition, extremely short probes, which typically

**Table 1**
**Nearest neighbor thermodynamic parameters for complementary dinucleotides in 1 M NaCl**

| Dinucleotide | $\Delta H°$ (kcal/mol)[1] | $\Delta H°$ (kcal/mol)[2] | $\Delta S°$ (e.u.[3])[1] | $\Delta S°$ (e.u.)[2] |
|---|---|---|---|---|
| AA | -8.4 | -7.9 | -23.6 | -22.2 |
| AT | -6.5 | -7.2 | -18.8 | -20.4 |
| TA | -6.3 | -7.2 | -18.5 | -21.3 |
| CA | -7.4 | -8.5 | -19.3 | -22.7 |
| GT | -8.6 | -8.4 | -23.0 | -22.4 |
| CT | -6.1 | -7.8 | -16.1 | -21.0 |
| GA | -7.7 | -8.2 | -20.3 | -22.2 |
| CG | -10.1 | -10.6 | -25.5 | -27.2 |
| GC | -11.1 | -9.8 | -28.4 | -24.4 |
| GG | -6.7 | -8.0 | -15.6 | -19.9 |

[1]Values from (16)[1] and (15)[2] are provided. In our study of optimized microarray design, we used values from (16), but the values provided in (15) are improved estimations of the parameters. [3]Entropy units, which are equal to 1 Cal/K/mol

have an unusually high GC content, or extremely long probes, which have an unusually high AT content, are likely to have high signal variance in experiments. These probes typically have low sequence complexity and should be removed.

*3.1.2. Probe Design for SNP Identification*

1. Define the genomic region of interest. For microbial species with small genomes (<20 Mb), it is possible to design microarrays against the entire genome sequence (For example, with an average of 12-base spacing, a 20-Mb genome can be tiled with ~1.7 million overlapping probes). For larger genomes, a targeted approach is recommended, for example designing probes corresponding to the coding fraction of the genome.
2. Remove low complexity and repetitive DNA sequence elements from the genomic sequence. This includes telomeric DNA, retrotransposon sequence, and ribosomal DNA. SNP variation cannot be reliably detected in these regions using DNA microarrays.
3. Initiate the first probe sequence from 5′ end of selected genomic sequence. Continue incrementing probe sequence until the estimated melting temperature of the probe is minimally different from the target melting temperature (see an example of the probe selection process in Note 2).
4. Initiate the next tiled probe from the site corresponding to the center of the previous probe (see Note 3).
5. Continue probe design in this way until the region is completely covered with overlapping tiled probes of a uniform melting temperature.

*3.1.3. Probe Design for SNP Genotyping*

1. Identify genomic coordinates and the two alleles for each SNP. For biallelic polymorphisms, it is necessary to have two independent probes that differ at a single base complementary to the SNP. The local sequence flanking ~20 bases on each side of the probe must be known.
2. Initiate probe design from the SNP site incrementing the probe on alternating 5′ and 3′ sides of SNP until the estimated melting temperature of the probe is minimally different from the target melting temperature (see example in Note 4).
3. Repeat this procedure for the alternative allele for each SNP (as described in Note 4).

### 3.2. Hybridization Experiments

The hybridization method for performing SNP discovery or genotyping is based on a standard Agilent comparative genomic hybridization (CGH) protocol. High-quality DNA is purified and randomly fragmented using sonication. Labeling by incorporation of a cyanine-3 or cyanine-5 labeled nucleotide is performed using the Klenow DNA polymerase. The labeling reaction is performed at a temperature that limits the processivity of the polymerase resulting in a uniform population of small fragment size. Short DNA fragments of <300 bp are required for efficient duplex formation. This labeling procedure results in an amplification of the sample DNA by approximately sevenfold. In my experience, this method does not result in biased amplification so long as the sample DNA has been randomly fragmented.

Two-color DNA microarray platforms allow for cohybridization of two samples enabling a variety of experimental designs. For mutation discovery, cohybridization of genomic DNA from a sample of known sequence (typically the sequence that was used for the microarray design) with a sample of unknown sequence is a common experimental design. For genotyping arrays two strains that are polymorphic at the targeted SNPs can be cohybridized. For bulk segregant mapping, one label should be used for the mixed sample and one label should be used for a heterozygous strain to enable comparison of the population allele frequency with a 50:50 allele frequency.

*3.2.1. Preparation of Genomic DNA*

1. Prepare genomic DNA using Qiagen Genomic Tip 100 following manufacturer's protocol (see Note 5).
2. Dilute 5 µg of sample genomic DNA in a total volume of 200 µl $dH_2O$ (see Note 6).
3. Sonicate the DNA. We use the settings of power = 1, duration = 0.5 s, total = 15 s on a Misonix Sonicator 4000 Homogenizer.
4. Run 15 µl on a 1% agarose gel to confirm that the sonicated product is sufficiently fragmented. There should be a broad distribution of DNA fragments with a median size of ~600 bp.
5. Concentrate the DNA in a DNA Clean and Concentrator-5 column. Add 1 ml of DNA binding buffer to 200 µl of sonicated genomic DNA and load 600 µl onto column. Perform a quick hard spin (see Note 7), discard the flow-through, and repeat with the additional 600 µl.
6. Elute DNA from the column in 25 µl $H_2O$.
7. Determine the DNA concentration using a fluorometer (see Note 8). You should expect around 2 µg of DNA. You need at least 1 µg of fragmented DNA to proceed with labeling.

*3.2.2. Labeling DNA with Cyanine-Labeled Nucleotides*

1. In a 200 µl PCR tube bring 1,000 ng of DNA to 72 µl in $H_2O$. Place the tube in ice and add 60 µl 2.5× random primer solution, which is provided in the BioPrime Array CGH Genomic Labeling System.
2. Denature the DNA by heating for 8 min at 99°C in PCR block, then fast ramp cool down to 4°C for 8 min. Centrifuge briefly to recover all liquid.

3. Add 13 μl of 10× dUTP mixture (provided in the kit) to the tube followed by 2 μl Cy-labeled dUTP. Mix briefly. Add 3 μl of Klenow fragment and mix gently but thoroughly by pipetting.
4. Incubate at 25°C for 16 h in a PCR machine.
5. Add 15 μl of stop buffer (provided in the kit) to inactivate the reaction.
6. Transfer the solution to a 1.5-ml tube and add 16 μl of 3 M sodium acetate (pH 5.2). Mix the contents of the tube and then add 400 μl of ice-cold ethanol. Mix by inverting the tube and then place it at −20°C for 1–2 h.
7. Centrifuge at maximum speed for 10 min to pellet the precipitated DNA. Carefully remove the supernatant and then wash the pellet with 500 μl of 80% ethanol at room temperature. Centrifuge at maximum speed for 10 min and then carefully remove the supernatant.
8. Dry the pellet at room temperature by keeping the lid of the tube open (see Note 9).
9. Resuspend the pellet in 50 μl $H_2O$. Mix well by vortexing. It may be necessary to disturb the pellet with a pipette tip to ensure full resuspension.
10. Run 5 μl on a 2% agarose gel to confirm tightly distributed band around ~100 bp (Fig. 1). If the labeled sample does not resemble the example, repeat the labeling procedure.

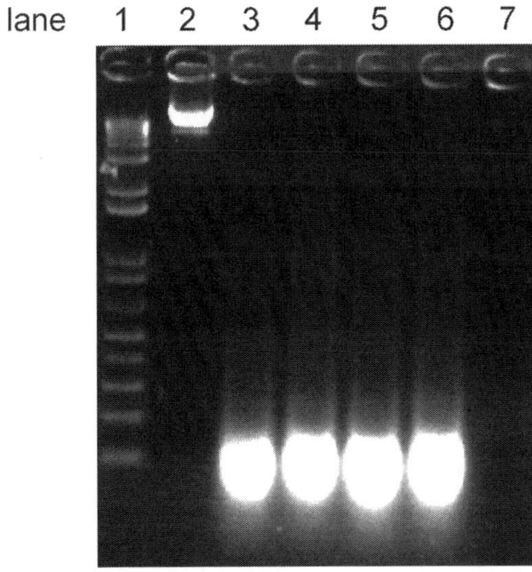


Fig. 1. Cyanine-dUTP labeling using Klenow enzyme at 25°C. Genomic DNA (lane 2) is fragmented using sonication to a median size of ~600 bp (not shown). The labeling procedure generates short fragments distributed around ~100 bp. Products from four independent labeling procedures are shown in lanes 3–6. Lane 1 contains a 1-kb ladder. Lane 7 is a blank control in which no template DNA was added to the labeling reaction.

11. Quantify the DNA using a fluorometer. You should expect a yield of approximately 5–7 μg.
12. The dye incorporation should be determined using a Nanodrop ND-1000, a spectrophotometer capable of quantifying cyanine-3 and cyanine-5 levels on the basis of absorbance. Our dye incorporation is typically greater than 10 pmol/μg DNA.
13. Store the labeled sample at –20°C.

*3.2.3. Performing Microarray Hybridization*

1. Add 1,350 μl of distilled water to the lyophilized pellet of 10× blocking agent. Leave for 60 min at room temperature to reconstitute. Store at –20°C thereafter. The solution can be reused.
2. For each hybridization reaction, add to a 1.5-ml tube 200 ng of each labeled DNA sample and water to a total volume of 208 μl (ensure that there are at least 2 pmol of dye in each channel). Then, add 52 μl of 10× Blocking Agent and 260 μl of 2× Hi-RPM Hybridization Buffer for a final volume of 520 μl. Mix sample well by vortexing. Heat at 95°C in a heat block for 5 min. Then, incubate at 37°C for 30 min. Perform a quick spin to collect the sample at bottom of tube.
3. Slowly dispense 490 μl of hybridization mixture onto a gasket slide (see Note 10).
4. Place a microarray slide on top of the gasket slide and create an enclosed reaction volume using the Agilent hybridization chambers.
5. Place the hybridization chamber in the hybridization oven at the appropriate hybridization temperature (e.g., hybridization should be performed at 62–65°C for a 60°C isothermal probe design) and a rotation speed of 20 rpm.
6. Allow hybridization to occur for 20 h.

*3.2.4. Washing Microarray*

1. Prepare four wash chambers, each containing a magnetic stirbar and place them on magnetic stirplates. Fill the first two chambers with wash A, the third chamber with wash B, and the fourth chamber with acetonitrile. Place the slide rack in the second chamber.
2. Disassemble each hybridization chamber one at a time. Place the microarray and gasket slide into the first chamber of Wash A. Use the plastic tweezers to gently wedge open the sandwich while keeping the microarray slide submerged in Wash A. You can allow the gasket slide to fall to the bottom of the wash chamber. Transfer microarray slide to the slide rack in the second Wash A chamber. Leave a gap between each slide and between the slides and the wall of the slide rack.

3. Once all the slides are in the rack, stir for 1 min in wash A. For all stirring steps, the wash liquid should be visibly turbulent so that a small vortex is visible. Make sure that the entire slide is submerged at all times.
4. Transfer the rack into Wash B and stir for exactly 1 min.
5. Transfer the rack into the acetonitrile. Leave submerged for 30 s. Slowly and evenly pull the rack out of the acetonitrile ensuring that all liquid drains from the slide
6. Dab microarray slide with a kimwipe to remove any remaining liquid.
7. Load the slides into scanning cartridges, with the Agilent name facing up and out. Do not touch anywhere except the edges of the slide and the bar code.

### 3.3. Data Analysis

#### 3.3.1. Recommended Control Experiments

1. DNA-microarray-based SNP discovery is based on a relative decrease in hybridization efficiency with respect to that obtained for perfectly complementary DNA. Repeated hybridization experiments of a strain identical to the genome sequence used to design the microarray provide a means of establishing the expected signal at each probe for perfectly matched DNA.
2. Genotyping individuals on biallelic genotyping microarrays requires knowledge of the expected intensity at each allele-specific probe. Cohybridization of genomic DNA from two samples that are homozygous and carry the alternate allele at each locus provides the ideal means of determining these expected intensities.
3. Bulk segregant mapping requires estimation of allele frequencies in mixed populations on the basis of hybridization signal. By hybridizing a strain that is heterozygous at each locus, in addition to strains that are homozygous at each locus (in two different experiments), it is possible to generate a three-point calibration of the expected intensity at each probe for 0, 50, and 100% allele frequencies.

#### 3.3.2. Detection of Point Mutations Using Tiled Overlapping Isothermal-Melting Probes

1. We have previously analyzed data for the purpose of mutation discovery using a likelihood ratio-based approach. This method requires a training dataset that consists of multiple hybridizations of the perfectly matched genome (to determine a mean and variance for each probe) and at least one hybridization experiment of a genome containing numerous known SNPs (several thousand) to train the algorithm. This method is analytically straightforward and readers should consult our previous publications for information on implementing this algorithm (7, 9).
2. If the aim is to identify SNPs for subsequent use as genetic markers, and, therefore, a level of false negatives can be toler-

ated, then a simple statistical test is likely to suffice for determining whether a hybridization signal from a sample of unknown genotype at a given probe is likely to be the result of imperfectly matched DNA sequence. One strategy entails comparing the hybridization signal at each probe to the triplicate hybridization data from the nonpolymorphic reference genome. This approach has been used for identifying single-feature polymorphisms (SFPs) (11, 12), and the reader should consult these references for details on this strategy.

#### *3.3.3. Analysis of Genotyping Data*

1. For each pair of probes interrogating a biallelic SNP, the aim is to assess whether an individual is homozygous for either allele or heterozygous at the locus. Several statistical procedures have been developed for this purpose including likelihood-based (13) and classification-based methods (14).
2. For bulk segregant mapping, the relative intensity at the two allele-specific probes for each locus can be converted to an estimated allele frequency. The reader should consult (10) for details on this method of anaylsis.

## 4. Notes

1. Agilent microarrays are designed to work with Agilent hybridization chambers and oven. I have not tested whether other hybridization chambers and ovens are compatible with Agilent microarrays.
2. An example of the method for identifying a tiling DNA microarray probe, for the purpose of SNP discovery, with a $T_m$ nearest to 60°C given the target sequence: ATGGATTCTGAGGTTGCTGCTTTGGTTATTGATAACG. The $T_m$ for each candidate probe is calculated by summing all the nearest neighbor values to calculate the total enthalpy and entropy of the DNA sequence using the values from (15). This calculation is performed iteratively for each candidate probe until the probe that is closest to the desired $T_m$ is identified. In this particular example, the candidate probe of 23 nucleotides long should be selected because the $T_m$ of this probe (59.4°C) is closer to the target $T_m$ than the 24-nucleotide candidate probe (61.08°C).

| Candidate probe sequence | Probe length (nucleotides) | Total $\Delta H°$(kcal/mol) | Total $\Delta S°$ (e.u.) | $T_m$ (°C) |
|---|---|---|---|---|
| ATGGATTCTGAGGTTG | 16 | -120.3 | -324.1 | 41.13 |
| ATGGATTCTGAGGTTGC | 17 | -130.1 | -348.5 | 46.37 |
| ATGGATTCTGAGGTTGCT | 18 | -137.9 | -369.5 | 48.91 |
| ATGGATTCTGAGGTTGCTG | 19 | -146.4 | -392.2 | 51.55 |
| ATGGATTCTGAGGTTGCTGC | 20 | -156.2 | -416.6 | 55.50 |
| ATGGATTCTGAGGTTGCTGCT | 21 | -164 | -437.6 | 57.31 |
| ATGGATTCTGAGGTTGCTGCTT | 22 | -171.9 | -459.8 | 58.40 |
| ATGGATTCTGAGGTTGCTGCTTT | 23 | -179.8 | -482 | 59.40 |
| ATGGATTCTGAGGTTGCTGCTTTG | 24 | -188.3 | -504.7 | 61.08 |

3. We have found that to maximize the sensitivity of overlapping tiling arrays for detection of SNPs it is necessary that every nucleotide fall within the internal 70th percentile of at least one probe. To achieve this a good rule of thumb is to start the subsequent probe from the center of the previous probe. In the example provided in Note 2, the subsequent probe should be initiated at the twelfth nucleotide of the 23-mer probe that was identified as having a $T_m$ closest to the target $T_m$ of 60°C. By following the same design guidelines the subsequent probe is the 25-mer GGTTGCTGCTTTGGTTATTGATAAC, which has a $T_m$ of 59.23°C. The next probe should now commence at the 13th base of this probe and so on.

4. An example of the method for identifying two probes with melting temperatures nearest to 60°C, when the SNP and adjacent sequence are known, is shown below. The example sequence is: ATGGATTCTGAGGTTGC[G/T]GCTTTGG-TTATTGATAACG. The nearest neighbor parameters from (15) were used.

| Allele | Candidate probe sequence | Probe length (nucleotides) | Total $\Delta H°$(kcal/mol) | Total $\Delta S°$ (e.u.) | $T_m$ (°C) |
|---|---|---|---|---|---|
| G | AGGTTGC*G*GCTTTGGT | 16 | -127.3 | -334.5 | 50.62 |
| | GAGGTTGC*G*GCTTTGGT | 17 | -135.5 | -356.7 | 53.06 |
| | GAGGTTGC*G*GCTTTGGTT | 18 | -143.4 | -378.9 | 54.56 |
| | TGAGGTTGC*G*GCTTTGGTT | 19 | -151.9 | -401.6 | 56.87 |
| | TGAGGTTGC*G*GCTTTGGTTA | 20 | -159.1 | -422.9 | 57.22 |
| | CTGAGGTTGC*G*GCTTTGGTTA | 21 | -166.9 | -443.9 | 58.94 |
| | CTGAGGTTGC*G*GCTTTGGTTAT | 22 | -174.1 | -464.3 | 59.75 |
| | TCTGAGGTTGC*G*GCTTTGGTTAT | 23 | -182.3 | -486.5 | 61.24 |
| T | AGGTTGC*T*GCTTTGGT | 16 | -125 | -331.1 | 47.54 |
| | GAGGTTGC*T*GCTTTGGT | 17 | -133.2 | -353.3 | 50.17 |
| | GAGGTTGC*T*GCTTTGGTT | 18 | -141.1 | -375.5 | 51.83 |
| | TGAGGTTGC*T*GCTTTGGTT | 19 | -149.6 | -398.2 | 54.29 |
| | TGAGGTTGC*T*GCTTTGGTTA | 20 | -156.8 | -419.5 | 54.76 |
| | CTGAGGTTGC*T*GCTTTGGTTA | 21 | -164.6 | -440.5 | 56.59 |
| | CTGAGGTTGC*T*GCTTTGGTTAT | 22 | -171 | -460.9 | 57.9 |
| | TCTGAGGTTGC*T*GCTTTGGTTAT | 23 | -180 | -483.1 | 59.09 |
| | TCTGAGGTTGC*T*GCTTTGGTTATT | 24 | -187.9 | -505.3 | 60.02 |
| | TTCTGAGGTTGC*T*GCTTTGGTTATT | 25 | -195.8 | -527.5 | 60.88 |

In the case of the G allele-specific probe, the 22-mer probe (CTGAGGTTGC*G*GCTTTGGTTAT) should be chosen. For the T allele-specific probe, the 24-mer probe (TCTGAGGTTGC*T*GCTTTGGTTATT) should be selected.

5. The DNA columns invariably become clogged. Use of a modified rubber stopper with a single inlet to apply gentle air pressure (from house air or a syringe) expedites the flow.
6. All water used in this protocol is distilled and autoclaved.
7. All spins in this protocol are performed in a microcentrifuge at the maximum speed (e.g., 14,000 × *g*).
8. Measuring DNA concentrations using a fluorometer is much more accurate than on a spectrophotometer, which cannot distinguish DNA and contaminating RNA. A fluorometer should always be used in this protocol.
9. The dye cyanine-5 is particularly susceptible to degradation by ozone at levels as low as 5–10 parts per billion. This problem varies between labs and locations. The problem is particularly acute when the dried slide is exposed to ozone after the washes. A commercially available plastic barrier (Ozone Barrier Slide Cover; Agilent) can be placed over the slide once it is in the scanner cartridge to provide some protection from atmospheric ozone. An ozone-free workspace for washing and handling microarrays and labeled samples can be established using a NoZone WS Workpace (SciGene), which consists of a benchtop polycarbonate enclosure with an external ozone filtration system. If rapid degradation of cyanine-5 continues to be a problem,

potential solutions include the installation of carbon filters into the laboratory air handling system or the use of alternative dyes.

10. This protocol describes a hybridization reaction for a single microarray per glass slide. If other formats are used such as the 4 × 44 k or 8 × 15 k platforms, the total reaction volume should be scaled according to the reaction volume guidelines provided by Agilent. The amount of DNA should also be reduced by the appropriate factor.

## Acknowledgments

I thank the labs of David Botstein, Leonid Kruglyak, Maitreya Dunham, and Justin Borevitz where many of these methods were developed. I also thank Bo Curry, Leonardo Brizuela, and Ben Gordon at Agilent Technologies for participation in the initial study of microarray design.

### References

1. Maskos U, Southern, EM (1993) A novel method for the parallel analysis of multiple mutations in multiple samples. Nucleic Acids Res **21**:2269–2270
2. Gresham D, Dunham MJ, Botstein D (2008) Comparing whole genomes using DNA microarrays. Nat Rev Genet 9:291–302
3. DeRisi JL, Iyer VR, Brown PO (1997) Exploring the metabolic and genetic control of gene expression on a genomic scale. Science **278:**680–686
4. Lieb JD, Liu X, Botstein D et al (2001) Promoter-specific binding of Rap1 revealed by genome-wide maps of protein-DNA association. Nat Genet **28**:327–334
5. Pollack JR, Perou CM, Alizadeh AA, et al (1999) Genome-wide analysis of DNA copy-number changes using cDNA microarrays. Nat Genet **23**:41–46
6. Pinkel D, Segraves R, Sudar D, et al (1998) High resolution analysis of DNA copy number variation using comparative genomic hybridization to microarrays. Nat Genet **20**:207–211
7. Gresham D, Ruderfer DM, Pratt SC, et al (2006) Genome-wide detection of polymorphisms at nucleotide resolution with a single DNA microarray. Science **311**:1932–1936
8. Ronald J, Akey JM, Whittle J, et al (2005) Simultaneous genotyping, gene-expression measurement, and detection of allele-specific expression with oligonucleotide arrays. Genome Res **15**:284–291
9. Gresham D, Curry B, Ward A, et al (2010) Optimized detection of sequence variation in heterozygous genomes using DNA microarrays with isothermal-melting probes. Proc Natl Acad Sci USA **107**:1482–1487
10. Ehrenreich IM, Torabi N, Jia Y, et al (2010) Dissection of genetically complex traits with extremely large pools of yeast segregants. Nature **464**:1039–1042
11. Winzeler EA, Richards DR, Conway AR, et al (1998) Direct allelic variation scanning of the yeast genome. Science **281**:1194–1197.
12. Borevitz JO, Liang D, Plouffe D, et al (2003) Large-scale identification of single-feature polymorphisms in complex genomes. Genome Res **13**:513–523
13. Cutler DJ, Zwick ME, Carrasquillo MM, et al (2001) High-throughput variation detection and genotyping using microarrays. Genome Research **11**:1913–1925
14. Liu WM, Di X, Yang G, et al (2003) Algorithms for large-scale genotyping microarrays, Bioinformatics **19:**2397–2403
15. SantaLucia J (1998) A unified view of polymer, dumbbell, and oligonucleotide DNA nearest-neighbor thermodynamics. Proc Natl Acad Sci USA **95**:1460–1465
16. SantaLucia J, Allawi HT, Seneviratne PA (1996) Improved nearest-neighbor parameters for predicting DNA duplex stability. Biochemistry **35**:3555–3562

# Chapter 11

# Genotyping with Sequenom

Martina Bradić, João Costa, and Ivo M. Chelo

## Abstract

Often in evolutionary genetics research, one needs to analyze polymorphisms in populations for which cost-efficient high-throughput arrays are nonexistent, either because the species is not a model organism or because the populations have been subjected to such specific conditions that their base variation is almost unique. In this situation, custom-made genotyping assays are required.

Sequenom's MassARRAY® genotyping platform is a powerful and flexible method for assaying up to a few thousand markers and up to thousands of individuals. It is based on distinguishing allele-specific primer extension products by mass spectrometry (MALDI-TOF). Most stages of the experimental protocol reflect adaptations of established PCR protocols to multiplexing, which allows the simultaneous amplification and detection of multiple markers per reaction.

**Key words:** Genotyping, SNP, MALDI-TOF, Sequenom, MassARRAY®

## 1. Introduction

SNP genotyping with Sequenom's iPLEX® Gold and MassARRAY® technology permits assays of as many as 40 markers per reaction on genomic DNA (or cDNA) of single individuals. This is particularly suitable for projects where a large number of individuals (up to several thousand) need to be genotyped in a medium-sized panel (tens to a few thousand) of polymorphisms. It is based on scoring biallelic markers such as Single-Nucleotide Polymorphisms (SNPs) but can also be used to genotype insertion/deletion polymorphisms. Sequenom technology is commonly used to fine-map specific regions or to provide genome-wide coverage of diversity measures (1, 2) but has also been often used in association studies (3).

The genotyping method relies on distinguishing alternative alleles by the different masses of primer extension products (4).

Virginie Orgogozo and Matthew V. Rockman (eds.), *Molecular Methods for Evolutionary Genetics*,
Methods in Molecular Biology, vol. 772, DOI 10.1007/978-1-61779-228-1_11, © Springer Science+Business Media, LLC 2011

The use of a region-specific template enrichment reaction together with mass spectrometry-based detection allows for very sensitive and specific assays to be developed. Every procedural step is performed by adding reagents to previously obtained products: thus, yield losses due to purification and transfer steps are reduced to a minimum.

The experimental procedure can be subdivided into three different steps (see Fig. 1), with two intermediate cleaning reactions, before detection of the extension products. Target regions where the markers of interest are located are amplified first [*polymerase chain reaction (PCR) amplification*] to increase the quantity of specific template DNA. After inactivating unincorporated dNTPs with Shrimp alkaline phosphatase (SAP) (*PCR reaction cleanup*), a primer extension (*iPLEX*) reaction is done with mass-modified ddNTPs. The reaction incorporates different nucleotides according to the allele that is present immediately downstream of the 3′ end of the primer. After treating the extended primers with resin (*iPLEX reaction cleanup*) to optimize detection, and then spotting them into a chip that contains a specific matrix (*transfer of the*

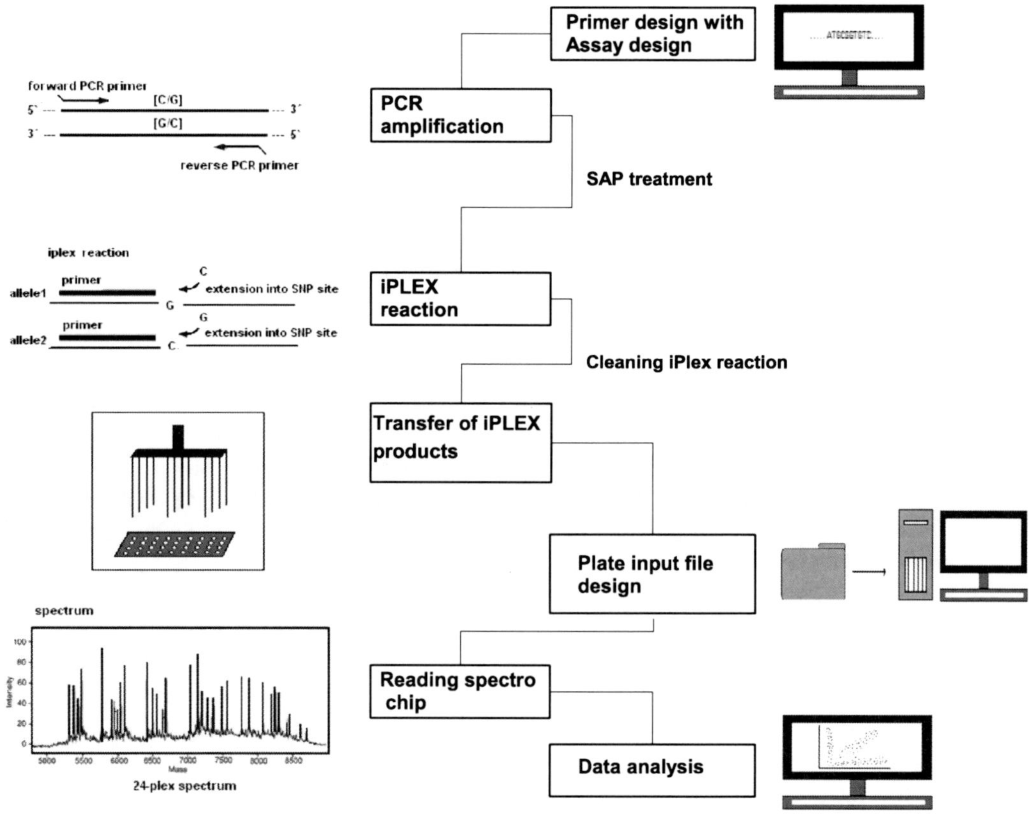


Fig. 1. Summary of genotyping with the Sequenom method.

*iPLEX reaction products*), the resulting products are analyzed by *MALDI-TOF MS* (matrix-assisted laser desorption/ionization time-of-flight mass spectrometry). In each assay, the specific ddNTP that was incorporated can be identified by the increase in mass of the primer. MALDI-TOF MS with the current analysis software distinguishes molecules that differ by at least 10 Da. The MALDI-TOF MS mass detection range and precision currently set the limit of 40 assays per reaction. The peak spectrum resulting from MALDI-TOF MS analysis can be analyzed with software that traces back primer masses to assayed alleles. Primer design and initial genotyping quality analysis can also be done with the software available from Sequenom.

The design of new assays in Sequenom's iPLEX® genotyping depends only on the ability to find a suitable set of primers in the regions where the SNPs of interest are located. This, together with the ease with which one can scale up the number of samples to be genotyped, makes it very flexible and particularly suited to analyze genetic variation in many contexts of evolutionary interest. At the same time, this genotyping method is always dependent on a previous knowledge regarding the location of polymorphisms in the populations being studied. Previous sequencing is, thus, required (either on single individuals or pooled DNA) in related populations or reference genomes whose divergence is thought to encompass the variation present in the populations to be genotyped. Ascertainment bias needs to be taken in consideration when analyzing such data to account for possible nonrandom sampling of the total variation. One other limitation of this method, which is common to many other genotyping procedures, is that it only returns genotypic data. Because of this, analyses that relate more than one SNP, such as linkage disequilibrium or haplotype diversity, require the most likely haplotypes to be inferred.

## 2. Materials

### *2.1. PCR Amplification (see Note 1)*

1. DNA samples at a working concentration of 5–10 ng/μl are placed on a 384-well PCR plate (ABgene PCR plates, Thermo Scientific). PCR-quality DNA should be in ultrapure PCR-grade water or Tris–HCl solution (pH 8.0) (see Notes 2 and 3). Store at −20°C.
2. 100 μM Amplification primers. Store in aliquots at −20°C.
3. 10× PCR buffer (500 mM KCl, 100 mM Tris–HCl (pH 8.3), 15 mM $MgCl_2$). Store at −20°C.
4. 25 mM $MgCl_2$. Store at −20°C.
5. 25 mM dNTPs. Store at −20°C.

6. 5 U/μl PCR Enzyme (DNA polymerase). Store at −20°C.
7. Ultrapure PCR-grade water.

### 2.2. PCR Reaction Cleanup with SAP

1. 10× SAP buffer. Store at −20°C (see Note 4).
2. 1.7 U/μl SAP. Store at −20°C.
3. Ultrapure PCR-grade water.

### 2.3. Primer Extension (iPLEX Reaction)

1. 500 μM Extension primers (see Note 5). Store in aliquots at −20°C.
2. 10× iPLEX Buffer Plus. Store at −20°C (see Note 4).
3. iPLEX Termination Mix. Store at −20°C.
4. iPLEX enzyme. Store at −20°C.
5. Ultrapure PCR-grade water.

### 2.4. iPLEX Reaction Cleanup with Resin

1. Clean Resin (see Note 4). Store at room temperature.
2. Ultrapure PCR-grade water.
3. 384 Dimple plate.
4. Plastic scraper.

### 2.5. Data Collection and Analysis

1. SpectroChip®. Store at room temperature (see Note 4).
2. Three-point calibrant. Store at −20°C.
3. 100% ethanol and 50% ethanol (dissolved in distilled water).
4. MassARRAY® Nanodispenser Samsung instrument and software (Sequenom).
5. MassARRAY® mass spectrometer (Bruker-Sequenom).
6. MassARRAY® TYPER software.

## 3. Methods

### 3.1. Primer Design with Assay Design (see Note 6)

The design of extension primers and the adjustment of primer concentrations in the primer mix are critical for the assay to work successfully. Since allele detection will be based on the distinction of the molecular weights of alternative extension products, extended primers should be between 4,500 and 9,000 Da (within the detection window), differing by at least 30 Da for different SNP assays and by 5 Da within each assay. These parameters can be defined and adjusted in SEQUENOM Assay Design software.

1. Input file format.
   SNP sequences must be arranged a TAB delimited text file (.txt). The file should contain two columns: one (headed

"SNP_ID") that will contain the SNP names, and the other (headed "Sequence") with the sequences of interest.

Sequences should be 300–400 bp in length and should contain no spaces or characters other than A, G, C, T, and N. All known SNPs other than the SNP of interest should be replaced with "N." Allele nucleotide variants should take the following format "[A/T]," and if the SNP is a one base insertion/deletion, it should take the form "[A/–]".

2. Running Assay Design.
   In the *Assay Design* window, after selecting the input file containing all the sequences of interest, confirm all available options and make sure that SBE (Single Base Extension) Mass Extend option is selected (see Note 7).

   Click *Run*.
3. Output.
   The output of the assay design is composed of several files:
   (a) A design report file with the description of the several plexes that were successfully designed (see Note 8).
   (b) A failed strands report file showing the SNPs for which no working assay could be designed, and reasons for those failures.
   (c) An Excel file with detailed information (see Note 9) on each of the successfully designed assays. This file can be used to order primers. It is also needed for the analysis software.

### 3.2. PCR Amplification

The purpose of this stage is to provide a specific enrichment of template DNA containing the SNPs to be genotyped. This is done in a single multiplex reaction (see Note 10).

1. For each plex, mix and dilute primers to a working concentration of 0.5 μM for each primer. See Table 1 for an example with 35 assays. For different number of primers/plex, the $H_2O$ volume needs to be adjusted.

**Table 1**
**Amplification primer mix preparation**

| | |
|---|---|
| Number of primer pairs in plex | 35 |
| $H_2O$ | 325 μl |
| Each Primer (100 μM) | 2.5 μl |
| Total volume | 500 μl |

**Table 2**
**PCR mix preparation (see Note 11)**

| | |
|---|---|
| Water | 1.8 μl |
| PCR Buffer (10×) | 0.5 μl |
| $MgCl_2$ (25 mM) | 0.4 μl |
| dNTP mix (25 mM each) | 0.1 μl |
| Primer mix (0.5 mM) | 1 μl |
| PCR Enzyme (5 U/ml) | 0.2 μl |
| Total volume | 4 μl |

2. Prepare the PCR mix according to Table 2. Volumes for a 384-well microplate should include 20% excess volume (this corresponds to 460 reactions) to account for volume loss with pipetting.
3. Add 4 μl of PCR mix reaction to each well of the sample plate (see Note 12).
4. Seal the microplate, mix briefly in a vortex (5 s), and spin down in a centrifuge (see Note 13).
5. Put the plate into an appropriate thermal cycler and use the following conditions:

| | |
|---|---|
| 94°C – 4 min | |
| 94°C – 20 s<br>56°C – 30 s<br>72°C – 60 s | 45× |
| 72°C – 3 min | |
| 6°C – hold | |

Amplification requires approximately 4 h.

### 3.3. PCR Reaction Cleanup with SAP

In this step SAP is used to neutralize unincorporated dNTPs from PCR amplification products by cleavage of the 5′ phosphate group.

1. Prepare SAP mix solution according to Table 3. Use a 20% excess (460 reactions for a 384-well plate).

**Table 3**
**SAP mix solution preparation**

| | |
|---|---|
| Water | 1.53 µl |
| SAP buffer 10× | 0.17 µl |
| SAP | 0.3 µl |
| Total volume | 2 µl |

2. Add 2 µl of SAP solution to each well of the 384-well plate (see Note 12).
3. Seal the microplate and spin down in a centrifuge (see Note 13).
4. Put the plate into an appropriate Thermal cycler and use the following conditions:

   37°C – 20 min

   85°C – 5 min

   6°C – hold

### *3.4. Primer Extension (iPLEX Reaction)*

In this stage, mass-modified ddNTPs are incorporated into SNP-specific oligos (primers) in an allele-specific fashion (primer extension reaction). Since all molecules within a given mass range will be detected, possible sources of contamination must be controlled. Therefore, it is suggested that extension primers are HPLC-purified and MALDI-TOF checked (see Note 5).

Furthermore, due to an inverse relationship between detection intensity and analyte mass in MALDI-TOF mass spectrometry, different primer concentrations are required in the same extension primer mix, with the lighter primers being less concentrated. To account for this, different primer working concentrations should be used for different primers. Dividing extension primers of each plex into four groups according to their molecular masses provides a practical way to implement this. Here, we give an example of the multiplex reaction with 35 assays where we have divided primers of each plex into four groups as follows: 9 (lowest mass group), 9, 9, and 8 (highest mass group) primers according to their unextended masses (see Note 14). Primer concentrations should then be adjusted based on the assays that are used in the genotyping. Prepare the iPLEX reaction according to the following steps:

1. For each plex, mix and dilute primers to working concentrations. See Table 4 for an example with a plex with 35 primers. An excess of 38% (530 reactions) will be used.

**Table 4**
**Extension primer mix preparation**

| | Number of primers | Stock concentration | Volume/primer (1 reaction)[a] | Final concentration[a] | Primer volume/plate (530 reactions) | Group volume/plate |
|---|---|---|---|---|---|---|
| GROUP I | 9 | 500 μM | 0.01674 μl | 0.93 μM | 0.01674 μl × 530 = 8.9 μl | 9 × 8.9 μl = 80.1 μl |
| GROUP II | 9 | 500 μM | 0.0225 μl | 1.25 μM | 0.0225 μl × 530 = 11.9 μl | 9 × 11.9 μl = 107.1 μl |
| GROUP III | 9 | 500 μM | 0.0288 μl | 1.6 μM | 0.0288 μl × 530 = 15.3 μl | 9 × 15.3 μl = 137.7 μl |
| GROUP IV | 8 | 500 μM | 0.0378 μl | 2.1 μM | 0.0378 μl × 530 = 20.0 μl | 8 × 20 μl = 160 μl |
| Total | 35 | – | – | – | – | 484.9 μl |

[a]Volume of primer and final concentration for the four groups are proposed by Sequenom, so the primer concentration adjustment is based on the number of primers

**Table 5**
**iPLEX mix preparation (see Note 15)**

| | Volume 1 reaction | ×530 reactions |
|---|---|---|
| Water | – | 341.9 µl |
| iPLEX Buffer Plus 10× | 0.2 µl | 106 µl |
| iPLEX Termination Mix | 0.2 µl | 106 µl |
| Primer mix | – | 484.9 µl |
| iPLEX enzyme | 0.04 µl | 21.2 µl |
| Total | | 1,060 µl |

2. Mix components of the iPLEX reaction according to Table 5. Use an excess of 38% (530 reactions) (see Note 15).
3. Add 2 µl of the primer extension mix to each well of the 384-well plate (see Note 12).
4. Seal the microplate and spin down on a centrifuge (see Note 13).
5. Centrifuge the plate for 1 min at 425×*g* at room temperature.
6. Put the plate into an appropriate thermal cycler and use the following conditions (see Note 1):

| | |
|---|---|
| 94°C – 30 s | |
| 94°C – 5 s<br>52°C – 5 s<br>80°C – 5 s<br>52°C – 5 s<br>80°C – 5 s<br>52°C – 5 s | 40× |
| 80°C – 5 s | |
| 72°C – 3 min | |
| 6°C – hold | |

Primer extension requires approximately 3.5 h.

### 3.5. iPLEX Reaction Cleanup with Resin

The presence of salts from previous reactions leads to an increased background noise in the mass spectrometry analysis. Thus, iPLEX reaction products are treated with a cationic resin (Clean resin) to remove salts as follows:

1. Fill all the holes of a 384 dimple plate with the resin (each hole takes 6 mg). Use the plastic scraper to spread the resin evenly through the dimple plate and also to remove the excess resin.
2. Place the 384-well plate with the iPLEX reaction products, upside down, onto the dimple plate (see Note 16).
3. Flip the plates over one another so that the dimple plate now stays on top of the 384-well plate. Tap the dimple plate to make the resin fall into the wells with the iPLEX reaction products (see Note 17).
4. Add 16 μl of ultrapure water to each well of the 384-well plate (see Note 12).
5. Rotate plate for 10 min along its main axis on a plate rotator.
6. Centrifuge the 384-well plate for 5 min at ~1,950 × *g*.

### 3.6. Transfer of the iPLEX Reaction Products onto a SpectroChip

The remainder of the protocol involves the use of the MassARRAY® specific workstation and MassARRAY® software. Thus, we will be walking through each of the steps required by the operator to perform the genotyping. If any additional details are needed, the user should consult the MassARRAY® Guide.

This step describes transfer of the extended/desalted iPLEX reaction products onto a SpectroChip® from a 384-well plate. SpectroChip®is a pad for the analysis of DNA samples by MALDI-TOF mass spectrometry, supplied in 384-well format and prespotted with a specially formulated MALDI matrix. The MassARRAY® Nanodispenser station for spotting of a 384 microtiter plate iPLEX reaction onto a SpectroChip® is used in this section.

A small volume (25 nl) of the reaction is dispensed onto the matrix spots on the SpectroChip using the following steps in the software that navigates the MassARRAY® Nanodispenser station:

1. Before beginning, make sure that the tank reservoirs (distilled water tank and the 50% ethanol tank) are filled and that the waste tank is empty.

*Preconditioning the spotting pins* (see Note 18).

2. On the nanodispensing software, select the *Pin conditioning* tab (/Operation/Status/Home Machine/Pin Conditioning).
3. Fill the sonicator with 100% ethanol.
4. Start pin conditioning of the main head (24 pins). Run for 30 min.

5. Repeat the pin conditioning but now for the single head (one pin).
6. Drain the sonicator by selecting the *Drain Sonicator* button.
7. Select the *Fill sonicator* button to refill the sonicator reservoir with 50% ethanol.

*Dispensing quality check.*

8. Place the 384-well plate and an old SpectroChip (a test Chip) on the deck of the MassARRAY® Nanodispenser.
9. Under *Load Method*, choose *System*, change the file type from *.tmf to *.vmf, and select the file *Volume384.vmf*, which is present in the "Volume" folder.
10. Run the volume check to adjust the dispense speed.
11. In the *Run Setup* tab, load the file *iPLEX*, change the dispense speed to that one which gave the best results in the volume check.

*Final dispensing.*

12. Replace the test Chip with a new one.
13. Select the *Status* tab and click *Start*. A few nanoliters (approximately 15 nl) of the samples are transferred onto the SpectroCHIP.
14. Add 70 µl calibrant to the calibrant reservoir on the MassARRAY® Nanodispenser.
15. In the *Run Setup* tab, load the file *Calibrant dispense* and select the *Start* button in the *Status* tab.

### 3.7. Design of Plate Input File

In order to connect the data that will be read from the chip with the sample and marker information, special file inputs should be created and loaded into the Sequenom software before the run. Here, we describe the necessary files and steps to be followed to load the files. Prepare a sample list file (.txt) with the samples' names in a single column ordered by their positions in the 384-well plate (A1...P24). The Excel design output file that contains details of termination chemistry and primer/assay information (see Subheading 3.1) is also required. Proceed to the following steps:

1. Open the MassARRAY® typer software and choose *plate* in Plate editor.
2. Create a new project and add a new plate within the project.
3. Move to Sample and in sample group add new sample group.
4. In the dialog box, give the name to the group ID, choose the open folder button, and select your sample list file.

5. Go back to the MassARRAY® typer home window and choose Assay editor.
6. Create a new project with all the assay information (the Excel design output file).
7. In the plate editor, choose your plate and select all the wells in the plate.
8. Choose the sample group that you have created for that plate and select apply samples.
9. Apply your assays by selecting the wells for each assay as used in the experimental procedure (see Note 19).
10. Check that all the samples and assays are correctly assigned to the plate by moving the cursor over the plate wells (see Note 20).

### 3.8. Acquisition of Spectrum Profiles Generated by MALDI-TOF MS

Using the MassARRAY® mass spectrometer, the masses of the products resulting from the experimental steps will be analyzed in real-time. Follow these steps of the Sequenom-provided software to initialize reading of the chip.

1. Make sure that *FLEXControl* and *ServerControl* programs are running.
2. Check that the correct *Method* (*iPLEX.par*) and *Sample Carrier* (*SequenomChip384C*) are loaded in *FLEXControl.*
3. Check if MassARRAY® CALLER is running.
4. In the Plate Editor, create a new chip run with assays and samples.
5. In the MassARRAY® Typer folder, select *ChipLinker.*
6. Connect to the database, providing access to the plate design and assay design that have been previously loaded.
7. Select the plate to be analyzed and enter an *Experiment Name* and the *Chip Barcode.*
8. Under *Dispenser* select *Nanodispenser S.*
9. Under *Process Method* select *Genotype.*
10. Enter the Chip Barcode.
11. Click *Add.*
12. Click *Create.*
13. Click *Done* and exit the *ChipLinker.*
14. Go to the SpectroAQUIRE and in the *Auto Run Set Up* tab under *Barcodes* enter the name of the SpectroCHIP.
15. Make sure that the *Parameter file* iPLEX is loaded.
16. Place the Chip on the chip holder.

17. Introduce target in the MassARRAY® READER with the *In/Out* function on the Autoflex instrument.
18. In SpectroAQUIRE in the *Auto Run Set Up* tab switch on the high voltage.
19. Click the *Auto Run* tab and under *Run* select *Start Auto Run*. The results will be automatically loaded into the database when the run is finished.

### 3.9. Analyzing Results on the MassARRAY® TYPER 4.0

Experimental data analysis can be performed in MassARRAY® TYPER 4.0 – Typer analyzer. This software allows the user to visualize the results of all assays simultaneously or to focus on single assays with a more detailed analysis. This provides a first step into quality control, as it allows identification and removal of nonworking assays and checking of the default genotype-calling thresholds. In order to read and analyze the data, proceed to the following steps of the Sequenom MassARRAY® TYPER 4.0 software:

1. Open the MassARRAY® TYPER 4.0 program and choose Typer Analyzer section.
2. Load data into the Typer Analyzer.
3. Go to the view option and create your own set of results visualization panes (see Note 21).
4. Select the experiments for the analysis from the *Project explorer* menu.
5. Check the success of your experiment by looking at *Traffic light* window that offers the visualization of the entire plate (see Note 22).
6. Check the *Automated data error* window that shows if there is any incongruence among repeats or water samples.
7. Check the individual marker success for each assay in *Histogram plot* window (see Note 23).
8. Check the *Call cluster plot* window showing the clustering of the individual genotypes based on the calls for each marker (see Note 24, see Fig. 2).
9. Check the *Details window*, which shows mass spectrometry detection peaks for each sample and primer extension products (occasionally unextended primer leftovers can also be seen) (see Note 25).
10. When finished with editing, save any changes (see Note 26).
11. Export all the information. Choose *Save all wells to file*, which will create a *.xml* file (see Note 27).

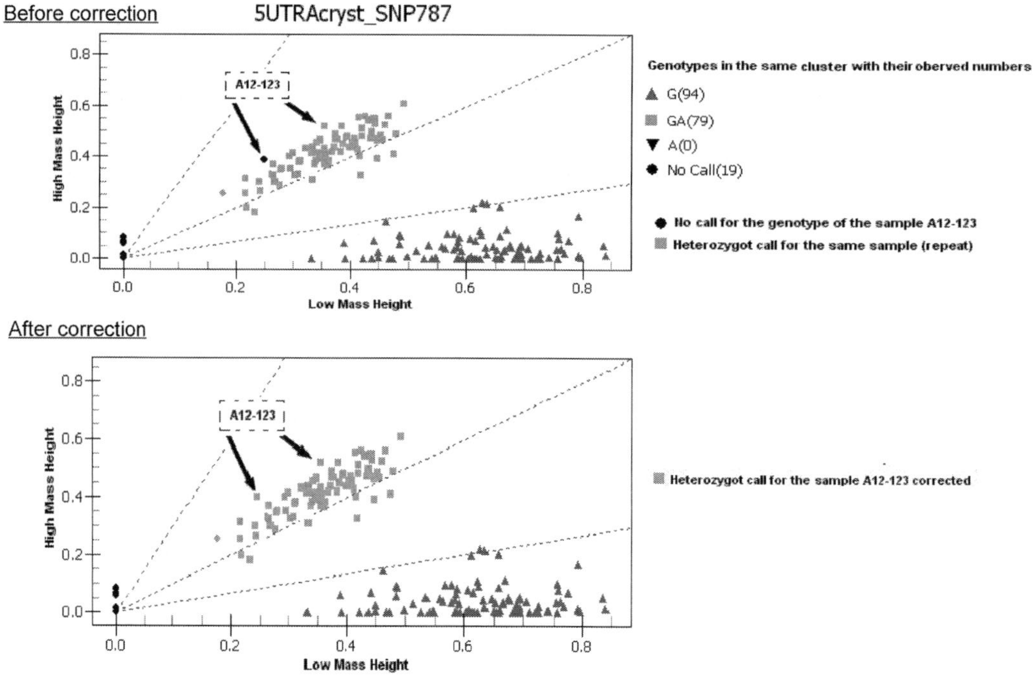


Fig. 2. Manual correction in the Call Cluster plot. Manual correction of a No Call sample in a Call Cluster plot analysis for single SNP assay (SNP ID:5UTRAcryst_ SNP787), inferring the genotype based on the membership in cluster and repeated sample information.

## 4. Notes

1. PCR reagents (buffer, dNTPs, $MgCl_2$, and polymerase) come as part of the SEQUENOM's "Complete Genotyping set" ready-to-use kit. Alternatively, other solutions can be used, but comparable results have only been obtained with "hot start" PCR amplification.

   Note that the PCR programs are designed for 384-Well Dual Gene Amp® PCR System 9700 (Applied Biosystems), with a maximum block ramp rate of 2.2°C/s. Equipment details are available here: http://www.biocompare.com/ProductDetails/481423/GeneAmp-PCR-System-9700-Base-Module.html

2. For long-term storage or transportation, DNA samples (up to 3 μl) can be dried directly on the plate by keeping it for 15–30 min on a thermocycler at a constant temperature of 60°C. For this purpose, the plate should be uncovered while drying in a sterile and DNA-free room to prevent contamination. In any case, it is recommended that 2–3 wells be reserved as blank controls (no DNA) and when possible a few wells should be used as replicates.

3. It is extremely important to check if the 384-well plates (or 96-well plates) are suited for all the stages of the process, which include not only the dispensing steps in automated stations and their fit into the thermal cyclers but also their fit into the dimple plate.
4. SAP reagents, iPLEX reagents, the “Clean resin,” the SpectroChip®, and the calibrant are provided in the SEQUENOM’s “Complete Genotyping Reagent Kit for MassARRAY® Compact 384” or “iPLEX Gold Reagent and Chip & Resin Kit.”
5. Although HPLC purification of extension primers is advised, in our experience primers with standard desalted purity work well.
6. MassARRAY® Assay Design software can be either installed or used on Sequenom’s Web site https://www.mysequenom.com/default.aspx by Sequenom’s customers.
7. Assay Design software provides users with control over many options regarding PCR amplification, primer extension conditions, or mass spectrometry detection limits by setting parameter values that will influence the sequence and localization of the primers to be designed. A careful study of the Assay Design Guide is recommended before the first use of this software. One option is worth special mention. There is a *Replex* option that instead of doing a de novo design from the input sequences uses information of previous design sessions to redesign primers. There are several alternative ways (accessed through suboptions) of using this process and its main advantage is that it allows the optimization of previous plexes by adding new assays or replacing nonworking assays. Nevertheless, we have generally found it difficult to significantly increase the number of assayed SNPs this way when the number of assays already in the plex is above 32–33.
8. The design report file (.trs) keeps a record of the general options used in the Assay Design run and gives information about the expected quality of the designed primers and plexes.
9. The Excel file returned from the Assay Design gives, for each assay, the primer sequences (amplification primers and iPLEX reaction primers) and primers’ molecular masses (including masses for the two possible extended primers) among other information. It can be seen in this file that the optimization of primer masses for the initial amplification reactions and for the efficient use of the available spectrum for mass spectrometry detection is done by adding defined 5′ tags with a specific number of nucleotides.
10. Plexes with more than 30 SNPs that are not previously tested can give up to 10% nonworking assays. It is possible to test

**Table 6**
**Single-region PCR amplification**

| | Volume (µl) for 1 sample | Final concentration |
|---|---|---|
| Water | 7.08 | |
| 10× PCR buffer (with 15 mM $MgCl_2$) | 1 | 1× |
| MgCl2 (25 mM) | 0.4 | 1 mM |
| dNTPs (6.25 mM each) | 0.32 | 0.2 mM |
| F Primer (25 µM) | 0.08 | 0.2 µM |
| R Primer (25 µM) | 0.08 | 0.2 µM |
| Taq (Hotstart) (5 U/µl) | 0.04 | 0.2 U |
| DNA | 1 | – |
| Total volume | 10 | |

separately for the amplification of single regions by doing a PCR reaction using the following protocol (Table 6) and the cycling conditions defined in step 5 of Subheading 3.2. This will test the efficiency of each reaction even if it does not guarantee its success in the multiplex reaction.

Products should be run on a 2.5% agarose gel (in 1× TAE) at 150 mV for 40 min.

11. It is assumed that 1 µl of DNA solution will be used and is already present in the 384-well plate. For different DNA solution volumes the water volume needs to be adjusted. Note that if a plex with fewer than 27 assays is used, the quantity of PCR Enzyme can be reduced to half (0.1 U/reaction).
12. The process of dispensing any solution into the 384-well plate should be optimized. Specific methods are available with automated workstations such as the MassARRAY® Liquid Handler. Alternatively, multichannel pipettes can also be used. See the iPLEX GOLD® Application Guide.
13. It is very important that the PCR sealing sheet is well placed and tight. Make sure that there are no bubbles in the wells after the spin-down, or at least that they are not in the bottom of the wells.
14. When it is not possible to have the same number of primers in the four groups, the "extra" primers should be part of the lower mass groups. For example, in a 32-primer plex the groups would have 8/8/8/8 primers (lower mass group first), but in

a 33-primer plex the distribution would be 9/8/8/8 and in a 34 plex, 9/9/8/8. Note also that because the differences in the required amounts of primers are compounded by the differences in the efficiency of primer synthesis according to their molecular masses, one should order larger amounts of primers belonging to the two highest mass groups.

15. Since in the iPLEX mix the total concentration of primers to be used depends on the number of primers in the plex, the volume of water needs to be adjusted for each plex.
16. When placing the 384-well plate onto the dimple plate, there is a small rounded post on the dimple plate that is used to match wells on both plates. The 384-well plate should rest against it.
17. Sometimes it may be difficult to pour all the resin into the 384-well plate, but this can be overcome by applying a more vigorous tapping on the dimple plate.
18. For further details, please check the MassARRAY® Nanodispenser Guide.
19. It is possible to have several different plexes being used in the same experiment. In the extreme, one could have up to 384 different plexes being run in the same plate.
20. When a mistake occurs at this stage, it is not always the case that error messages will be shown or that they will be clear in revealing the true nature of the problem.
21. Different layouts can be created and used according to one's preferences. The layout can be saved, exported, and loaded every time when needed.
22. Each well is individually typed for the markers of the assay, with an overall quality assessment being given by different colors: green, good; yellow, moderate; red, bad.
23. The proportions of the colors in the histogram reflect the observed frequencies of both homozygous and heterozygous genotypes, as well as the proportion of failed calls (no calls).
24. Careful inspection of the *Call cluster plot* window is advised. Cluster boundaries (or individual calls) for the three different genotypes can be changed, according to the researcher's criteria. This procedure can be used to rescue previously discarded data or remove less obvious genotype calls. Caution and objective criteria should always be used.
25. The *Details window* is very helpful for troubleshooting, as several different problems occurring during the experimental procedure can be recognized here. For instance, the presence of a large unextended primer peak with very small analyte peaks usually indicates that PCR was not very efficient. If only unextended primer peaks are observed, this may mean that there was a

failure of the iPLEX reaction or that the iPLEX mix was not well dispensed.

26. After saving any changes, the original data can always be restored if needed. The workspace defined by the plates that were loaded and edited can be saved as a *Session* and recalled to the Typer when needed.
27. Specific information can be exported from each pane by selecting the icon *copy to the clipboard*. Genotype data are stored in the pane called *Plate*, so one can copy them and paste them into an Excel sheet.

## Acknowledgments

We thank to Henrique Teotónio and Richard Borowsky for their support and useful comments and everyone at the Instituto Gulbenkian de Ciência Genomics Unit, especially Isabel Marques for the help with the overall procedure and data analysis.

### References

1. Gabriel SB, Schaffner SF, Nguyen H et al (2002) The structure of haplotype blocks in the Human genome. Science **296**: 2225–2229
2. Teotónio H, Chelo IM, Bradic M et al (2009) Reverse evolution reveals natural selection on standing genetic variation. Nat Genet **41**:251–257
3. Ayodo G, Price AL, Keinan A et al (2007) Combining evidence of natural selection with association analysis increases power to detect malaria-resistance variants. Am J Hum Genet **81**:234–242
4. Tang K, Fu D, Julien D et al (1999) Chip-based genotyping by mass spectrometry. Proc Natl Acad Sci USA **96**:10016–10020

# Chapter 12

# Isolating Microsatellite Loci: Looking Back, Looking Ahead

José A. Andrés and Steven M. Bogdanowicz

## Abstract

Microsatellite DNA loci are tandemly repeated simple sequence repeats (SSRs) that are ubiquitous in eukaryotic genomes. When flanked by unique sequences, length variation (driven by high rates of strand slippage during DNA replication) at a given repeat locus can be assayed by PCR and electrophoretic separation of the resulting DNA fragments (representing alleles defined by fragment size or repeat number at that locus). In nonmodel organisms that do not have sequence information at SSR loci (or at SSRs in a closely related taxon), microsatellites must be isolated and sequenced de novo. Traditionally, this has been accomplished with cloning of genomic DNA fragments enriched for SSRs, a protocol described in detail here. PCR primers flanking microsatellite repeats can be used to assay repeat length variation among individuals (typically through fluorescent labeling of one strand and capillary electrophoresis), useful for questions related to population variation, individual assignment, mating studies, selection scans, mapping, and phenotypic traits. High-throughput next-generation sequencing will likely supplant traditional cloning methods for the discovery of microsatellite loci.

**Key words:** Microsatellite, Cloning, SSR, Next-generation sequencing, Genotyping

## 1. Introduction

Microsatellites (or simple sequence repeats, SSRs) are tandem repeats of short nucleotide motifs ubiquitous in eukaryotic genomes. Because of their high levels of polymorphism, associated with high mutation rates ($10^{-2}$ to $10^{-6}$ (1)), they have been widely used in a broad range of evolutionary/genetic studies. Microsatellite loci have proven to be exceptionally valuable tools for investigating population variation and structure, individual assignment, pedigree and parentage analyses, and mapping studies. High mutation rates driving high numbers of alleles per locus give microsatellites a powerful window into relatively recent evolutionary processes,

Virginie Orgogozo and Matthew V. Rockman (eds.), *Molecular Methods for Evolutionary Genetics*,
Methods in Molecular Biology, vol. 772, DOI 10.1007/978-1-61779-228-1_12, © Springer Science+Business Media, LLC 2011

including selection scans (2), human diseases (3), variation in gene expression (4), and a host of other traits. Limitations of microsatellite loci include the presence of homoplasic (identical in size but not by descent) and null (nonamplifying) alleles. Microsatellite loci are thought to mutate mainly by slippage of DNA polymerase during replication, resulting in gains or losses of single repeat units (5–8). Although high-throughput analyses of single nucleotide polymorphism (SNPs) will continue to compete with microsatellites in population genetic/genomic studies as well as in genome-wide association experiments, microsatellites will remain a marker of choice whenever large numbers of alleles per locus are deemed useful. In this chapter, we describe both traditional and "next-generation" protocols for isolating microsatellite loci from eukaryotic genomes.

## 2. Materials

### *2.1. Enrichment, Capture, and Amplification of Genomic Fragments*

1. Molecular Biology grade water (MBG-water).
2. Mineral oil.
3. Distilled or deionized water (D-water) from a building/laboratory distillation or deionization system.
4. DNeasy Blood and Tissue Kit (and/or DNeasy Plant Mini Kit), (Qiagen, Valencia, CA).
5. Restriction enzymes *BsaAI*, *HincII*, and *PmeI* (New England Biolabs, Beverly, MA).
6. 10× NEBuffer 4: 500 mM potassium acetate, 200 mM Tris–acetate, 100 mM magnesium acetate, 10 mM dithiothreitol (pH 7.9) (New England Biolabs, supplied with *PmeI*).
7. 100× BSA (10 mg/ml) (New England Biolabs).
8. T4 DNA ligase (New England Biolabs).
9. Streptavidin-coated magnetic beads (New England Biolabs).
10. ATP (10 mM) (New England Biolabs).
11. 10 mM dNTPs (dilution of deoxynucleotide set, New England Biolabs). To make a working stock of 10 mM each dNTP, combine 10 μl of each 100 mM dNTP stock with 60 μl MBG-water (100 μl total volume). Store at −20°C.
12. Dynal MPC-S magnet (Invitrogen, Carlsbad, CA).
13. SPRIplate 96-Ring magnet (Beckman Coulter Genomics, Beverly, MA).
14. Biotinylated oligonucleotides for enrichment (Integrated DNA Technologies, Coralville, IA). Each of the following oligonucleotides should be synthesized with a 3′ Biotin-TEG group

(100 nmole synthesis scale): $(GT)_8$, $(TC)_{9.5}$, $(TTC)_7$, $(GTA)_{8.33}$, $(GTG)_{4.67}$, $(TCC)_5$, $(GTT)_{6.33}$, $(TTTC)_6$, $(GATA)_7$, $(TTAC)_{6.75}$, $(GATG)_{4.25}$, $(TTTG)_{5.25}$. Fractional repeat lengths indicate the addition of a partial repeat at the 3′ end of the oligonucleotide; for example, the sequence $(GATG)_{4.25}$ is GATGGATGGA TGGATGG (see Note 1).

15. Oligonucleotide enrichment mixes. We use five unique mixes of the 3′-biotinylated oligonucleotides for enrichment. Mix 1 = $(GT)_8$, 5 μM, mix 2 = $(TC)_{9.5}$, 5 μM, mix 3 = $(TTC)_7$ + $(GTA)_{8.33}$ + $(GTG)_{4.67}$ (each at 1.67 μM, total concentration = 5 μM), mix 4 = $(TCC)_5$ + $(GTT)_{6.33}$ (each at 2.5 μM, total concentration 5 μM), and mix 5 = $(TTTC)_6$ + $(GATA)_7$ + $(TTAC)_{6.75}$ + $(GA\ G)_{4.25}$ + $(TTTG)_{5.25}$ (each at 1 μM, total concentration 5 μM). Oligonucleotides are diluted in Qiagen AE buffer (0.5×), and mixed in the concentrations indicated (see Note 2).
16. Phosphorylated NP forward primer: 5′-pGTTTCTTCAGT-GCTAGCAGTTT-3′ (*p* = 5′ phosphate group) (Integrated DNA Technologies, Coralville, IA).
17. Phosphorylated NP reverse primer: 5′ pAAACTGCTAGCACT-GAAGAAACAAAA-3′ (Integrated DNA Technologies).
18. Double-stranded (ds) NP linker: 5′-pGTTTCTTCAGT*GCTA GC*AGTTT-3′

    3′-AAAACAAAGAAGTCA*CGATCG*TCAAAp-5′

    Dissolve NP forward and reverse oligonucleotides to 250 μM in 1× NEBuffer 3 (New England Biolabs). Combine 20 μl of each oligonucleotide, incubate at 80°C for 5 min, let stand at room temperature for 30 min to anneal. Add 460 μl of 1× NEB buffer 3 to the annealed oligonucleotides. The final concentration (working stock) of the ds linker is 10 μM. Store at −20°C. The restriction site for *NheI* is in italics (see Note 3).
19. 20× SSC: 3 M sodium chloride, 0.3 M citric acid (trisodium salt) (Sigma Chemicals). Dissolve 175.3 g sodium chloride and 88.2 g citric acid in 1 l D-water. Do not adjust the pH of, or autoclave, 20× SSC.
20. 12× SSC: combine 600 μl 20× SSC with 400 μl MBG-water and mix.
21. 6× SSC: combine 300 μl 20× SSC with 700 μl MBG-water and mix.
22. 20% (w:v) sodium dodecyl sulfate (Sigma Chemicals). Dissolve 20 g sodium dodecyl sulfate in 100 ml MBG-water. Dissolution can be speeded up by swirling the bottle of SDS in warm tap water while mixing.
23. 2× SSC/0.1% SDS: Combine 100 μl 20× SSC and 5 μl 20% SDS with 895 μl MBG-water and mix.

24. 0.5× AE buffer: Mix equal amounts of buffer AE from a Qiagen Blood and Tissue kit and MBG-water.
25. Platinum *Taq* DNA polymerase (Invitrogen).
26. PCR buffer (10×): 200 mM Tris–HCl (pH 8.4), 500 mM potassium chloride (Invitrogen, supplied with the Platinum *Taq*).
27. Magnesium chloride (50 mM) (Invitrogen, supplied with the Platinum *Taq*).
28. QIAquick PCR purification kit (Qiagen).

### 2.2. Cloning of Enriched PCR Products

1. MBG-water.
2. D-water from a building/laboratory distillation or deionization system.
3. Plasmid pUC19 (New England Biolabs).
4. Restriction enzymes *XbaI* and *NheI* (New England Biolabs).
5. NEBuffer 2, 10× (New England Biolabs, supplied with both *Nhe I* and *Xba I*): 500 mM sodium chloride, 100 mM Tris–HCl (pH 7.9 at 25°C), 100 mM magnesium chloride, 10 mM dithiothreitol.
6. 100× BSA (10 mg/ml) (New England Biolabs).
7. ATP (10 mM) (New England Biolabs).
8. Shrimp Alkaline Phosphatase (GE Healthcare, Piscataway, NJ).
9. QIAquick PCR purification kit (Qiagen).
10. *XbaI*-digested, dephosphorylated pUC19: In a 50 μl total volume, digest 10 μg of pUC19 with at least 20 U of *XbaI*, following the manufacturer's instructions. Incubate at 37°C for 2 h. Add 45 μl of 1× digestion buffer and 5 μl (=5 U) of Shrimp Alkaline Phosphatase. Incubate at 37°C for an additional 2 h. Purify the reaction with a QIAquick PCR purification kit and elute in 50 μl of EB buffer. Read the concentration on a spectrophotometer or fluorometer and adjust to 100 ng/μl with EB buffer. Store at −20°C.
11. T4 DNA ligase (New England Biolabs).
12. Adenosine triphosphate (ATP, 10 mM) (New England Biolabs).
13. Electromax DH5α-E electrocompetent cells (Invitrogen).
14. X-gal (Invitrogen).
15. SOC medium (Invitrogen).
16. Eppendorf 2510 Electroporator and cuvettes (1 mm gap width) (Fisher Scientific).
17. Ampicillin (50 mg/ml): Dissolve 500 mg ampicillin in 10 ml MBG-water. Sterilize with a syringe filter and store 1–2 ml aliquots at −20°C.

18. Luria agar (Sigma Chemicals).
19. Sterile 14-ml polypropylene snap-cap culture tubes (Laboratory Products sales, Rochester, NY).
20. 90- and 150-mm sterile polystyrene petri dishes (Fisher scientific).

***2.3. Replication and Hybridization of Colonies with Repeats***

1. MBG-water.
2. Mineral oil.
3. D-water from a building/laboratory distillation or deionization system.
4. SOC medium (Invitrogen).
5. 150-mm LB/agar plate containing 50 μg/ml ampicillin.
6. 137 mm Magna Lift nylon transfer membranes (GE Osmonics, Minnetonka, MN).
7. 18-gauge hypodermic needles (Fisher Scientific).
8. 80°C oven.
9. Rotating hybridization oven.
10. 20× SSC (see Subheading 2.1).
11. FisherBrand thick chromatography paper, 46 × 57 cm (Fisher Scientific).
12. Hybridization bottles (30 × 3.5 cm) (Fisher Scientific).
13. Disposable 50-ml polypropylene screw cap centrifuge tubes (Fisher Scientific).
14. Oven mesh sheets (22 × 22 cm) (Fisher Scientific).
15. 20% (w:v) sodium dodecyl sulfate (see Subheading 2.1).
16. 0.5 M EDTA solution, pH 8.0 (Sigma Chemicals).
17. Membrane scrub buffer (1 l): 2× SSC, 0.5% SDS. Add 100 ml 20× SSC and 25 ml 20% SDS to 875 ml D-water. Mix well with a magnetic stir bar.
18. Prehybridization and hybridization buffer (50 ml): 5× SSC, 0.5% SDS, 1 mM EDTA pH 8.0, 0.1% (w:v) bovine serum albumin. Combine and mix 36.15 ml MBG-water, 12.5 ml 20× SSC, 1.25 ml 20% SDS, 0.1 ml 0.5 M EDTA (pH 8.0), and 0.05 g bovine serum albumin.
19. Probe wash buffer (500 ml): 4× SSC, 0.5% SDS, 1 mM EDTA. Add 100 ml 20× SSC, 12.5 ml 20% SDS and 1 ml 0.5 M EDTA (pH 8) to 886.5 ml D-water. Mix well with a magnetic stir bar.
20. Bovine Serum Albumin (Sigma).
21. Kodak BioMax MR35 single emulsion film (Sigma).
22. Oligonucleotide probe solution: mix equal volumes of the five oligonucleotide enrichment mixes (Subheading 2.1).

23. ATP, [γ-$^{33}$P]- 3,000 Ci/mmol, 10 mCi/ml (PerkinElmer, Waltham, MA).
24. T4 polynucleotide kinase (New England Biolabs).
25. 35×43 cm pieces of thin cardboard.

#### 2.4. Plasmid DNA Extraction from Positive Clones

1. MBG-water.
2. 2× YT buffer: 16 g tryptone, 10 g yeast extract, 5 g sodium chloride per liter of MBG-water. Sterilize by autoclaving and store at room temperature. Immediately before use, add ampicillin (sterile 50 mg/ml stock) to a final concentration of 50 μg/ml in the 2× YT. We make multiple 50–100 ml aliquots of 2× YT buffer (a 96-well plate of colonies would consume about 40 ml, at 400 μl YT buffer/well), since the ampicillin is only stable in the 2× YT buffer for about a week at 4°C.
3. Ampicillin (50 mg/ml) (see Subheading 2.2).
4. Sterile (autoclaved) 10 μl pipette tips (Fisher scientific).
5. 2.2-ml storage plate and gas-permeable seals (Thermo Fisher Scientific, Waltham, MA).
6. CosMCPrep kit, 4×96 and CleanSEQ (Agencourt, Beverly, MA).

#### 2.5. Sanger Sequencing of Plasmid Clones and Data Analysis

1. MBG-water.
2. M13 forward primer: 5′-CCCAGTCACGACGTTGTAAAACG-3′, M13 reverse primer: 5′-AGCGGATAACAATTTCACACAGG-3′ (Integrated DNA Technologies).
3. BigDye Version 3.1 cycle sequencing kit (Applied Biosystems, Foster City, CA).
4. CleanSEQ (Beckman Coulter genomics).
5. 3100 and/or 3730 DNA Analyzers (Applied Biosystems).
6. Assembly/alignment software (CodonCode Aligner, Codon Code Corporation, Dedham, MA, and/or SeqMan Pro, DNASTAR, Madison, WI).

#### 2.6. Designing and Ordering Genotyping Primers

1. BatchPrimer 3 Web interface. (http://probes.pw.usda.gov/cgibin/batchprimer3/batchprimer3.cgi).
2. Fasta file of aligned/assembled reads from Subheading 3.5, Step 4.
3. Integrated DNA Technologies (IDT) Web site (http://www.idtdna.com).
4. 0.5× AE buffer (see Subheading 2.1).

#### 2.7. Primer Testing 1- Two Primer PCR

1. DNeasy Blood and Tissue Kit (and/or DNeasy Plant Mini Kit), (Qiagen, Valencia, CA).

2. Working stocks (10 μM) of forward and reverse primers for each microsatellite locus of interest. Each reverse primer should have the sequence GTTTCTT attached to the 5′ end.
3. 0.5× AE buffer: Mix equal amounts of buffer AE from a Qiagen Blood and Tissue kit and MBG-water.
4. Platinum *Taq* DNA polymerase (Invitrogen).
5. PCR buffer (10×): 200 mM Tris–HCl (pH 8.4), 500 mM potassium chloride (Invitrogen, supplied with the Platinum *Taq*).
6. Magnesium chloride (50 mM) (Invitrogen, supplied with the Platinum *Taq*).
7. MBG-water and mineral oil.

### 2.8. Primer Testing II- Three Primer PCR

1. DNeasy Blood and Tissue Kit (and/or DNeasy Plant Mini Kit), (Qiagen, Valencia, CA).
2. Working stocks (10 μM) of forward and reverse primers for each microsatellite locus of interest. Each forward primer should have a long tag (5′-CGAGTTTTCCCAGTCACGAC-3′) attached to its 5′ end; each reverse primer should have the sequence GTTTCTT attached to the 5′ end.
3. FAM-labeled long-tag (Integrated DNA Technologies): 5′-(6-FAM)-CGAGTTTTCCCAGTCACGAC-3′. Working stock is 10 μM.
4. 0.5× buffer AE: Mix equal amounts of buffer AE from a Qiagen Blood and Tissue kit and MBG-water.
5. Platinum *Taq* DNA polymerase (Invitrogen).
6. PCR buffer (10×): 200 mM Tris–HCl (pH 8.4), 500 mM potassium chloride (Invitrogen, supplied with the Platinum *Taq*).
7. Magnesium chloride (50 mM) (Invitrogen, supplied with the Platinum *Taq*).
8. MBG-water and mineral oil.
9. Hi-Di Formamide (Applied Biosystems).
10. Genescan LIZ-500 size standard (Applied Biosystems).
11. ABI 3100 and/or 3730 Genetic Analyzer (Applied Biosystems).

### 2.9. Genotyping by Multiplex PCR

1. DNeasy Blood and Tissue Kit (and/or DNeasy Plant Mini Kit) (Qiagen).
2. Working stocks (10 μM) of forward and reverse primers for each microsatellite locus of interest. Each forward primer should have a 5′ dye label (6-FAM, PET, NED, or VIC) attached to its 5′ end; each reverse primer should have the sequence GTTTCTT attached to its 5′ end.

3. Type-It Microsatellite PCR kit, 70 or 200 reaction size (Qiagen).
4. MBG-water and mineral oil.
5. Hi-Di Formamide (Applied Biosystems).
6. Genescan LIZ-500 size standard (Applied Biosystems).
7. ABI 3100 and/or 3730 Genetic Analyzer (Applied Biosystems).

## 3. Methods

A "traditional" method for discovering and genotyping microsatellites (described in detail, below and based on (9)) involves the following steps: Extracted genomic DNA is digested with two restriction enzymes (*BsaAI* and *HincII*) and ligated to NP ds linkers (named for a restriction enzyme used for vector cloning, *NheI*, and a second enzyme for the digestion of linker-linker dimers, *PmeI*) using T4 DNA ligase. Ligated fragments are then enriched for microsatellites by hybridization to biotinylated dimeric, trimeric, and tetrameric nucleotide repeats. Single-stranded DNA is recovered using streptavidin-coated magnetic beads and the enriched fragments are made double-stranded by a polymerase chain reaction (PCR) using an NP forward primer. The PCR products are digested with the restriction enzyme *NheI* and ligated to *XbaI*-digested, dephosphorylated pUC19 plasmid vector The NP linker has *Nhe I* sites that generate an overhang (5′CTAG-3′) compatible with *XbaI*-digested pUC19. These recombinant plasmids are then used to transform DH5α *E. coli* cells. Transformed cells are then plated on Luria–Bertani agar plates containing ampicillin. Colonies are transferred to nylon membranes and hybridized with $^{33}$P radiolabeled probes. Plasmid DNA from positive colonies is isolated, grown in minicultures, purified, and Sanger-sequenced using M13-primers. Finally, allele sizes at microsatellite loci are determined by PCR with locus-specific forward and reverse primers (one of which typically carries a 5′-dye label). Capillary electrophoresis is used to separate fluorescently labeled products, and peak-detection software is used to call the allele sizes.

Alternatively, high-throughput sequencing can be used to isolate microsatellite loci. The Roche GS-FLX Titanium Series (454 Life Sciences, Branford, CT, USA), utilizing pyrosequencing technology, is currently capable of producing 400–600 million high quality bases per run with a read length averaging over 400 bp. Massive amounts of data afforded by this technology allows for the efficient identification of many more microsatellite loci than the traditional method. Because microsatellite loci are relatively common in genomes, shotgun sequencing of standard (nonenriched) genomic DNA libraries, followed by bioinformatics detection of SSRs, can result in the isolation of microsatellite loci (10–13). The utility of this approach may be relatively taxon-specific, and it relies critically on both the depth of coverage and the frequency of microsatellites in the genome of interest. Much higher isolation efficiencies are likely to be realized from libraries enriched for SSRs (14). Enrichment can also be more cost-effective; as the proportion of reads containing microsatellites increases, a smaller fraction of a sequencing run needs to be employed in the search for loci. The use of molecular identifier tags (MIDs, short unique DNA sequences that appear at the end of each read) allow one to pool unique genomic libraries in the same run; we have gotten good results pooling up to 12 enriched libraries per half 454 run. While a single 454 read may be less accurate in general than single Sanger read (particularly in homopolymeric regions), the large numbers of reads per library generated by the 454 means that many microsatellite loci will be "covered" by multiple 454 reads, increasing the accuracy of the consensus generated. This raises some tensions when performing 454 runs for microsatellite discovery; steps taken to maximize the number of unique loci found (increasing the number of unique oligonucleotides during enrichment, for example), would tend to lower the average number of reads per locus (which may impact consensus accuracy and associated primer design). Moreover, any assembly of 454 sequence data from a repeat-enriched library runs the risk of assembling contigs based on the repeats themselves, which may generate chimeric consensus sequences from different (noncontiguous) loci in the genome. Assembly of 454 data should be stringent enough (when considering assembly parameters such as minimum match length and percentage) to minimize assemblies based on the repeats alone, and consensus sequences used for primer design should be scrutinized to verify that this has not in fact occurred.

Currently, read lengths afforded by the 454 (in the neighborhood of hundreds of nucleotides, on average) make it the next-generation platform of choice for microsatellite discovery. While the total sequencing output from Illumina platforms is orders of magnitudes higher than 454 (when comparing full runs), Illumina read lengths are quite a bit shorter, which may further confound the read assembly issues described above. As Illumina read lengths continue to increase, however, this platform should become a viable alternative to 454 for microsatellite discovery.

Next-generation sequencing technologies also raise possibilities for massively parallel genotyping. Given current technology, it would be possible (for example) to enrich multiple individuals for a single repeat type, tag each sample with a 454 MID, and collect allelic variation at hundreds or even thousands of unique loci. Obviously, read coverage per locus would be a primary consideration in an experiment such as this, and resolving orthologous reads from closely related paralogs could be problematic. Nonetheless, in instances where assaying large numbers of loci (rather than large numbers of individuals) is desirable, the potential for an experiment like this exists. Given the pace of technological advance of next-generation platforms, we likely cannot yet fathom the possibilities for locus discovery and genotyping that will almost certainly be available in upcoming years (if not months).

The GS FLX Titanium 454 Enriched Library Preparation Protocol is the same as the traditional method through the library enrichment step (Subheading 3.1 below). The enriched fragments are then ligated to Titanium 454 Rapid Library adapters, size-selected by gel-extraction, and then sequenced following Roche/454 protocols, beginning with the Library Quantitation step of the Rapid Library Preparation Manual (revised January 2010).

### 3.1. Enrichment, Capture, and Amplification of Genomic Fragments

1. In separate reactions, digest 200–800 ng of genomic DNA with the restriction enzymes *BsaAI* and *HincII* (0.75 μl each, 4–8 U of each enzyme) in 1× NEBuffer 4 and 100 μg/ml BSA. The total volume of each digest should be 20 μl. Incubate at 37°C for 1 h and then let stand at room temperature (20–23°C) for 10 min.
2. Add 2 μl 10 mM ATP, 3 μl NP linker (10 μM working stock), 0.75 μl *PmeI*, and 0.75 μl T4 DNA ligase to each reaction. Incubate at room temperature for 4–20 h.
3. Combine the two samples and mix gently. Add 8 μl of this mix to each of five wells of a microtitre plate, along with 2.25 μl MBG-water, 12.5 μl 12× SSC, 1.25 μl 1% SDS, and 1 μl each 3′-biotinylated oligonucleotide enrichment mix. A master mix can be made of the combined digests, water, 12× SSC, and 1% SDS, for ease of pipetting.
4. Cover each well with a drop of mineral oil (or use a heated lid function) and incubate in a thermal cycler at 98°C for 5 min and then at 56°C for 20 min.
5. When there are about 5 min left in the 56°C incubation, wash 50 μl of resuspended streptavidin-coated magnetic beads twice with 6× SSC (50 μl per wash). Capture the beads between washes on a Dynal MPC-S magnet. After the second wash, resuspend the beads in 50 μl of 6× SSC.
6. At the conclusion of the 56°C incubation step, change the thermal cycler to 45°C and add 10 μl of washed beads to each enrichment reaction. Incubate for 30 min at 45°C, mixing the beads in each reaction with a pipette tip (stirring and/or pipetting the solutions up and down repeatedly) about halfway through the incubation.
7. Capture the beads on a SPRIplate 96-Ring magnet for 3–5 min. During this time, set the thermal cycler to 50°C.

8. Remove and discard the supernatants and add 100 µl 2× SSC/0.1% SDS to each sample. Resuspend the beads by pipetting the solutions up and down repeatedly Incubate at 50°C for 5 min. Repeat this wash (steps 7 and 8) once more, for a total of two washes.
9. During the second magnetic capture above, set the thermal cycler to 95°C and add 50 µl of 0.5× AE buffer to each sample. Incubate at 95°C for 5 min. Capture beads on the SPRIplate 96-Ring magnet for 3–5 min and remove the supernatant to a clean microcentrifuge tube. Store samples at −20°C.
10. PCR-amplify each enrichment elution in a 50 µl total volume with Platinum *Taq* DNA polymerase. Each PCR reaction contains 36.5 µl water, 3 µl enriched DNA from the previous step, 5 µl 10× PCR buffer, 2 µl 50 mM magnesium chloride, 1 µl 10 mM dNTPs, 2 µl NP forward primer, and 0.5 µl (2.5 U) Platinum *Taq* polymerase. Cycle the reactions 35 times at 94°C for 50 s, 55°C for 45 s, and 72°C for 1 min.
11. Analyze 3 µl of each PCR on a 1% agarose gel. Ideally, one hopes to see a smear of PCR product, with few strong/discrete bands.
12. Combine reactions within each repeat class (di, tri, tet), purify with a QIAquick PCR purification kit, and elute with 32 µl of EB buffer.

### 3.2. Cloning of Enriched PCR Products

1. For each repeat class, combine 30 µl of enriched, PCR-amplified DNA with 4.6 µl of MBG-water, 4 µl of 10× NEBuffer 2, 0.4 µl of 100× BSA, and 1 µl (10 U) of *NheI*. Incubate at 37°C for 2 h.
2. Purify with a QIAquick PCR purification kit and elute with 40 µl of EB buffer. Determine the concentration with a spectrophotometer or fluorometer.
3. For each repeat class, combine 0.6 µl (60 ng) of *XbaI*-digested, dephosphorylated pUC19 (from Subheading 2.2), 130 ng of DNA from step 2, 2 µl of 10 mM ATP, 2 µl of 10× NEBuffer 2, 0.5 µl of T4 DNA ligase (200 cohesive end units), 0.2 µl of *NheI* (2 U) and MBG-water to a volume of 20 µl. Incubate at room temperature for at least 2 h.
4. Purify with a QIAquick PCR purification kit and elute with 30 µl of EB buffer.
5. Cast 90 mm LB agar plates with D-water containing 50 µg/ml ampicillin. You will need a plate for each experimental sample you want to transform, as well as a positive and negative control. After hardening, coat each plate with 25 µl of X-gal (50 mg/ml stock). Allow the X-gal to evaporate for about 1 h in a 37°C incubator, with the plate lid ajar.

6. Transform 16 μl of Electromax DH5α-E cells with 1 μl of purified ligation from step 4, above. Set the Eppendorf 2510 electroporator to 1,900 V. Use cuvettes with a 1 mm gap width and chill (place on ice while still in wrapper) prior to use. Transform 10 μl of cells with 1 μl intact (nonrecombinant) pUC19 (10 pg/ml) as a positive control. Transform 10 μl of cells with 1 μl water as a negative control. If you do not want to consume an electroporation cuvette, grow 10 μl of non-transformed cells in step 7, below. Either type of negative control will confirm the activity of the ampicillin in the plates (the drug should kill nontransformed cells, resulting in clear LB plates after overnight incubation in step 8).
7. Following electroporation, add 300 μl of room temperature SOC medium to each cuvette (or negative control) and flush cells out of the chamber by pipetting up and down repeatedly. Recover the mixture to a 14-ml polypropylene snap-cap tube and incubate in a shaking (225 rpm) 37°C water bath for 1 h, and then at 4°C for approximately 30 min.
8. Mix 2 μl of each experimental transformation with 98 μl of room temperature SOC medium; spread 20 μl of each mixture on a 90 mm LB/ampicillin/X-gal plate. Plate 20 μl, undiluted, of each positive and negative control. Incubate the plates overnight (18–20 h) at 37°C. Store the remaining transformations at 4°C.
9. Verify that (a) there is no growth on the negative control plate (proof that the ampicillin is killing nontransformed colonies), (b) all colonies on the positive control plate are blue (proof that X-gal is indicating nonrecombinant colonies), and (c) the majority of the colonies on the experimental plates are white (only recombinant colonies can harbor inserts with microsatellite loci). Estimate the volume of transformed cells needed to generate 1,400–1,800 total colonies (white plus blue) on each experimental plate. Cast six 150-mm LB/agar plates with 50 μg/ml ampicillin, two for each enrichment type. You may choose to cast additional 150-mm plates as backup for the next step. There is no need to add X-gal to the 150-mm plates.

### 3.3. Replication and Hybridization of Colonies with Repeats

1. Label each LB/agar plate with its ID, date, and enrichment type. For each enrichment transformation (di, tri, tet), combine the volume needed for 1,400–1,800 total colonies with SOC medium to a total volume of 100 μl. Mix gently and plate 50 μl onto each 150-mm LB/agar plate. Grow at 37°C overnight (18–20 h).
2. Place a 137-mm MagnaLift nylon transfer membrane onto each plate. It is best to slightly fold the membrane in the middle, align with the plate until it starts to moisten near the fold, then let each half slowly moisten toward each edge of the LB/

agar plate. Let the membrane stay in contact with the plate for 3–5 min (there is no detriment to letting the membrane stay on the plate for a few minutes longer than this).

3. With a new 18-gauge needle, make three or four asymmetric orientation holes through the membrane and LB/agar plate. Hold the membrane down with a pair of forceps as you withdraw the needle from each hole; otherwise, there is a risk of dislodging the membrane.
4. Remove each membrane and place colony side up onto 46×57 cm thick chromatography paper that has been folded in half. You should be able to get six of the 137-mm membranes onto one half of the folded chromatography paper sheet.
5. Incubate the original LB/agar plates at 37°C until the colonies are visible again. This should take 8–12 h but monitor the plate rejuvenation closely so that the colonies do not overgrow (and crowd each other). Store the LB plates at 4°C until they are needed to pick positive colonies (Subheading 3.4).
6. Fold the chromatography paper so that the membranes are covered and autoclave (5 min sterilization, 5 min drying on a "dry" or "flash" cycle). After autoclaving, place the membranes in an 80°C oven for 1 h. The membranes can then be stored at room temperature until hybridization.
7. Make 500 ml of membrane scrub buffer. Pour 250 ml of this into a plastic tray or round tub only slightly larger in area than each membrane. Wet each membrane one at a time by placing in the tray, with colony side up. Moisten a few Kimwipes in the tray, and wipe the colony side of each membrane with the Kimwipes; this step helps remove cellular debris and will not smear the colonies. Once wiped, place the membranes into a second tray with the remaining membrane scrub buffer. Pour off the buffer, leaving the membranes in the second tray.
8. Place three membranes colony side down against a 22 cm×22 cm oven mesh sheet, and the other three membranes colony side up. Roll up the membranes and sheet and put in a large (30 cm×3.5 cm) hybridization bottle. Add 35 ml of prehybridization buffer and incubate the bottle in a rotating oven at 50°C for 2–4 h. Make sure the filters unroll during rotation; if they roll up into a tighter tube, simply reverse the orientation of the bottle on the rotating rack. Incubate the remaining 15 ml of hybridization buffer in a disposable 50-ml screw cap centrifuge tube at 50°C.
9. Make a radiolabeled probe by combining (in a 0.2- or 0.5-ml tube) 4 μl MBG-water, 1 μl 10× T4 polynucleotide kinase buffer, 2 μl oligonucleotide probe solution (equal volumes of the five oligonucleotide mixes used for the enrichment step,

Subheading 2.1), 2 μl $^{33}$P-ATP (20 mCi), and 1 μl (10 U) T4 polynucleotide kinase. Cover with two drops of mineral oil and incubate at 37°C for 45 min.

10. Discard the prehybridization buffer from the bottle and add the entire labeled probe to the 15 ml of hybridization buffer, preheated to 50°C. Pour this into the bottle, cap, and incubate the bottle in a rotating oven at 50°C for 18–24 h.
11. Pour off and save the radioactive hybridization buffer into a glass bottle. To wash the membranes, make 500 ml of probe wash buffer. Wash the membranes three times in the hybridization bottle. Preheat the probe wash buffer in a microwave (be careful not to exceed 50°C) and use 25 ml of probe wash buffer per wash, incubating at 50°C for 10–15 min with the hybridization bottle rotating in the hybridization oven.
12. After the third wash in the hybridization bottle, remove the membranes and wash twice in a plastic tray set in a shaking water bath set to 50°C. Preheat 200 ml of probe wash buffer to 50°C and shake the membranes for 10–15 min per wash.
13. Air-dry the membranes on paper towels (colony side up), then tape to 35 × 43 cm pieces of thin cardboard (the spacers from the Kodak BioMax MR box work well here). Add some asymmetry to the membrane placement, and be careful to tape only the very edges of each filter with three or four small pieces of Scotch tape; $^{33}$P is a weak emitter and even a thin piece of tape will diminish signal on the X-ray film. Cover the entire sheet of taped membranes/cardboard with a layer of plastic wrap and expose to BioMax MR film in a metal film cassette for 1–2 days.
14. Develop the film with manual or automatic film processing, and use the faint outlines of each filter on the developed film to orient the film with its corresponding membranes taped to cardboard. Mark the orientation holes from each membrane onto the film with an indelible marker (you may need a magnifying glass and some backlighting to find all the holes) and label each membrane on the film as well.

### 3.4. Plasmid DNA Extraction from Positive Clones

1. Retrieve the 150-mm LB agar plates from step 4 in Subheading 3.3 and warm them at 37°C for 30 min. For each positive clone to be grown, dispense 400 μl of 2× YT buffer containing 50 μg/ml ampicillin into each well of a Thermo 2.2-ml square-well storage plate.
2. Align the warmed plate with its corresponding autoradiographic image. The colonies on the LB plate should unambiguously align with the developed spots (colonies) on the X-ray film.
3. With a small (10 μl) sterile pipette tip, touch a positive (corresponding to a dark spot on the film) bacterial colony on the

LB plate and drop into a unique well containing the 2× YT buffer. Leave the pipette tip in the Thermo plate to mark the wells that have been inoculated.

4. After the desired number of colonies has been transferred to the Thermo plate, remove the pipette tips from each well, being careful not to cross-contaminate the wells.
5. Cover the Thermo plate with a gas-permeable adhesive seal and grow cultures for approximately 17 h at 37°C, shaking at 250 rpm.
6. Extract the plasmid DNA from the Thermo plate with a CosMcPrep kit, following the kit protocols. The 400 μl of 2× YT is a half-sized culture; kit reagents should be scaled down accordingly).
7. Elute the plasmid DNA with 22 μl of RE1 buffer, transfer 20 μl of the elutions to a sterile PCR plate, cover with a drop of mineral oil, and store at −20°C (see Note 4).

### 3.5. Sanger Sequencing of Plasmid Clones and Data Analysis

1. In each well of a 96-well PCR plate, combine 2.6 μl MBG-water, 0.75 μl 5× ABI sequencing buffer (supplied with BigDye kit), 0.15 μl 10 μM M13 forward primer, 0.5 μl BigDye version 3.1 ready reaction mix, and 1 μl eluted plasmid DNA from step 7 in Subheading 3.4.
2. Cycle the sequencing reactions at 90°C for 2 min, then 35 cycles at 94°C for 50 s, 56°C for 20 s, and 60°C for 4 min.
3. Remove unincorporated dye-labeled terminators with CleanSEQ magnetic beads, elute with 37 μl of water and transfer 30 μl of the elution to a 96-well plate suitable for loading onto ABI 3100 or ABI 3730 Genetic Analyzers.
4. Trim vector and linker sequences and assemble sequences with suitable alignment software (CodonCode Aligner, SeqMan Pro are two examples), to determine which clones (if any) are similar or identical in sequence (no point in designing PCR primers independently to similar or identical sequences). Clones with long inserts (where the sequence quality may degrade before the entire insert is read or a microsatellite is encountered) can be resequenced from the other direction with the M13 reverse primer. Export/save sequences as fasta files.

### 3.6. Designing and Ordering Genotyping Primers

There are many commercial and open source programs for PCR primer design; we have successfully used PrimerSelect (DNAStar, Madison, WI), Primer 3 (Whitehead Institute and Howard Hughes Medical Institute), and BatchPrimer 3 (University of California, Davis). The three most important considerations when designing primers for genotyping microsatellites are (1) complete trimming of all vector and linker sequences from the sequence data, (2) avoiding potentially chimeric inserts (see Note 5), and (3) designing primers in regions of high read quality. Points 1 and 3 are (relatively) easily addressed through the assembly/alignment software; point 2 can present more cryptic problems (although chimeric inserts are typically the exception, not the rule, for the cloning protocols described here. The primer design protocol here utilizes the BatchPrimer3 software/Web interface (http://probes.pw.usda.gov/cgi-bin/batchprimer3/batchprimer3.cgi); this program will analyze and design primers for multiple sequences simultaneously.

1. On the BatchPrimer3 (v 1.0) home page, choose a Primer Design Server (for example, choose Primer Design Server 1, Albany).
2. In the "Choose Primer Type" window, choose "SSR Screening and primers".
3. Browse/upload or copy/paste the sequences of interest into the Input Sequences Window. Make sure both the "Pick left primer…"and "Pick right primer…" boxes are checked.
4. In the SSR Screenining window, select the Pattern types to be screened (Di, Tri, Tetra, etc.) and the Minimum number of SSR pattern repeats for each pattern type.
5. In the General Settings for Generic primers window, set the Product Sizes to 125 (min), 0 (opt) and 400 (max). If you would like the program to return more than one pair of primers, you can increase the Number to Return, although this will increase analysis time for large projects.
6. Reduce the Max Tm Difference box to 5.0 and the Max Primer size to 25 (if designing primers for three-primer PCR in 3.8). These parameters can be changed in subsequent runs, depending on the results of initial primer searches.
7. Leave all the other settings as defaults, verifying a setting of 50 for the Salt Concentration box.
8. Click on the "Pick Primers" button near the top of the page (to the right of the "Choose Primer type" pull down menu). The resulting Report has many options for viewing and saving the output from the primer design search. Saving the output as an excel file allows for rapid ordering of large numbers of primers from the IDT Web site.
9. Log in to the IDT Web site and under "Quick Select' choose to order your primers one at a time, ten per page, or by pasting an excel sheet. Be aware that not all modifications are available at all synthesis scales (for example, 5′ fluorescent dyes are not available at the 25 nmole scale, only at 100 nmole and larger).
10. Primers are shipped dry from IDT and should be diluted to 500 mM in 0.5× Qiagen AE buffer (Item 16, Subheading 2.1). This represents a 50× stock (the typical working stock for

primers is 10 mM). Concentrated stocks of primers can be stored frozen in 0.5× AE buffer at –20°C for at least a year; if one wishes to preserve more expensive (dye-labeled) primers for longer periods it is best to aliquot known amounts (10–100 nmoles) into multiple microcentrifuge tubes, dry in a rotary evaporator, and store at –20°C.

### *3.7. Primer Testing I: Two-Primer PCR*

In most cases, allele sizes at microsatellite loci are determined by PCR with a 5′-dye labeled primer, a reverse primer that is "pig-tailed" (15) by the addition of the sequence GTTTCTT to its 5′ end, and capillary electrophoresis to separate the fluorescently labeled products. The pig-tailed primer reduces PCR stutter and facilitates electrophoretic allele-size discrimination. Synthesizing PCR primers with 5′ fluorescent dyes is relatively expensive, and rarely done for untested loci without first exploring PCR success through less expensive options.

In the "two primer" testing method, primers found by design software are synthesized (by IDT or another commercial source) and tested on small numbers of DNA samples, and PCR products are analyzed on agarose gels. Loci exhibiting discrete bands have one primer resynthesized with a 5′-dye for genotyping. One advantage of this scenario (relative to testing by three-primer PCR, below) is that longer primers can be designed, if necessary (most companies require expensive purification techniques for primers above a certain length). Another advantage is that agarose electrophoresis is less expensive and time-consuming than capillary electrophoresis. One disadvantage is that agarose gels are poor indicators of both allelic stutter and polymorphism: it is possible to invest in 5′ dye-labeled primers that amplify messy or (more rarely) monomorphic PCR fragments upon capillary electrophoresis. This can be at least partially addressed by employing high-resolution agarose (Sigma #A4718, for example), or vertical polyacrylamide electrophoresis when analyzing the PCR products.

1. Using a Qiagen animal or plant DNA extraction kit, extract genomic DNA from a small number (3–5) of individuals from the taxon of interest.
2. For each microsatellite locus, set up PCRs (10 μl total volume) containing 6.9 μl MBG-water, 1 μl 10× PCR buffer, 0.4 μl 50 mM magnesium chloride, 0.2 μl forward primer, 0.2 μl reverse primer, 0.2 μl 10 mM dNTPs, and 0.1 μl (0.5 U) Platinum *Taq* polymerase.
3. Incubate PCR plate or tubes at 90°C for 2 min, then cycle at 94°C (denature) for 50 s, 55°C (anneal) for 45 s, and 70°C (extend) for 1 min. Repeat this cycling profile 35 times. Or perform a "touchdown" cycling protocol, with an initial elevated annealing tempertaure (for example, 60°C) for the first cycle that then drops one degree per cycle for the first seven or

eight cycles, then a constant (50°C) annealing temperature for the remaining 27 or 28 cycles. A touchdown profile like this may be better compromise when simultaneously attempting to amplify multiple primer pairs with variable annealing temperatures.

4. Analyze 3 μl of each PCR products by agarose electrophoresis. Loci that exhibit robust, discrete bands can have the forward primer resynthesized from IDT with an appropriate 5′ fluorescent dye for multiplex genotyping (see Subheading 3.9).

### 3.8. Primer Testing II: Three-Primer PCR

In this protocol (based on (16)), a 20-base "long tag" (for example. 5′-CGAGTTTTCCCAGTCACGAC-3′, but other sequences will work as well) is added to the 5′ end of either locus-specific primer; the other primer is "pig-tailed" as in Subheading 3.7. A third primer (a 6-FAM labeled long tag) is included with each pair of locus-specific primers. The primary advantage of this three-primer system is that a single dye-labeled long tag can be used to fluorescently label any locus of interest, for analysis by capillary electrophoresis. This allows for the ascertainment of both locus *quality* (presence/absence of allelic stutter and multiple PCR products) and *polymorphism* (allelic size differences) that may not be apparent upon agarose electrophoresis after two-primer PCR. The disadvantage is that at least one of the locus-specific primer sequences typically must be no more than 24 bases long (no more than 44 when the tag is added) to avoid expensive purification. This can often be achieved by simply choosing the shorter of the two primers found by the primer design software for long tag addition, or by limiting maximum primer lengths in the primer design parameter settings.

1. Using a Qiagen animal or plant DNA extraction kit, extract genomic DNA from a small number (3–5) of individuals from the taxon of interest.
2. For each microsatellite locus, set up PCRs (10 μl total volume) containing 6.9 μl MBG water, 1 μl 10× PCR buffer, 0.4 μl 50 mM magnesium chloride, 0.05 μl tagged forward primer, 0.2 μl reverse primer, 0.15 μl FAM tag, 0.2 μl 10 mM dNTPs, and 0.1 μl (0.5 U) Platinum *Taq* polymerase.
3. Incubate PCR plate or tubes at 90°C for 2 min, then cycle at 94°C (denature) for 50 s, 55°C (anneal) for 45 s, and 70°C (extend) for 1 min. Repeat this cycling profile 35 times. Or, perform a "touchdown" cycling protocol, with an initial elevated annealing temperture (for example, 60°C) for the first cycle that then drops one degree per cycle for the first seven or eight cycles, then a constant (50°C) annealing temperature for the remaining 27 or 28 cycles. A touchdown profile like this may be better compromise when simultaneously attempting to amplify multiple primer pairs with variable annealing temperatures.

4. Dilute PCR products in water. The dilution factor needs to be determined empirically and will likely have a locus-specific component, but 1:5 is a good starting point. Combine 1.5 μl of diluted PCR product with 18 μl Hi-Di Formamide and 0.2 μl LIZ-500 size standard. Collect fluorescent fragment data on 36 cm or 50 cm capillaries, following ABI protocols. Loci exhibiting discrete, variable alleles are candidates for resynthesis of forward primers with 5′ fluorescent dyes.

### 3.9. Genotyping by Multiplex PCR

One can collect data with the three-primer PCRs described above (in theory, one could synthesize four unique long tags, each with a different dye label, for multiplexing upon PCR or upon loading). But it is hard to beat the fluorescent intensities afforded by 5′ dyes, which allow one to combine multiple loci (multiple PCR primer pairs) in a single PCR reaction. As long as alleles of the same colors are nonoverlapping in size, they can be analyzed in the same capillary.

Multiplexing upon loading (separate PCR reactions for each locus that are then combined before electrophoresis and data collection) is a given when attempting to genotype large numbers of samples at multiple loci, but multiplexing upon PCR (combining multiple loci in a single PCR reaction) is the real time/money saver (consider that the ability to amplify even a pair of loci at once cuts your PCR effort in half). We have successfully used Qiagen Type-It Microsatellite PCR kits for multiplex PCR of up to ten loci in a single reaction.

After PCR, multiplex products are diluted in water (this needs to be determined empirically for each multiplex set, but a 1:15 dilution is a good starting point). Data are collected on ABI Genetic Analyzers, using either 36 cm or 50 cm capillary arrays. It is best to stay with one machine for the duration of a large study since allele size calls can vary quite a bit across different machines (and, to a lesser extent, temporally for the same machine). It is often a good idea to carry a "standard" (the same sample loaded across multiple runs) to monitor machine drift in calling alleles.

1. Using a Qiagen animal or plant DNA extraction kit, extract genomic DNA from the individual organisms of interest. Analyze a subset of samples on a spectrophotometer or fluorometer to determine a common dilution factor for the eluted DNAs that will give a concentration typically between 5 and 50 ng/ml. Dilute an aliquot of all samples by this dilution factor, and store the rest of the undiluted DNA sample at –20°C.
2. For PCR, follow the instructions in the kit handbook. Scale down reactions to 10 μl total volume. A typical reaction contains 1 μl RNase-free water (a kit component), 5 μl 2× Type-It Multiplex PCR Master Mix, 2 μl 5× Q solution, 1 μl 10× primer mix (2 μM each primer), and 1 μl DNA sample (5–50 ng).

3. Cycle samples with an initial activation step of 95°C for 5 min, followed by 28 cycles of 95°C for 30 s, 60°C (or 57°C, see kit handbook) for 90 s, 72°C for 30 s. After the 28th cycle is complete, perform a final extension at 60°C for 30 min.
4. Dilute PCR products 1:15 in MBG water. Combine 1.5 μl diluted PCR product with 18 μl Hi-Di Formamide and 0.2 μl LIZ-500 size standard. Collect fluorescent fragment data on 36-cm or 50-cm capillaries, following ABI protocols.
5. For best results, relative fluorescent units should be in the range of 500–2,000 for each locus, although alleles can be scored when they are outside of this range. Often, primer mixes have to be adjusted after initial runs (add less primer for the loci that fluoresce the strongest); the optimal dilution factor for the multiplex PCR usually needs to be adjusted as well.

## 4. Notes

1. The same pool of biotinylated oligonucleotides (oligos) is used to both enrich genomic DNA fragments for repeats and radioactively probe membranes replicated with bacterial colonies containing recombinant plasmids. These pools of different oligonucleotides should have melting temperatures that are highly similar; otherwise, certain oligos may not contribute to the either process. The Tm (annealing/melting temperature) of an oligo is largely a function of its length, G+C content, concentration of monovalent cations (usually sodium or potassium) in solution, and temperature of the medium. These oligos all have Tms around 65°C, as determined by the OligoAnalyzer tool on the IDT Web site.
2. A relatively small number of oligos can enrich and probe for a large number of unique repeats. Consider the enrichment/probe oligo $(GTA)_{8.33}$. This oligo will both enrich for and detect via radiolabeled hybridization the unique trimers GTA, TAG, AGT and their complements CAT, ATC, and TCA (during radiolabeled hybridization, both strands of DNA on the membrane are available to the oligo probes). For these reasons of "frame" and "complementarity," one could enrich for (and detect by radiolabeled hybridization) all 60 possible trimers (excluding homopolymers) with ten unique oligos. The same principles hold true for other repeat types as well.
3. The restriction enzymes *NheI* (used to trim the enriched PCR fragments in Subheading 3.2) and *XbaI* (used to digest the plasmid pUC19) each generate the same 4-base overhang (5′-CTAG-3′) that allows for efficient ligation of the genomic fragments to the vector. The original ds linker described by

Hamilton et al. (10) was called SNX, since it contained restriction enzyme sites for *StuI* and *NheI*, and *XmnI* was used to prevent the formation of linker–linker dimers. *XmnI*, a six-cutter, would also digest the genomic DNA fragments in the reaction, creating the possibility for *XmnI*+*BsaAI* or *XmnI*+*HincII* chimeric fragments after the ligation step. By redesigning the linker so that *PmeI* (an 8-cutter) is used to prevent the formation of linker dimers, this problem is minimized; there should be fewer *PmeI* sites in genomic DNA (relative to *XmnI*), by a factor of 16.

4. One could also PCR-amplify the insert DNAs from positive colonies with M13 primers that flank the *XbaI* cloning site of pUC19, and sequence these products. The sample prep is easier (colonies can be touched into 50 ml of 0.5× AE buffer and heated for a few minutes at 95°C to liberate the plasmid DNA from the cells), but the sequencing is less reliable. Sequences generated from these "boiling preps" often fail at the microsatellite repeat, since the PCR process often generates fragments that vary in length at the repeat itself. Problematic clones can be sequenced from both directions (with M13 forward and reverse primers) to obtain the necessary flanking sequence information; one has to decide whether the simplicity of the boiling prep is worth this extra sequencing effort.

5. Encountering an internal NP linker sequence in a Sanger read is a sure sign of a chimera; chimeric fragments generated by splicing are less common and a bit harder to detect (especially since *BsaAI* and *HincII* accept degenerate nucleotide positions in their respective recognition sites).

## References


1. Yinglei L and Fengzhu S (2003) The relationship between microsatellite slippage mutation rate and the number of repeat units. Mol Biol Evol **20**:2123–2131
2. Kauer MO, Dieringer D, and Schlötterer C (2003) A microsatellite variability screen for positive selection associated with the "out of Africa" habitat expansion of *Drosophila melanogaster*. Genetics **165**:1137–1148
3. Oda S, Maehara Y, Ikeda Y et al (2005) Two modes of microsatellite instability in human cancer: differential connection of defective DNA mismatch repair to dinucleotide repeat instability. Nucleic Acids Research **33**:1628–1636
4. Vinces MD, Legendre M, Caldara M et al (2009) Unstable tandem repeats in promoters confer transcriptional evolvability. Science **324**:1213–1216
5. Weber JL and Wong C (1993) Mutation of human short tandem repeats. Hum Mol Genet **2**:1123–1128
6. Primmer CR, Saino N, Møller AP et al (1996) Directional evolution in germline microsatellite mutations. Nat Genet **13**:391–393
7. Wierdl M, Dominska M, Petes TD (1997) Microsatellite instability in yeast: dependence on the length of the microsatellite. Genetics **146**:769–779
8. Schlötterer C (2000) Evolutionary dynamics of microsatellite DNA. Chromosoma **109**:365–371
9. Hamilton MB, Pincu EL, Fiore AD et al (1999) Universal linker and ligation procedures for construction of genomic DNA libraries enriched for microsatellites. BioTechniques **27**:500–507

10. Abdelkrim J, Robertson BC, Stanton J-AL, et al (2009) Fast, cost-effective development of species-specific microsatellite markers by genomic sequencing. BioTechniques **46**:185–192
11. Allentoft ME, Schuster SC, Holdaway RN et al (2008) Identification of microsatellites from an extinct moa species using high-throughput (454) sequence data. BioTechniques **46**:195–200
12. Castoe TA, Poole AW, Gu W et al (2009) Rapid identification of thousands of copperhead snake (*Agkistrodon contortrix*) microsatellite loci from modest amounts of 454 shotgun genome sequence. Mol Ecol Resour **10**:341–347
13. Csencsics D, Brodbeck S, Holderegger R (2010) Cost-effective, species-specific microsatellite development for the endangered Dwarf Bulrush (*Typha minima*) using next-generation sequencing technology. J Hered **101**: 789–793
14. Santana QC, Coetzee MPA, Steenkamp ET et al (2009) Microsatellite discovery by deep sequencing of enriched genomic libraries. BioTechniques **46**:217–223
15. Brownstein MJ, Carpten D, Smith JR (1996) Modulation of non-templated nucleotide addition by Taq DNA polymerase: primer modifications that facilitate genotyping. BioTechniques **20**:1004–1010
16. Schuelke, M (2000) An economic method for the fluorescent labeling of PCR fragments. Nature Biotechnology **18**:233–234

# Chapter 13

# Design of Custom Oligonucleotide Microarrays for Single Species or Interspecies Hybrids Using Array Oligo Selector

**Amy A. Caudy**

## Abstract

New technologies for DNA sequencing have made it feasible to determine the genome sequence of any organism of interest. This sequence is the resource required to create tools for downstream studies, including DNA microarrays. A number of vendors can produce DNA microarrays containing customer-specified sequences, allowing investigators to design and order arrays customized for any species of interest. Freely available, user-friendly computer programs are available for designing microarray probes. These design programs can be used to create probes that distinguish between two related genomes, allowing investigation of gene expression or gene representation in intra- or interspecies hybrids or in samples containing DNA from multiple species.

**Key words:** Microarray, Array CGH, Gene expression, Interspecies hybrids

## 1. Introduction

DNA microarrays have a large number of applications, including the quantification of gene expression, measurement of DNA copy number change, and genotyping (reviewed in ref. 1). The growing accessibility of whole-genome DNA sequencing makes it possible to plan genomic experiments in nearly any organism of interest. However, the throughput, expense, and availability of ultrahigh-throughput sequencing do not currently match the cost and accessibility of DNA microarrays for many users (see Note 1). Fortunately, with only a genome sequence and list of genes, it is now possible to design and purchase custom microarrays for use in expression or comparative genomic hybridization.

Many vendors offer custom DNA array synthesis. The technologies used by some vendors permit orders as small as a single array. For instance, Agilent Technologies synthesizes DNA directly

Virginie Orgogozo and Matthew V. Rockman (eds.), *Molecular Methods for Evolutionary Genetics*,
Methods in Molecular Biology, vol. 772, DOI 10.1007/978-1-61779-228-1_13, © Springer Science+Business Media, LLC 2011

on a glass slide by printing out each base on each array feature with an inkjet printer (2). Roche NimbleGen uses a photoactivated synthesis in which the location of each base is specified by the path of light reflected onto the array surface by digitally controlled micromirrors (3). In both of these manufacturing approaches, each slide is the result of a separate printing process, and so each array can be an independently designed set of sequences. Affymetrix uses a photolithographic manufacturing approach that has a high cost for initial design and setup, but a low incremental cost per array (4). This can be economical if a large number of identical arrays are required.

Although most array vendors provide microarray design tools for commonly used genomes, designing a microarray for nonstandard or unsupported genomes requires the use of specialized computer programs. In addition, designing a custom array provides flexibility for targeted uses, such as creating arrays for strains with significant divergence at the nucleotide level, or designing arrays that distinguish between orthologous genes to measure gene expression in interspecies hybrids (5, 6). This chapter describes the use of the freely available software Array Oligo Selector (7) for designing arrays that can be used for measuring either gene expression or DNA copy number. Instructions are provided for designing arrays that can distinguish species, including the appropriate controls to validate multispecies arrays. There are a variety of other software programs available for array design (systematically compared in (8)); the general principles and advice presented here should be useful even if a different program is used.

The Array Oligo Selector program consists of two scripts. The first, a probe generation script, outputs a list of all candidate probes for a set of target sequences. Then, for each of the candidate probes, the next most similar sequence is identified in the genome, and the binding energy of the probe with this related sequence is calculated. In addition, the first Array Oligo Selector script calculates the self-hybridization potential of the probe, the GC content of the probe, and the lossless compression score (a measure of sequence complexity). These measurements of probe uniqueness and hybridization potential form the input for the second probe selection script, which identifies the best scoring probe for each target sequence.

The Array Oligo Selector software compares candidate regions from the genes file to all sequences present in the "genome" file, ultimately selecting the probes that are the most unique in comparison to the compilation of all sequences. By providing two or more genomes as a background set, Array Oligo Selector can identify probes that are as unique as possible in all genomes. If only a single-species input is provided for background comparison, it is possible that selected probe sequences are present in multiple genomes.

## 2. Materials

1. Genome sequence of your organism of interest in FASTA format (see Note 2). The genome sequence does not need to be entirely complete; a partially assembled genome as a list of "contigs" is adequate for the design of useful arrays (see Note 3).
2. Gene sequences for your organism of interest in a FASTA format (see Note 4). These sequences could be the result of purely computational prediction, the output of EST/cDNA sequencing, or a combination of efforts. For design of expression arrays, the gene sequences must be in the sense orientation so that the designed probes are compatible with RNA labeling protocols. The methods for both the "direct" labeling of cDNA and the "cRNA" approach to RNA labeling yield nucleic acids labeled that correspond to the antisense strand of transcripts. (If the array will be used only for hybridization of genomic DNA, both strands are labeled and the strand represented on the array will not affect the results). If the intended use of the array is CGH or chromatin IP rather than gene expression, complete coverage of the genome can be achieved by dividing the genome sequence into windows of the desired length (see Note 5). These tiled windows are then presented to Array Oligo Selector as the "genes."
3. (Optional) If designing an interspecies array, obtain the genome sequence of the other organism(s) of interest in FASTA format. Make a combined file containing the whole-genome sequences of all of the organisms.
4. Login access to a Unix/LINUX server (available at nearly any university; contact your system administrator for information). It is also possible to run the program on a Mac OS (see Note 6).
5. Information on target probe length and total number of probes, obtained from custom array manufacturer.

## 3. Methods

### 3.1. Microarray Probe Design

1. Download the current version of Array Oligo Selector from http://sourceforge.net/projects/arrayoligosel/ (see Note 7).
2. Transfer the downloaded Array Oligo Selector file to your Unix system. For most systems, you will use an sftp (secure file transfer protocol) program to upload the file. Your system administrator can recommend a free sftp client to transfer files from your computer to the Unix system.

3. On the Unix system, type the following command to extract the compressed archive, creating a new directory, ArrayOligoSelector, containing the files (change the "N" placeholders in the command to match the version of the downloaded file):

   ```
   tar -zxvf ArrayOligoSelectorN.N.N.tar.gz
   ```

4. Enter the newly extracted software directory (`cd` means change directory):

   ```
   cd ArrayOligoSelector
   ```

5. Test your installation of the program using the files included in the install. Run the following test command for the probe generation script (the parameters are described in detail below), which generates candidate probe sequences and calculates the uniqueness, complexity, and binding energy of the probes:

   ```
   ./Pick70_script1_contig test_input test_genome
   70 yes blat
   ```

   If there is an error of "`command not found`," try adding the directory to your executable path, which is the list of directories that have programs that can be run on the system. First, locate your directory within the Unix system by typing `pwd` (a command that returns the present working directory). This will give an output something like `/username/ArrayOligoSelector`. Add this location to your path by typing the following command (replace the location below with the output of pwd on your system):

   ```
   PATH=$PATH:/username/ArrayOligoSelector
   ```

6. The program will run, printing output to the screen as each sequence in the input file is split into all possible 70 nucleotide fragments, and these are compared to the genome sequence. The program will finish with the notification "`OLIGO program has successfully finished. The output files are output0, output1,…`" If this does not appear, delete the Array Oligo Selector directory and associated files and repeat the download and install process.

7. Test the second script, oligo selection, by typing the following command:

   ```
   ./Pick70_script2 28 70 1 -30 20 AT 0.1
   ```

8. Run `Pick70_script_1_contig`, the probe generation script, on your data, altering the command as indicated:

   (a) The fasta file of your genes should be inserted as "genes."

   (b) The fasta file of your genome should be listed as "genome." If designing probes to distinguish between two genomes, the "genome" file should be a composite fasta file combining both genomes. (You can generate this composite genome by running the following command to concatenate separate genome files: `cat genome1.fa genome2.fa > genome_composite.fa`)

(c) For design of Agilent arrays, the maximum probe length for standard synthesis is 60 nucleotides. If your vendor or experimental plans require a different length, replace the 60 with the appropriate integer to design probes of that length.

(d) The argument "yes" or "no" is used to exclude lowercase letters in the fasta file from design. Unless you have used some other program to mask specific regions of the genome, chose "no" so that all sequences are included in the design (see Note 8).

(e) The last argument dictates the algorithm used for alignment of each candidate probe from the genes file to the genome. It can be `blast`, `blat`, or `gfclient`. The command `blat` is approximately 100 times more rapid than `blast`, while `blast` is capable of recognizing homology between more distant mismatches. In practice, very similar probes pose the greatest risk of cross-hybridization, and we have found `blat` yields completely satisfactory results. `gfclient` requires significant configuration. Linux executables are provided by the ArrayOligoSelector.tar.gz file; use on other platforms will require installation of the relevant alignment application.

A typical command would be:

```
./Pick70_script1_contig genes genome 60 no blat
```

9. Wait for the probe generation script to finish (this is typically several hours on most systems, and is dependent on genome/transcriptome sizes and available computing resources). The notification of successful completion will appear as mentioned in step 6. For Unix/Linux systems, the use of the program `screen` (http://www.gnu.org/software/screen/) will allow you to logout and leave Array Oligo Selector running.

10. Run the oligo selection script, with the appropriate command line options for your data (see Note 9). Note that the output of `Pick70_script1_contig` (written to files `output0`, `output1`, etc.) is not affected by the oligo selection, and the oligo selection program can be run repeatedly. The program will overwrite the contents of the output `oligo_fasta` file; previous results can be saved by renaming this file.

(a) The first input is the target GC percentage, expressed as a number, such as 37.5 for 37.5%. Probe performance depends on GC percentage; a target percentage of 35–45% has been observed to yield probes with high specificity for their targets (9).

(b) The length of the oligo must match the length used in the first script, expressed as an integer.

(c) The number of oligos selected per gene. The choice of this value depends on the number of features desired on the array. For instance, when designing probes for 18,000 genes for an array containing 40,000 features, there would be sufficient space on the array to design two probes per gene, allowing measurement of two probes per gene.

A typical command would be:

```
./Pick70_script2 37.5 60 2
```

11. When the oligo selection script completes, notifications will appear for any genes failing the selection process. The output will indicate "`the following genes were not designed for oligos because their sequences have too much low complexity regions,`" followed by a list of genes failing the selection process due to low complexity sequence. It is worth noting any such genes, to examine them and attempt redesign if possible. Any other genes failing the selection process are written to a file named "nodesign" that appears in the ArrayOligoSelector directory. Frequently, these are genes that have very similar paralogs within the genome (or similar orthologs in the second genome, for the design of dual-species arrays). In other cases, these may be genes with unusual GC content. If these genes are of interest for the array design, Array Oligo Selector can be rerun with just this subset of genes, with relaxed parameters for probe uniqueness (see Note 10). If less stringent design parameters are used for a subset of probes, this should be noted in subsequent array analysis as these probes may be more likely to reflect cross-hybridization.
12. The probe sequences will have been written to a file called "`oligo_fasta`." The location of each probe within the gene is indicated by a number appended at the end of the sequence name. For example, _40 indicates that the probe sequence begins at nucleotide 40 in the fasta sequence. Provide this file to the array vendor for production of the custom array.

### 3.2. Validating Probe Specificities with Hybrid Organisms

1. To identify probes that cross-hybridize in hybrid organisms (or mixtures of organisms), obtain DNA from both inbred, homozygous parents.
2. For two-color based array platforms, label the DNA from one parent with one color and the DNA from the other parent with the opposite color. Hybridize these samples together to the same array. The majority of probes should be either one color or the other, with cross-hybridizing probes showing hybridization from both parents. For single color array platforms, hybridize the DNA from each parent to separate arrays and compare the probe intensities; specific probes will have significant

hybridization intensities on one array and low intensities on the other.

3. Prepare a list of probes to use in subsequent analyses of hybrid data, excluding those showing significant cross-hybridization. Appropriate cutoffs for cross-hybridization depend on the intended application of the data; typically, a four to tenfold difference in hybridization will allow sensitive differentiation of the data. Cross-hybridization between probes depends on the degree of complementarity and is best described by the number of contiguous complementary bases shared by two sequences (10). In practice, Array Oligo Selector outputs the most divergent probes for a sequence of interest. For genomes with low divergence, other methods are available for designing SNP-specific probes (see Chapter 10, this volume).

## 4. Notes

1. At the time of this writing, the cost per sample, including library prep, for one lane of RNA sequencing using the Illumina technology is approximately $1200. By contrast, the cost per sample for an Agilent microarray, including labeling, is approximately $250 for an array with 44,000 sequences, and approximately $150 for an array with 15,000 sequences represented. In addition, the bioinformatics tools and expertise for analysis of array data are more mature than the tools for analysis of sequence data. Also, if the desired application is array CGH, sequence coverage adequate to detect copy number variation or the presence/absence of genes can require many lanes of sequence depending on genome size, while the same information can be acquired from a single array.
2. The fasta format consists of a header, demarcated with a > symbol at the beginning, on the first line. The sequence data begins on the second line and continues until the next instance of >, indicating the header at the beginning of a new sequence.
3. If only gene sequences are available, these can be used as the genome file. In this case, the same parameter will be used for both the gene and the genome filename.
4. The completeness of the gene file is of paramount importance. Any gene missing from the target file will be absent from the array design. Time invested in hand-checking genes of particular interest can prevent the disappointment of a favorite gene being left off of the arrays designed.
5. The optimum size for tiling applications varies depending on the intended application. For chromatin immunoprecipitation, the average length of genomic fragments following shearing is

typically 400–500 bp. Consequently, to provide several probes per fragment, windows of 100–300 bp are typical. For use in array CGH, the length of target regions depends on the desired resolution. When an array is used for a mapping experiment, a window length of 10–50 kbp might be appropriate.

6. If running Array Oligo Selector on a Macintosh, the blast package from NCBI needs to be installed and made executable by adding it to the system path. Array Oligo Selector expects an older version of blast, 2.2.10. This version can be downloaded from NCBI at ftp://ftp.ncbi.nlm.nih.gov/blast/executables/release/2.2.10/. Also, several lines in the Python code need to be updated to use current system calls. In short, using the pre-compiled executables on a Linux system is preferable for most users of Array Oligo Selector.
7. To learn more about Array Oligo Selector, view the README.html file included in the downloaded software package. To open this file, decompress the Array Oligo Selector file on your desktop/laptop machine (a wide variety of programs can uncompress this type of file; on a Mac, double-clicking the compressed file will be sufficient to open it.) Use File/Open in a Web browser to open the README.html file in the Array Oligo Selector folder.
8. Array Oligo Selector can be set to ignore lowercase sequences. This option can be used to mask repetitive regions of the genome with a tool such as RepeatMasker (11), which compares the genome sequence to a library of repetitive elements and outputs a version of the genome where regions similar to repetitive elements are converted to lowercase letters. RepeatMasker can be used with known repetitive elements, or the user can provide a custom list of repetitive element sequences.
9. Four additional options are available for the second Array Oligo Selector script, which chooses oligonucleotides for each gene. Following the first three required inputs (target GC percentage, oligo length, and number of oligos per gene), the options are a user-defined binding energy cutoff, and the bases, length, and tolerance for simple nucleotide repeats. The binding energy is calculated from the theoretical energy of binding between the probe and its next-most-similar sequence (as identified by `blat` or `blast` comparison) in the genome. If the user does not provide an energy cutoff for this binding parameter, a default cutoff is defined as the top (least stable) 5% of binding energies for probes for that sequence. Using this default metric is recommended, because it flexibly alters the binding energy cutoff for the group of probes targeting each individual sequence. This flexibility permits more stringent probe selection when the available probes have less similarity to the genome. The masking sequences can be used to exclude stretches of sequence with specific nucleotide compositions. For example, to exclude

sequences with more than 20 bp of AT dinucleotide pairs and less than 10% of non-AT nucleotides, the input should be 20 AT 0.1. N can be used as a masking sequence, allowing the removal of probes containing ambiguous sequences.

10. If sequences fail the selection process, the design can be rerun using relaxed parameters. Adjusting the binding energy cutoff (see Note 9) by increasing its value or adjusting the target GC percentage typically results in selected probes. In cases of extremely similar genes in two genomes, Array Oligo Selector can be rerun using just one genome as background. Such probes are very likely to cross-hybridize. However, the benefit of the information gained from a probe, even if the signal represents cross-hybridization, is typically preferred to blinding the experiment to both paralogs entirely.

## Acknowledgments

Maitreya Dunham's original design of *Saccharomyces bayanus* probes for a dual species *S. bayanus–S. cerevisiae* array was the original source of experience and insight for several subsequent generations of custom oligonucleotide arrays. John Matese provided helpful guidance on the use of Array Oligo Selector. The students and teaching staff of QCB301, Experimental Project Laboratory gave useful feedback on course exercises using Array Oligo Selector. Many thanks are due to Adam Rosebrock for thoughtful comments on this manuscript.

### References

1. Dufva M (2009) Introduction to microarray technology. Methods Mol Biol **529**:1–22
2. Blanchard A, Kaiser R, Hood L (1996) High-density oligonucleotide arrays. Biosensors and bioelectronics **11**:687–690
3. Singh-Gasson S, Green RD, Yue Y et al (1999) Maskless fabrication of light-directed oligonucleotide microarrays using a digital micromirror array. Nat Biotechnol **17**:974–978
4. Pease AC, Solas D, Sullivan EJ et al (1994) Light-generated oligonucleotide arrays for rapid DNA sequence analysis. Proc Natl Acad Sci USA **91**:5022–5026
5. Horinouchi T, Yoshikawa K, Kawaide R (2010) Genome-wide expression analysis of *Saccharomyces pastorianus* orthologous genes using oligonucleotide microarrays. J Biosci Bioeng **11**:602–607
6. Muller L, McCusker J (2009) A multispecies-based taxonomic microarray reveals interspecies hybridization and introgression in *Saccharomyces cerevisiae*. FEMS Yeast Research **9**:143–152
7. Bozdech Z, Zhu J, Joachimiak MP et al (2003) Expression profiling of the schizont and trophozoite stages of *Plasmodium falciparum* with a long-oligonucleotide microarray. Genome Biol **4**:R9
8. Sophie L, Florence C, Stephane L (2009) An evaluation of custom microarray applications: the oligonucleotide design challenge. Nucleic Acids Res **37**:1726–1739
9. Sharp A, Itsara A, Cheng Z et al (2007) Optimal design of oligonucleotide microarrays for measurement of DNA copy-number. Hum Mol Genet **16**:2770
10. Chen Y, Chou CC, Lu X et al (2006) A multivariate prediction model for microarray cross-hybridization. BMC Bioinformatics **7**:101
11. Smitl A, Hubley R, Green P (1996–2010) RepeatMasker Open-3.0. http://www.repeatmasker.org

# Part IV

## Obtaining Candidate Gene Sequences

# Chapter 14

# Identification of Homologous Gene Sequences by PCR with Degenerate Primers

**Michael Lang and Virginie Orgogozo**

## Abstract

Degenerate primers are mixtures of similar oligonucleotides that are used in a PCR, so-called degenerate PCR, to amplify unknown DNA sequences, typically coding sequences of genes. Degenerate primers are designed based on sequence data of related and already sequenced gene homologs. This method is useful for identifying new members of a gene family or orthologous genes from different organisms where genomic information is not available. We describe here how to design degenerate primers, set up the PCR (with genomic DNA or cDNA as a template), clone the resulting PCR fragments, and sequence them. Since this method only yields partial coding sequences, complete gene sequences must then be achieved by other approaches such as inverse PCR (see Chapter 16), 5′ RACE, 3′ RACE, or circular RACE (see Chapter 15).

**Key words:** PCR, Degenerate primers, Degenerate PCR, Homologous genes, Cloning, Partial coding sequences, Multiple alignments

## 1. Introduction

When testing whether a candidate gene is responsible for a given evolutionary change or when examining the evolution of a gene of interest across several species, one might want to recover gene sequences from organisms where genomic information is not available.

If the organism of interest is very closely related to a species with available sequence information, the gene might simply be amplified by PCR and sequenced using oligonucleotides designed on the data of the known sequence. Unfortunately, synonymous mutations are frequent, and a single-nucleotide change in the region where the specific oligonucleotide is supposed to anneal is often sufficient to prevent correct primer annealing and PCR product formation.

If the budget is significant, a fast and prolific approach is to sequence the entire species' genome or transcriptome (see Chapters 5–8), with the hope that the gene of interest will be part of the

Virginie Orgogozo and Matthew V. Rockman (eds.), *Molecular Methods for Evolutionary Genetics*,
Methods in Molecular Biology, vol. 772, DOI 10.1007/978-1-61779-228-1_14, © Springer Science+Business Media, LLC 2011

sequence data. However, if the gene of interest must be sequenced from multiple species, or if budget or time is limited, other classical methods do exist.

If the DNA sequence is known only from one related species, then cloning techniques involving preparation and screening of genomic libraries should be considered. Nowadays, with the ever-growing sequence data, sequences of homologous genes from multiple related species are often available. One can, thus, use degenerate PCR to amplify similar sequences in related species. First, sequences of the protein of interest from multiple related species are aligned to search for conserved regions. Then, degenerate oligonucleotides (i.e., a mixture of similar but not identical primers) are designed to allow the amplification of part of the gene of interest in related species by PCR. The template can be genomic DNA (PCR) or cDNA prepared from RNA (RT-PCR). Then, PCR fragments are cloned into PCR cloning vectors and are finally sequenced. This method only yields partial coding sequences. Complete gene sequences are easily achieved by other approaches such as inverse PCR (see Chapter 16), 5′ RACE, 3′ RACE, or circular RACE (see Chapter 15). In this chapter, we describe the design of degenerate oligonucleotides, the degenerate PCR itself, PCR fragment cloning, and sequencing.

## 2. Materials

### 2.1. Design of Degenerate Oligonucleotides

1. DNA sequence editor, e.g., BioEdit (Windows) (1), SeaView (Windows, Mac, Linux) (2).
2. Multiple alignment program, e.g., ClustalW, Mafft, DialignTX, Muscle, PROBCONS, T-Coffee (3–8).
3. Online primer design program to check for internal stability and dimers of primer pairs, e.g., Perlprimer (9).

### 2.2. Degenerate PCR

1. GoTaq Green Master Mix (Promega).
2. Genomic DNA or cDNA.
3. Forward degenerate oligonucleotide (10 μM).
4. Reverse degenerate oligonucleotide (10 μM).
5. PCR-grade $ddH_2O$.
6. Thermocycler, e.g., Gene Amp 2700 (Applied Biosystems).
7. Gel Electrophoresis system.
8. Gel-Electrophoresis-grade agarose (e.g., Promega).
9. DNA Molecular weight standard, e.g., 1 kb DNA ladder (Promega).

10. Gel Electrophoresis Buffer, e.g., TBE (89 mM Tris–borate, 2mM EDTA, pH 8.3) or TAE (40 mM Tris–acetate, 1 mM EDTA, pH 7.6).

#### 2.3. PCR Cloning and Sequencing

1. pGEM-T Easy PCR cloning kit (Promega).
2. JM109 competent cells (Promega).
3. SOC medium (Invitrogen).
4. LB-Agar plates containing 100 μg/ml ampicillin, with 100 μl of 100 mM IPTG and 20 μl of 50 mg/ml X-Gal spread over the surface for blue/white screening.
5. Bacterial incubator shaker set up at 37°C.
6. LB Broth containing ampicillin (50 μg/ml).
7. GoTaq Green Master Mix (Promega).
8. SP6 primer (ATTTAGGTGACACTATAG), 10 μM.
9. T7 primer (TAATACGACTCACTATAGGG), 10 μM.
10. PCR-grade $ddH_2O$.
11. Thermocycler, e.g., Gene Amp 2700 (Applied Biosystems).
12. Gel Electrophoresis system.
13. Gel-Electrophoresis-grade agarose (e.g., Promega).
14. DNA Molecular weight standard, e.g., 1 kb DNA ladder (Promega).
15. Glycerol (autoclaved).
16. TBE buffer or TAE buffer (see Subheading 2.2).
17. Plasmid Mini Kit I (E.Z.N.A, Omega bio-tek).

## 3. Methods

#### 3.1. Design of Degenerate Primers

The design of degenerate primers is probably the most crucial factor for the success of the experiment. Designing degenerate primers is a compromise between increased sequence ambiguities and sufficient sequence specificity. The more degenerate the primers, the more likely they will anneal to the sites of interest. However, a gain in degeneracy will also increase the likelihood that they anneal to nonspecific sites, raising background amplification.

1. Download as many DNA sequences as possible of the gene of interest from the DNA sequence databases (NCBI, UCSC browser, ENSEMBL, etc.) (10–12).
2. Gather all the protein or DNA sequence data within a single sequence file using a DNA sequence editor.
3. Translate DNA sequences to protein sequences with the DNA sequence editor.

4. Align protein sequences with a multiple alignment program (see Note 1).
5. Label each conserved amino-acid position in the alignment with its corresponding degeneracy (use Table 1).

**Table 1**
**The standard genetic code, with degenerate sequences described using nomenclature recommended by the International Union of Biochemistry (14). Note that a few species have evolved genetic code differences (15)**

| Amino acid | Code | Codon triplets (5′-3′) | Corresponding degenerate sequence | Degeneracy of the corresponding sequence |
|---|---|---|---|---|
| Serine | S | TCA, TCC, TCG, TCT<br>AGC, AGT | WSN | 16 |
| Arginine | R | CGA, CGC, CGG, CGT<br>AGA, ACG | MGN | 8 |
| Leucine | L | CTA, CTC, CTG, CTT<br>TTA, TTG | YTN | 8 |
| Alanine | A | GCA, GCC, GCG, GCT | GCN | 4 |
| Glycine | G | GGA, GGC, GGG, GGT | GGN | 4 |
| Proline | P | CCA, CCC, CCG, CCT | CCN | 4 |
| Threonine | T | ACA, ACC, ACG, ACT | ACN | 4 |
| Valine | V | GTA, GTC, GTG, GTT | GTN | 4 |
| Isoleucine | I | ATA, ATC, ATT | ATH | 3 |
| Asparagine | N | AAC, AAT | AAY | 2 |
| Aspartic acid | D | GAC, GAT | GAY | 2 |
| Cysteine | C | TGC, TGT | TGY | 2 |
| Glutamic acid | E | GAA, GAG | GAR | 2 |
| Glutamine | Q | CAA, CAG | CAR | 2 |
| Histidine | H | CAC, CAT | CAY | 2 |
| Lysine | K | AAA, AAG | AAR | 2 |
| Phenylalanine | F | TTC, TTT | TTY | 2 |
| Tyrosine | Y | TAC, TAT | TAY | 2 |
| Methionine | M | ATG | ATG | 1 |
| Tryptophan | W | TGG | TGG | 1 |
| Terminator | . | TAA, TAG, TGA | TRR | 4 |

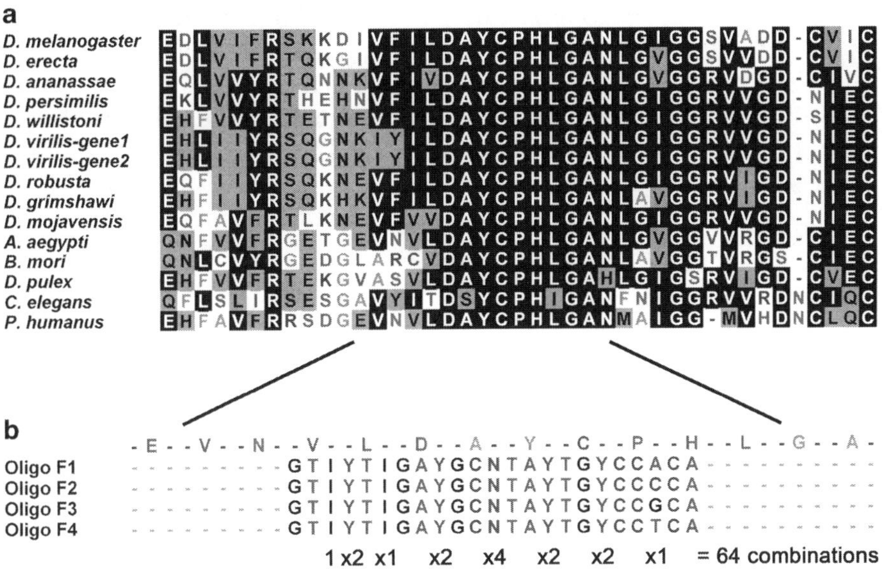


Fig. 1. Primer design in a conserved region of the Neverland protein. (**a**) Alignment of partial Neverland sequences from some insect species, *Daphnia pulex*, and *Caenorhabditis elegans*. (**b**) Primer design of one forward degenerate primer to amplify *Neverland* homologs in other insect species. Four degenerate primers are designed to reduce degeneracy in the 3′ end. The number of oligonucleotide combinations is calculated by multiplying the numbers of possible sequences at each position.

6. Choose regions of 7–8 amino acids with the lowest total number of corresponding DNA sequence combinations, i.e., with the lowest degeneracy, for primer annealing sites (see Fig. 1 as an example). The length of the expected amplicon should be between 200 bp and 1 kb (see Note 2). Sometimes, it is more judicious to choose regions with less conserved amino acids whose degeneracy is low than regions with highly conserved amino acids whose degeneracy is high. In general, avoid regions with arginine (R), leucine (L) or serine (S) amino acids and favor regions with methionine (M) or tryptophane (W). Since most codons encoding a particular amino acid are often identical at their first and second position, include these two positions if possible into the 3′ end region covered by the primers. Each degenerate primer should be approximately 20–23 nucleotides long.
7. In our hands, primers with 128-fold degeneracy or less have been more successful than primers with higher degeneracy (see Note 3). If no region with such a low degeneracy can be found, try to design two or more pools of primers over a particular stretch of codons. Each pool will have a lower degeneracy than a single pool including all of the same codons. The pools are then used separately to carry out PCR reactions (see Note 4).
8. If step 7 still does not yield a sufficiently low degeneracy, include inosine (I) at primer positions where any of the four bases might be required. Each use of inosine can, thus, reduce the degeneracy fourfold and, thus, the number of combinations of different

oligonucleotide variants (see Note 3). Inosine is a purine base that forms stable base pairings with adenine, thymine, and cytosine. However, possible I:G mismatches may hamper successful PCR amplification, unless exact base pairing at other positions in the primer can overcome the mismatch. Therefore, try to avoid inosine in the last five nucleotide positions at the 3′ end of the degenerate primer. Try also not to include more than three inosines in a degenerate primer because increasing the number of inosines raises the likelihood of nonspecific PCR product amplification and I:G mismatches. Most oligonucleotide synthesis facilities can make inosine-containing oligonucleotides.

9. Try also to design primers with at least three nondegenerate nucleotides at their 3′ end, to limit nonspecific PCR amplification. Repeat steps 6–8 if necessary.
10. Use the degenerate base code shown in Table 2 to write both degenerate primer sequences. Using the sequence editor program, reverse complement the degenerate sequence located most 3′ in the gene as this will form the reverse primer.

**Table 2**
**Single letter codes for nucleic-acid bases (14)**

| Symbol | Base |
|---|---|
| G | Guanine |
| A | Adenine |
| T | Thymine |
| C | Cytosine |
| I | Inosine |
| R | G or A |
| Y | T or C |
| M | A or C |
| K | G or T |
| S | G or C |
| W | A or T |
| H | A or C or T |
| B | G or T or C |
| V | G or C or A |
| D | G or A or T |
| N | G or A or T or C |

11. Examine both oligonucleotides with a primer evaluation program to check for dimerization and hairpin formation. The melting temperatures of the two primers should preferentially be similar.
12. Order both degenerate primers from an oligonucleotide synthesis facility, using standard purification.

### 3.2. Degenerate PCR

Degenerate PCR can use either genomic DNA or cDNA as a template. Genomic DNA has the advantage that all members of a gene family are present in equimolar amounts and that genomic DNA is easily prepared from any sample. However, the obvious disadvantage is that introns may disrupt primer sites, or may create a long PCR product that it is not amplified efficiently relative to shorter nonspecific PCR products. cDNA templates, although harder to obtain, can overcome this problem because desired PCR products should be of a known size.

Genomic DNA can be extracted manually or with commercial kits (e.g., DNeasy Blood & Tissue kit, QIAGEN). Protocols for genomic DNA preparation are described in Chapters 16 and 23. Preparation of cDNA involves RNA extraction and reverse-transcription (see Chapters 6, 15, 17 and 18 for detailed protocols).

1. Prepare a mix containing:

   25–50 ng of genomic DNA or cDNA

   12.5 µl of GoTaq Green Master Mix (see Note 5)

   0.75 µl of the10 mM stock solution of forward degenerate primer

   0.75 µl of the 10 mM stock solution of reverse degenerate primer

   $ddH_2O$ to bring the final reaction volume to 25 µl.
2. Mix gently and incubate in a PCR thermocycler with the following program: initial denaturation at 94°C for 2 min, 35 cycles of (denaturation at 94°C for 30 s, primer annealing at 47°C for 30 s, extension at 72°C for 1 min) and final extension at 72°C for 5 min.
3. Analyze 5 µl of the degenerate PCR on a 1.5% agarose gel. If a smear or several bands are observed, try increasing annealing temperature to reduce nonspecific band production. If no band is observed, try lower annealing temperatures (see Note 6).

### 3.3. PCR Cloning and Sequencing

Degenerate primers can usually not be used for direct sequencing of the PCR fragments because they generate multiple overlapping peaks in the chromatogram. Therefore, PCR products must be cloned into a plasmid vector and the primers used for sequencing should anneal to the insert-flanking vector sequence (see Note 7). Cloning of PCR products is highly simplified by a variety of available kits.

Usually, a molar ratio of insert:vector DNA of 1:1 to 3:1 is optimal for PCR cloning. PCR products of 1 kb or less can be easily cloned into the pGEM-T Easy vector with the following protocol.

1. Set up a 5 μl-cloning reaction in a 1.5-ml or 2-ml tube:

   1.5 μl of fresh nonpurified PCR product (see Note 8)

   2.5 μl of 2× ligation buffer (vortex before use)

   0.5 μl of pGEM-T Easy vector solution (50 ng)

   0.5 μl of T4 DNA ligase.
2. Mix very gently with the pipet tip and incubate overnight at 4°C (see Note 9).
3. Defrost JM109 competent cells on ice.
4. Add 40 μl of competent JM109 bacteria to each cloning reaction. Do not mix up and down.
5. Incubate for 20 min on ice.
6. Put LB-agar Petri plates with Amp, IPTG, and X-gal at room temperature (one per transformation mix).
7. Heat-shock the cloning reaction and bacteria at 42°C in a stationary water bath for exactly 45 s and then chill the mix rapidly on ice for 2 min.
8. Add 250 μl of SOC medium and close the tube tightly.
9. Shake tubes horizontally at 37°C for 1 h to 1 h 30 min at 200–250 rpm.
10. Spread 200 μl of the transformation mix onto the plates.
11. Incubate plates overnight at 37°C for colony growth.
12. If plasmid DNA preparations are desired, then follow steps 18–34. If the only desired result is the PCR fragment sequence(s), then follow steps 13–17, in which inserts will be amplified by PCR and directly sent for sequencing.
13. Prepare the following PCR mix (for each tube) (see Note 10):

    12.5 μl of GoTaq Green Master Mix

    11 μl of $ddH_2O$

    0.75 μl of the T7 primer solution

    0.75 μl of the SP6 primer solution.
14. Isolate single white clones with sterile toothpicks or pipette tips and inoculate the PCR mix.
15. Incubate in a PCR thermocycler with the following program: initial denaturation at 94°C for 2 min, 35 cycles of (denaturation at 94°C for 30 s, primer annealing at 50°C for 30 s, extension at 72°C for 1 min) and final extension at 72°C for 5 min.

16. Analyze 5 μl of the PCR on a 1.5% agarose gel. Make sure that a single band is observed. If not, adjust PCR conditions.
17. Send the unpurified PCR product directly for sequencing (see Note 11).
18. Isolate single white clones with sterile toothpicks or pipette tips and transfer to 4.5 ml of LB-broth containing ampicillin (see Note 10).
19. Incubate cultures overnight at 37°C with shaking at 225 rpm.
20. Prepare liquid culture of clones of interests for storage at −80°C: draw out 450 μl of the liquid bacterial culture and add 50 μl of autoclaved glycerol. Mix well. Such cultures can be stored at −80°C for approximately 10 years.
21. Centrifuge the remaining liquid culture for 10 min at 4,500 × *g*.
22. Remove as much supernatant as possible.
23. The following steps describe plasmid DNA extraction using the E.Z.N.A Plasmid Mini-Kit I (see Note 12). Re-suspend the bacterial pellet in 250 μl of Solution I.
24. Add 250 μl of Solution II and carefully mix solution 4–6 times (see Note 13).
25. Add 350 μl of Solution III and mix immediately 4–6 times. Chromosomal DNA and cell debris will form white precipitate.
26. Centrifuge samples at 13,000 × *g* for 10 min at room temperature.
27. Add 100 μl of equilibration buffer in the empty HiBind DNA MiniPrep column. Centrifuge at 13,000 × *g* for 60 s. Discard the flow-through liquid.
28. Apply the cleared supernatant to the spin column. Avoid carrying over white precipitates. Spin columns at 20,000 × *g* for 1 min. Discard flow-through.
29. Wash the column with 500 μl of HB Buffer. Repeat centrifugation and discard flow-through.
30. Wash the column with 700 μl of DNA Wash Buffer. Repeat centrifugation and discard flow-through.
31. Repeat centrifugation for 2 min at maximum speed. Make sure that the column matrix is dry.
32. Place the column into a clean 1.5-ml tube. Add 100 μl of Elution Buffer to the column matrix. Incubate 1 min at room temperature. Centrifuge for 1 min at full speed.
33. Examine 1 μl of plamid solution on a 1% agarose gel.
34. Send the plasmid DNA for sequencing with the SP6 and T7 universal primers.

## 4. Notes

1. Although an accurate alignment is helpful, the software choice is not very important here since only highly conserved protein regions are of interest and those usually align well with any program.
2. The longer the expected PCR product, the more likely shorter nonspecific PCR fragments will take over. We recommend 400 bp-fragments if possible, so that a sufficiently large region is sequenced to facilitate primer design for subsequent RACE or inverse PCR.
3. Designing a degenerate oligonucleotide with an "R" at a certain position means that half of the primers will contain an A (Adenine) at this position and the other half a G (Guanine). Increasing degeneracy in the oligonucleotide sequence thus increases the total number of sequence variants. This in turn lowers the concentration of specific primers and dilutes them out within the pool of unspecific variants.
4. Try not to use more than four pools for each region, as this drastically increases the number of PCRs. For example, 16 PCRs with different primer pairs will have to be performed if four pools are designed for the forward and for the reverse primers.
5. If another polymerase is used, make sure that it is capable of synthesizing DNA over an inosine-containing template and that it allows subsequent T/A cloning.
6. PCR amplification might be inhibited by primer dimer formation. In this case, it is useful to vary primer concentrations and to check for optimal amplification results. These tests can be done with a control template of an already known gene homolog. The optimal primer annealing temperature can also be optimized with an already known gene homolog as template.
7. An alternative is to include the M13 or T7 sequence at the 5′ end of the degenerate primers. In this case, M13 or T7 primers can be directly used for sequencing the PCR fragments. We have no experience with this strategy.
8. If several bands are observed on the gel, note that the smaller fragments will be preferentially cloned. If PCR products are purified using a spin column purification kit and resuspended in EB buffer, use 0.5 μl of PCR solution and 1.5 μl of $ddH_2O$ because the cloning reaction does not work well with EB buffer.
9. A 1-h incubation at room temperature is also possible but the resulting cloning will not be as efficient as an overnight incubation at 4°C, especially for fragments larger than 500 bp.

10. A "correct" sized band amplified from a cDNA template may be a complex mixture of products from many gene family members. It is thus advisable to analyze several clones generated from such a band.
11. Nowadays, most sequencing companies accept nonpurified PCR products and perform the purification step prior to sequencing.
12. Plasmids can also be prepared using a standard manual Miniprep protocol (13). However, manual plasmid preparations are apparently contaminated with inhibiting substances and give shorter sequence reads than spin-column-purified plasmid DNA. In our hands, the E.Z.N.A. Plasmid Mini Kit I yields approximately twice more DNA than MiniPrep kits from QIAGEN or Promega.
13. Do not shake vigorously, as it will shear chromosomal DNA and lower plasmid purity. Do not allow the lysis reaction to exceed 5 min.

## Acknowledgments

Our work is supported by an ATIP-AVENIR grant to VO and by a postdoctoral fellowship from the French Foreign Ministry to ML.

### References

1. Hall T (2005) BioEdit Sequence Alignment Editor for Windows 95/98/NT/XP. http://www.mbio.ncsu.edu/BioEdit/bioedit.html. Accessed 2010 Oct 20
2. Gouy M, Guindon S, Gascuel O (2010) SeaView Version 4: A Multiplatform Graphical User Interface for Sequence Alignment and Phylogenetic Tree Building. Molecular Biology and Evolution **27**:221–224
3. Thompson JD, Higgins DG, Gibson TJ (1994) CLUSTAL W: improving the sensitivity of progressive multiple sequence alignment through sequence weighting, position-specific gap penalties and weight matrix choice. Nucleic Acids Research **22**:4673–4680
4. Subramanian A, Kaufmann M, Morgenstern B (2008) DIALIGN-TX: greedy and progressive approaches for segment-based multiple sequence alignment. Algorithms for Molecular Biology **3**:6
5. Katoh K, Misawa K, Kuma K et al (2002) MAFFT: a novel method for rapid multiple sequence alignment based on fast Fourier transform. Nucleic Acids Res **30**:3059–3066
6. Edgar R (2004) MUSCLE: Multiple sequence alignment with high score accuracy and high throughput. Nucleic Acids Res **32**:1792–1797
7. Do CB, Mahabhashyam MS, Brudno M et al (2005) ProbCons: Probabilistic consistency-based multiple sequence alignment. Genome Research **15**:330–340
8. Notredame C, Higgins D, Heringa J (200) T-Coffee: a novel algorithm for multiple sequence alignment. J Mol Biol **302**:205–217
9. Marshall OJ (2005) PerlPrimer: cross-platform, graphical primer design for standard, bisulphite and real-time PCR. Bioinformatics **20**: 2471–2472
10. EMBL, EBI, Wellcome Trust Sanger Institute (2010) Ensembl release 59. http://www.ensembl.org/index.html. Accessed 2010 Oct 20
11. U.S. National Library of Medicine (2010) Nucleotide home. http://www.ncbi.nlm.nih.gov/nuccore. Accessed 2010 Oct 20
12. University of California Santa Cruz Genome Bioinformatics (2010) UCSC Genome Browser. http://genome.ucsc.edu/index.html. Accessed 2010 Oct 20

13. Sambrook J, Russell DW (2000) Molecular cloning: a laboratory manual. 3 éd. New York: Cold Spring Harbor Laboratory Press
14. Nomenclature Committee of the International Union of Biochemistry (NC-IUB) (1985) Nomenclature for incompletely specified bases in nucleic acid sequences. Biochem J **229**: 281–286
15. Moura GR, Paredes JA, Santos MA (2010) Development of the genetic code: Insights from a fungal codon reassignment. FEBS Letters **584**:334–341

# Chapter 15

# Characterizing cDNA Ends by Circular RACE


## Patrick T. McGrath



## Abstract

Rapid amplification of cDNA ends (RACE) is a widely used PCR-based method to identify the 5′ and 3′ ends of cDNA transcripts from partial cDNAs. While conceptually simple, this method often requires substantial optimization before accurate end identification is achieved. This is due in part to the anchoring of a universal primer to a cDNA or mRNA for PCR, which can lead to the generation of nonspecific amplification. Here, we describe an improvement of the original RACE method, circular RACE, which can be used to simultaneously identify both the 5′ and 3′ end of a target cDNA.



**Key words:** 5′ UTR, 3′ UTR, Circular RACE


## 1. Introduction

The complete isolation of a full-length gene transcript is an important step in studying a gene function, yet can be difficult even in well-studied model organisms. In eukaryotes, coding regions are divided between multiple exons, which are separated by noncoding introns. The complexity of transcription initiation, termination, and splicing makes ab initio gene prediction from sequence extremely challenging. As an orthogonal approach, expressed sequence tag (EST) libraries containing cDNA fragments can be used to identify short (~500 bp) portions of expressed genes. Typically, these libraries will not completely cover the entire transcriptome – ESTs are often biased to the 3′ end of transcripts and transcripts with low to medium levels of transcription often will not be completely covered. Even in organisms with high-quality genome sequence and large numbers of EST sequences, such as the nematode *Caenorhabditis elegans*, it has been estimated


Virginie Orgogozo and Matthew V. Rockman (eds.), *Molecular Methods for Evolutionary Genetics*,
Methods in Molecular Biology, vol. 772, DOI 10.1007/978-1-61779-228-1_15, © Springer Science+Business Media, LLC 2011

that 20% of the genome is incorrectly annotated (1) and many gene predictions lack 5′ and 3′ UTR regions.

Rapid amplification of cDNA ends (RACE) was originally developed in the late 1980s as a method to clone unknown flanking cDNA sequences for a particular gene of interest when a small amount of cDNA sequence is either already known or can be confidently predicted (2–4). A universal anchor sequence is attached to the 5′ or 3′ end of RNA or cDNA that has been isolated from an organism of interest. Then, PCR using a primer specific to the anchor sequence and a primer specific to the known sequence of the transcript of interest is used to amplify the region 5′ or 3′ of the gene specific primer. This product can then be cloned or sequenced to identify the unknown sequence 5′ or 3′ of the known sequence.

As originally described, RACE is often fraught with technical difficulties and can require substantial optimization before the desired result is achieved (5). A number of modifications have been developed to overcome some of these difficulties. Here, we describe one of these methods, circular RACE, that offers a few advantages over traditional RACE. Because no universal adaptor needs to be ligated to a cDNA in circular RACE, multiple gene-specific primers can be used to increase the specificity of the PCR reaction. Additionally, this strategy also allows the simultaneous identification of both the 5′ and 3′ ends of the target transcript by inverse PCR. While circular RACE can also describe a technique where mRNA-derived cDNAs are circularized and used as templates for inverse PCR (6), the protocol described here (adapted from Mandl et al. (7)) involves first circularizing RNA and then generating cDNA to use as template for inverse PCR. We prefer this second protocol as it allows for a powerful control to distinguish between inverse PCR products that are generated from intramolecularly ligated intact mRNAs (the goal) and PCR products that are generated from nonspecific amplification or degraded or incompletely processed mRNAs (the contamination). Before mRNAs can be intramolecularly ligated, or circularized, they must first be "decapped" by removing the 5′-terminal methylated guanine nucleotide. Thus, by running a reaction without decapping the mRNAs, one can identify the PCR products that are generated from nonspecific hybridization or mRNA degradation products.

## 2. Materials

### 2.1. Decapping the RNA

1. High quality total RNA from your species of interest.
2. Tobacco acid pyrophosphatase (TAP) (10 U/μl) (Epicentre, Madison, WI).
3. 10× TAP buffer (Epicentre).

4. Nuclease-free water (Ambion, Austin, TX).
5. RNAse*ZAP* wipes (Ambion).
6. RNAse-free microfuge tubes (Ambion).
7. RNAse-free tips (Ambion).

#### 2.2. Circularizing the RNA

1. Decapped RNA from previous step.
2. T4 RNA ligase (20 U/μl) (New England Biolabs, Ipswitch, MA).
3. 10× T4 RNA ligase buffer (New England Biolabs).
4. RNAse-free microfuge tubes (Ambion).
5. RNAse-free tips (Ambion).

#### 2.3. Reverse Transcribing the Circularized RNA into cDNA

1. Circularized RNA from previous step.
2. Superscript III RT (200 U/μl) (Invitrogen, Carlsbad, CA) (items 2–8 can be purchased as the Superscript III First-Strand Synthesis System for RT-PCR).
3. RNaseOUT recombinant RNAse inhibitor (40 U/μl) (Invitrogen).
4. 5× First-strand buffer (Invitrogen).
5. 0.1 M DTT (Invitrogen).
6. 10 mM dNTP mix (Invitrogen).
7. Random hexamers (50 ng/μl) (Invitrogen).
8. RNAse H (2 U/μl) (Invitrogen).
9. Gene-specific primer (1 μM).
10. Thin-walled RNAse-free PCR tubes (Ambion).
11. Nuclease-free water (Ambion).

#### 2.4. Nested PCR

1. cDNA from previous step.
2. Outer and inner gene-specific primers (10 μM).
3. PfuUltra II Fusion HS DNA polymerase (Agilent Technologies, Santa Clara, CA).
4. 10× PfuUltra II buffer (Agilent).
5. 10 mM dNTP mix (Invitrogen).
6. De-ionized water.
7. Zymoclean Gel DNA Recovery Kit (Zymo Research, Orange, CA).

## 3. Methods

A schematic of the overall protocol is shown in Fig. 1. The protocol assumes that the user has already purified total RNA from their sample of interest. RNA can be extracted using a Trizol-based

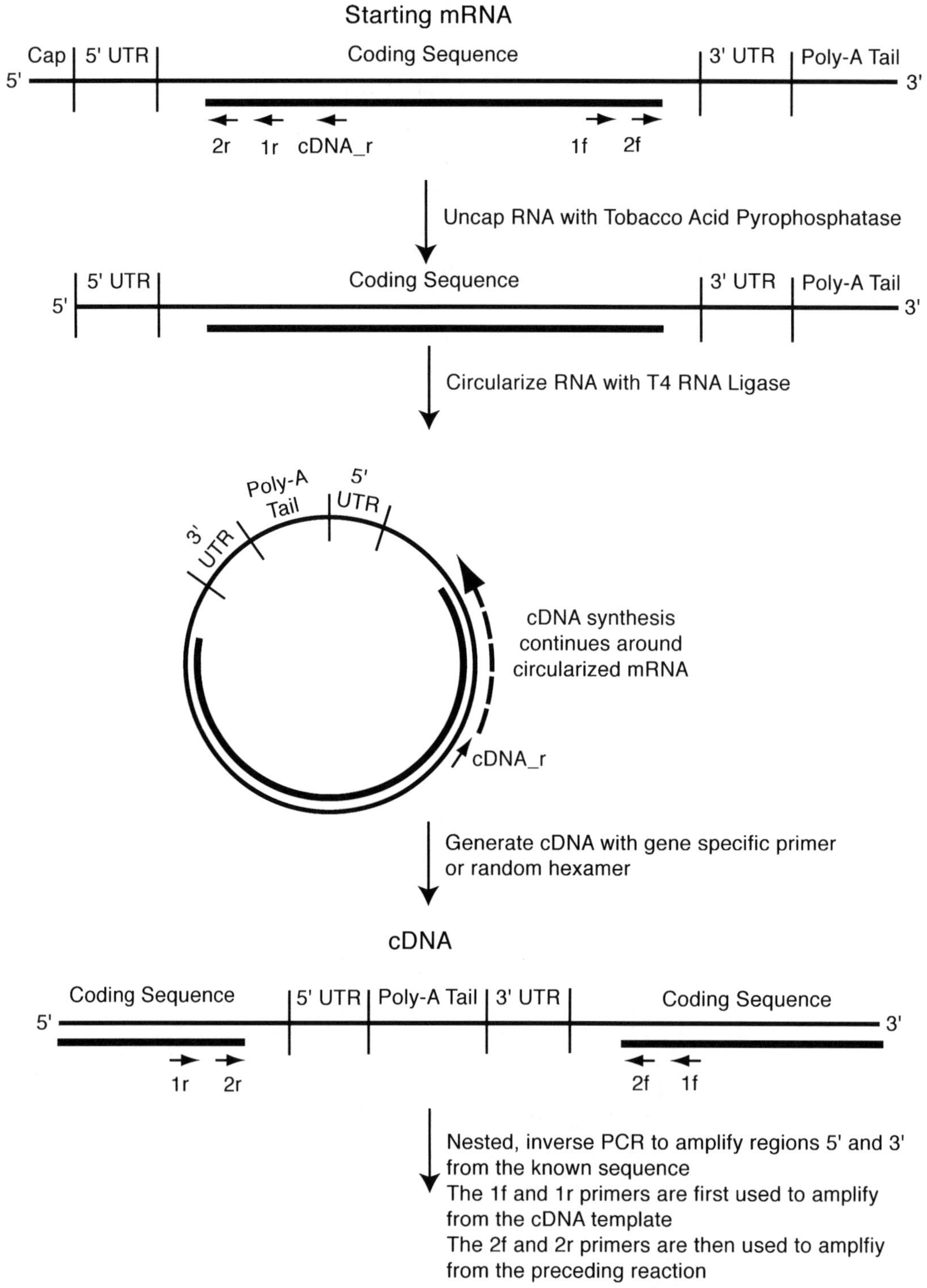


Fig. 1. Schematic depicting the overall strategy of circular RACE, starting from total RNA isolated from a sample. The final PCR product should be sequenced to identify the 5′ and 3′ ends of the transcript. While primers are not used in the first step of mRNA uncapping, we show them with respect to the mRNA to aid in primer design. The *black bar* underneath the mRNA indicates the region of the transcript already identified by ESTs or can be confidently predicted computationally. Please note that random hexamers can be used to generate cDNA in place of the cDNA_r gene-specific primer.

protocol or one of the many commercially available RNA purification kits. The RNA is then decapped with TAP (a control reaction without TAP will also be run). TAP cleaves the pyrophosphate bond of the 5′-terminal methylated guanine nucleotide "cap" of eukaryotic messenger RNAs. The decapped RNA can then be intramolecularly ligated with T4 RNA ligase to create circularized RNA, whereby the 5′ and 3′ ends of the RNA are joined. At this point, the circularized RNA is reverse transcribed using either a gene-specific primer or random hexamers to create a cDNA containing the 5′–3′ junction. Finally, two nested PCR reactions are run from this cDNA template to amplify a PCR product containing the junction for the user's gene of choice. This product can then be cloned and or sequenced to identify the 5′ and 3′ ends of the transcript.

The initial quality of the RNA sample is essential to the success of the protocol. Since RNA can be easily degraded, standard RNA handling techniques should be applied. A cleaved mRNA can still be intramolecularly ligated and used as a template for the cDNA synthesis, creating a band that could be interpreted as a 5′ end of the transcript.

### 3.1. Decapping the RNA

1. To prevent RNA degradation, gloves should always be worn, nuclease-free water should be used for reactions, and bench area/equipment should be wiped down with RNAse*ZAP* wipes (see Notes 1 and 2 for information on how to assess RNA quality).
2. For the +TAP reaction, in an RNAse-free microfuge tube, combine 500 ng of total RNA (or 125 ng of mRNA, see Note 3), 1 μl of TAP, 2 μl of 10× TAP Reaction buffer, and enough nuclease-free water to bring the total reaction volume to 20 μl.
3. Spurious PCR products in downstream steps can also result from degraded or incompletely processed transcripts, or cross-contamination from other uncircularized RNA species. PCR of these spurious bands will not require the addition of TAP. Therefore, as a control, in a second RNAse-free microfuge tube, combine 500 ng of total RNA (or 125 ng of mRNA), 2 μl of 10× TAP Reaction buffer, and enough nuclease-free water to bring the total reaction volume to 20 μl.
4. Incubate both reactions at 37°C for 2 h.

### 3.2. Circularizing the RNA

1. The decapped RNA is used as a substrate for the next reaction (see Note 4). For the +TAP and –TAP reactions, combine 17 μl of +TAP or –TAP RNA with 2 μl of 10× Reaction buffer, and 1 μl of T4 RNA ligase.
2. Incubate both reactions at 37°C for 2 h.
3. Inactivate the T4 RNA ligase by incubating at 65°C for 15 min.

### 3.3. Reverse Transcribing the Circularized RNA into cDNA

1. In order to create a template for PCR, the circular RNA must first be reverse transcribed into linear cDNA. The exact location where linearization occurs is determined by the location of the primer and must not be near the 5′–3′ junction. Note that this means that a poly-T primer cannot be used for the RT reaction. Rather, a gene-specific primer must be chosen in a particular region of the predicted sequence (illustrated in Fig. 1). This primer will be the reverse complement to part of the known mRNA sequence, and should be ~200 bp downstream of the unknown 5′ sequence. Alternatively, random hexamers can also be used to generate cDNA. For most genes, template generated from random hexamers is sufficient to identify the 5′ and 3′ ends of a transcript. Since cDNA generated from random hexamers can be used as a template for any gene of interest, we recommend using random hexamers. If difficulty is encountered in subsequent steps, we then recommend switching to a gene-specific primer for the reverse transcription reaction.
2. It is recommended to follow the protocol for RT-PCR exactly to ensure long extensions and sufficient yield. While not necessary, performing the following reaction in a PCR machine is encouraged to ensure accurate incubation times and temperatures. In two nuclease-free PCR tubes, add 10 μl of circularized RNA from the +TAP or –TAP reactions, 2 μl of random hexamers or 2 μl of gene-specific primer, 1 μl of 10 mM dNTP mix, and nuclease-free water to 13 μl. Heat mixture to 65°C for 5 min and then incubate on ice for at least 1 min.
3. To these tubes, add 4 μl 5× First-Strand Buffer, 1 μl 0.1 M DTT, 1 μl RNaseOUT Recombinant Rnase Inhibitor, and 1 μl of SuperScript III RT.
4. Mix by pipetting up and down. When using random hexamers, incubate the tubes at 25°C for 5 min. Then, incubate the tubes at 50°C for 45 min, followed by 55°C for 45 min. Inactivate the reaction by heating at 70°C for 15 min. This can be a useful place to stop for the day (see Note 5).
5. Amplification of some targets may require the removal of the complementary RNA. We recommend adding 1 μl (2 Units) of RNAse H to each tube and incubating at 37°C for 20 min.

### 3.4. Nested PCR

1. A PCR product containing unknown regions 5′ and 3′ from the transcript sequence can now be amplified from the preceding product. Since many transcripts will be found at low levels either due to low expression or limited expression in a subset of tissues, we recommend performing a nested PCR reaction to improve specificity. In nested PCR, the target DNA undergoes the first round of amplification using the outer primers (1f and 1r in Fig. 1). This step will amplify DNA from the target cDNA as well as additional nonspecific, unwanted PCR products. A second round of amplification uses two new primers internal

to the outer primers used in the first step (2f and 2r in Fig. 1). Note, that the inner primers should not overlap with the outer primers. These inner primers will again amplify from the target DNA, but it is unlikely any nonspecific, contaminating transcripts amplified from the first PCR reaction will contain binding sites for the new inner primers.

2. The inner and outer primers should be chosen from the region of known sequence, as shown in Fig. 1. If the primers are at least 50 bp away from the boundary between known and unknown sequence, the final product can be sequenced directly. Alternatively, the PCR product can be cloned into a sequencing vector. The primers should be chosen as close to the boundary between known and unknown sequence as possible. This will lead to a shorter PCR product and higher chance of success in amplifying product from the transcript of interest. However, care should be taken in selecting the sequence of the primers. We recommend using Primer3 software (http://frodo.wi.mit.edu/primer3/) to choose primers with a melting temperature of around 60°C.

3. While most DNA polymerases can be used, we recommend using PfuUltra II due to its high specificity and processivity. In two 200 μl thin-walled PCR tubes, combine 2 μl of cDNA template from the previous reaction, 39.5 μl of distilled water, 5 μl of 10× PfuUltra II reaction buffer, 1.5 μl of dNTP mix, 1 μl of outer primer 1f (at 10 μM), 1 μl of outer primer 1r (at 10 μM), and 1 μl of PfuUltra II fusion HS DNA polymerase. Mix gently by pipetting up and down.

4. We recommend using a touchdown PCR to reduce amplification of nonspecific sequence. A typical cycling protocol for PCR primers with a 60°C melting temperature would be:

| | |
|---|---|
| Denature: | 95°C for 1 min |
| Touchdown cycle: | Denature at 95°C for 20 s<br>Anneal primers at 65°C for 20 s<br>Primer extension at 72°C for 30 s<br>Cycle seven times, decreasing the temperature for annealing primers by 1°C each cycle |
| Subsequent cycle: | Denature at 95°C for 20 s<br>Anneal primers at 58°C for 20 s<br>Primer extension at 72°C for 30 s<br>Cycle 30 times |
| Final extension: | 72°C for 3 min |

5. Often, a single PCR reaction will not generate enough specific product for sequencing or cloning. Dilute a 2 μl aliquot of the +TAP and −TAP PCR products into 48 μl of de-ionized water or TE buffer. In two 200 μl thin-walled PCR tubes, combine

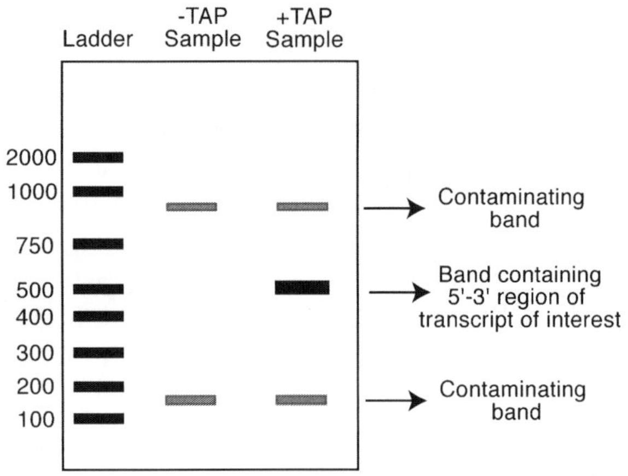


Fig. 2. A characteristic agarose gel electrophoresis result from circular RACE. Bands observed in the −TAP control reaction are likely contaminating bands. Any bands that are observed in the +TAP reaction lane should be isolated, purified, and sequenced.

2 μl of diluted PCR product from the previous reactions, 39.5 μl of distilled water, 5 μl of 10× PfuUltra II reaction buffer, 1.5 μl of dNTP mix (10 mM each dNTP), 1 μl of inner primer 2f (at 10 μM), 1 μl of inner primer 2r (at 10 μM), and 1 μl of PfuUltra II fusion HS DNA polymerase. Mix gently by pipetting up and down.

6. Run a touchdown PCR identical to the previous reaction.
7. The PCR product for the +TAP and –TAP reactions should be analyzed using agarose gel electrophoreses.
8. Any bands observed in the +TAP reaction but not the –TAP reaction should be cut out and purified using the gel purification kit (Fig. 2 and see Note 6). These products can be sequenced using the 2f and 2r inner primers (see Note 7). Because of the presence of the poly-A tail within this PCR product, which is difficult to sequence, it will likely be necessary to sequence the PCR products from both ends to identify the 5′ and 3′ ends.

## 4. Notes

1. RNA degradation can be a serious issue for this protocol. The amount of degradation in an RNA sample can be estimated using agarose gel electrophoresis. The 28S and 18S rRNA products can be visualized by running a total RNA sample, and should appear as two clear bands. If smearing is observed, RNA should be re-isolated.
2. To ensure that the transcript of interest is present in the RNA sample, a Northern blot can be performed.

3. For most genes, total RNA can be used as a starting point for circular RACE. However, rRNAs and incompletely processed transcripts can increase background amplification in later PCR reactions. For extremely rare transcripts, it is recommended that mRNA be purified using one of the many commercially available kits. In this case, 125 ng of purified mRNA should be used in place of the 500 ng of total RNA for the decapping reaction.
4. TAP does not need to be deactivated before proceeding with the circularizing reaction.
5. The decapping, circularization, and reverse transcription reactions (up to the RNAse H treatment) should be run on the same day. At this point, the cDNA template can be stored indefinitely at −20°C.
6. If no bands are detected after the second round of PCR, it is useful to start troubleshooting with the nested PCR step. Using a positive control, typically a transcript in which the circular RACE protocol had been previously successfully applied to, can be particularly helpful in testing the successes of the preceding reactions. If the positive control works, then standard troubleshooting measures following the guidelines of the DNA polymerase manufacturer typically resolve the issue. New nested primers can also be tried.
7. A poly-A tail should be identified between the 5′ and 3′ ends of the transcript in the final sequencing reaction.

## Acknowledgment

We thank Andres Bendesky for critical reading of this protocol.

### References

1. Salehi-Ashtiani K, Lin C, Hao T et al (2009) Large-scale RACE approach for proactive experimental definition of *C. elegans* ORFeome. Genome Res **19**:2334–2342
2. Frohman MA, Dush MK, Martin GR (1988) Rapid production of full-length cDNAs from rare transcripts: amplification using a single gene-specific oligonucleotide primer. Proc Natl Acad Sci USA **85**:8998–9002
3. Loh EY, Elliott JF, Cwirla S et al (1989) Polymerase chain reaction with single-sided specificity: analysis of T cell receptor delta chain. Science **243**:217–220
4. Ohara O, Dorit RL, and Gilbert W (1989) One-sided polymerase chain reaction: the amplification of cDNA. Proc Natl Acad Sci USA **86**:5673–5677
5. Schaefer BC (1995) Revolutions in rapid amplification of cDNA ends: new strategies for polymerase chain reaction cloning of full-length cDNA ends. Anal Biochem **227**: 255–273
6. Maruyama IN, Rakow TL, and Maruyama HI (1995) cRACE: a simple method for identification of the 5′ end of mRNAs. Nucleic Acids Res **23**:3796–3797
7. Mandl CW, Heinz FX, Puchhammer-Stockl E et al (1991) Sequencing the termini of capped viral RNA by 5′-3′ ligation and PCR. Biotechniques **10**:484, 486

# Chapter 16

# Identification of DNA Sequences that Flank a Known Region by Inverse PCR

## Anastasios Pavlopoulos

## Abstract

The Polymerase Chain Reaction (PCR) with its multiple applications in molecular genetic analysis is the cornerstone of modern basic and applied biomedical research. This chapter focuses on the inverse PCR technique that has been used widely over the last two decades in genotyping and chromosome walking applications for the isolation of unknown DNA sequences upstream and downstream of a known DNA region. The method is based on the use of circularized templates and primers facing outward from the known sequence, rather than primers facing each other used in conventional PCR. As a result, the original genome sequence is rearranged, and stretches of known sequence end up flanking the unknown DNA sequence in the inverse PCR product. I also discuss the special case of using outward facing primers to isolate the intergenic region between genes clustered in tandem or inverted arrangement, since it can hugely simplify the cloning of *cis*-regulatory sequences in new species of interest.

**Key words:** Inverse PCR, Chromosome walking, Genotyping, Gene cloning, *Cis*-regulatory sequences, Promoter, Enhancer, Gene clusters

## 1. Introduction

Even in our postgenomic era, almost every molecular genetic laboratory is facing the need of isolating the unknown sequence to one or both sides of a known DNA region, for example to recover the integration site of transgenesis vectors in the sequenced genomes of model species, or to clone coding or gene regulatory sequences from unsequenced nonmodel species. A variety of approaches have been developed to isolate unknown sequences from genomic DNA or cDNA templates, including library screening, rapid amplification of cDNA ends (RACE), and inverse Polymerase Chain Reaction (iPCR).

Virginie Orgogozo and Matthew V. Rockman (eds.), *Molecular Methods for Evolutionary Genetics*,
Methods in Molecular Biology, vol. 772, DOI 10.1007/978-1-61779-228-1_16, © Springer Science+Business Media, LLC 2011

This chapter describes the iPCR method that was developed in the late eighties (1–3) and has found wide use for routine genotyping and chromosome walking applications. Starting from a DNA stretch of known sequence, iPCR involves the circularization of restriction fragments containing the region of interest (Fig. 1a).

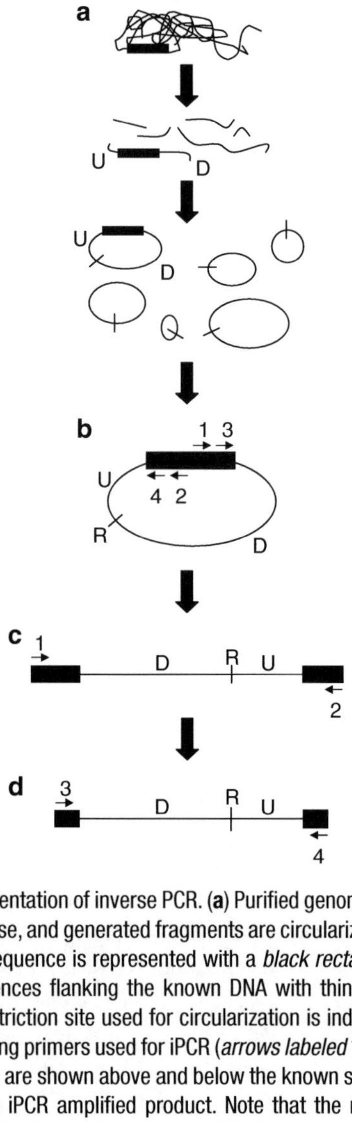


Fig. 1. Schematic representation of inverse PCR. (**a**) Purified genomic DNA is digested with a restriction endonuclease, and generated fragments are circularized with DNA ligase. The DNA region of known sequence is represented with a *black rectangle*, and the upstream and downstream sequences flanking the known DNA with thin lines labeled U and D, respectively. (**b**) The restriction site used for circularization is indicated with R. The positions of the outward facing primers used for iPCR (*arrows labeled* 1 *and* 2) and nested PCR (*arrows labeled* 3 *and* 4) are shown above and below the known sequence. (**c**) The inside-out arrangement of the iPCR amplified product. Note that the relative positions of the regions immediately upstream and downstream of the known stretch of DNA has changed compared to their original genomic arrangement. (**d**) Nested PCR product with similar arrangement generated with second pair of primers (*arrows labeled* 3 *and* 4) that bind outside the first pair of iPCR primers (*arrows labeled* 1 *and* 2) on the known DNA fragment (compare with (**b**)).

The second step involves the use of outward facing primers (hence inverted relative to conventional PCR) that will amplify around the circularized template, outward from the known DNA into the unknown flanking sequence and back into the known DNA (Fig. 1b). The original DNA sequence is rearranged in the resulting iPCR amplicon, in the sense that the unknown DNA sequence is flanked by stretches of known sequence (Fig. 1c). The actual structure of this inside-out arrangement of amplified iPCR fragments depends on the position of the restriction sites used for circularization. If no iPCR product is evident, conventional nested PCR (with a second pair of outward facing primers that bind outside of the first pair of primers on the known DNA) can be performed with the initial iPCR reaction as template (Fig. 1b, d).

A common task in Evolutionary Developmental Biology is the use of iPCR for the isolation of promoter and other *cis*-regulatory elements in diverse species of interest, especially in species that are amenable to functional approaches. In addition to the standard iPCR methodology, it can be very effective to use outward facing primers to isolate *cis*-regulatory sequences from genes that are physically linked in the genome, in particular duplicated genes organized in clusters. Clustered paralogous genes can also be homogeneous in nucleotide sequence due to gene conversion (4), and their intergenic sequence can be recovered rapidly in a simple PCR reaction (Fig. 2). Together with colleagues, we have used this approach successfully to isolate constitutive and heat-inducible *cis*-regulatory sequences for functional genetic studies in the crustacean *Parhyale hawaiensis*, a species with only limited genomic information available at present (5, 6).

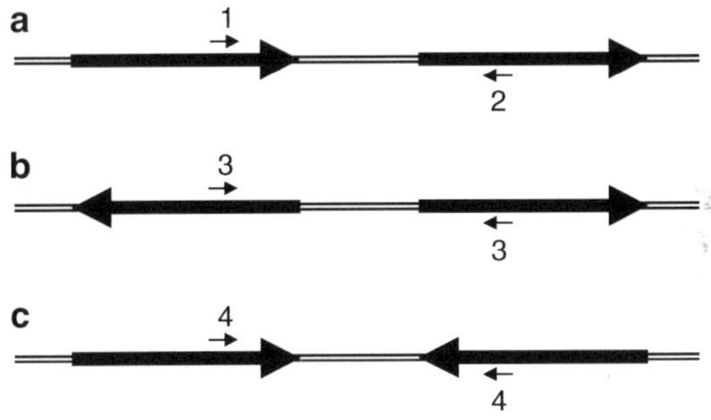


Fig. 2. Isolation of intergenic sequences from clustered genes. (**a**) Two outward facing gene-specific primers (*arrows labeled* 1 *and* 2) are required, if the duplicated genes are tandemly arrayed. (**b**, **c**) A single outward facing gene-specific primer can be enough, if the duplicated genes are very similar in nucleotide sequence and are arranged (**b**) in an inverted tail-to-tail configuration (*arrows labeled* 3) or (**c**) in an inverted head-to-head configuration (*arrows labeled* 4).

## 2. Materials

### *2.1. Purification of Genomic DNA*

1. Nuclease-free $ddH_2O$.
2. DNA purification kit, e.g., from Qiagen.
3. Lysis buffer (prepare fresh from stock solutions): 100 mM Tris–HCl pH 7.5, 100 mM EDTA pH 8, 100 mM NaCl, 0.5% SDS.
4. LiCl/KAc solution (prepare fresh from stock solutions): 2.5 parts 6 M LiCl, 1 part 5 M KAc.
5. Isopropanol.
6. 70% ethanol.
7. Disposable nuclease-free pestles and tubes, e.g., from Kontes.
8. Pasteur pipette with sealed tip (if necessary).

### *2.2. Template Preparation for iPCR*

1. NanoDrop/spectrophotometer.
2. High-fidelity restriction endonucleases and reaction buffers, e.g., from New England Biolabs (NEB).
3. RNase A.
4. T4 DNA Ligase (NEB).
5. T4 DNA Ligase Buffer (NEB), make small aliquots and use two to three times each.
6. Phenol:chloroform:isoamylalcohol 25:24:1.
7. Chloroform:isoamylalcohol 24:1.
8. Linear polyacrylamide, e.g., GenElute-LPA (Sigma).
9. 3 M sodium acetate, pH 5.2.
10. Absolute and 70% ethanol.

### *2.3. iPCR and Nested PCR Reactions*

1. PCR grade $ddH_2O$.
2. High-specificity/sensitivity *Taq* DNA polymerase and PCR buffer, e.g., AmpliTaq Gold 360 (Applied Biosystems), Platinum (Invitrogen).
3. Purified custom oligos, e.g., Pure and Simple Primers (Sigma).
4. 10 mM dNTP mix.
5. 50 mM $MgCl_2$.

### *2.4. Cloning and Sequencing*

1. PCR purification/gel extraction kit, e.g., QIAquick (Qiagen).
2. PCR fragment cloning kit, e.g., pGEM-T Easy (Promega), TOPO TA (Invitrogen).
3. High-fidelity proofreading DNA polymerase and buffer, e.g., Phusion (Finnzymes).
4. Regular DNA Taq polymerase.

#### 2.5. Isolation of Intergenic Sequences from Clustered Genes

1. Long PCR kit, e.g., Elongase amplification system (Invitrogen).

## 3. Methods

### 3.1. Purification of Genomic DNA

Isolate genomic DNA (or other DNA source) from the species/tissue/cell line of interest using either a commercial kit or the following quick protocol modified from the Berkley Drosophila Genome Project Web site (tested with many different arthropods):

1. Flash-freeze tissue in liquid nitrogen and grind with mortar and pestle if required.
2. Homogenize tissue for 1 min with disposable tissue grinder in about 5 volumes of lysis buffer.
3. Add 5 more volumes of lysis buffer and continue homogenization for 1 min.
4. Incubate for 30 min at 65°C.
5. Add 20 volumes of LiCl/KAc solution, incubate on ice for 20 min, and centrifuge at 13,000×*g* for 20 min at room temperature.
6. Transfer supernatant carefully to a new tube.
7. Add 0.6 volumes of isopropanol, mix well, and fish DNA out with a sealed Pasteur pipette (or spin immediately at 13,000×*g* for 20 min at room temperature to pellet DNA).
8. Wash DNA in 70% ethanol, air-dry briefly, and resuspend in $ddH_2O$.

### 3.2. Template Preparation for iPCR

1. Set up a number of parallel DNA digests with different restriction endonucleases (see Note 1). Digest DNA to completion with high-fidelity enzymes according to the instructions of the manufacturer. As a rule of thumb, incubate 5 μg of purified DNA for 1–3 h with 5 μl of enzyme (about 50 Units) in a final volume of 100 μl in appropriate buffer and temperature. Add RNase A to a final concentration 0.1 μg/μl for the last hour of incubation to remove RNA (not required for DNA prepared with commercial kits).
2. Extract digested DNA once with phenol–chloroform, once with chloroform, and precipitate/wash in ethanol. Resuspend DNA in $ddH_2O$ (about 10 μl/μg digested DNA).
3. Analyze 5 μl from each digest by agarose gel electrophoresis to confirm digestion, and measure concentration on a NanoDrop/spectrophotometer.

4. Circularize DNA fragments in 100–500 μl reaction volumes overnight at 16°C with T4 DNA ligase, using 1 Unit (0.015 Weiss Units) per μl of reaction in standard T4 DNA ligase buffer at low DNA concentration of 1–2 ng/μl (see Note 2).
5. Extract circularized DNA once with phenol–chloroform and once with chloroform. Add 5 μg of linear polyacrylamide per 300 μl as carrier and precipitate/wash in ethanol. Resuspend DNA in $ddH_2O$ (about 5 μl/100 ng of circularized DNA).

### 3.3. iPCR and Nested PCR Reactions

1. Depending on template complexity, incubate 1–500 ng of circularized (see Note 3) genomic DNA (use 100 ng or more for human genome templates) in iPCR reaction with 0.025 Units/μl of a high-specificity/sensitivity *Taq* DNA polymerase according to manufacturer's instructions (typically 50 μl reaction in 1× *Taq* buffer, 1.25 Units *Taq*, 200 μM each dNTP, 0.5 μM each primer and 1.5–2 mM $MgCl_2$).
2. Set the thermal cycling conditions according to manufacturer's recommendations (see Note 4). A standard cycling program can be as follows:

| | | |
|---|---|---|
| Initial denaturation: | | 95°C for 5 min |
| (and activation of *Taq* polymerase if required) | | |
| Main cycling program: | Denaturation | 95°C for 30 s |
| (30–35 cycles) | Annealing | Primer $T_m$ for 30 s |
| | Extension | 72°C for 2 min |
| Final extension: | | 72°C for 5 min |

3. Analyze 10 μl of each iPCR reaction by agarose gel electrophoresis.
4. If no amplification product is evident, proceed with nested PCR repeating steps 1–3 on a 1:100 to 1:1,000 dilution of the iPCR reaction. If multiple amplification products are present, try to adjust PCR conditions (see Note 4).

### 3.4. Cloning and Sequencing

1. If a single abundant iPCR or nested PCR amplification product is recovered, it can be purified with a PCR purification/gel extraction kit and sent out for sequencing with the same primers used.
2. If multiple amplification products are present, they should be first gel-purified with a PCR purification/gel extraction kit and cloned in a standard vector for PCR fragments, and then sequenced.
3. If necessary, more rounds of iPCR might be selected to further extend the known sequence by repeating all steps in Subheading 3.3 with new pairs of primers.
4. Once the flanking sequence is determined, the extended DNA sequence can be recovered with a proofreading DNA

polymerase from undigested genomic DNA with conventional primers amplifying convergently from the two ends (see Note 5). Use 1–500 ng of genomic DNA (e.g., ≥100 ng of human genomic DNA) as template in 50 μl-reaction with 1 Unit of Phusion plymerase, 1× HF buffer, 200 μM each dNTP, and 0.5 μM each primer, using the following cycling conditions (refer to the manufacturer's manual for optimization):

| | | |
|---|---|---|
| Initial denaturation: | | 98°C for 2 min |
| Main cycling program: | Denaturation | 98°C for 10 s |
| (30–35 cycles) | Annealing | Primer $T_m$ + 3°C for 20 s |
| | Extension | 72°C for 30 s/kb |
| Final extension: | | 72°C for 5 min |

5. Purify the amplified product with a PCR purification/gel extraction kit.
6. Proofreading DNA polymerases produce blunt-end fragments that must be A-tailed at their 3′ termini for TA-cloning in a PCR vector and sequencing. Treatment with a *Taq* DNA polymerase can add A-overhangs. Incubate the purified fragment in a 10 μl-reaction with 5 Units of *Taq* in 1× *Taq* buffer and 200 μM dATP at 72°C for 15 min. Proceed with cloning and sequencing of the A-tailed fragment.

### *3.5. Isolation of Intergenic Sequences from Clustered Genes*

The *cis*-regulatory sequences controlling expression of duplicated genes that remain clustered can be recovered easily from genomic DNA using a proofreading DNA polymerase suitable for amplifying long templates (see Note 6). If the duplicated genes are tandemly arrayed, two outward facing primers are used to amplify the intergenic region (Fig. 2a). If the duplicated genes are arranged in inverted configuration, a single outward facing primer is able to amplify the intergenic region (Fig. 2b, c).

1. Use 1–500 ng of genomic DNA (e.g., ≥100 ng of human genomic DNA) as template in 50 μl-reaction with 1 μl of Elongase, 1× buffer with 1.7 mM $MgSO_4$, 200 μM each dNTP, and 0.2 μM each primer, using the following cycling conditions (refer to manufacturer's manual for optimization):

| | | |
|---|---|---|
| Initial denaturation: | | 94°C for 2 min |
| Main cycling program: | Denaturation | 94°C for 30 s |
| (30–35 cycles) | Annealing | Primer $T_m$ for 30 s |
| | Extension | 68°C for 10 min (see Note 6) |
| Final extension: | | 68°C for 5 min |

2. Proceed as described in steps 5–6 in Subheading 3.4.

## 4. Notes

1. The restriction fragment to be amplified is constrained by a minimum size of about 0.3 kb required for efficient circularization and a maximum size of about 3 kb that can be amplified efficiently. In most cases, where the restriction map of the flanking sequences is not known, the choice of the restriction enzymes can be made probabilistically based on the GC content of the digested DNA and the size, degeneracy, and GC content of the restriction site. If the availability of DNA is not an issue, the size of the expected fragment produced with each digest can be determined beforehand with Southern blot analysis using the known DNA fragment as a probe. To identify the integration site of transgenesis vectors in species with sequenced genomes, in which case only a few flanking nucleotides are required, one typically uses restriction enzymes with 4-bp recognition sites that cut on average every $4^4$ or 256 bp in random DNA sequence.

   The choice of the restriction endonucleases is also influenced by the requirement to amplify sequences on both sides or on one side of the known DNA region. In the first case, the enzyme should not cut within the known sequence (as shown in Fig. 1b), while in the latter case the enzyme should cut within the known sequence (to the right of primer 1 if upstream sequence is desirable or to the left of primer 2 if downstream sequence is the target).
2. The ratio of intramolecular versus intermolecular ligation (i.e., circularization versus concatenation) is given by the expression $1974/L^{1/2} \times C$, where $L$ is the fragment length in bp and $C$ is the DNA concentration in ng/μl (7).
3. Some authors also recommend the relaxation of the circularized templates to improve the efficiency of iPCR (3, 8), but I have not found this step to be necessary. This can be done by linearization with a restriction enzyme that cuts between the two primers in the known DNA, by nicking with endonucleases or by denaturation with boiling.
4. A 2–3-kb plasmid containing the target sequence can be used as a positive control to optimize iPCR conditions. Take care to avoid contamination of reagents with this plasmid. A number of negative controls should be also included to check the specificity of the amplified iPCR products, including reactions without template, with uncircularized template, and with one primer only on the circularized template. The specificity of the iPCR and nested reactions can be improved following general PCR troubleshooting, such as optimizing the concentration of template, primers, and $MgCl_2$, and adjusting the length and temperature of cycling parameters.

5. This step is recommended for two reasons, first to control for specificity, and second to reconstruct a contiguous fragment if multiple rounds of iPCR were done.
6. This approach is based on the assumption that the clustered organization of duplicated genes found in other species is also present in the species of interest. It should be stressed that there is no a priori knowledge of the actual arrangement and distance of the duplicated copies in the hypothetical cluster. For this reason, a long extension step is selected first that can be decreased later if necessary.

## Acknowledgments

Some of the ideas and protocols described in this chapter have been developed in close interaction with my PhD supervisor and mentor Dr. Michalis Averof.

### References

1. Ochman H, Gerber AS, Hartl DL (1988) Genetic applications of an inverse polymerase chain reaction. Genetics **120**:621–623
2. Triglia T, Peterson MG, Kemp DJ (1988) A procedure for in vitro amplification of DNA segments that lie outside the boundaries of known sequences. Nucleic Acids Res **16**:8186
3. Silver J, Keerikatte V (1989) Novel use of polymerase chain reaction to amplify cellular DNA adjacent to an integrated provirus. J Virol **63**:1924–1928
4. Bettencourt BR, Feder ME (2002) Rapid concerted evolution via gene conversion at the *Drosophila* hsp70 genes. J Mol Evol **54**: 569–586
5. Pavlopoulos A, Kontarakis Z, Liubicich DM et al (2009) Probing the evolution of appendage specialization by Hox gene misexpression in an emerging model crustacean, Proc Natl Acad Sci USA **106**:13897–13902
6. Douris V, Telford MJ, Averof M (2009) Evidence for multiple independent origins of trans-splicing in Metazoa. Mol Biol Evol **27**:684–693
7. Sambrook J, Fritsch EF, Maniatis T (1989) Molecular Cloning: A Laboratory Manual, Cold Spring Harbor Laboratory Press, Cold Spring Harbor, New York
8. Jong AY, T'Ang A, Liu DP et al (2002) Inverse PCR. Genomic DNA cloning. Methods Mol Biol **192**:301–307

# Part V

## Analyzing Candidate Gene Transcripts

# Chapter 17

# Quantification of Transcript Levels with Quantitative RT-PCR

Karen L. Carleton


## Abstract

Differential gene expression is a key factor driving phenotypic divergence. Determining when and where gene expression has diverged between organisms requires a quantitative method. While large-scale approaches such as microarrays or high-throughput mRNA sequencing can identify candidates, quantitative RT-PCR is the definitive method for confirming gene expression differences. Here, we describe the steps for performing qRT-PCR including extracting total RNA, reverse-transcribing it to make a pool of cDNA, and then quantifying relative expression of a few candidate genes using real-time or quantitative PCR.


**Key words:** Gene expression, Messenger RNA, Quantitative RT-PCR, Real-time RT-PCR

## 1. Introduction

One of the goals of evolutionary genetics is to determine the molecular basis for differences in phenotypes. The two most common molecular mechanisms driving diversification and adaptation involve either differences in gene coding sequences, causing a change in protein function (1–3), or differences in gene expression, altering the timing, location, and amount of a particular gene and its associated protein (4–6). Numerous debates have arisen as to the relative importance of these two mechanisms for phenotypic evolution (7–9). However, these mechanisms are part of a continuum of molecular change (10, 11), requiring an integrative genomic approach (12).

In this chapter, we discuss one facet of these approaches, quantifying the relative amount of expressed transcripts using quantitative reverse transcription-polymerase chain reaction (qRT-PCR). This method, also called real-time RT-PCR, relies on PCR to quantify the relative amounts of a few genes and has been nicely

Virginie Orgogozo and Matthew V. Rockman (eds.), *Molecular Methods for Evolutionary Genetics*, Methods in Molecular Biology, vol. 772, DOI 10.1007/978-1-61779-228-1_17, © Springer Science+Business Media, LLC 2011

described in several review articles (13–15). This method is more limited than those that provide data for hundreds to thousands of genes, including microarray experiments (16, 17) or next-generation transcriptomics (18–20). However, qRT-PCR is the gold standard by which differences in transcript levels identified by other methods are confirmed (21, 22).

The key steps in this method are to isolate RNA (typically as total RNA) from a tissue and developmental stage of interest, quantify the RNA, reverse-transcribe the messenger RNA to make cDNA, and perform quantitative PCR (qPCR) on the expressed genes of interest (Table 1). This chapter describes each of these steps in detail.

There are several important decisions to make in designing a qRT-PCR experiment. The first decision is whether to do a one-step process where reverse transcription occurs in the same tube as the subsequent qPCR or whether to do a two-step experiment with reverse transcription done first, followed by qPCR. The one-step process is possible if the number of genes to be quantified is four or fewer, and if a multicolor qPCR machine is available that can separately follow all four transcripts. However, quantifying more than four transcripts typically requires a two-step process where cDNA is first prepared and then multiple genes are quantified in multiple wells.

The second decision is how to normalize the transcripts to make comparisons between different individuals or different treatments.

**Table 1**
**Key steps in the qRT-PCR process**

| Task | Steps |
|---|---|
| Total RNA isolation | Dissect tissue<br>Tissue disruption using micropestle tube<br>Tissue homogenization using QIAshredder column<br>Purification on RNA-binding column |
| RNA quantification of total RNA | Prepare RNA dilution<br>Measure $A_{260}$ and $A_{280}$ and calculate RNA concentration |
| Reverse transcription to make cDNA | Add primer to total RNA; heat to 65°C and quench on ice<br>Add RT enzymes and incubate at 42°C |
| qRT-PCR | Prepare cDNA master mixes<br>Prepare gene specific primer–probe master mixes<br>Pipette to plate and run on qPCR machine |
| Data analysis | Extract $C_t$'s for each sample<br>Determine PCR efficiencies from standard or dilution series<br>Calculate relative gene expression |

Some methods normalize gene expression relative to a housekeeping gene such as beta-actin or GAPDH. However, Bustin (14) argues that expression levels of housekeeping genes are often not constant, biasing the normalized results. Instead, he suggests that the best normalization method is to quantify total RNA and then to reverse-transcribe the same amount of total RNA for each individual or treatment for subsequent analyses.

The third decision is which chemistry to use for monitoring PCR products in the qPCR. The simplest chemistry is to use two primers and a dye that binds to double-stranded DNA (e.g., SYBR Green) to monitor PCR progress. While this is often successful, it can require optimization to minimize unwanted signal. Background signal can arise either from primer dimers or from any carried-over genomic DNA. (Nearly all RNA extraction methods carry over some amount of genomic DNA.) Careful checks need to be run to test for genomic DNA contamination by performing a control reaction using a sample that has not undergone reverse transcription. An alternative is to treat the RNA sample with DNase prior to reverse transcription. To avoid these potential problems, a qPCR chemistry such as TaqMan® can be used. In this chemistry, a dual labeled probe binds to a specific DNA sequence located between the two amplification primers. This probe is hydrolyzed during PCR, releasing a fluorescing dye from its quenching partner. The fluorescence of the released dye is proportional to the amount of PCR product generated. The binding site of this probe typically spans an exon–exon junction, preventing the probe from binding to genomic DNA. Therefore, only cDNA amplification is detected. Typically, this is sufficient to discriminate against any background genomic DNA so that DNase treatment is not required prior to reverse transcription. Further, there should be minimal background signal from primer dimers, since the TaqMan probe will not bind to the primer dimers.

The fourth and final decision that needs to be made is the number of biological and experimental replicates to perform. Biological replicates account for individual variation and should include two to four samples. This would, therefore, include multiple individuals for each comparison, be it developmental time points, tissues, treatments, or populations sampled. For experimental replicates, qPCR quantification is done two or three times for each biological sample. This is necessary because of the inherent exponential nature of PCR and the resulting errors that can accumulate through many rounds of PCR. Studies sometimes also repeat the reverse transcription step as well. In this case, a given biological RNA sample would be reverse-transcribed twice and each of these would then be quantified by qPCR at least twice. In our experience, most of the error is in the qPCR step, rather than the reverse transcription step, since the former is exponential and the latter is a linear process.

Quantification of the relative amounts of transcripts by qPCR assumes that products accumulate exponentially during the earlier cycles of PCR amplification. During this exponential phase, the amount of PCR product of gene i, $P_i$, is related to the initial amount of gene transcript, $T_i$, the PCR amplification efficiency of that gene, $E_i$, and the number of PCR cycles, $n$, by the following equation:

$$P_i = T_i(1 + E_i)^n \tag{1}$$

In the ideal situation, efficiency is 1 and PCR product doubles with each amplification cycle. In practice, it is necessary to quantify efficiency for each gene.

While it is possible to determine the absolute amount of initial gene transcript by comparison to a standard curve of samples with known copy number, this is not necessary if all that is desired is a comparison of one gene between two treatments or of two genes within an individual. In this case, it is possible to monitor PCR product, $P$, and then set a threshold level somewhere in the exponential amplification phase. At this point, the two samples have the same amount of PCR product ($P_i = P_j$) and the relative amounts of initial transcripts can be determined:

$$P_i = T_i(1 + E_i)^{C_{ti}} = P_j = T_j(1 + E_j)^{C_{tj}} \tag{2}$$

$$\frac{T_i}{T_j} = \frac{(1 + E_j)^{C_{tj}}}{(1 + E_i)^{C_{ti}}} \tag{3}$$

Here, i and j are either two treatments or two genes, and $C_t$ is the number of cycles at which each PCR reaches threshold, or the critical cycle number. The ratio of initial transcripts is then determined from the critical cycle numbers and the PCR efficiencies.

Determining PCR efficiencies can be done by many different methods. One of the easiest methods is to prepare a dilution curve of the template of interest and perform qPCR on this series of samples. The dilution series can be prepared from the actual cDNA sample itself containing the expressed gene, or it can use an amplified PCR product from the gene, or a plasmid containing the cloned gene of interest. In the latter two cases, the gene should be amplified from cDNA and not genomic DNA so that it has the same exonic structure as the expressed transcript. In considering Eq. 1, we note that at threshold, $P$ is equal to the constant threshold, and $n$ is equal to $C_t$. Therefore, we can take the natural log of both sides, set the log of the threshold level to be $K$, and rearrange Eq. 1 to get:

$$\ln T = K - C_t \ln (1 + E) \tag{4}$$

Therefore, a plot of $\ln T$ versus $C_t$, for the dilution series will yield a line with a slope of $-\ln(1 + E)$. Here, $T$ is the relative transcript concentration (e.g., 1×, 10×, 500×), and need not be an absolute amount.

The slope is determined from a linear least squares fit to the data and used to calculate efficiency from the following equation:

$$E = e^{-\text{slope}} - 1 \quad (5)$$

The following method is an example from our work to illustrate how these steps might proceed as well as some specific variations. Much of our work involves expression of opsin genes in fish retina (23, 24). Like most other fishes and vertebrates, cichlid fishes have cone opsin genes from the classes of short wavelength sensitive (SWS), rhodopsin-like (RH2) and long-wavelength-sensitive (LWS) opsin genes (25, 26). Specifically, cichlids have seven different genes, which fall in six different classes and cover the full spectral range: SWS1 (ultraviolet), SWS2B (violet), SWS2A (blue), RH2B (blue-green), RH2A (green), and LWS (red). To quantify the relative expression of these six opsin gene classes, we use TaqMan® chemistry, with a forward and reverse primer for each gene as well as a gene-specific probe. Although there are different forms of the RH2A gene, RH2Aα and RH2Aβ genes (24) are genetically so similar that the same set of primers and probe amplify both forms. They can be distinguished by moving the forward primer further upstream where the gene sequences diverge (27), though we typically quantify them together and deal only with six cone opsin gene classes.

We use the dilution method to obtain the absolute efficiency of one gene of interest, for example the RH2A gene. This typically involves making a dilution series covering three orders of magnitude in concentration. Comparisons are then made between samples with $T$ set to nine different relative concentrations: 1×, 2×, 5×, 10×, 20×, 50×, 200×, 500×, and 1,000×. These nine samples are then run to obtain $C_t$'s and estimate $E$ for this gene from the slope of the $\ln T$ versus $C_t$ plot.

In order to determine the relative PCR efficiencies of the other five gene classes, we made a gene construct in which the key parts of each of the six gene classes are ligated together (24). This construct, therefore, contains each of six genes in a fixed 1:1:1:1:1:1 ratio (see Note 1). Therefore, we can get the relative efficiency of each gene to any other. To solve for this efficiency relationship, we start with Eq. 2 where we know that at threshold, the amount of each gene PCR product is equal. Then, we note that in the construct, the initial amount of each gene is identical, since they are ligated together. By setting $T_i = T_j$, we can simplify Eq. 2 to get:

$$(1 + E_i)^{C_{ti}} = (1 + E_j)^{C_{tj}} \quad (6)$$

Then, we use Eq. 6 to solve for the efficiency of any of the other genes from the RH2A expression, determined from the dilution series. In Eq. 6, we substitute $E_j = E_{RH2A}$ and $C_{tj} = C_{tRH2A}$ so that:

$$(1 + E_i)^{C_{ti}} = (1 + E_{RH2A})^{C_{tRH2A}} \quad (7)$$

We are typically most interested in the expression level of each opsin gene relative to the total opsin levels present in the retina so that we can determine which opsins are present and which are not. We are not so concerned with the absolute levels. We, therefore, determine the amount of transcript of each opsin relative to the total opsin genes from:

$$\frac{T_{\mathrm{i}}}{\sum T_{\mathrm{i}}} = \frac{\dfrac{1}{(1+E_{\mathrm{i}})^{C_{\mathrm{ti}}}}}{\sum \dfrac{1}{(1+E_{\mathrm{i}})^{C_{\mathrm{ti}}}}} \tag{8}$$

Using the efficiencies determined from the construct, we can solve for the relative expression of any of the genes in a sample normalized to total cone opsin expression using the $C_t$'s determined in the qPCR step.

## 2. Materials

In performing RNA isolation and reverse transcription, it is important to take precautions to minimize the presence of RNase which can degrade RNA. Chemicals should be set aside and used just for RNA procedures. Typically, this means using newly opened bottles of chemicals and wearing gloves whenever handling them. Do not use general lab chemicals, which are not assured of being RNase-free. RNase-free water can either be purchased or be prepared by treatment with diethylpyrocarbonate (DEPC). All plastics and glassware should be RNase-free. Plastics can be purchased that are guaranteed RNase-free, while glassware can be acid-washed and baked at 180°C for four hours prior to use. Gloves should be worn and changed frequently to prevent contamination with RNases. Once past the reverse transcription step (Subheading 3.3), it is no longer necessary to maintain RNase-free conditions. At that point, plasticware and water should be DNase-free as is typical for most other molecular biology experiments.

### 2.1. RNA Extraction

1. 1.5-ml micropestle tubes and pestles (Kontes through VWR) (see Note 2).
2. RNeasy mini kit (QIAGEN, Valencia, CA). This kit includes buffers RLT, RW1, and RPE, as well as RNA binding columns. Ethanol needs to be added to buffer RPE prior to its use.
3. QIAshredder columns (QIAGEN, Valencia, CA). These columns provide tissue homogenization following disruption, which reduces solution viscosity.

4. β-Mercaptoethanol (Sigma Aldrich, St. Louis, MO).
5. 70% Ethanol, made up fresh from ethanol and RNase-free water.

### 2.2. RNA Quantification

1. RNase-free water.
2. Small volume (50 μl) UV transmissive cuvette.

### 2.3. Reverse Transcription

1. Total RNA, extracted and quantified.
2. Superscript III reverse transcriptase (Invitrogen, Carlsbad, CA).
3. RNaseOUT, recombinant ribonuclease inhibitor (Invitrogen, Carlsbad, CA).
4. polyT primer, 10 μM primer made up in RNase-free water. We use a $polyT_{17}$ primer with a unique sequence on the 5′ end: $GCGAATTCGTCGACAAGGCT_{17}$.
5. dNTPs, 10 mM each. These are made from 100 mM stocks (USB, Cleveland, OH). Add 30 μl of each of ATP, CTP, GTP, and TTP to 180 μl of RNase-free water. Keep frozen in an RNase-free O-ring-sealed tube at –20°C.

### 2.4. qRT-PCR

1. qPCR machine (see Note 3).
2. PCR plate that fits the qPCR machine along with sealing tape.
3. TaqMan universal PCR master mix (Applied Biosystems, Carlsbad, CA).
4. Primers and probes for each gene to be studied (see Note 4). This includes a forward primer (3 μM), a reverse primer (3 μM), and a dual labeled probe (2 μM). These gene-specific primers and probes can be designed using Primer Express (Applied Biosystems, Carlsbad, CA) with the probe spanning an exon–exon junction. If using a single-color qPCR machine, the probe is typically 5′ labeled with 6′FAM and 3′ labeled with TAMRA and then HPLC-purified. The primers need to be desalted.
5. cDNA mixture from reverse transcription step.
6. Positive control, which could be a plasmid containing the gene or genes of interest.

## 3. Methods

### 3.1. RNA Extraction

There are many methods for RNA isolation (see Note 5). The following RNA extraction method follows QIAGEN's instructions for the RNeasy kit with the addition of the QIAshredder column.

*3.1.1. Tissue Disruption and Homogenization*

1. Prepare the tissue of interest either from a fresh dissection or by removing it from an RNA preserving solution (e.g., RNAlater).
2. Place in a micropestle tube containing 600 μl of buffer RLT and 6 μl of β-mercaptoethanol (see Notes 6 and 7). β-Mercaptoethanol and buffer RLT are harmful and should be used in a hood while wearing gloves and protective clothing.
3. Disrupt the tissue by fine grinding using the micropestle (see Note 2).
4. Homogenize the solution by pipetting it onto the QIAshredder column and spinning at 12,000 ×*g* for 2 min.
5. Remove the QIAshredder column and cap the tube. Spin for an additional 3 min at maximum speed.

*3.1.2. Purification on RNA Column*

1. Add 600 μl of 70% ethanol to a clean 1.5-ml tube. Transfer the solution spun through the QIAshredder column to the 70% ethanol and mix by pipetting (see Note 8).
2. Transfer half of this new mixture to the RNA binding column in a 2-ml collection tube. Centrifuge at 8,000 ×*g* for 15 s.
3. Pour off the flow-through and add the other half of the solution to the RNA column and spin again for 15 s. Discard flow-through.
4. Add 500 μl of buffer RW1 to the column and spin at 8,000 ×*g* for 15 s.
5. Transfer the RNA column to a clean collection tube. Add 500 μl of buffer RPE and spin at 8,000 ×*g* for 15 s. Discard flow-through and add another 500 μl of buffer RPE and spin at 8,000 ×*g* for 1 min. Discard the flow-through.
6. Place the RNA column back in the collection tube and spin for another 2 min to dry the column and remove any traces of ethanol.
7. Place the RNA column into a clean, RNase-free tube. Add 30–50 μl of RNase-free water and let the column sit for 1 min. Spin at 12,000 ×*g* for 1 min. Add another 30–50 μl of water and repeat letting it sit and then spin to elute the RNA.

**3.2. RNA Quantification**

Quantify the total RNA isolated with the QIAGEN RNeasy kit by measuring the ratio of absorbance at 260 nm, $A_{260}$, to that at 280 nm, $A_{280}$ (see Note 9).

1. Zero the spectrometer at 260 and 280 nm by taking a blank using pure water.
2. Dilute a small quantity of the RNA, such as 4 μl diluted to 60 μl of RNase-free water, and place in a 50-μl cuvette.

3. Measure the absorbance of the diluted RNA sample at 260 and 280 nm.

4. Calculate the RNA concentration. In the ideal case, the $A_{260}/A_{280}$ ratio is 2 and there is no protein contamination. RNA concentration can then be determined using $A_{260} = eC$ where $A_{260}$ is the absorption at 260 nm, $e$ is the RNA extinction coefficient which is 25 μl/μg at 260 nm, and $C$ is the concentration. (This all assumes a 1-cm cell path length.) However, for other $A_{260}/A_{280}$ ratios, a correction should be made for contributions of protein to the absorption, using the method of Glasel (28). In this case:

$$N = \frac{Re_{280,P} - e_{260,P}}{(e_{260,N} - e_{260,P}) - R(e_{280,N} - e_{280,P})} \tag{9}$$

$$C_N = \frac{NA_{260}}{Ne_{260,N} + Pe_{260,P}} \tag{10}$$

where $N$ is the ratio of nucleic acids (RNA in this case) to the sum of nucleic acids plus protein, $P$ is the ratio of protein to the sum (so that $P = 1 - N$), $C_N$ is the concentration of nucleic acid (RNA), $R$ is the $A_{260}/A_{280}$ ratio, and the $e$ are the extinction coefficients of RNA and protein at the two wavelengths ($e_{260,N} = 25$ μl/μg; $e_{260,P} = 0.57$ μl/μg; $e_{280,N} = 12.5$ μl/μg; $e_{280,P} = 1$ μl/μg; (28)). $N$ can be calculated from Eq. 9 using $R$ and the extinction coefficients. $P$ is then calculated as $1 - N$. These are then used in Eq. 10 with the absorption at 260 nm ($A_{260}$) to get the RNA concentration, $C_N$.

5. The concentration of the initial RNA solution is calculated from that of the diluted sample by multiplying by one over the dilution factor. For the dilution above, where 4 μl is diluted to 60 μl, the measured (diluted) concentration should be multiplied by 15 to obtain the initial concentration.

6. Calculate the volume of RNA required to add 0.5 μg of RNA to the reverse transcription (RT) reaction.

### 3.3. Reverse Transcription

1. Prepare the initial additions to the reverse transcription reaction including 0.5 μg of total RNA, 2.5 μl of 10 μM polyT primer, 1.25 μl of 10 mM each dNTPs, and enough RNase-free water to bring the volume to 15.6 μl in an RNase-free tube. It is easiest to add the water, then 3.75 μl of a master mix of polyT primer and dNTPs to each tube, and finally the individual total RNA.

2. Heat this mixture to 65°C for 5 min and then quench on ice for 1 min. This reduces secondary structure to ensure transcription of full-length cDNAs.

3. Prepare a master mix of 5 μl of 5× first-strand buffer, 2.5 μl of 0.1 M DTT, and 0.65 μl of RNaseOUT (25 U) for all the samples and then add 8.15 μl of master mix to the total RNA mixture.
4. Spin down and incubate at room temperature for 2 min.
5. Add 1.25 μl (250 U) of Superscript III, bringing the total volume to 25 μl.
6. Briefly vortex, spin down, and incubate at room temperature for 10 min.
7. Incubate at 42°C for 50 min.
8. Heat-inactivate at 70°C for 15 min (see Note 10) and then store at –20°C. In the subsequent qPCR step, we typically use 0.5 μl of this cDNA mixture in each qPCR reaction. If each gene is quantified in a separate qPCR, and each gene is measured twice, the 25 μl of cDNA mixture is enough to quantify 25 different genes, with replicates. If genes are multiplexed with more than one primer–probe mixture per tube, more genes could be measured from this volume of cDNA.

### 3.4. qRT-PCR

The qRT-PCRs are prepared using master mixes. These include one master mix for each individual or cDNA and one for each gene's primer–probe combination (see Note 11). One method of arranging things is for the individuals to be divided across the rows and then each gene added down a column of a plate.

1. For each individual or cDNA, make a master mix containing 10 μl of 2× TaqMan universal PCR buffer, 3.5 μl of water, and 0.5 μl of cDNA mixture. This is multiplied by however many genes are to be quantified plus 10% for pipetting losses. Mix the three reagents in one tube, vortex, spin down, and aliquot 14 μl into each well of the qPCR plate, possibly along one row.
2. Make a master mix for each gene containing 2 μl each of the forward primer, reverse primer, and probe. This is multiplied by however many individuals are to be quantified plus 10% for pipetting losses. The primer master mix is vortexed, spun down, and then 6 μl is aliquoted into each well of the qPCR plate, possibly along one column. This step can be nicely done with a multichannel pipettor if the primers lay out in a simple fashion. It is helpful to mix with the pipettor as the primer–probe mixture is added to the TaqMan/cDNA mixture in each well.
3. Seal the qPCR plate with sealing tape and then lightly spin down in a centrifuge.
4. Run the plate on a quantitative or real-time PCR machine for at least 40 cycles (see Note 12 for cycling parameters, Note 13 for replicate plate layouts, and Note 14 for factors affecting qPCR reproducibility).
5. Determine the critical cycle numbers for each sample (see Note 15).

### 3.5. Calculating PCR Efficiencies and Data Analysis

It is common to first perform a dilution curve for a particular primer–probe combination. This confirms that the qPCR result is proportional to template concentration and also provides the PCR efficiency for a particular primer–probe combination. This PCR efficiency is specific to the actual primer–probe concentrations and is typically measured every time a new batch of primers and probes are made up.

1. Prepare a set of dilutions. The DNA used can be a plasmid containing the gene of interest or cDNA from an individual known to express the gene. The dilutions should cover at least three orders of magnitude in concentration (e.g., 1×, 2×, 5×, 10×, 20×, 50×, 200×, 500×, and 1,000×).
2. Prepare a qPCR plate containing a dilution series for each gene being studied and run them together on one plate.
3. Extract the critical cycle numbers from the PCR machine using any of several fitting approaches (see Note 15).
4. Plot $\ln T$ versus $C_t$, obtain the slope, and calculate the PCR efficiency for each gene, using Eq. 5. For the data shown in Fig. 1, the RH2A slope is $-0.708 \pm 0.023$. Here, 0.023 is the standard error in the slope, obtained from the linear regression. The resulting PCR efficiency is $1.03 \pm 0.1$ (see Note 16). Larger PCR efficiencies suggest the gene of interest is amplifying well and should provide data proportional to transcript concentration. The other two genes shown in Fig. 1, SWS1 and LWS, have efficiencies that are not quite so high. Their slopes are $-0.626 \pm 0.021$ and $-0.605 \pm 0.16$, which give PCR efficiencies of $0.87 \pm 0.08$ and $0.83 \pm 0.06$, respectively. These are typical values for short 70–80 bp amplicons. Longer amplicons typically have lower efficiencies.

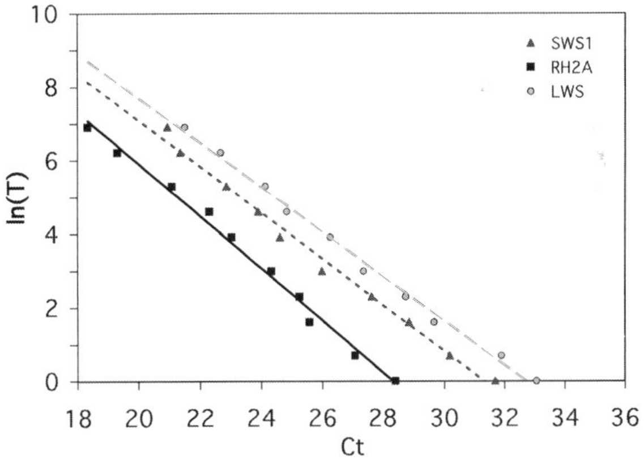


Fig. 1. Dilution series for several opsin gene templates. qPCRs with decreasing amounts of template are prepared and run. The resulting $C_t$ values are then plotted versus the natural log of the relative concentration ($\ln T$). The slope of this plot is related to PCR efficiency as given in Eq. 5.

5. For the opsin work, we can also use the multigene construct to obtain relative PCR efficiencies and then tie this to the RH2A efficiency determined from the dilution curve (Eq. 7). When we do this, we get slightly tighter estimates of PCR efficiencies as evidenced by smaller error bars. For example, PCR efficiencies estimated from the construct for the SWS1 and LWS genes are $0.909 \pm 0.024$ and $0.878 \pm 0.035$. These more accurate efficiencies enable a slightly better estimate of gene ratios.
6. Use the PCR efficiencies to determine the ratios between genes according to Eq. 3. If all of the opsin genes are measured, these can be normalized relative to the sum, using Eq. 8. Sample amplification curves are shown in Fig. 2a with the corresponding normalized gene expression ratios shown in Fig. 2b.

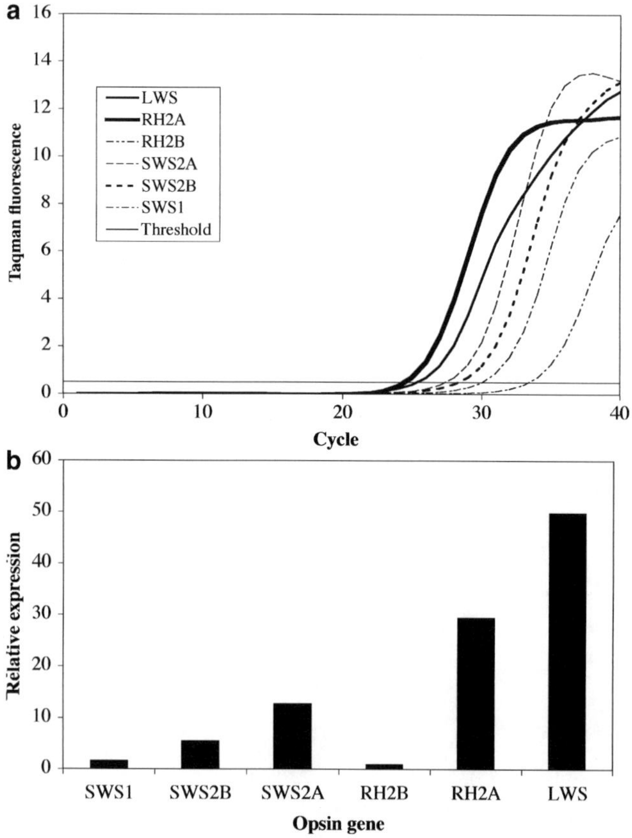


Fig. 2. (**a**) Sample amplification curves determined by TaqMan fluorescence monitored versus the number of PCR cycles. There can be significant variation in the overall shape because of random differences in amplification. The threshold method is used here to determine the critical cycle number for each gene. The threshold is set where amplification is in the exponentially increasing phase. If fluorescence were plotted on a logarithmic scale, this would be a linear region. (**b**) The relative gene expression for six opsin genes is determined from the critical cycle numbers using PCR efficiencies and Eq. 8. Note that even though $C_{tLWS}$ is higher than $C_{tRH2A}$, LWS gene transcripts are more abundant than RH2A transcripts because $E_{LWS}$ is lower than $E_{RH2A}$.

7. For final results, replicates of an individual sample can be averaged together. The individual results can then be averaged across individuals of a species (23), or developmental time points (27) or treatments (e.g., rearing temperature). Alternatively, the individuals might be used as separate data points in an ANOVA to compare species, developmental time points, or treatments (29).

## 4. Notes

1. The construct assures that the gene ratios are fixed. However, this approach could also use a mixture of gene products or plasmids made up with known relative concentrations.
2. The micropestle tubes work well for breaking up soft tissue such as retina. However, harder tissues should be disrupted using a rotor–stator tissue homogenizer to ensure that the tissue is thoroughly dissected and separated into cells.
3. There are numerous qPCR machines available. These differ primarily in the optical set up and in the software. Because PCR products are monitored by fluorescence, light must be sent to each well to excite a probe and then the emitted light is collected. In order to multiplex the detection of multiple genes, different dyes are used for each gene. These must then be spectrally separated during detection. Excitation typically uses either a spectrally broad lamp (tungsten–halogen or xenon) in combination with band-pass filters, or a spectrally narrower light-emitting diode or laser. Emitted light is typically separated by filters to isolate fluorescence from different dyes, which label different genes. Machines differ in how many emission signals they can separate from just one to four or more. Detection can be done one well at a time using a photomultiplier tube or photodiode. The detector is then scanned across each well of the qPCR plate to quantify each sample. Alternatively, light from the entire plate can be collected by a charge-coupled device (CCD) to detect and quantify PCR amplification in all wells simultaneously. Any of these machines can do the job as long as the fluorescent dyes are selected to match the excitation and emission wavelengths available for a given machine.
4. The primers and probes for qPCR can be made up using DNase-free water as these reactions work on cDNA and not RNA. We typically make primers up in TE/10 [1 mM Tris (pH 8.0) 0.1 mM EDTA]. Some manufacturers, such as Applied Biosystems (ABI), recommend testing a range of primer–probe concentrations to determine the optimal concentrations. We have not found this necessary and have used the concentrations listed here, which occupy the midpoint of the range suggested by ABI.

5. There are cheaper methods than ones using a kit to extract total RNA. These use a reagent such as TRIzol® (Invitrogen, Carlsbad, CA) or TRI reagent (Molecular Research Center, Cincinnati, OH) to isolate the RNA, followed by an RNA precipitation step. While these methods often work well, there can be problems with occasionally losing RNA pellets and difficulty with RNA resuspension. We have found the QIAGEN kit to be robust and reproducible across many different users in the lab.
6. QIAGEN has also developed an alternate method that uses 2% dithiothreitol (12 μl of 2 M DTT in 600 μl of buffer RLT), instead of 1% β-mercaptoethanol (6 μl of β-ME per 600 μl of buffer RLT), during lysis.
7. No more than 30 mg of tissue should be used, as the mini column can only capture 100 μg of RNA. See the QIAGEN manual for estimated amounts of RNA obtained from various kinds of tissue. Larger kits are available that can handle more tissue.
8. After spinning retina through the QIAshredder, there may be a dark layer in the bottom of the tube. This layer may contain proteins and retinal pigment and is typically brown to black in color. It often is quite loose and stringy and so is easily caught up during pipetting. It should be avoided, as it decreases the quality of RNA (based on the $A_{260}/A_{280}$ ratio).
9. If there is significant pigment carryover into the RNA (e.g., from melanin in the retinal pigment epithelium), this will provide significant absorbance background such that the $A_{260}/A_{280}$ ratio will not provide a good estimate of RNA concentration. In this case, it is better to use a fluorescent quantification method based on a dye such as RiboGreen (Invitrogen, Carlsbad, CA).
10. We often skip the heat inactivation step following the reverse transcription reaction. The first step of the qPCR is a 95°C hold for 10 min which should easily inactivate any remaining RT enzyme.
11. Genes could be multiplexed, combining several primer–probe mixes in the same tube. This requires labeling probes for different genes with different dyes, and having a qPCR machine that can resolve multiple dyes.
12. The thermal cycling parameters depend somewhat on the primer–probe design characteristics. Often, the probe is designed to anneal 10°C higher than the primers. It is common to use a two-step cycle with a 95°C denaturation step and a 60°C annealing and extension step. However, we have also used 95°C denaturation step for 15 s, a 55°C annealing step for 30 s and a 65°C extension step for 1 min with good success.

13. In performing qPCR replicates, the best replicates will be obtained if the same individual is prepared using enough master mix for both replicates and then run on the same qPCR plate. However, this may not provide the best estimate of qPCR errors. It is probably more realistic to prepare separate master mixes for each replicate and run them on different qPCR plates to get an actual estimate of the instrumental and pipetting errors that go into estimates of transcript expression. This will provide better comparisons with the individual to individual variation that is being quantified.
14. One factor that has a significant impact on $C_t$ reproducibility is probe concentration, as it impacts PCR efficiency. A factor of two in probe concentration can cause a $C_t$ shift of one cycle or more. We, therefore, make up a large enough batch of primer–probe mixture for an entire experiment. An experiment would include dilution curves for each gene plus all the individuals and replicates for that data set. So, if we wanted to examine ten individuals of ten species, we would make up enough primer–probe mixture (forward primer, reverse primer, and probe) for 2 replicates of 100 reactions plus another 20 reactions to measure the dilution series at the beginning and again at the end. This would then require 220 reactions worth of the primer–probe mixture for each gene. We have also noticed problems with extensive freeze thawing of primer–probe mixtures where $C_t$ tends to increase over time. Therefore, we either make up a large primer–probe aliquot and store it in the refrigerator and use it over a 1- or 2-week period, or we make up aliquots of a size needed to prepare one qPCR plate and store them in the freezer so that each aliquot is thawed only once.
15. The critical cycle number is determined based on a threshold value, which is determined differently on different qPCR machines. The threshold value can be determined by setting a standard threshold for all reactions (ABI), by determining the noise level of the background signal and setting the threshold at several times above this noise level (Stratagene), or by using the second derivative to determine the cycles at which the PCR product is most rapidly increasing (Roche). We have repeated samples on an ABI machine using a set threshold and on a Roche machine using second derivatives and have gotten comparable results by these two methods.
16. Theoretically, the PCR efficiency can never be greater than 1, as PCR products can only double from one cycle to the next. However, there is always experimental error in determining the slope of the dilution curve. When we get PCR efficiencies slightly greater than 1, we typically set them to 1.

## Acknowledgments

The author would like to thank Tyrone Spady for help with the development of the multigene construct for measuring PCR efficiencies and Christopher Hofmann for helpful comments to improve this manuscript. This work was supported with funding from NSF (IOS-0841270).

### References

1. Jessen TH, Weber RE, Fermi G et al (1991) Adaptation of bird hemoglobins to high altitudes: demonstration of molecular mechanism by protein engineering. Proc Natl Acad Sci USA **88**:6519–6522
2. Yokoyama S, Yokoyama R (1996) Adaptive evolution of photoreceptors and visual pigments in vertebrates. Annual Review of Ecology and Systematics **27**:543–567
3. Hoekstra HE, Hirschmann RJ, Bundey RA et al (2006) A single amino acid mutation contributes to adaptive beach mouse color pattern. Science **313**:101–104
4. King MC, Wilson AC (1975) Evolution at two levels in humans and chimpanzees. Science **188**:107–116
5. Shapiro MD, Bell MA, Kingsley DM (2006) Parallel genetic origins of pelvic reduction in vertebrates. Proc Natl Acad Sci USA **103**: 13753–13758
6. Prud'homme B, Gompel N, Rokas A et al (2006) Repeated morphological evolution through cis-regulatory changes in a pleiotropic gene. Nature **440**:1050–1053
7. Hoekstra HE, Coyne JA (2007) The locus of evolution: evo devo and the genetics of adaptation. Evolution Int J Org Evolution **61**:995–1016
8. Carroll SB (2008) Evo-devo and an expanding evolutionary synthesis: a genetic theory of morphological evolution. Cell **134**:25–36
9. Wray GA (2007) The evolutionary significance of cis-regulatory mutations. Nat Rev Genet **8**:206–216
10. Oakley TH (2007) Today's multiple choice exam: (a) gene duplication; (b) structural mutation; (c) co-option; (d) regulatory mutation; (e) all of the above. Evol Dev **9**:523–524
11. Stern DL, Orgogozo V (2008) The loci of evolution: how predictable is genetic evolution? Evolution **62**:2155–2177
12. Hawkins RD, Hon GC, Ren B (2010) Next-generation genomics: an integrative approach. Nat Rev Genet **11**:476–486
13. Bustin SA (2000) Absolute quantification of mRNA using real-time reverse transcription polymerase chain reaction assays. J Mol Endocrinol **25**:169–193
14. Bustin SA (2002) Quantification of mRNA using real-time reverse transcription PCR (RT-PCR): trends and problems. J Mol Endocrinol **29**:23–39
15. Liu W, Saint DA (2002) A new quantitative method of real time reverse transcription polymerase chain reaction assay based on simulation of polymerase chain reaction kinetics. Anal Biochem **302**:52–59
16. Gibson G (2002) Microarrays in ecology and evolution: a preview. Mol Ecol **11**:17–24
17. Zhou XJ, Gibson G (2004) Cross-species comparison of genome-wide expression patterns. Genome Biol **5**:232
18. Marguerat S, Bahler J (2009) RNA-seq: from technology to biology. Cell Mol Life Sci **67**:569–579
19. Marioni JC, Mason CE, Mane SM et al (2008) RNA-seq: an assessment of technical reproducibility and comparison with gene expression arrays. Genome Res **18**:1509–1517
20. Wang Z, Gerstein M, Snyder M (2009) RNA-Seq: a revolutionary tool for transcriptomics. Nat Rev Genet **10**:57–63
21. Rajeevan MS, Ranamukhaarachchi DG, Vernon SD et al (2001) Use of real-time quantitative PCR to validate the results of cDNA array and differential display PCR technologies. Methods **25**:443–451
22. Rajeevan MS, Vernon SD, Taysavang N et al (2001) Validation of array-based gene expression profiles by real-time (kinetic) RT-PCR. J Mol Diagn **3**:26–31
23. Hofmann CM, O'Quin KE, Marshall NJ et al (2009) The eyes have it: Regulatory and structural changes both underlie cichlid visual pigment diversity. PLoS Biol **7**:e1000266
24. Spady TC, Parry JW, Robinson PR et al (2006) Evolution of the cichlid visual palette through

ontogenetic subfunctionalization of the opsin gene arrays. Mol Biol Evol **23**:1538–1547

25. Hofmann CM, Carleton KL (2009) Gene duplication and differential gene expression play an important role in the diversification of visual pigments in fish. Integrative and Comparative Biology **49**:630–643
26. Yokoyama S (2008) Evolution of dim-light and color vision pigments. Annu Rev Genomics Hum Genet **9**:259–282
27. Carleton, K.L., Spady TC, Streelman JT et al (2008) Visual sensitivities tuned by heterochronic shifts in opsin gene expression. BMC Biol **6**:22
28. Glasel, J.A. (1995) Validity of nucleic acid purities monitored by 260nm/280nm absorbance ratios. Biotechniques **18**:62–63
29. Hofmann CM, O'Quin KE, Smith, A.R et al (2010) Plasticity of opsin gene expression in cichlids from Lake Malawi. Mol Ecol **19**: 2064–2074

# Chapter 18

# Using Pyrosequencing to Measure Allele-Specific mRNA Abundance and Infer the Effects of *Cis*- and *Trans*-regulatory Differences

Patricia J. Wittkopp

## Abstract

Changes in gene expression are an important source of phenotypic differences within and between species. Differences in RNA abundance can be readily quantified between genotypes using a variety of tools, including microarrays, quantitative real-time PCR, cDNA sequencing, and in situ hybridization, but determining the genetic basis of heritable expression differences has historically been less straightforward. Genetic changes that affect RNA abundance can be broadly classified into two groups depending on how they affect gene expression: *cis*-acting changes affect expression of a single allele in a diploid cell and are typically located close to the affected gene in the genome, whereas *trans*-acting changes affect expression of both alleles of a gene in a diploid cell and can be located virtually anywhere within a genome. By comparing relative expression of two alleles in an $F_1$ hybrid with relative expression between the two parental genotypes, the net effects of *cis*- and *trans*-acting changes can be discerned. Here, I describe how pyrosequencing can be used to obtain relative gene-specific and allele-specific expression. I also describe how such data can be used to infer the relative contribution of *cis*- and *trans*-acting changes to expression differences between genotypes.

**Key words:** Gene regulation, Allelic imbalance, Gene expression, Pyrosequencing, Quantitative, mRNA transcripts, Divergence, Polymorphism, Evolution

## 1. Introduction

Quantifying allele-specific expression is a powerful way to examine the regulation of gene expression and determine how this process differs between individuals and between species. For example, measurements of allele-specific expression can be used to test for genomic imprinting (e.g., (1, 2)), for expression divergence between paralogous genes (e.g., (3)), and for differences in *cis*- and *trans*-regulation within and between species (e.g., (4–8)). Pyrosequencing

Virginie Orgogozo and Matthew V. Rockman (eds.), *Molecular Methods for Evolutionary Genetics*,
Methods in Molecular Biology, vol. 772, DOI 10.1007/978-1-61779-228-1_18, © Springer Science+Business Media, LLC 2011

is a time- and cost-effective technique for quantifying allele-specific expression of single genes in a high-throughput manner. Here, I describe the protocols used in my laboratory for obtaining measurements of relative gene expression between two genotypes and relative allelic expression between two alleles within a single heterozygous genotype. These methods have been shown to produce estimates of relative gene expression that are consistent with microarrays (2), quantitative reverse transcriptase PCR (qRT-PCR) (2), and (most recently) cDNA sequencing (9).

Pyrosequencing is a method of DNA sequencing that couples primer extension with light production (10): each time a nucleotide is added to a 3′ end of DNA by DNA polymerase, a constant amount of light is produced. This light is captured by a camera monitoring each well of a 96-well plate and the amount of light produced in each well is recorded in a "pyrogram" (a sample of which is shown in Fig. 3a). The height of "peaks" observed in the pyrogram provides a quantitative readout of the number of nucleotides added to 3′ ends of DNA within a well at a particular time. This quantitative readout of primer extension makes pyrosequencing well suited not only for genotyping individuals but also for quantifying relative abundance in samples of DNA (or cDNA) containing more than one allele.

Pyrosequencing has many applications; however, this chapter focuses solely on using pyrosequencing to measure differences in transcript abundance between genotypes and between different alleles in heterozygous cells. Such data can be used to distinguish between *cis*- and *trans*-acting changes that contribute to expression differences between genotypes (6). Total expression differences are measured between two genotypes, and then relative allelic expression is measured in $F_1$ hybrids produced by crossing the two genotypes. These $F_1$ hybrids carry one *cis*-regulatory allele from each of the parental genotypes within the same cell, providing a direct readout of relative *cis*-regulatory activity because the two alleles are exposed to a common *trans*-regulatory environment. Any differences in allelic expression within these heterozygous genotypes must, therefore, be caused by differences in *cis*-regulatory activity (4). Any expression difference between parental genotypes for that gene that is in excess of the *cis*-regulatory difference observed in the $F_1$ hybrids is attributed to changes in *trans*-regulation (6). Differences in the activity or abundance transcription factors as well as differences in the environment and/or abundance of cell types will all be detected as *trans*-regulatory effects with this assay. The methods used to obtain such measures of transcript abundance are described below, divided into the following sections: (a) designing a pyrosequencing assay, (b) extraction of genomic DNA and RNA, (c) cDNA synthesis, (d) pyrosequencing, (e) experimental design, and (f) data analysis and interpretation.

## 2. Materials

### *2.1. Designing a Pyrosequencing Assay*

1. At least 50 bp of aligned, transcribed, exonic sequence from two alleles of each gene (or exon) of interest, containing at least one single-nucleotide polymorphism (SNP).
2. PyroMark Assay Design Software 2.0 (Qiagen). This software is recommended, but not essential (see step 3 in Subheading 3.1).

### *2.2. Extraction of Genomic DNA and Total RNA from Biological Tissue*

1. Tissue samples to be analyzed. This may include samples from two (preferably inbred) genotypes and/or samples from a single heterozygous genotype. For the inference of *cis*- and *trans*-regulatory differences between genotypes, one sample should contain an approximately equal mix of tissue from the two genotypes of interest and another should contain tissue from $F_1$ heterozygotes produced by crossing the two genotypes of interest.
2. SV Total RNA Isolation Kit (Promega) containing: Spin Columns, Waste Collection tubes, Elution tubes, RNA Lysis Buffer, RNA Dilution Buffer, β-mercaptoethanol (BME, 48.7%), DNase I (lyophilized), $MnCl_2$, 0.09 M Yellow Core Buffer, DNase Stop Solution, RNA Wash Solution, and Nuclease-Free Water.
3. 95% ethanol, prepared with RNAse-free water.
4. 70% ethanol, chilled to −20°C, does NOT need to be prepared with RNAse-free water.

### *2.3. cDNA Synthesis*

1. RNA from tissue(s) of interest.
2. RNAse-free DNAse (Promega).
3. Primer for reverse transcription (500 μg/ml). A "poly-T" primer such as 5′-TTTTTTTTTTTTTTTTTT-3′ or 5′-TTTT TTTTTTTTTTTTTVN-3′ is most often used; however, a gene-specific primer could be used if the researcher is only interested in assaying expression of a single gene.
4. dNTP mix containing dATP, dCTP, dTTP, and dGTP at 10 mM each.
5. RNAsin (Promega).
6. Moloney Murine Leukemia Virus Reverse Transcriptase (M-MLV-RT, Promega), which is shipped with 5× First-Strand Buffer [250 mM Tris–HCl, pH 8.3 at room temperature, 375 mM KCl, 15 mM $MgCl_2$] and 0.1 M DTT. SuperScript™ II Reverse Transcriptase with its associated buffer (Invitrogen) has also been used with success.

### 2.4. Pyrosequencing

1. Nucleic acid template (genomic DNA or cDNA).
2. 10× PCR buffer: 100 mM Tris–HCl, 500 mM KCl, 15 mM $MgCl_2$, pH 8.3 at 25°C.
3. dNTP mix containing dATP, dCTP, dTTP, and dGTP at 1.5 mM each.
4. 10 μM solution of biotinylated PCR primer, see (1) in Fig. 1.
5. 10 μM solution of nonbiotinylated PCR primer, see (2) in Fig. 1.
6. *Taq* or equivalent thermostable DNA polymerase.
7. Sterile water.
8. Glassware for solutions, rinsed with deionized water to eliminate residual phosphate from detergent.
9. Pyrosequencing primer (100 μM), see (3) in Fig. 1, for each assay.
10. Streptavidin Sepharose, High Performance (GE Healthcare).
11. 70% ethanol.
12. 4 M hydrochloric acid and 1 M acetic acid for pH adjustments.
13. Binding Buffer: 10 mM Tris–HCl, 2 M NaCl, 1 mM EDTA, 0.1% Tween 20, pH 7.6.
14. Denaturing Buffer: 0.2 M NaOH.
15. Wash Buffer: 10 mM Tris–acetate, pH 7.6.
16. Annealing Buffer: 20 mM Tris–acetate, 2 mM Mg–acetate, pH 7.6.
17. PyroMark Q96 Vacuum Prep Troughs (Qiagen).
18. PyroMark Q96 Plate Low (Qiagen).
19. PyroMark Q96 Cartridge (Qiagen).
20. Pyro Gold Reagents or Pyro Gold SQA Reagents (Qiagen), containing: Enzyme mixture (DNA polymerase, ATP-sulfurylase, luciferase, and apyrase), Substrate mixture (luciferin, adenosine 5′ phosphosulfate), Nucleotides (dATP αS, dCTP, dGTP, and dTTP, separately).

```
      (1) Biotinylated PCR primer           focal SNP
5'-*ATCGTGTGCGTCGAGATACA-3                     ↓
  5'-ATCGTGTGCGTCGAGATACACTACTGA G/C TtgcactattgctcatAGCAACCTCTAGTATAGCGTAATCTG-3'
                                    3'-acgtgataacgagta-5'3'-GAGATCATATCGCATTAGAC-5'
                                    (3) Pyrosequencing primer          (2) PCR primer
```

Fig. 1. Overview of primers and sequence components of a pyrosequencing assay. Three primers are required for each pyrosequencing assay: two primers (1 and 2) that are used for PCR amplification of a region including the focal SNP (*arrow*) and an internal primer that is used for pyrosequencing (3). The PCR primer (1) that is on the opposite strand from the pyrosequencing primer (3) is labelled with a biotin molecule (*asterisk*) at its 5′ end.

21. PyroMark Vacuum Prep Tool (Qiagen).
22. PyroMark Vacuum Prep Tool Filter Probes (Qiagen).
23. PyroMark Q96 ID machine (Qiagen), or a predecessor such as the PSQ 96 machine (Biotage), with accompanying operating software and computer.

## 3. Methods

### 3.1. Designing a Pyrosequencing Assay

Pyrosequencing determines the relative abundance of alternative mRNA transcripts by using a SNP to discriminate between two alleles. Selection of the SNP to be assayed is, therefore, critical to the success of the experiment. Pyrosequencing assay design begins with at least 50 bp of transcribed, exonic sequence from each allele for a gene of interest (see Note 1). If not already available, allele-specific sequences can typically be obtained with traditional Sanger sequencing of PCR products produced from genomic DNA or cDNA. Using these sequences, three primers must be designed for each pyrosequencing assay, all centered around the chosen focal SNP (Fig. 1): two primers will be used to amplify a 50–200-bp region of sequence containing the focal SNP via PCR and the third primer will be annealed within 1–3 bp of the focal SNP and used for pyrosequencing.

1. Align sequences from the alleles to be compared and identify all SNPs and other sequence differences. This can easily be done in most sequence analysis programs.
2. Examine each SNP to identify the one(s) that are best suited to pyrosequencing, considering the following criteria:
   (a) At least 15 bp of sequence immediately adjacent to the SNP on at least one side must be identical between the two alleles. There must also be two regions of identical exonic sequence flanking the focal SNP that are located 50–200 bp apart, each at least 20 bp long, to allow for annealing of PCR primers (Fig. 1). To allow the direct comparison of amplicons from genomic DNA and cDNA, the amplified fragment (containing the focal SNP) should come from a single exon.
   (b) Try to avoid SNPs that are part of homopolymers, which are strings of two or more consecutive, identical nucleotides (e.g., GG or TTT), in either allele. All consecutive bases of the same type are incorporated at the same time in a pyrosequencing reaction, and the accuracy of such aggregate peaks is lower than peaks reflecting the incorporation of a single base in each sequence. If homopolymers cannot be avoided completely, choose a SNP in which one allele

forms a homopolymer not more than two nucleotides long (e.g., G/TG, where G/T are the alternate alleles of the SNP and the following G is present in both alleles) (see Note 2).

(c) Give highest priority to G/C SNPs, next highest priority to G/A, G/T, C/A, and C/T SNPs, and lowest priority to A/T SNPs. This is because the incorporation of dATP during pyrosequencing (which cannot be avoided for A/T SNPs) produces more light than the incorporation of dTTP, dGTP, or dCTP, requiring the use of a correction factor (see Note 3) that can increase the variance of replicate measurements.

(d) If a "poly T" primer will be used for the production of cDNA, give preference to SNPs located near the 3′ end of the transcribed region to maximize the likelihood that the focal SNP is contained within each cDNA molecule synthesized from the mRNA of interest.

3. Design PCR and pyrosequencing primers to interrogate focal SNP. The easiest way to do this is to use the PyroMark Assay Design Software 2.0 (http://www.pyrosequencing.com/DynPage.aspx?id=7257) with the "allele quantification" option selected. This software allows multiple assays to be designed in a high-throughput, "batch processing" manner. If this proprietary software is not available, however, the three primers required for each pyrosequencing assay can be designed manually using a freely available primer design program such as Primer3 (11). Care must be taken to check all primers and the PCR product for hairpins and complementary sequences within and between primers that could cause unintended nucleotide bases to be added to 3′ ends of DNA during pyrosequencing. Because the pyrosequencing reaction occurs at 28°C, complementary sequence of as few as four 3′ bases of DNA can prime DNA synthesis. Such extension introduces background signal that can interfere with the accurate quantification of alleles at the focal SNP. Additional tips for designing primers well suited for pyrosequencing are available from the technical support division of Qiagen.

4. Synthesize the three primers designed for each assay, adding a biotin molecule to the 5′ end of the PCR primer that anneals to the opposite strand from the pyrosequencing primer (Fig. 1). Most commercial suppliers of oligonucleotides (e.g., Integrated DNA Technologies) will add a 5′ biotin molecule to an oligonucleotide for an additional fee.

### 3.2. Extraction of Genomic DNA and Total RNA from Biological Tissue

This chapter specifically describes analysis of the two types of biological samples required to infer the relative effects of *cis*- and *trans*-regulatory variation: a mixed sample of tissue from two highly inbred "parental" genotypes and a tissue sample from the heterozygous $F_1$ hybrid genotype produced by crossing the two parental genotypes together (see Note 4). For the mixed parental tissue sample, and in any case where expression is compared between two genotypes, similar amounts of tissue from the two genotypes should be used. For the hybrid tissue sample, and in any case where only a single genotype is examined, all of the tissue is derived from the same (heterozygous) genotype. Genomic DNA and total RNA are extracted from each tissue sample. Genomic DNA and RNA should always be extracted from the same homogenate of a mixed tissue sample to allow the relative abundance of both cells and RNA from each genotype to be determined. The extraction of genomic DNA and RNA from the same tissue homogenate is not essential for samples containing only a single genotype, but is recommended for consistency if comparing to mixed tissue samples. Regardless of extraction method, pyrosequencing analysis of genomic DNA from heterozygous cells is critical to measure and control for any inequality in PCR amplification and/or pyrosequencing detection of the two alleles (5, 6).

A protocol for extracting genomic DNA and total RNA from a single tissue homogenate is described below. It was developed for use with the SV Total RNA isolation kit from Promega (Madison, WI), and was modified from (12). It has been tested most extensively with *Drosophila* (fruit fly) species, but should also be suitable for tissue from most multicellular eukaryotes. The protocol is divided into three sections: tissue homogenization (steps 1–8), RNA extraction (steps 9–22), and genomic DNA extraction (steps 23–29). The genomic DNA and RNA recovery can proceed in parallel; however, if they are processed in series, RNA recovery (steps 9–22) should be completed first to minimize the likelihood of degradation.

1. Collect tissue, freeze in liquid nitrogen, and store at –80°C until ready for extraction.
2. Homogenize ~15 mg of tissue (see Note 5) in 175 μl SV RNA Lysis Buffer with BME added. Add 350 μl of SV RNA Dilution Buffer and vortex at least for 1 min.
3. Centrifuge for 10 min on maximum speed at room temperature.
4. Transfer supernatant to RNAse-free microcentrifuge tube and add 75 μl of 95% ethanol (RNAse-free).
5. Mix by inverting ten times.
6. Transfer to SV Total RNA Spin Column Assembly and let stand for 5 min at room temperature. Genomic DNA binds to the column resin during this step.

7. Centrifuge for 1 min on maximum speed at room temperature.
8. Transfer flow-through, which contains RNA and proteins, to a clean RNAse-free microcentrifuge tube.
9. Add 300 μl of RNAse-free 95% ethanol to the flow-through from step 8 above.
10. Mix gently by inversion.
11. Transfer solution to a *new* SV Total RNA Spin Column Assembly and let stand for 1 min at room temperature. RNA binds to the column resin during this step.
12. Centrifuge on high speed for 1 min. Discard the flow-through.
13. Apply 600 μl of SV RNA Wash solution to the column. Centrifuge on high for 1 min. Discard the flow-through.
14. Mix 40 μl of Yellow Core buffer, 5 μl of 0.09 M $MnCl_2$, 5 μl of DNAse (in this order), and pipette mixture onto the column. Be sure to cover column surface completely.
15. Let stand for 15 min at room temperature.
16. Add 200 μl of SV DNAse Stop Solution, let stand at room temperature for 1 min, and then centrifuge for 1 min on high speed. Discard the flow-through.
17. Apply 600 μl of SV RNA Wash solution to the column. Centrifuge on high for 1 min. Discard the flow-through.
18. Apply 250 μl of SV RNA Wash solution to column. Centrifuge on high for 1 min. Discard the flow-through.
19. Centrifuge again for 1 min to remove any residual wash solution. Discard the flow-through.
20. Place Spin Column into sterile Elution tube. Add 100 μl of Nuclease-free water to column, covering surface completely. Let stand at room temperature for 5 min. Centrifuge on high for 1 min. This eluate contains total RNA.
21. Quality and quantity can be crudely examined using agarose gel electrophoresis. Strong bands corresponding to 18S and 28S rRNA should be clearly visible along with faint a "smear" of RNA of other lengths.
22. RNA samples should be stored at –80°C until used for cDNA synthesis to avoid degradation.
23. Add 700 μl of cold 70% ethanol to the Spin Column used for steps 1–8. Let stand for 1 min at room temperature. Centrifuge on high for 1 min. Discard the flow-through.
24. Repeat previous step.
25. Centrifuge for 1 min on high to remove any residual ethanol. Discard the flow-through.

26. Place Spin Column into a sterile Elution tube. Add 100 μl of nuclease-free water to the Spin Column. Let stand at room temperature for 5 min. (Heating the column to 55–60°C while standing increases recovery, but can also increase degradation.) Centrifuge on high for 1 min. This eluate contains the genomic DNA.
27. Repeat previous step and combine eluates.
28. Quality and quantity of genomic DNA can be crudely examined using agarose gel electrophoresis. A large, single band should be most prominent.
29. Genomic DNA should be stored at either –20°C or –80°C until needed.

### 3.3. cDNA Synthesis

Prior to pyrosequencing, the RNA must be converted into (single- or double-stranded) cDNA. Any cDNA synthesis protocol can be used for this purpose. "Poly T" primer, which will allow cDNA to be synthesized from all polyadenylated mRNA, or one or more gene-specific primers can be used depending on the number of genes that will be examined. A DNAse treatment of the RNA template immediately prior to cDNA synthesis is strongly recommended to remove any genomic DNA that survived the DNAse treatment administered during RNA extraction.

1. Combine 8.0 μl (~1.5 μg) total RNA extracted as described in Subheading 3.2, 8.4 μl of 5× First-Strand Buffer, and 2.0 μl of DNAse. Incubate at 37°C for 1 h.
2. Heat to 65°C for 15 min to inactivate the DNAse.
3. Add 5.4 μl (500 μg/ml) of primer for reverse transcription and slowly cool to 37°C for over 10 min.
4. Add 4.2 μl of dNTP mix (10 mM per nucleotide), 1 μl of RNAsin, and 1.2 μl of M-MLV-RT and incubate at 37°C for 1 h. (Inclusion of 3 μl of DTT is optional).
5. Dilute as appropriate. We typically add 69.8 μl of nuclease-free water to dilute the 30.2 μl of cDNA synthesis reaction to 100 μl total. For most genes, 1–2 μl of this diluted single-stranded cDNA is sufficient to produce a strong PCR product suitable for pyrosequencing (see below). For lowly expressed genes, increasing the amount of cDNA used may help to achieve a strong PCR product.

### 3.4. Pyrosequencing

Pyrosequencing involves three major steps: PCR amplification of sequence containing the focal SNP, recovery of single-stranded PCR product with the pyrosequencing primer annealed, and pyrosequencing, which is the real-time monitoring of a controlled primer extension reaction by a machine such as the PyroMark Q96 ID (Qiagen) or PSQ 96 (Biotage).

#### 3.4.1. PCR Amplification of Sequence to Be Analyzed

Virtually any PCR protocol that produces a single amplified product with no evidence of primer dimers or residual primers can be used for pyrosequencing. Each pair of PCR primers may require some optimization (e.g., by changing the annealing temperature, extension time, and/or amount of DNA or cDNA template) to obtain a single amplified product that produces enough material for pyrosequencing. Starting conditions used for testing each new pair of PCR primers for pyrosequencing in my laboratory follow:

- 2 μl of nucleic acid template (i.e., genomic DNA or cDNA, ~0.1–10 ng).
- 5 μl of 10× PCR buffer (including 15 mM $MgCl_2$).
- 5 μl of dNTP mix (i.e., dATP, dCTP, dTTP, and dGTP, each at 1.5 mM).
- 2 μl of 10 μM biotinylated PCR primer, (1) in Fig. 1.
- 2 μl of 10 μM nonbiotinylated PCR primer, (2) in Fig. 1.
- 0.2 μl of *Taq* polymerase (5 units/μl) (or equivalent thermostable DNA polymerase).
- 33.8 μl of sterile water.

This 50-μl reaction is subject to 35–50 cycles of 94°C for 30 s, 55–68°C (depending on primer sequences) for 30 s, and 72°C for 15–60 s (depending on length of PCR product). These cycles are preceded by heating the reaction to 94°C for 3 min and followed by cooling the reaction to 4°C. The amount of PCR product is assessed by running 5 μl of the completed PCR reaction on an agarose gel. An easily visible band containing at least 30 ng of DNA should be observed. PCR products must be arrayed in a 96-well plate format for pyrosequencing, and it is easiest to simply perform the PCR reactions in a 96-well plate.

#### 3.4.2. Recovery of Single-Stranded PCR Product with Pyrosequencing Primer Annealed

Prior to pyrosequencing, the double-stranded PCR product must be denatured and the strand that is not complementary to the pyrosequencing primer removed. The pyrosequencing primer is then annealed to the remaining, complementary strand. Recovery of the appropriate strand is mediated by the interaction between biotin (which is located at the 5′ end of the appropriate PCR primer (Fig. 1)) and streptavidin-coated sepharose. The most efficient way to process a 96-well plate of samples is to use the PyroMark Vacuum Prep Tool (Qiagen), as described below. This hand-held vacuum device is fitted with 96 PyroMark Vacuum Prep Tool Filter Probes, which allow liquids, but not the streptavidin sepharose, to pass through. A protocol for using this tool to prepare a 96-well plate of PCR products for pyrosequencing follows. An alternative protocol using magnetic beads instead of the PyroMark Vacuum Prep Tool is available from Qiagen.

1. Preheat a heating block that holds a 96-well plate to 90°C.
2. Add 3 μl of streptavidin sepharose and 40 μl of Binding Buffer to each PCR product (which should be 40–45 μl after analysis of 5 μl by gel electrophoresis), and cover tightly (see Note 6).
3. Vortex the plate containing PCR products and streptavidin sepharose at maximum speed for 10 min at room temperature to maximize binding between the biotinylated strands of PCR products and the streptavidin sepharose.
4. While the plate is shaking, do the following:
   (a) Fill five PyroMark Q96 Vacuum Prep Troughs with the following solutions, arranging the trays from left to right in the following order: deionized water, 70% ethanol, Denaturing Buffer, Wash Buffer, and deionized water.
   (b) Prepare a PyroMark Q96 Plate Low (which is a specially sized 96-well plate) for pyrosequencing by adding 40 μl of 0.5 μM pyrosequencing primer diluted in Annealing Buffer (20 mM Tris–Acetate, 2 mM Mg–Acetate, pH 7.6) to each well. The pyrosequencing primer in each well should match the PCR product in the corresponding well of the original PCR plate.
   (c) Add 620 μl of water to the Pyro Gold (or Pyro Gold SQA) Reagent vial labelled "Enzyme". Mix thoroughly by shaking.
   (d) Add 620 μl of water to the Pyro Gold (or Pyro Gold SQA) Reagent vial labelled "Substrate". Mix thoroughly by shaking.
   (e) Pipet all 620 μl of the resuspended "Enzyme" and "Substrate" solutions as well as 200 μl of each nucleotide into the PyroMark Q96 Cartridge as shown in Fig. 2 (see Note 7).
   (f) Allow solutions to warm completely to room temperature.

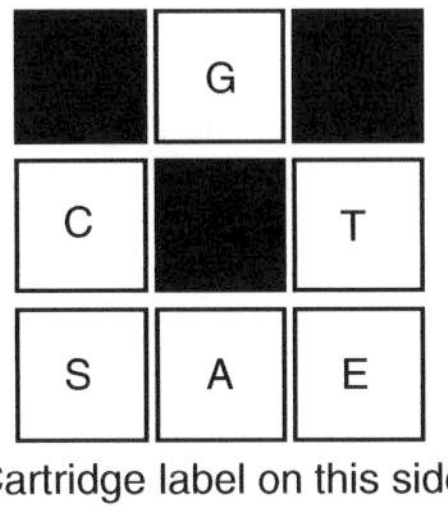


Fig. 2. Placement of enzyme (E), substrate (S), and nucleotides (A, C, G, T) in the PyroMark Q96 Cartridge. Arrangement shown is looking down at the top of the cartridge with the label closest to the researcher, as indicated.

5. Remove the plate containing PCR products and streptavidin beads from the vortex. Remove plate cover carefully to avoid contamination of neighboring wells. Turn on vacuum so that air is being drawn through the PyroMark Vacuum Prep Tool Filter Probes of the PyroMark Vacuum Prep Tool. Place in the left-most trough containing water for 30 s, drawing water through the pins.
   (a) Move the PyroMark Vacuum Prep Tool into the 96-well plate containing the PCR products and streptavidin beads for 2–3 s, moving it up and down. The goal is to capture all of the beads from each well on the bottom of a Vacuum Prep Tool Filter Probe.
   (b) Move the PyroMark Vacuum Prep Tool into the second trough (ii) containing 70% ethanol for 5–10 s.
   (c) Move the PyroMark Vacuum Prep Tool into the third trough (iii) containing Denaturing Buffer for 5–10 s.
   (d) Move the PyroMark Vacuum Prep Tool into the fourth trough (iv) containing Wash Buffer for 5–10 s.
   (e) Remove the PyroMark Vacuum Prep Tool from the fourth trough and (after all of the liquid has been pulled away from the sepharose), *turn off the vacuum*, holding the PyroMark Vacuum Prep Tool in the air (ideally, just above the PyroMark Q96 Plate Low). Make sure the suction has stopped completely prior to proceeding with the next step.
   (f) Carefully place the PyroMark Vacuum Prep Tool into the PyroMark Q96 Plate Low containing the pyrosequencing primers in annealing buffer. Be sure to line up the pins and wells correctly such that the beads originally collected from well A1 in the PCR plate match up with the pyrosequencing primer for well A1 in the PyroMark Q96 Plate Low.
   (g) Gently swirl the PyroMark Vacuum Prep Tool in the PyroMark Q96 Plate Low to shake off sepharose.
   (h) Place the PyroMark Q96 Vacuum Prep Tool into the fifth trough (v) containing water and shake to further remove any remaining sepharose.
   (i) Transfer the PyroMark Q96 Plate Low to a heat block at 90°C and let it stand for 2 min.
   (j) Remove the PyroMark Q96 Plate Low from the heating block and allow to cool slowly to room temperature (10–15 min). This plate contains the single-stranded PCR product with the pyrosequencing primer annealed and is ready to be used for pyrosequencing.

6. Clean the PyroMark Q96 Vacuum Prep Tool by turning the vacuum on and allowing it to sit in the first trough (i) containing clean water for 30 s. With the vacuum still running, carefully lift the PyroMark Q96 Vacuum Prep Tool out of the trough and shake in the air for 30 s to remove any excess water. Store on a piece of dry paper towel (see Note 8).

#### *3.4.3. Pyrosequencing*

Before pyrosequencing can be performed, each assay must be programmed into the software and the arrangement of assays within a plate must be entered into the operating software. For each assay, the following information must be entered:

- "Sequence to analyze", which is the sequence immediately following the pyrosequencing primer, including the focal SNP. For the assay shown in Fig. 1, the sequence to analyze is 5′-AG/CTCAGTAGT-3′. Note that this is the reverse complement of the sequence shown in Fig. 1 because of the strand that anneals to the pyrosequencing primer.
- "Dispensation order", which is the order in which nucleotides will be dispensed. For the assay shown in Fig. 1, one possible dispensation order is tAGCaTCAGTAGT. The lower case "t" and "a" nucleotides are not expected to be added to the growing oligonucleotide chain, but rather are used to detect background signal in the assay. The PyroMark operating software will determine the dispensation order based on the sequence to analyze; however, the user can also manually edit the dispensation order and may want to do so in some cases (see Note 9).

Place PyroMark Q96 Plate Low containing streptavidin beads bound to biotinylated single-stranded PCR product with pyrosequencing primer annealed and the PyroMark Q96 Cartridge filled as described in Subheading 3.4.2 step 4(e) into the pyrosequencing machine and run as instructed in the operating manual. At the end of a pyrosequencing run, which takes approximately 15 min for a single 96-well plate, the results from each well are provided graphically in a pyrogram (Fig. 3a). The height of each nucleotide specific peak can also be exported in a tabular format (Fig. 3b). For large projects involving many different assays and/or many different biological samples, custom programs can be written to most efficiently calculate relative allele-specific expression levels using the table of peak height information (see Note 10).

### *3.5. Experimental Design*

This section deals with the most effective experimental design for inferring *cis*- and *trans*-regulatory differences between genotypes, including critical controls, an optional titration series analysis, and considerations for levels of replication required to obtain reliable data.

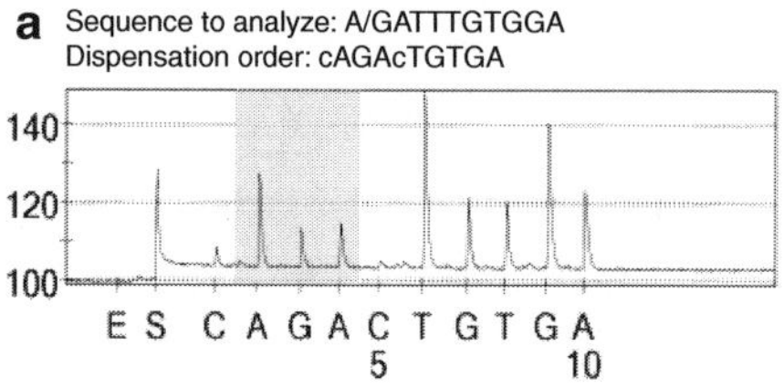


**b**

| Disp. | 1 | 2 | 3 | 4 | 5 | 6 | 7 | 8 | 9 | 10 |
|---|---|---|---|---|---|---|---|---|---|---|
| Well | C | A | G | A | C | T | G | T | G | A |
| | 4.96 | 24.11 | 9.66 | 11.05 | 1.76 | 45.25 | 18.05 | 17.1 | 37.09 | 19.87 |

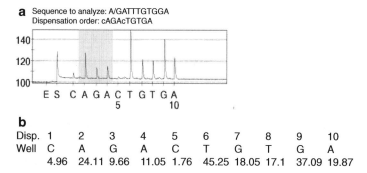

Fig. 3. Sample output from pyrosequencing. (**a**) A "pyrogram" showing the peaks reflecting the amount of light produced following the addition of the enzyme (E), substrate (S), and individual nucleotides (C, A, G, A, C, T, G, T, G, A) to the pyrosequencing reaction. The sequence to analyze and dispensation order are also shown. *Lower case bases* are not expected to be incorporated. Note the presence of some background signal when the first cytosine was added to the reaction. Also note that this assay involves a homopolymer (AA) in one of the two alleles. The dispensation order was altered from the default suggested by the pyrosequencing software to completely separate peaks from the two alleles. In this case, the software recommended a dispensation order of "cGAc", whereas the dispensation order used was "cAGAc". This change allows the first A peak to represent only one allele (AATTTGTGGA), whereas the G and second A represent only the other allele (GATTTGTGGA). The rationale for this modification is further described in Note 2. *Peaks* reflecting incorporation of nucleotides corresponding to the alternate alleles are *shaded gray*. The *first A peak* represents incorporation of two successive A nucleotides. (**b**) *Peak heights* (PH) shown in the tabular output format. In panel (**a**), the percentage of the molecules attributed to the A allele of the SNP reported by the pyrosequencing software (using its proprietary formulas) was 51.5%. Using the data from the peak heights table and the default correction factor for each adenine of 0.86, the percentage of molecules attributed to the A allele of the SNP is $(0.86 \times 24.11)/((0.86 \times 24.11) + 9.66 + (0.86 \times 11.05)) = 52\%$.

#### 3.5.1. Controls

Prior to the use of any new pyrosequencing assay to collect biologically relevant data, there are three important control pyrosequencing reactions that must be run:

- *Confirm allele-specific genotypes*: Pyrosequencing reactions should be run to analyze PCR products derived from each individual genotype examined to confirm the focal SNP alleles that the assay was designed to detect.
- *Template only*: A reaction should be performed by replacing the annealing buffer containing the pyrosequencing primer in the PyroMark Q96 Plate Low with annealing buffer alone. Any signal pyrosequencing signal observed in this reaction is attributed to a hairpin forming at the 3′ end of the single-stranded PCR product that primes DNA synthesis (see Note 11).
- *Pyrosequencing primer only*: A reaction should be performed in which the PCR product is replaced with water. Sepharose from this well should be transferred to a well in the PyroMark Q96 Plate Low containing the pyrosequencing primer for each assay

in annealing buffer. Any pyrosequencing signal observed in this reaction is attributed to the pyrosequencing primer hybridizing to itself (in either a hairpin or primer dimer) at the 3′ end that primes DNA synthesis (see Note 11).

*3.5.2. Titration Series (Optional)*

Analysis of a titration series is recommended for first-time users and for trouble-shooting; however, it is not strictly required for all assays once the protocol has been well established in a laboratory. It can be performed as follows:

1. Use PCR primers for a given assay to amplify each of the alleles to be compared in separate PCR reactions, as described for the "*confirm allele-specific genotypes*" control reaction in the preceding section.
2. Dilute both PCR products to approximately 1 ng/μl. Estimates based on the intensity of bands on an agarose gel are sufficient for this purpose.
3. Perform serial dilutions with each PCR product to get a range of concentrations. For example, to examine a titration series from 70:30 to 30:70, with steps of ~10%:
   (a) Combine 16 μl of original PCR product and 4 μl water to get dilution #1, and then combine 16 μl of dilution #1 and 4 μl of water to get dilution #2. Repeat this process five more times to produce dilutions #1–7 for each PCR product.
   (b) Combine 3 μl of dilution #3 from PCR product A with 3 μl of dilution #7 from PCR product B to generate a solution that is 70.94% PCR product A by volume. Add 0.6 μl water to dilute DNA concentration to be equal to the 50% sample described in step (d) below.
   (c) Combine 3 μl of dilution #4 from PCR product A with 3 μl of dilution #6 from PCR product B to generate a solution that is 60.98% PCR product A by volume. Add 0.15 μl water to dilute DNA concentration to be equal to the 50% sample.
   (d) Combine 3 μl of dilution #5 from PCR product A with 3 μl of dilution #5 from PCR product B to generate a solution that is 50% PCR product A by volume.
   (e) Combine 3 μl of dilution #6 from PCR product A with 3 μl of dilution #4 from PCR product B to generate a solution that is 39.02% PCR product A by volume. Add 0.15 μl of water to dilute DNA concentration to be equal to the 50% sample.
   (f) Combine 3 μl of dilution #7 from PCR product A with 3 μl of dilution #3 from PCR product B to generate a

solution that is 29.06% PCR product A by volume. Add 0.6 μl of water to dilute DNA concentration to be equal to the 50% sample.

(g) For each of these five combinations of PCR products, use 2 μl as the template for new PCR reactions and analyze the PCR products with pyrosequencing.

4. A PCR/pyrosequencing reaction should also be performed in parallel using genomic DNA from cells known to be heterozygous for the two alleles under study. This provides a pyrosequencing measurement for a template that is known to contain exactly 50% of each allele and measures the relative PCR amplification efficiency of the two alleles.
5. Using the peak heights from the focal SNP from each pyrosequencing reaction, divide the peak height from the nucleotide present in allele 1 by the peak height from the nucleotide present in allele 2.
6. Compare these ratios from the heterozygous DNA pyrosequencing reaction and the 50:50 PCR product pyrosequencing reaction by dividing the allele 1–allele 2 ratio from the 50:50 DNA sample by that from the heterozygous DNA sample. This value is called "*C*", and represents the concentration of PCR product 1 at the beginning of the serial dilutions relative to the concentration of PCR product 2 at the beginning of the serial dilutions. The 50:50 DNA sample is affected by the same (if any) PCR amplification bias between alleles observed in the heterozygous DNA sample, which is cancelled out by taking the ratio, leaving only the relative concentration of the starting PCR products used to construct the titration series (6).
7. To compare the pyrosequencing estimates of relative allelic abundance in the titration series to the "true" relative allele abundance in each sample, the volume-based proportions of the two alleles must be adjusted for concentration differences between the two PCR products used to construct the titration series. These adjusted values are calculated as: (proportion by volume of allele $1 \times C$)/(proportion by volume of allele $1 \times C +$ proportion by volume of allele 2). For example, in the sample containing 30% by volume of allele 1, the "true" proportion of allele 1 in the mixed sample (by number of molecules) would be $(0.3 \times C)/((0.3 \times C) + 0.7)$.

Figure 4 shows a theoretical and an empirical example of results from a titration series.

#### 3.5.3. Replication

To obtain the most reliable estimates of relative allelic expression, an experiment should include replicate biological samples as well as replicate pyrosequencing measurements of each biological sample. The most appropriate amount and type of replication will vary

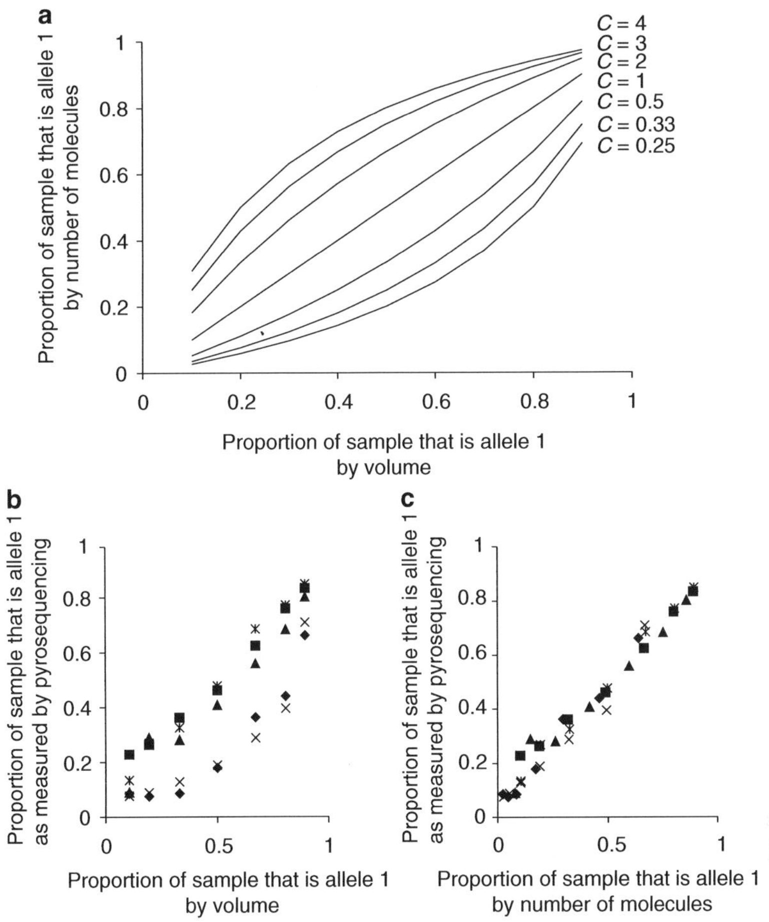


Fig. 4. Theoretical and empirical results for titration series analysis of allele abundance using pyrosequencing. (**a**) Theoretical relationship between the relative abundance of alleles in mixed samples constructed by volume and the relative abundance of the same allele in the same mixed samples after adjusting for differences in the starting concentrations of samples used to construct the titration series. Relative concentrations (*C* = allele 1/allele 2) ranging from 0.25 to 4 (i.e., 1/4 to 4/1) are shown. For real samples, *C* can be calculated empirically as described in step 6 of Subheading 3.5 of the main text. (**b**) Measurements of relative allele abundance determined by pyrosequencing are compared to the relative volume of each allele combined for the titration series. (**c**) Measurements of relative allele abundance determined by pyrosequencing are compared to the relative number of molecules from each type of allele as determined by the volume of each allele combined for the titration series as well as the empirically determined relative concentration *C*, as described in step 7 of Subheading 3.5 of the main text. Data shown in (**b**) and (**c**) are from a titration series performed for pyrosequencing assays used to analyze five *D. melanogaster* genes (for more details, *see* the Supplementary Information section in ref. 6).

according to the researcher's experimental design. In my experience working with genomic DNA and cDNA samples from *Drosophila* species, the overwhelmingly largest source of variance is replicate samples of biological tissue, with replicate RNA samples having greater variance than replicate genomic DNA samples; replicate samples containing tissue from two different genotypes nearly always show greater variance than replicate samples containing a single genotype. Of the technical sources of variance, cDNA synthesis, PCR, and pyrosequencing reactions, in this order, usually have progressively decreasing contributions to variance. A typical experiment performed in my laboratory will include analysis of both genomic DNA and cDNA from at least three replicate biological tissue samples. cDNA synthesis is performed in duplicate at least for each RNA sample, and PCR reactions for each genomic DNA or cDNA sample are performed in triplicate at least. Each PCR product is analyzed in a single pyrosequencing reaction.

### 3.6. Data Analysis and Interpretation

Before calculating any summary statistics, the pyrogram from each pyrosequencing reaction should be examined manually to identify and exclude any obviously failed reactions (e.g., pyrograms with no peaks), reactions with background signal contaminating the peaks for the focal SNP nucleotides, and cases where the peak heights are outliers (i.e., either very high or very low compared to most other reactions). From the remaining wells, the relative expression of the two alleles is calculated as the ratio of peak heights resulting from the incorporation of alternative nucleotides at the SNP. The percentages of each allele reported by the pyrosequencing software can also be used in some cases without further calculation.

To test for (a) a significant expression difference between genotypes, (b) a significant expression difference between alleles in $F_1$ hybrids, and (c) a significant difference in relative expression between the parental genotypes and between alleles in the $F_1$ hybrids, we fit the data to a mixed general linear model in SAS using proc MIXED that incorporates the replication structure of the experiment and performs the pairwise *t*-tests used to infer *cis*- and *trans*-regulatory differences (for examples of appropriate models, see refs. 5, 7). A significant difference in expression between two genotypes is interpreted as divergent expression. A significant difference in expression between alleles in $F_1$ hybrids is interpreted as evidence for *cis*-regulatory differences between the two parental alleles. And a significant difference in relative expression between parental genotypes and between alleles in $F_1$ hybrids is interpreted as evidence for *trans*-regulatory differences between the two parental genotypes.

## 4. Notes

1. Because pyrosequencing uses a single SNP to compare expression of two alleles, measurements reflect expression only of the exon containing this focal SNP. If this exon is not present in all isoforms of mRNA transcribed from the gene (e.g., because of alternative splicing), the estimate of relative transcript

abundance in a cDNA pool provided by a single pyrosequencing assay may not accurately reflect the relative abundance of all exons of the gene.

2. Longer homopolymers or more complex SNP sequence contexts can be used (usually with an increased variance of replicate measurements) if the user can find a way to estimate the proportion of one or more peaks attributable to each allele. For example, if allele 1 contains the sequence GGG and allele 2 contains the sequence TGG, a dispensation order of GTG could be used in which the first peak would measure the incorporation of the three consecutive Gs from allele 1, the second peak would measure the incorporation of the T from allele 2 and the third peak would measure the incorporation of the two Gs following the T in allele 2. In this case, the relative abundance of allele 1 to allele 2 could be calculated as the height of peak 1 divided by the combined heights of peaks 2 and 3.
3. The manufacturers of pyrosequencing machines recommend the use of 0.86 as a correction factor for the incorporation of dATP αS. That is, the height of a peak produced by the addition of adenine to the pyrosequencing primer should be multiplied by 0.86 to make its height equal to a peak reflecting incorporation of the same number of molecules of dCTP, dGTP, or dTTP. This correction factor can also be determined empirically for a given reaction by comparing the peak height resulting from an A that is present in both allele sequences to the peak height for a C, T, or G that is present in both allele sequences, assuming that none of the nucleotide peaks examined is part of a homopolymer.
4. If a researcher is interested only in testing for *cis*-regulatory differences between alleles in a heterozygous genotype, only tissue from this genotype is required. This is the most common experimental design used for analysis of human genes, since tissue from only a single heterozygous individual is typically available (e.g., (13)). To compare expression between recently duplicated ("paralogous") genes within a genome (e.g., (3)), tissue is also needed from only one genotype. To test for genomic imprinting, two heterozygous genotypes should be examined separately that are produced by performing reciprocal crosses between two parental genotypes (e.g., (1, 2)).
5. For *Drosophila melanogaster*, 15 whole adult flies can be easily homogenized by hand in a microfuge tube using a pestle homogenizer. For other tissue types, different homogenization tools may be more suitable. Regardless of the method used, samples should be kept on ice (ideally dry ice) until homogenization to prevent the degradation of RNA. The recommended 15 mg of tissue is based on *Drosophila*. Other amounts of tissue

may be appropriate for other species, but care should be taken to avoid saturating the SV Total RNA Isolation spin columns; additional guidelines are provided in (12).

6. For extremely abundant PCR products, a subset of the PCR reaction should be used. The ideal amount can be determined empirically by examining a pyrogram peak resulting from a nucleotide found in both alleles that is not part of a homopolymer. If this peak height is <10 units, greater variance among replicate reactions is often observed; if it is >50 units, the amount of light produced may be detected in neighboring wells, artificially inflating their peak heights, again increasing variance among replicate reactions.
7. Volumes given are for analysis of a full 96-well plate of PCR products. If a partial plate is analyzed, smaller volumes of Enzyme, Substrate, and nucleotides can be loaded into the cartridge. Formulas for determining the required amounts are provided in the reagent use guide included with the Pyro Gold (or Pyro Gold SQA) Reagents kit. Any unused Enzyme, Substrate, or nucleotides can be stored for at least 6 months at −20°C. All components should be warmed to room temperature before use, and the resuspended Enzyme and Substrate should not be refrozen once thawed.
8. If preparing more than one 96-well plate for pyrosequencing in the same session, you do not need to perform this full cleaning step between plates. Simply, leave the PyroMark Vacuum Prep Tool in the fifth trough containing water between plates, completing the full cleaning and drying protocol after the last plate.
9. The default dispensation order determined by the pyrosequencing machine is generally adequate, but I often prefer to alter the dispensation order to maximize use of all nucleotides (i.e., choose nucleotides that are most rare in the sequence to analyze as the unincorporated bases at the start of the sequence and following the SNP) and to separate base incorporation at and near the SNP as completely as possible. For example, the software typically suggests a dispensation order of "CG" to assay the sequence G/CG. This dispensation order results in a peak from the incorporation of C that reflects only one allele, but a peak from the incorporation of G that includes the G following the C in one allele as well as the two consecutive Gs in the other allele. By comparison, a dispensation order of "GCG" will result in the first G peak reflecting only one allele and the following two peaks (C and G) reflecting the other allele.
10. Custom programs can be written in languages such as Perl or Python that can easily parse the exported file containing a table of peak heights for each well. The "notes" section of the

pyrosequencing software can also be used to provide descriptive information for the sample in each well, which can then be extracted from exportable summary files that allow automated data processing and analysis. Any such program will need to be customized to fit the researcher's needs.

11. If the source and sequence of any background signal can be determined, it may be possible to adjust the dispensation order of nucleotides for the assay to prevent the extension of hairpins and primer dimers. If this can be done, it is still possible to obtain reliable data from the focal SNP in reactions containing both the PCR template and pyrosequencing primer.

## References


1. Wang X, Sun Q, McGrath SD et al (2008) Transcriptome-wide identification of novel imprinted genes in neonatal mouse brain. PLoS One **3**:e3839
2. Wittkopp PJ, Haerum BK, Clark AG (2006) Parent-of-origin effects on mRNA expression in *Drosophila melanogaster* not caused by genomic imprinting. Genetics **173**: 1817–1821
3. Anderson DW, Evans BJ (2009) Regulatory evolution of a duplicated heterodimer across species and tissues of allopolyploid clawed frogs (*Xenopus*). J Mol Evol **68**:236–247
4. Cowles CR, Hirschhorn JN, Altshuler D et al (2002) Detection of regulatory variation in mouse genes. Nat Genet **32**:432–437
5. Landry CR, Wittkopp PJ, Taubes CH et al (2005) Compensatory *cis-trans* evolution and the dysregulation of gene expression in interspecific hybrids of *Drosophila*. Genetics **171**:1813–1822
6. Wittkopp PJ, Haerum BK, Clark AG (2004) Evolutionary changes in *cis* and *trans* gene regulation. Nature **430**:85–88
7. Wittkopp PJ, Haerum BK, Clark AG (2008) Regulatory changes underlying expression differences within and between *Drosophila* species. Nat Genet **40**:346–350
8. Tung J, Primus A, Bouley AJ et al (2009) Evolution of a malaria resistance gene in wild primates. Nature **460**:388–391
9. McManus CJ, Coolon JD, Duff M et al (2010) Regulatory divergence in *Drosophila* revealed by mRNA-Seq. Genome Research **20**:826–25
10. Ahmadian A, Gharizadeh B, Gustafsson AC et al (2000) Single-nucleotide polymorphism analysis by pyrosequencing. Anal Biochem **280**:103–110
11. Rozen S, Skaletsky HJ (2000) Primer3 on the WWW for general users and for biologist programmers, in Bioinformatics Methods and Protocols: Methods in Molecular Biology. (Krawetz S, Misener S, Eds.), pp 365-386, Humana Press, Totowa, NJ
12. Otto P, Kephart D, Bitner R et al (1998) Separate isolation of genomic DNA and total RNA from single samples using the SV Total RNA Isolation System. Promega Notes **69**:19
13. Wang H, Elbein SC (2007) Detection of allelic imbalance in gene expression using pyrosequencing. Methods Mol Biol **373**:157–176

# Chapter 19

# Whole-Mount In Situ Hybridization of Sectioned Tissues of Species Hybrids to Detect *Cis*-regulatory Changes in Gene Expression Pattern

**Ryo Futahashi**


## Abstract

To distinguish whether differences in gene expression between species or between individuals of the same species are caused by *cis*-regulatory changes or by distribution differences in *trans*-regulatory proteins, comparison of species-specific mRNA expression in an F1 hybrid by whole-mount in situ hybridization is a rarely used yet very powerful tool. If asymmetric expression pattern is observed for the two alleles, this implies a *cis*-regulatory divergence of this gene. Alternatively, if symmetric expression pattern is observed for both alleles, the change in expression of this gene is probably caused by changes in the distribution of *trans*-regulatory proteins. In this chapter, I describe how to prepare RNA probes, tissue samples and how to detect mRNA expression pattern using in situ hybridization. Although I choose to present here the detection of *yellow-related gene* (*YRG*) expression pattern in the larval epidermis of swallowtail butterflies, this protocol can be adapted to other species and tissues. *YRG* mRNA expression is correlated with interspecific differences of yellow and green larval color pattern such as V-shaped markings in swallowtail butterflies. F1 hybrids show an intermediate color pattern between parental species. In this case, both species-specific *YRG* mRNA showed a similar expression pattern in F1 hybrids, suggesting that the change in expression of *YRG* is mainly caused by changes in the distribution of *trans*-regulatory proteins.


**Key words:** *Cis*-regulatory changes, *Trans*-regulatory changes, F1 hybrid, Whole-mount in situ hybridization, Species-specific probes

## 1. Introduction

A key challenge in evolutionary biology is to understand the molecular basis of phenotypic diversity. Many examples have been reported in which differences in gene expression are a major cause of interspecific differences (1–3). Differences in specific gene expression can arise from modifications of *cis*-regulatory sequences or from the differential deployment or activity of the transcription

Virginie Orgogozo and Matthew V. Rockman (eds.), *Molecular Methods for Evolutionary Genetics*,
Methods in Molecular Biology, vol. 772, DOI 10.1007/978-1-61779-228-1_19, 

factors that act upon these sequences, or both. The *cis*- and *trans*-regulatory changes can be distinguished by comparing the expression of differentially expressed orthologous genes in a common genetic background. One powerful method for making such comparisons is to analyze the F1 hybrid specimen (4–7). If the modifications of the *cis*-regulatory sequences are responsible for interspecific differences in orthologous gene expression, then the gene from each species are expected to be regulated differently in the F1 hybrid, and to show asymmetric expression pattern, which should coincide with the parental pattern (Fig. 1). Alternatively, similar allelic expression in F1 hybrid should be observed if the *trans*-regulation has diverged between these species (Fig. 1). If divergent expression patterns are caused by both *cis*- and *trans*-regulatory evolution, then expression pattern is expected to be intermediate between the above two cases. In this chapter, I describe how to prepare RNA probes, tissue samples and how to detect mRNA expression pattern using in situ hybridization. This protocol

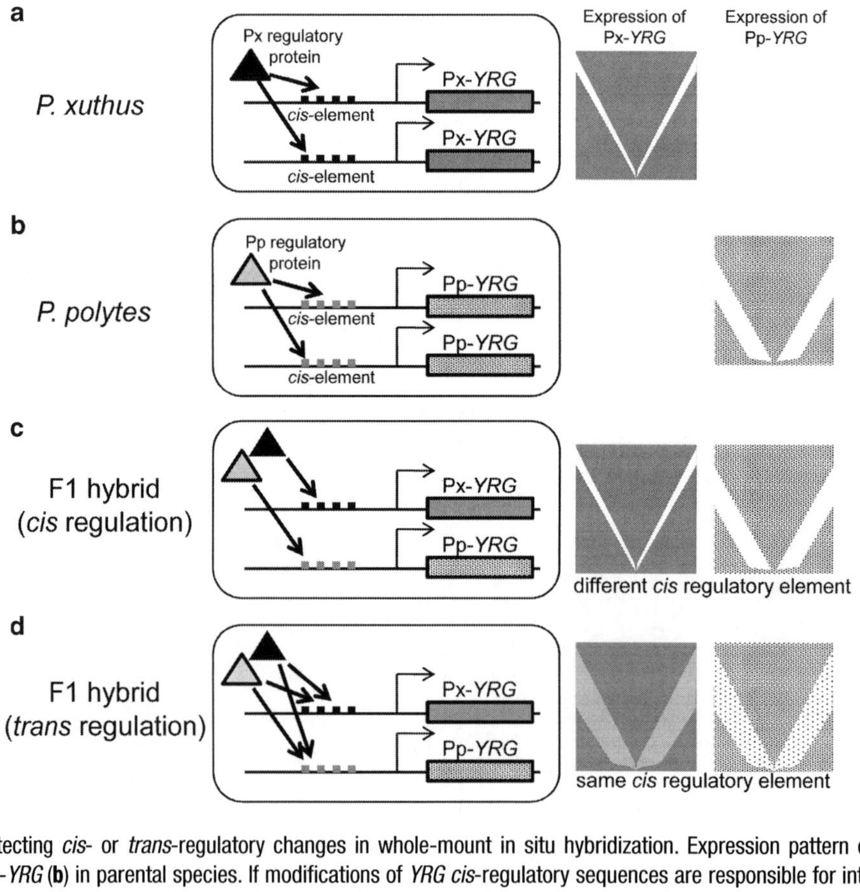


Fig. 1. Detecting *cis*- or *trans*-regulatory changes in whole-mount in situ hybridization. Expression pattern of Px-*YRG* (**a**) and Pp-*YRG* (**b**) in parental species. If modifications of *YRG cis*-regulatory sequences are responsible for interspecific differences in *YRG* expression, Px-*YRG* (*gray*) and Pp-*YRG* (*dotted*) are expected to be differentially expressed in F1 hybrid (**c**). If the distribution differences of *trans*-regulatory proteins are solely responsible for interspecific differences in *YRG* expression, both Px-*YRG* and Pp-*YRG* are expected to show the same expression pattern in F1 hybrid (**d**). Note also that hybrids may show a *YRG* expression pattern different from both parents (as in **d**), possibly because of interactions of *trans* factors between species or because of the presence of only one copy of each species-specific allele.

focuses on the detection of *yellow-related gene* (*YRG*) expression pattern in the larval epidermis of swallowtail butterflies, but it can be easily adapted to other species and tissues. In the larval epidermis of the swallowtail butterflies *Papilio xuthus* and *P. polytes*, the expression pattern of *YRG* correlates with differences in yellow and green color pattern between these two species (7, 8). In *P. xuthus*, *YRG* is broadly expressed except for the boundary of V-shaped markings, whereas in *P. polytes*, *YRG* is not expressed within the V-shaped markings (see Figs. 1 and 3c). The larval color pattern is intermediate in F1 hybrids (Fig. 3a). The *YRG* mRNA region with lowest sequence identity between *P. xuthus* and *P. polytes* is the 3′UTR (Fig. 2). Species-specific *YRG* probes that detect

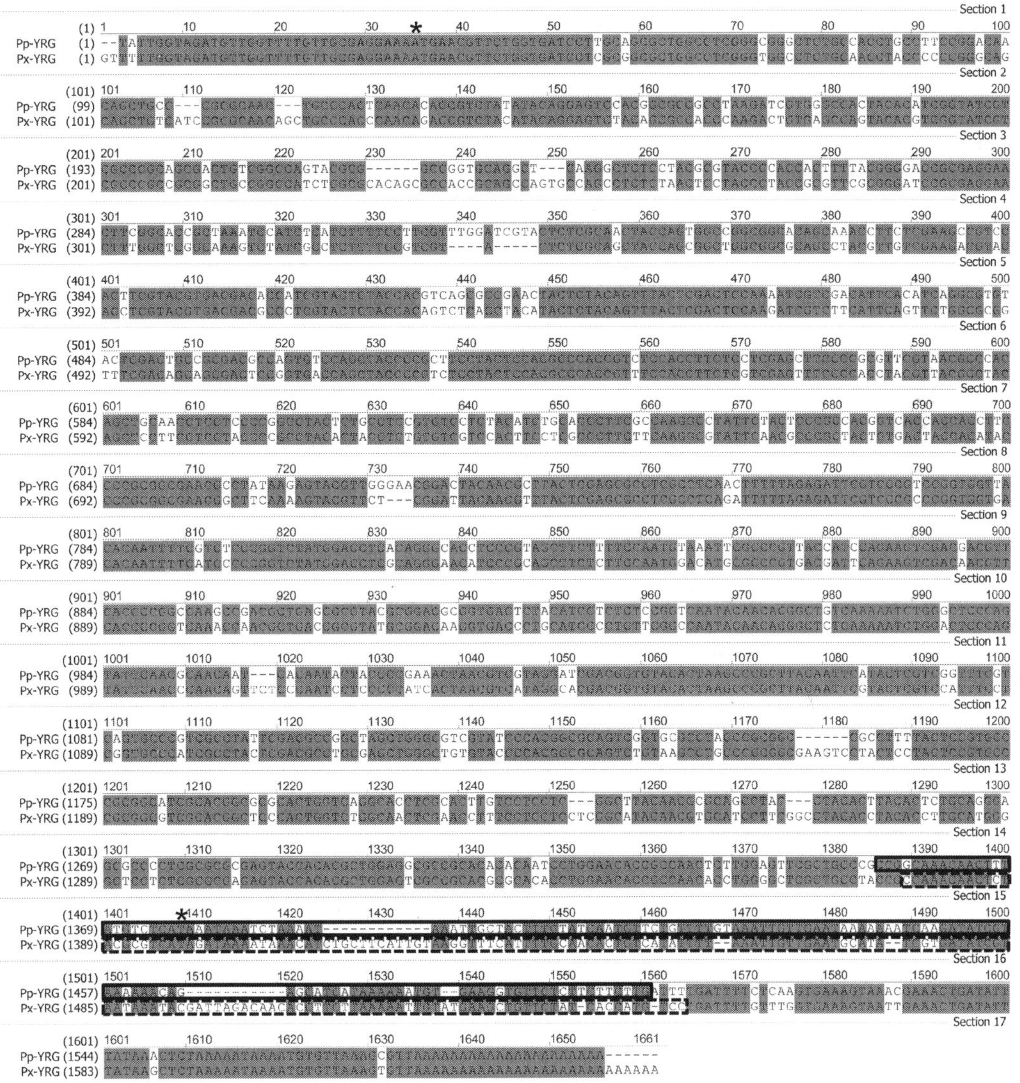

Fig. 2. Position of species-specific probes for *YRG* of *P. polytes* (*solid boxes*) and *P. xuthus* (*dotted boxes*). The nucleotide identity of this region is 53.4%. *Asterisks* indicate start and stop codon position. The nucleotide sequences of Px-*YRG* and Pp-*YRG* were deposited in GenBank under accession numbers AB264650 and AB525748, respectively.

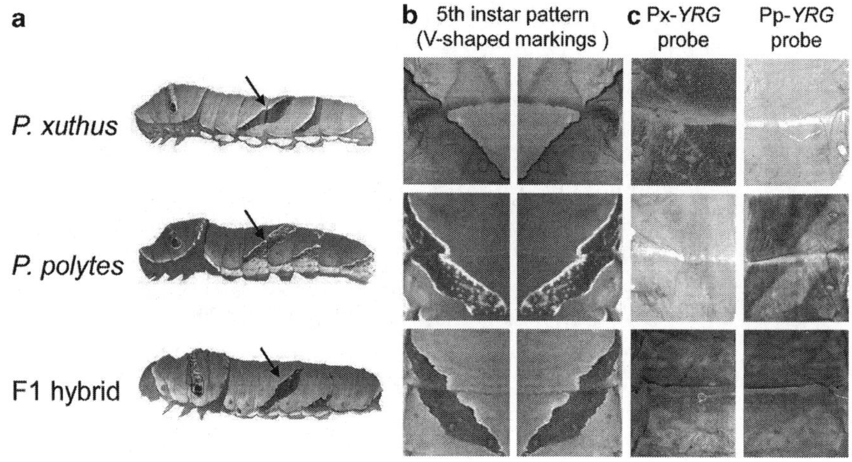


Fig. 3. (**a**) Lateral view of final instar larva of *P. xuthus*, *P. polytes*, and an F1 hybrid. *Red arrows* indicate V-shaped markings. (**b**) Dorsal view of V-shaped markings of *P. xuthus*, *P. polytes*, and an F1 hybrid. (**c**) Results of species-specific *YRG* expression by whole-mount in situ hybridization. Probe for Px-*YRG* only detects *P. xuthus* mRNA (*upper row*) and probe for Pp-*YRG* only detects *P. polytes* mRNA (*middle row*). Expression pattern of Px-*YRG* and Pp-*YRG* is similar in hybrid specimen (*bottom row*). All samples were dissected at 13 h after HCS during the fourth molt (modified from ref. 7).

only its own mRNA (Fig. 3c) were designed in the 3′UTR region. By dividing the F1 larval epidermis in half along the midline and comparing the expression pattern between sides, species-specific *YRG* mRNA expression was examined. Px-*YRG* and Pp-*YRG* showed a similar expression pattern in F1 hybrid (Fig. 3c), suggesting that the change in expression of *YRG* between *P. xuthus* and *P. polytes* is caused mainly by changes in the distribution of *trans*-regulatory proteins.

## 2. Materials

### *2.1. RNA Probe Preparation*

1. Gene- and species-specific primers.
2. PCR buffer (ExTaq, Takara Shuzo, Japan).
3. dNTP.
4. ExTaq polymerase (Takara Shuzo, Japan).
5. QIAquick PCR purification columns (Qiagen).
6. pGEM-T-easy vector system (Promega), containing ligase and ligase buffer.
7. Spectrophotometer.
8. T7 RNA polymerase and its associated buffer (Takara Shuzo, Japan).
9. RNase Inhibitor (Takara Shuzo, Japan).

10. 0.1 M DTT (Roche).
11. 10× DIG-labeling Mix: 10 mM ATP (Roche), 10 mM GTP (Roche), 10 mM CTP (Roche), 6.5 mM UTP (Roche), and 3.5 mM DIG UTP (Roche).
12. Recombinant DNase I (RNase-free, Takara Shuzo, Japan).
13. 0.5 M EDTA.
14. Electrophoresis system apparatus.
15. 0.8% agarose gel.
16. 1× TBE.
17. Loading buffer.
18. Loading dye.
19. 3 M sodium acetate.
20. 100% ethanol.
21. 80% ethanol.

#### 2.2. Preparation of Samples for In Situ Hybridization

1. PBS.
2. Forceps.
3. Microscissors.
4. Fixation buffer: 4% paraformaldehyde in PBS.
5. 100% methanol.

#### 2.3. Detection of Species-Specific mRNA Expression by In Situ Hybridization

1. Fixation buffer: 4% paraformaldehyde in PBS.
2. PBT: 0.1% Tween 20 in PBS.
3. Proteinase K solution: 20 μg/ml proteinase K (Merck) in PBT. If precipitate is present, vortex vigorously before use.
4. Prehybridization buffer: 50% formamide, 5× SSC (1× SSC is 0.15 M sodium chloride and 0.15 M sodium citrate, pH 7.4), 5× Denhardt's solution (0.2% each of bovine serum albumin (BSA), Ficoll, and polyvinylpyrrolidone), 25 μg/ml sonicated salmon sperm DNA (Funakoshi), and 0.1% Tween 20.
5. Hybridization buffer: Add 1 μg of digoxigenin-labeled RNA probe per 1 ml of Prehybridization buffer.
6. Wash buffer I: 50% formamide, 2× SSC with 0.1% SDS.
7. Wash buffer II: 2× SSC with 0.1% SDS.
8. Wash buffer III: 0.2× SSC with 0.1% SDS.
9. Blocking buffer: 1% blocking reagent (Roche) in PBS.
10. Antibody: anti-DIG-alkaline-phosphatase-conjugated antibody (Roche).
11. Detection buffer: 100 mM Tris–HCl, 100 mM NaCl, 50 mM $MgCl_2$, pH 9.5.

12. Developing solution (light sensitive): 3.5 μl/ml 5-bromo-4-chloro-3-indolyl-phosphate, 4-toluidine salt (BCIP; Roche), and 4.5 μl/ml nitroblue tetrazolium chloride (NBT; Roche) in detection buffer.
13. Mounting medium: 50% glycerol.
14. 48-well plates, multidish, round wells (Nunc CN-150687).

## 3. Methods

### 3.1. RNA Probe Preparation

1. Align the orthologous gene sequences and search for low conserved region to determine the best region to use for species-specific probe (see Fig. 2, Note 1).
2. Design species-specific primers and amplify both orthologous regions, either by PCR using genomic DNA (see Chapters 16 and 23 for genomic DNA preparation protocols) or by RT-PCR using total mRNA if the region of interest spans across introns (see Chapters 6, 15, 17 and 18 for detailed protocols).
3. Subclone the PCR product into pGEM-T-easy vector according to the manufacturer's protocol (see Chapters 14 and 23 for detailed subcloning protocols).
4. Confirm the subcloned sequence and orientation by sequencing the vector insert.
5. PCR-amplify the insert using a vector primer containing the T7 polymerase promoter sequence at its 5′ end (see Note 2), and a gene-specific primer to produce a template for in vitro transcription (see Note 3).
6. Purify the PCR product using QIAquick PCR purification columns according to the manufacturer's protocol. Elute DNA using deionized distilled $H_2O$ ($ddH_2O$).
7. Measure DNA concentration with a spectrophotometer.
8. Prepare the transcription reaction mixture (10 μl): 1 μl of 10× DIG-labeling Mix, 1 μl of 10× T7 polymerase buffer, 1 μl of 0.1 M DTT, 1 μl of T7 RNA polymerase, 0.5 μl of RNase Inhibitor, and template DNA (500 ng in 5.5 μl $ddH_2O$) (see Note 4).
9. Mix thoroughly by pipetting and incubate at 37°C for 2 h.
10. Remove DNA template by adding 1 μl of DNase I and mix well. Incubate at 37°C for 20 min.
11. Stop the reaction by adding 1 μl of 0.5 M EDTA.
12. Check if the transcript is present by running 0.5 μl of the sample on a 0.8% agarose gel in 1× TBE for 30 min at 100 V.

13. Add 1 μl (0.1× vol.) of 3 M sodium acetate and 27.5 μl of 100% ethanol (2.5× new vol.) to the probe labeling reaction, mix by pipetting, and allow precipitation overnight at −20°C.
14. Pellet RNA by spinning for 20 min at (15,300 × *g*) in a microcentrifuge at 4°C. Remove supernatant taking care not to disturb the pellet. The pellet should be very obvious.
15. Wash pellet once with 80% ethanol, centrifuge again for 20 min at (15,300 × *g*) at 4°C, and dissolve pellet in 10 μl of $ddH_2O$.
16. If your probe is longer than 1 kb, it is better to alkaline-hydrolyze the RNA probes to an average of 100–200 bp (see Note 5).

### 3.2. Preparation of Samples for In Situ Hybridization

1. Obtain F1 hybrids at the correct developmental stage (see Notes 6 and 7). Dissect the whole dorsal integument from the thoracic 2 segment to the abdominal 7 segment from a larva in PBS.
2. Carefully remove the fat body and muscle attached to the epidermis (see Note 8).
3. Immediately fix in fixation buffer for at least 12 h at 4°C.
4. Store the samples in 100% methanol at −30°C until use.
5. Before starting in situ hybridization, divide the samples in half along the midline using microscissors.

### 3.3. Detection of Species-Specific mRNA Expression by In Situ Hybridization

1. Move the samples to PBT in wells of 48-well culture plate at room temperature (see Note 9).
2. Wash the epidermal samples in PBT three times, 5 min each.
3. Incubate the samples in Proteinase K solution for 20 min (see Note 10).
4. Refix the samples in Fixation Buffer for 20 min (see Note 10).
5. Wash the samples in PBT three times, 5 min each.
6. Incubate the samples in Prehybridization buffer for at least 1 h at 55°C.
7. Heat Hybridization buffer (including RNA probe) at 68°C for 10 min for denaturation. Use Digoxigenin-labeled antisense RNA probes for mRNA detection, and Digoxigenin-labeled sense probes as negative control.
8. Incubate the samples in Hybridization Buffer for at least 16 h at 55°C. To detect the species-specific mRNA expression, use probes derived from different species for left- and right-side samples (i.e., Px-*YRG* probe in the left-side samples, and Pp-*YRG* probe in the right-side samples, see Fig. 3c, Note 1).
9. Wash the samples in Wash buffer I at 60°C twice, 20 min each time.

10. Wash the samples in Wash buffer II at 60°C twice, 20 min each time.
11. Wash the samples in Wash buffer III at 60°C twice, 20 min each time.
12. Incubate the samples in blocking buffer for 1 h.
13. Incubate the samples in the anti-DIG antibodies solution (1:1,200 dilution in PBS) overnight at 4°C, or for 2 h at room temperature.
14. Wash the samples in PBT four times, 15 min each time.
15. Rinse the samples in Detection buffer for 5 min.
16. Develop samples in 1 ml of Developing Solution. Since the Developing Solution is light-sensitive, the plates should be wrapped in foil to prevent light exposure when not checking samples. Time of development must be monitored each time (generally check after 5–10 min and then increase intervals up to overnight). Developing times can change even when using the same probes and developing solution.
17. Rinse the samples in PBT three times, 5 min each time.
18. Mount samples into 50% glycerol.
19. Compare expression patterns between sides. An example result is shown in Fig. 3c (see Note 11).

## 4. Notes

1. Check the probe specificity by using host species samples as shown in Fig. 3, before using hybrid samples.
2. The following primers containing T7 promoter sequences: T7-S: 5′-TAATACGACTCACTATAGGGAGACCGCGGGA ATTCGAT-3′ and T7-AS: 5′-TAATACGACTCACTATAGGG AGAGAATTCACTAGTGAT-3′ can be used with pGEM-T Easy.
3. If your fragment is inserted in the pGEM-T Easy plasmid as follows, then PCR by forward primer and T7-AS primer will generate a template for antisense probe, and PCR by reverse primer and T7-S primer will generate a template for sense probe.

   T7---(T7-S primer binding site) forward primer »»» reverse primer (T7-AS primer binding site)---SP6
4. For RNA work, always wear disposable gloves while handling samples and reagents. Avoid touching your skin or hair during the procedures, as they contain RNAse. Decontaminate the bench area, pipettes, and tube stands with RNase Away Spray

Bottle (Molecular BioProducts/Thermo Fisher). Use RNase-free, filtered pipette tips.

5. Digoxigenin-labeled RNA probes were hydrolyzed in alkaline solution (40 mM $NaHCO_3$, 60 mM $Na_2HCO_3$) at 60°C. Time for hydrolysis was calculated using the equation:

$$T = L_0 - L_f / L_0 \times L_f \times K,$$

where $T$ is time in min, $L_0$ is the initial length of probe in kb, $L_f$ is the desired length of probe in kb, and $K$ is the number of strand scissions per kb per min and is approximately equal to 0.11. For example, if the initial length of probe is 1 kb and desired length of probe is 0.2 kb, then

$$T = 1 - 0.2 / 1 \times 0.2 \times 0.11 = 0.8 / 0.022 = 36\text{min}.$$

6. F1 hybrids between *P. polytes* females and *P. xuthus* males are obtained by hand-pairing (9). Male butterflies should be 3 days old before hand-pairing. Freshly emerged females can be used when hand-pairing. Butterflies should be held carefully with their wings over their backs and tips of abdomens together until coupling occurs. When the male is actually pairing, his claspers will grasp the female's abdomen. They become docile and stop moving as soon as they couple.
7. For in situ hybridization, the staging of molting period is critical. The staging of molting period is based on the time when head capsule slippage (HCS) occurs, as well as spiracle index, which represents the characteristic sequence of new spiracle formation (7, 10, 11).
8. Be careful to keep materials RNase-free before hybridization step. Use disposable plastic. Serological pipettes are very useful for making up solutions. Diethyl pyrocarbonate (DEPC) treatment is a very effective (but not essential) way to treat solutions that will contact RNA. Add DEPC to a 0.1% final volume and shake solutions vigorously overnight. DEPC must be removed from solutions by autoclaving or heating at 100°C for 15 min.
9. This is a very delicate and difficult procedure. Although attached fat body and muscle reduce signal, the damage of epidermis increases nonspecific signals. Do not be discouraged if it takes many experiments to obtain good samples.
10. The Proteinase K concentration and the length and temperature of digestion should be optimized for each species or stage. To examine highly expressed genes in *P. xuthus* and *P. polytes* during the latter half of molting period, both steps can be omitted.
11. If needed, embed epidermal pieces in paraffin and section at 5 μm for more detailed observations.

## Acknowledgments

I would like to thank Dr. Mizuko Osanai-Futahashi for her critical reading of the manuscript.

### References

1. Carroll SB (2008) Evo-devo and an expanding evolutionary synthesis: a genetic theory of morphological evolution. Cell **134**:25–36
2. Monteiro A, Podlaha O (2009) Wings, horns, and butterfly eyespots: how do complex traits evolve? PLoS Biol 7:e37
3. Stern DL, Orgogozo V (2009) Is genetic evolution predictable? Science **323**:746–751
4. Wittkopp PJ, Haerum BK, Clark AG (2004) Evolutionary changes in cis and trans gene regulation. Nature **430**:85–88
5. Wittkopp PJ, Haerum BK, Clark AG (2008) Regulatory changes underlying expression differences within and between *Drosophila* species. Nat Genet **40**:346–350
6. Jeong S, Rebeiz M, Andolfatto P et al (2008) The evolution of gene regulation underlies a morphological difference between two *Drosophila* sister species. Cell **132**:783–793
7. Shirataki H, Futahashi R, Fujiwara H (2010) Species-specific coordinated gene expression and trans-regulation of larval color pattern in three swallowtail butterflies. Evol Dev **12**:305–314
8. Futahashi R, Fujiwara H (2008) Identification of stage-specific larval camouflage associated genes in the swallowtail butterfly, *Papilio xuthus*. Dev Genes Evol **218**:491–504
9. Clarke CA, Sheppard PM (1956) Hand-pairing of butterflies. Lepid News **10**:47–53
10. Kiguchi K, Agui N (1981) Ecdysteroid levels and developmental events during larval moulting in the silk worm, *Bombyx mori*. J Insect Physiol **27**:805–812
11. Futahashi R, Fujiwara H (2005) Melanin-synthesis enzymes coregulate stage-specific larval cuticular markings in the swallowtail butterfly, *Papilio xuthus*. Dev Genes Evol **215**: 519–529

# Chapter 20

# Identifying Fluorescently Labeled Single Molecules in Image Stacks Using Machine Learning

Scott A. Rifkin

## Abstract

In the past several years, a host of new technologies have made it possible to visualize single molecules within cells and organisms (Raj et al., Nat Methods 5:877–879, 2008; Paré et al., Curr Biol 19:2037–2042, 2009; Lu and Tsourkas, Nucleic Acids Res 37:e100, 2009; Femino et al., Science 280:585–590, 1998; Rodriguez et al., Semin Cell Dev Biol 18:202–208, 2007; Betzig et al., Science 313:1642–1645, 2006; Rust et al., Nat Methods 3:793–796, 2006; Fusco et al., Curr Biol 13:161–167, 2003). Many of these are based on fluorescence, either fluorescent proteins or fluorescent dyes coupled to a molecule of interest. In many applications, the fluorescent signal is limited to a few pixels, which poses a classic signal processing problem: how can actual signal be distinguished from background noise?

In this chapter, I present a MATLAB (MathWorks (2010) MATLAB. Retrieved from http://www.mathworks.com) software suite designed to work with these single-molecule visualization technologies (Rifkin (2010) *spotFinding Suite*. http://www.biology.ucsd.edu/labs/rifkin/software.html). It takes images or image stacks from a fluorescence microscope as input and outputs locations of the molecules. Although the software was developed for the specific application of identifying single mRNA transcripts in fixed specimens, it is more general than this and can be used and/or customized for other applications that produce localized signals embedded in a potentially noisy background. The analysis pipeline consists of the following steps: (a) create a gold-standard dataset, (b) train a machine-learning algorithm to classify image features as signal or noise depending upon user defined statistics, (c) run the machine-learning algorithm on a new dataset to identify mRNA locations, and (d) visually inspect and correct the results.

**Key words:** Single molecule, FISH, Machine learning, MATLAB, mRNA, Microscopy, Biological image informatics

## 1. Introduction

*S*ingle *m*olecule RNA *f*luorescence *i*n *s*itu *h*ybridization (smFISH) is a relatively new technique that enables visualization of transcripts in fixed cells or organisms. Several varieties of the technique have

Virginie Orgogozo and Matthew V. Rockman (eds.), *Molecular Methods for Evolutionary Genetics*,
Methods in Molecular Biology, vol. 772, DOI 10.1007/978-1-61779-228-1_20, © Springer Science+Business Media, LLC 2011

been demonstrated in the literature, which all yield the same general kind of data: groups of pixels (*spots*) of relatively high intensity against a background field of lower intensity (1–5).

Measurements of variation in gene expression have become quite common in the literature of comparative biology. In evolutionary-developmental biology, they often take the form of traditional in situ assays for a set of homologous genes in different species, which give qualitative information about spatial expression patterns but are not quantitative. Evolutionary genetic techniques include, for example, microarrays, RNA-Seq, and pyrosequencing, which are usually relative measures of expression and have no spatial information because they destroy the sample. smFISH yields absolute counts of mRNA abundances with high spatial resolution. The trade-offs are that it is relatively low throughput compared to genomic techniques, and the signals are weaker than those in traditional in situ assays. smFISH is appropriate for questions that require highly resolved measures of gene expression and/or an explicit spatial context. Furthermore, because it only requires sequence information, it can be used on nonmodel organisms as long as sequences are available.

The software (10) discussed in this chapter was developed using data from the technique of Raj et al. 2008 (1, 11), and so, I briefly describe the experimental technique below. A comprehensive description of the experimental protocol can be found in ref. 11 or online at http://www.singlemoleculefish.com. A set of thirty to fifty 20-mer oligo probes is designed to be complementary to a target transcript. These oligos are labeled at the 3′ end with a fluorophore. Probes are incubated with fixed samples (e.g., cells, tissue sections, organisms) in a formamide-based hybridization buffer, and then unbound probe is removed in a series of washes. Labeled samples can then be imaged under a fluorescence microscope. When bound to an mRNA in a fixed specimen, this set of oligos appears under the microscope as a diffraction-limited fluorescent spot (Fig. 1).

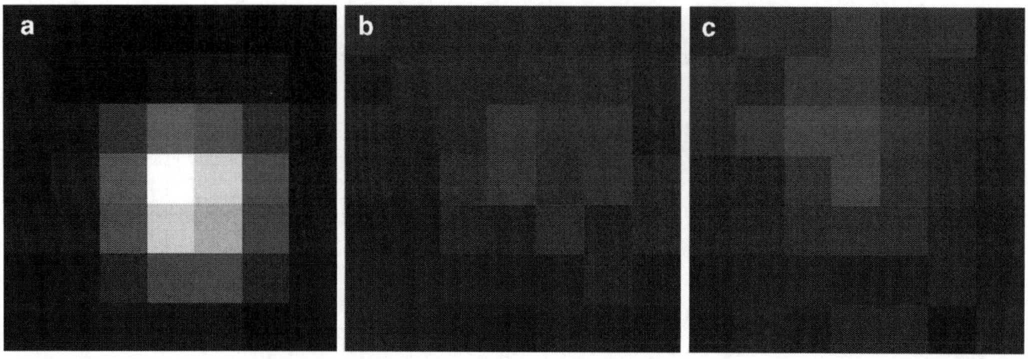


Fig. 1. Example of smFISH spots. (**a**) A 7 × 7 pixel box centered around a clear mRNA spot. (**b**) A local intensity maximum that is not an mRNA spot. (**c**) A marginal mRNA spot.

In my experience, using a wide-field epifluorescence microscope, a probe set of at least 21 oligos is necessary to be able to identify a localized signal above background. As a consequence of this requirement for multiple oligos to bind and the relative uniqueness of 20-mers in a genome, the technique is highly specific, although like many sequence-based techniques, extremely similar paralogs cannot be distinguished. Background fluorescence can come from a few oligos binding to other molecules, unbound fluorophores not being completely washed away, autofluorescence of the sample, or out-of-focus light. These factors can be controlled by checks during probe design, adjustments to the stringency of the washes, judicious use of fluorophores, or modifications to the microscopy setup. However, these modifications may involve tradeoffs that weaken the signal, and so, in many cases an appreciable degree of background noise will have to be tolerated.

In the following discussion, I assume that the microscopist has taken z-stacks through a sample, producing a series of two-dimensional slices that can be concatenated into a three-dimensional image. Furthermore, I leave it to the reader to segment the image stacks. The details of how to do this will depend upon the particular type of specimen – in particular on the contrast between the object boundary and everything outside, which may include other confluent objects. There is not a single solution that will work for everything, and reviewing various approaches is beyond the scope of this chapter. The starting data for the single molecule identification is an image stack and a segmentation mask that distinguishes pixels that belong to an object from those that do not (Fig. 2). For convenience in the discussion below, I refer to these objects as

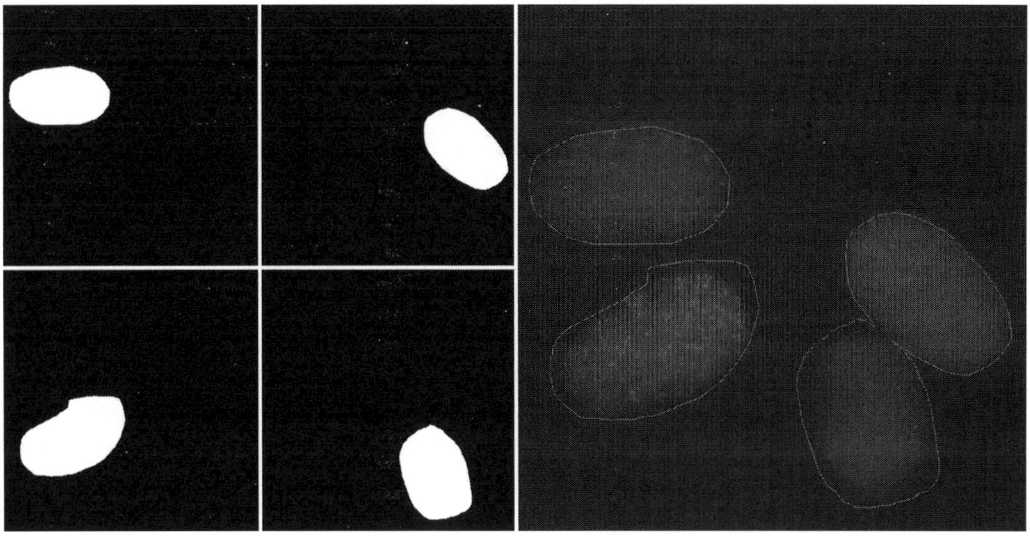

Fig. 2. An example of a series of segmentation masks for the image on the *far right*.

"*specimens*". They could be cells, small animals, anything. *Cell* is unfortunately a technical term in MATLAB and *objects* can be ambiguous, so I use *specimen* simply as a convenient specific identifier for these segmented objects. The intensity pattern from a single fluorescent molecule is called a *spot.*

The spot finding software is built around a machine learning core and consists of four parts which are covered in detail below: Subheading 3.2 – Manually annotate an image to create a gold-standard dataset; Subheading 3.3 – Use the gold-standard dataset to train a classifier to distinguish between spots representing mRNA signals and noise; Subheading 3.4 – Apply the classifier to a new image; Subheading 3.5 – Manually review and curate the results which may include re-rerunning the training and subsequent classification. This software is modular and flexible. The annotation component (Subheading 3.2) could be used on its own as a way to manually identify spots (e.g., if only a few images need to be processed). The machine learning component (Subheadings 3.3 and 3.4) uses the random forest algorithm (12–14), but this could straightforwardly be modified for the user's preferred classifier. The reviewing software (Subheading 3.5) relies only upon a particular data and file structure. As long as the output from a classification algorithm can be translated into this data format, the reviewing software can be used to manually review and correct the results from any spot-classification program.

## 2. Materials

1. Computer with sufficient RAM to process the image files.
2. MATLAB (http://www.mathworks.com).
3. spotFinding Suite (http://www.biology.ucsd.edu/labs/rifkin/software.html).
4. R (http://r-project.org).
5. randomForest R package (http://cran.r-project.org/web/packages/randomForest/).

   The following MATLAB packages can be downloaded individually but are also included with spotFinding Suite under the BSD license.
6. SC(http://www.mathworks.com/MATLABcentral/fileexchange/16233).
7. gfit2(http://www.mathworks.co.uk/MATLABcentral/fileexchange/22020).

The following MATLAB package can be downloaded individually but is also included with spotFinding Suite under the GNU GPL3 license.

8. tiffread (http://www.embl.de/~nedelec/misc/).

## 3. Methods

The software is designed to work in a single directory. All data and segmentation files, described in Subheading 3.1 below, should in the same directory, and all files that the software generates will be saved in this directory. The default file name for an image stack is (dye) (UniqueStackidentifier).tiff. For example, the third image stack labeled by the fluorescent dye TMR would be named tmr003.tiff where 003 is the unique stack identifier. The default for the segmentation file is segmenttrans(UniqueStackIdentifier).mat, e.g., segmenttrans003.mat. The software allows a user to enter image file names, segmentation file names, fluorophores, and unique stack identifiers at the command line, but it is much quicker and simpler (especially when processing many image stack files) to ensure that files are in the default format before starting.

On Unix-like systems (e.g., Linux, Mac OS X), no modifications are needed to call R. On Windows, the software by default assumes that the R executable is located at:

C:\\"Program Files"\\R\\R-2.9.0\\bin\\Rterm.exe.

If this is not correct, the user will need to locate this line in trainFISHClassifier.m and classifyFISHSpots.m and replace it with the correct location.

Matlab specific terms used in this chapter are defined in Table 1. More detailed information can be found in the Matlab help documents.

### 3.1. Correctly Format the Image and Segmentation Files

The software assumes that the segmentation and image files are in a specific format. Assume that the images are z-stacks of two-dimensional slices of size A × B pixels. The segmentation file is a MAT file consisting of a cell array that the program assumes is called currpolys. An entry in the cell array is an A × B pixel binary image with 1 s denoting a specimen of interest and 0 s denoting area outside the specimen. Often, a single image contains several specimens to segment. It is convenient to store the segmentation masks for each specimen together in a single file, each one being stored in a separate cell in the cell array.

The software comes configured to read multi-image TIFF files using the MATLAB function tiffread. An image stack consisting of MATLAB doubles is created with the following commands:

**Table 1**
**Matlab terms used in this chapter**

| | |
|---|---|
| MAT file | A binary, Matlab-specific data file format with the extension.mat |
| Cell array | A data structure that can hold an assorted collection of objects. Think of it as an integer-indexed set of bins (called cells) where any Matlab data structure can be placed in a cell |
| Double | A double precision floating point number |
| Struct | Stuctured array. A data structure where each entry (value) is indexed by text (field) and can be a cell array or number. These are especially useful for collecting assorted information about a particular object (see Tables 3 and 4) |
| Function calls | Matlab functions are called using the following format: outputArguments = functionName(inputArgument1, inputArgument2, ...). A semicolon at the end of a statement blocks output from being displayed on the screen |

```
stack = tiffread(stackFileName);
stack = double(stack.data);
```

If images cannot be saved in a tiffread compatible format, the user will need to find these lines in the code and modify them to read his or her particular image format. The subsequent program represents the data stack as a three-dimensional array of doubles.

During the process of finding spots, several files are created. The names of the training set files are based on the dye and the transcript. For example, if TMR is used to label the *C. elegans elt-2* transcript, the user might designate the dye as "tmr" and the gene as "C_el_elt2". The training set would then be stored in trainingSet_tmr_C_el_elt2.mat. Other files are associated with particular stacks via the unique stack identifier. For example, tmr003_wormGaussianFit.mat contains the results of the spot finding program run on the multi-image tiff file tmr003.tiff.

### 3.2. Creating a Training Set

Command:

```
trainingSet = createFISHTrainingSet(stackName, probeName);
```

Once the appropriate files are in place and properly formatted, the first step in finding spots is to annotate an smFISH image by identifying examples of true spots and examples of sets of pixels that are not spots. After the user identifies particular and segmentation files to use, a GUI window pops up, which allows the user to do this manual classification. However, some preprocessing must be done on the image to make this a manageable task. The size of spot will depend upon the microscope magnification and resolution; by default, the software assumes a spot in two-dimensions fits well within a $7 \times 7$ pixel square. A specimen of approximately $400 \times 250$ pixels will contain close to 100,000 of these $7 \times 7$ squares in each slice. It would be impossible to go through all of these manually, and so, preliminary ranking of the pixels is essential.

The software first identifies the local 3D intensity maxima in the image stack. The idea is that a single fluorescent molecule will appear as a diffraction-limited spot covering several pixels and that the intensities of these pixels will decay at a roughly Gaussian rate from the center. As a result, true spots will contain a central local maximum, and so, only pixels that are local maxima need to be considered. However, thousands of pixels will be local maxima. True spots should be more fluorescent than nonspots, and so, ranking by intensity is a natural way to order these maxima. However, some samples may have nonuniform background across the sample and may have more out-of-focus light in some slices. Instead of a straight ranking by intensity, the software corrects for local background by performing a morphological opening (see Note 1) and subtracting this opened image from the raw image. The size of the structuring element used for the opening is based upon the size of a spot in the user's microscopy setup; by default it is a disk of radius 7. Other local background correction procedures could be substituted if desired. The local maxima are then ranked by their background-subtracted intensities and presented to the user for evaluation. Although the pixel intensities in the image are manipulated in this step, all manipulations, whether local background subtraction or intensity scaling, are for the user interface only. All computational evaluations of the spots by the machine learning algorithm are performed on the unadulterated raw image. If there were a reason to adjust the images – for example to remove a systematic increase in average intensity with z-position of the slice – this could certainly be implemented (see Note 2).

The annotation GUI window called identifySpots3 (Fig. 3) has several components. On the left is a 16 × 16 pixel image with blue pixels (marked with "B" in the figure) against a background of gray pixels. For display, each slice of the stack is scaled such that the minimum pixel intensity is 0 and the maximum is 1, and the pixel intensities on the display image are the scaled intensities. As mentioned above, this scaling is for display only. The blue pixel in the ninth row, ninth column from the top is the local maximum at the rank indicated by the "Spot Rank" slider. Other blue pixels in the 16 × 16 field indicate other local maxima in the vicinity.

On the right-hand side of the window is a zoomed portion of the entire slice centered on the pixel of interest. By default, this is set to 512 × 512 pixels and is normalized for viewing such that the minimal pixel value of the slice is 0 and the maximal value is 1. It is sometimes useful to be able to see the pixel highlighted in blue on the left against a background of more of the specimen. The segmentation outline of the specimen is highlighted in yellow, and the 16 × 16 square on the left is outlined green.

Below this right-hand side image is a smaller image displaying the entire slice with segmented specimens highlighted in red and outlines of the areas depicted in the left and right larger images.

In the middle of the window is a stack of five 16 × 16 pixel surface plots. The height and color of a pixel reflects its intensity.

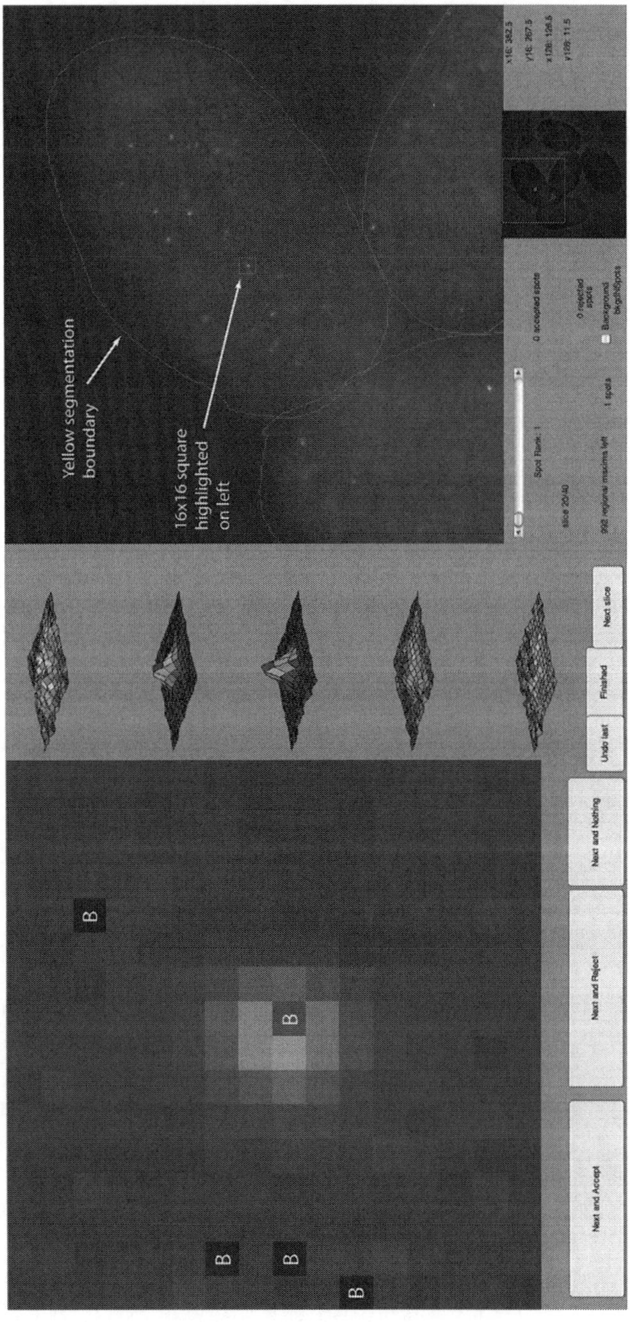


Fig. 3. The annotation GUI. For the purposes of this chapter, *blue* pixels in the *left panel* are marked with B. Other colors are as noted.

If the current slice is $n$, the surface plots are the $16 \times 16$ pixel area of the image on the left in (from bottom to top) slices $n-2$, $n-1$, $n$, $n+1$, $n+2$. It is good practice to take z-slices close enough together such that a spot will appear in at least two. This representation of five consecutive slices around a local maximum gives information about the three-dimensional context of the putative spot.

Along the bottom of the window are a series of push buttons that tell the software what should be done with the local maxima highlighted in the left image. The software will process local maxima in order of rank. The slider below the right-hand side image allows the user to jump to a particular rank. Finally, a series of text fields below the images give information on the current slice, the number of regional maxima (up to 1,000) that are left to evaluate, the number of potential spots (local maxima) in the current $16 \times 16$ field of view, and the number of local maxima that have been rejected or accepted so far. On the far right, the current coordinates for the upper left corners of the left and right images are listed for reference.

Collecting a training set entails assessing some number of these local maxima and either accepting them as spots or rejecting them. This consists of the following steps:

1. Evaluate the slice. Look at the right, large image. Are spots visible or does the entire image look fairly uniform? Slices at the top or bottom of the stack may be outside the boundary of the specimen and so may look rather uniform without clear spots or definition (see Note 3). In this case, it is worthwhile to press the *Next Slice* button. This will simply advance to the next slice up and will neither accept nor reject any of the blue local maxima in the current $16 \times 16$ field on the left. If spots are visible, implying that the slice is within the specimen, it is worthwhile to evaluate the local maxima.
2. Decide on an appropriate local maximum rank to look at. By default, the software starts with the top-ranked local maximum in the initial slice. If there are spots in a slice, this should be an unambiguous example of a true spot. After the user has accepted a good number of solid spots and rejected many non-spots, it might be worthwhile to include some more borderline ones. Adjusting the *Spot Rank* slider is a quick way to jump around the rankings to find intermediate cases. Jumping to a new rank is done by moving the slider and then pressing one of the *Next* buttons. This ranking is carried over between slices: if *Next Slice* is pressed with *Spot Rank* slider on 75, the focal local maximum in the next slice will be the one with rank 75.
3. Evaluate the local maxima in the $16 \times 16$ image. While the focal local maximum will be in the center, there may be other local maxima in the $16 \times 16$ image. True spots could be close together, in which case the $16 \times 16$ image would contain more than one true spot. Usually, however, the nonfocal blue pixels

are just noise – random local maxima in the background. Good spots generally show up in more than one slice (as long as the slices are close enough together, ~0.4 μm), are roughly Gaussian and regular in shape, and have a higher intensity than the local background. A candidate spot can be rejected by clicking on it. This turns it from blue to gray and also increases the rejected spot count by 1. If the user makes a mistake, the last action can be undone with the button *Undo last*. Clicking on a gray pixel will change it to blue, thereby designating it as a potential spot (see Note 4). When the user is satisfied that the blue pixels that remain mark true spots, clicking *Next and Accept* will store them, change their color to red, and increase the "accepted spot" count accordingly. In some cases, none of the blue pixels will mark real spots. Instead of clicking on each one, the whole lot can be rejected by clicking *Next and Reject*. Rejected pixels are changed to gray. If the remaining blue pixels are ambiguous, the user can remain agnostic so as not to contaminate the training set by clicking *Next and Nothing*. When a *Next* button is pressed, the software moves on to either the next ranked local maximum or the local maximum with rank indicated by the *Spot Rank* slider. Alternatively, the user can move the focus to a particular location within the specimen by clicking on it in the right-hand side image. The upper left corner of the 16×16 pixel square is moved to the clicked location.

4. Decide whether to move to a new slice. If there are just a few true spots in a slice, the user will quickly move through them and start rejecting local maxima that are not spots. While it is important to include local maxima that are not spots in the training set as negative examples, this is rather easy, and it does not make sense to process all 1,000 local maxima in a slice before moving on to a new slice. In addition, it is not necessary to include all the spots in a sample in the training set, and it makes sense to include spots from multiple slices of the sample, although whether this is strictly necessary is unclear. In practice, around 100 accepted and 100 rejected spots works well, especially because the training set can be augmented later on by corrections to a classification (Subheading 3.5). The user can switch to a new slice by clicking *Next Slice* and, if finished collecting the training set, can press *Finished* to move on to the next step.

### 3.3. Train the Classifier

Command:

trainingSet = trainFISHClassifier(trainingSet,0);

The output from the annotation is stored in two files. goldSpots_(dye)_(gene).mat contains an X-by-3 array of doubles where each row has the coordinates of one of the X accepted local maxima (row, column, slice) in the matrix representation of the image stack. rejectedSpots_(dye)_(gene).mat contains the rejected maxima coordinates. These coordinates, along with the raw image file are piped to a function that will calculate various statistics on the maxima and train a classifier based on these statistics.

Statistics, or observations, of the data are a crucial part of any classification scheme. Good statistics capture aspects of true spots that distinguish them from noise. Designing a statistic is something of an art, but the usefulness of a statistic can be evaluated post hoc based on how much importance the classifier assigns it. In this software, most statistics are calculated on a square of pixels centered around a local maximum. By default this is a $7\times7$ pixel square but the size can be adjusted depending upon the usual size of a spot in the user's particular microscopy/camera setup. A few of the default statistics use the $7\times7\times3$ pixel box around the maximum. Most of the default statistics are based on measuring how the pixel intensity drops off around the maximum under the prediction and observation that good spots have a Gaussian profile. Users can add their own statistical functions if desired. This requires writing a MATLAB function that takes a two- or three-dimensional array of doubles as input and outputs one or more statistics and corresponding names. Users can use default statistics in the folder spotFindingStatistics as templates and add the appropriate lines to the function calculateFISHStatistics.m.

The software calculates statistics on the maxima in the training set and outputs the results to a large matrix with one row for each maximum, one column for each statistic, and a final column with the classification index. This is then sent to the machine learning classifier. The software currently uses the R implementation of the random forest classifier called randomForest (12). In principle, the user could substitute any classifier with fairly minimal code modification. Random forests perform comparably to other machine learning classifiers or better, are fast, and are amenable to parallelization, which could be useful for processing large datasets. For complete details about the theory and implementation of random forests and in particular for information about how to set and interpret the parameters it takes, readers are encouraged to consult refs. 11–13. In brief, random forests are sets of decision trees that are built using subsets of the training data – about two third of the data end up being used for each tree. A tree consists of successive branch points at which the dataset is recursively partitioned based on a subset of the statistics with the goal of generating homogenous partitions. At each recursion, the random forest algorithm chooses a random subset of the statistics and finds a best partition of the remaining set of data. The algorithm stores exactly how the partition was made at each recursion in each tree. Classifying a new local maximum consists of running its statistics down each tree in the forest. Each branching point of each tree corresponds to a particular partition based on a subset of the statistics, and eventually the local maximum will reach a terminal leaf where it is labeled as either a spot or not. Each tree in the forest performs this classification with different combinations of subsets of the statistics and votes as to whether the local maximum is a spot or not. The majority decision is the final classification of the forest. Because only two third of the training data is used to generate any given tree, the remaining one third of the training data can be run down the tree to generate an independent estimate the error rate of the classification algorithm (12–14). The extent to which this error rate can be extrapolated to novel data depends upon how representative the training set is of the novel data. The initial training set is likely to be overrepresented for maxima where the classification is clear, and so, this initial error rate will underestimate the actual error rate on novel data. Subheading 3.5 describes two ways to estimate a more accurate error rate for the final dataset.

randomForest outputs several files (all prefixed by trainingSet_(dye)_(gene)) which can be used to assess the statistics and the likely classification error. Of these, the most useful are listed in Table 2.

Readers should consult refs. 12, 13 for other further randomForest options. These can be passed to the randomForest function via the tuneRF function call that can be found in trainFISHClassifier.m.

After the classifier is trained, the software stores all of the classification data including the training set and input and output to and from the random forest alogorithm in a structure called trainingSet stored in the file trainingSet_(dye)_(gene).mat.

**Table 2**
**Output files from randomForest**

| | |
|---|---|
| .randomForest | contains the trained classifier to be applied to novel data |
| _votes.txt<br>_margin.pdf | List and plot of the results of the voting across the forest for each maximum |
| _confusion.txt | Estimate of the error rate. The first row consists of maxima annotated as nonspots; the second row is for true spot annotations. The first column has numbers of maxima classified as nonspots; the second column numbers represent maxima classified as spots. The third column has rates of misclassification |
| _varImp.pdf | Plot of statistic importance. This plot portrays two measures of the importance of individual statistics to correct classification. Of the default statistics, intensity and goodness-of-fit to a Gaussian often dominate the classification |
| _MDS.pdf | Multidimensional scaling plot of the data classification. By default, this is a two-dimensional representation |

### 3.4. Apply the Classifier to a New Image

Commands:

worms = evaluateFISHImageStack(stackName,1);

worms = classifyFISHSpots(dye, uniqueStackIdentifier, probeName, optional(worms));

After the classifier is trained with the initial training data, it can be applied to novel data. As for the training data, this requires segmentation and image files in the proper format (Subheading 3.1). As before, local maxima are identified and ranked in the three-dimensional image according to their local background subtracted intensities. The number of local maxima depends upon many factors including the size of the image stack, the concentration of mRNA, and the microscopy setup, but it can run upward of 1% of the pixels. This could be tens of thousands of local maxima. Computing and evaluating statistics for each of these would be computationally intensive and completely unnecessary, since the vast majority is just spurious noise. The challenge lies in determining when to stop without imposing user-dependent thresholds or cutoffs (cf. (1)). The software takes the following approach:

1. Start with the highest ranked local maximum and proceed in rank order.
2. Calculate the statistics for the local maximum. These will be the same set of statistics used for the training set.
3. Extract the statistic that measures goodness-of-fit to a Gaussian (see Note 5) and store it in an array. Along with intensity, this is usually one of the most relevant statistics for classification.
4. Go to step 1 until the first 30 local maxima have been evaluated meaning that the goodness-of-fit array is of length 30.
5. Find the 60th percentile of this array.
6. If the goodness-of-fit statistic for the 60th percentile is below 0.9, stop. If not, then continue down the ranked list as in step 1, adding the goodness-of-fit statistic to the array. Maintain an array of length 30, i.e., if the software has just processed the local maximum with rank 45, then the goodness-of-fit array would contain statistics from ranks 16 to 45. If at any point the 60th percentile drops below 0.9, then stop (see Note 6).

Once the list of candidate local maxima has been identified, the software passes the randomForest R function a matrix comprised of their statistics along with the random forest file from the training set. The machine learning program runs the data from each maximum down the decision trees in the forest. Each tree classifies the local maximum as a spot or not, and the final classification is decided by a majority vote. The classification for all of the candidate maxima is passed back to MATLAB.

MATLAB generates several files in the course of evaluating these local maxima. They are uniquely labeled by the image stack

**Table 3**
**The fields in the struct worms{i}**

| | |
|---|---|
| mask | A binary image that is the segmentation mask for the specimen |
| boundingBox | A stuct containing the BoundingBox measurement from MATLAB's regionprops function |
| regMaxSpots | An Nx5 double array. Each row corresponds to a local maximum with the information: [row, column, slice, raw intensity, filtered intensity] |
| spotInfo | A cell array containing information about the local maxima evaluated |
| goodWorm | Indicates whether something is wrong with the specimen (0) or not (1) |
| spotsFixed | Indicates whether the spot classifications have been reviewed (see Subheading 3.5) |
| probeName | Name of the smFISH probe |
| RFNSpots | Number of local maxima classified as spots by the randomForest algorithm |
| trainingFileName | Name of the training set file used for the classification |
| nSpotsFinal | Final count of spots. Manual review and curation could change this |

name and the number of the specimen in the segmented image. For example, if the image stack contains five specimens, the naming convention might be RFtestdatamatrix_tmr003_w3.txt where tmr003 is the unique stack identifier and this is the statistics matrix for the third specimen. The classification is stored in a cell array of structs called worms in the file tmr003_wormsGaussianFit.mat. Results from each specimen in the image stack will have its own struct in the cell array, and further functions in the software work with this data structure (Table 3). The use of "worms" and "w" in file names and in the software itself reflects its history of being developed and tested with data from nematodes.

One of the fields, spotInfo, contains information specific to a local maximum (Table 4).

### *3.5. Manually Review and Curate the Classification*

Command:

reviewFISHSpotClassification(dye, uniqueStackIdentifier, worms);

The final step in identifying mRNA spots consists of reviewing the automated classification and refining the classifier. The initial training set is likely to have an overabundance of easily classified local maxima. As a result, the classifier will not do an optimal job of classifying borderline cases. The manual review component of the software allows the user to correct misclassified local maxima and to add these to the training set. A new classifier can then be trained based on the augmented training data and applied to the image to generate a revised classification. As might be expected, adding marginal local maxima to the training set quickly improves the accuracy of the classifier. Perfect automated classification,

**Table 4**
**Fields in worms{i}.spotInfo{j}**

| | |
|---|---|
| Locations | A struct containing [row, column, slice] location of the local maximum (a) in the entire stack and (b) relative to the BoundingBox of the specimen |
| rawValue | Raw intensity of the local maximum |
| filteredValue | Intensity of the local maximum after background subtractions |
| spotRank | Rank of the local maximum after background subtractions |
| dataMat | A square matrix of pixel intensities (default 7×7) centered on the local maximum |
| directory | A cell array containing the path to the working directory which contains the data and output files |
| dye | Fluorescent dye |
| stackSuffix | Unique identifier for the image stack |
| wormNumber | Specimen number (based on segmentation) within the image |
| statNames | The names of the statistics in the column order of the data |
| statData | The statistics calculated on the local maximum |
| machLearnResult | A quantitative measure of the machine learning classification. For the random forest algorithm, this is the fraction of trees that voted for spothood |
| classification | A struct containing the classification from the machine learning algorithm and the final classification, which could be modified after review |

while theoretically possible, should not be the goal. As mentioned in Subheading 3.3, the randomForest function returns an estimate of the error rate based on the training data. The error rate for any given specimen can be calculated directly using the GUI described in this section. If the error rate is reasonably low, the user can choose to correct misclassified spots manually using the GUI (presumably achieving a perfect classification, at least in the eye of the user) or to deem the error rate acceptable and account for it in subsequent analyses. The user should refer to step three in Subheading 3.2 for criteria to use in evaluating spots. It can also be useful to switch between maximum merge and individual slice views in the reviewing GUI (see below, Fig. 4) to compare spot intensities between slices. In many samples, the distinction between spots and nonspots is stark and easy to score. In others, there will be more ambiguity. It might be useful to look at many stacks to get a feel for the variation in spot morphology and intensity, including negative controls where potential spots simply reflect noise.

The reviewing GUI window contains several images, information fields, and buttons (Fig. 4). On the left is a 25×25 grid of

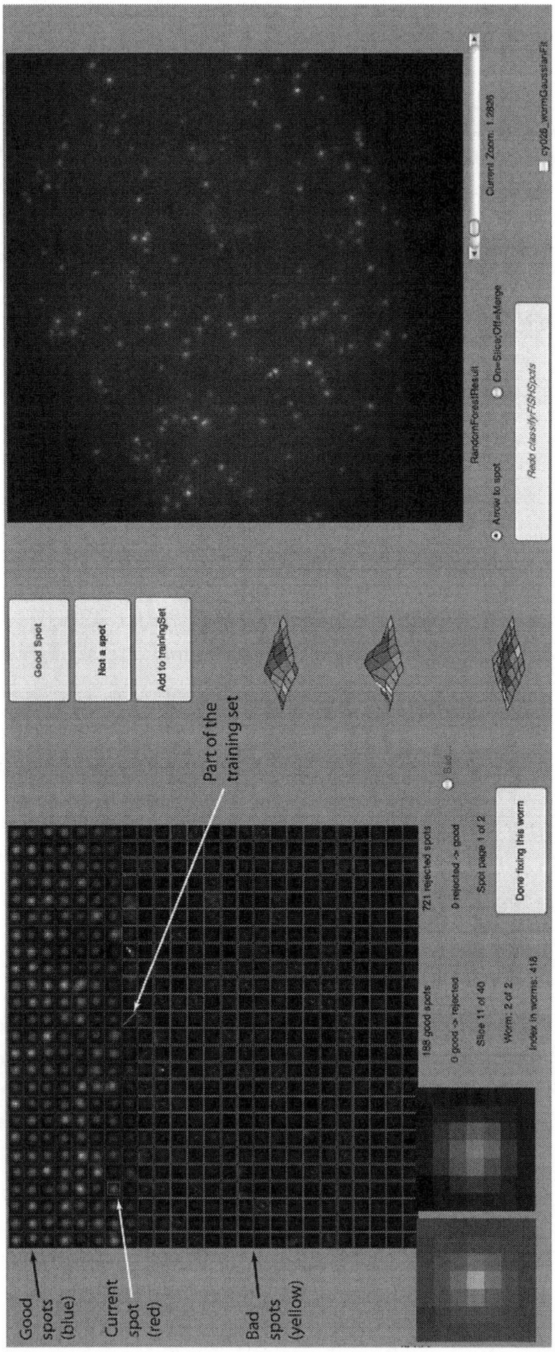


Fig. 4. The reviewing GUI. Colors in the actual display are as marked.

evaluated local maxima and their (by default) 7×7 pixel surroundings, extracted from the image slice they are found in after scaling all intensities to lie between 0 and 1. For compactness, I refer to this 7×7 box as the *spot box*. Each spot box is initially edged in blue or yellow. A blue border means that the local maximum was classified as an mRNA spot. A yellow border means that it was rejected. Local maxima that are included in the training set have diagonal lines across their spot boxes. The spot box in current focus is highlighted by a red boundary (the *focal maximum*). The user can navigate around this grid using the mouse by clicking on different spot boxes or by the arrow keys. Only 625 spot boxes fit on a screen; page up/down will scroll to the next set. The local maxima are arranged in order of the fraction of spot votes they received in the random forest voting, from those that were unanimously classified as true spots to those that were unanimously rejected. This results in questionable calls being primarily grouped near each other around the place where blue boundaries yield to yellow ones. The GUI opens with the most marginal good spot in focus.

Below the spot box grid are two 7×7 pixel images. These portray the spot box in current focus. In the left one, the raw pixel intensities are tinted blue with the regional maximum tinted pink. The right one is gray scale and is equivalent to the scaled spot box in the large left image.

On the right-hand side of the GUI window is a large image that shows the specimen. The focal maximum will generally be in the middle unless its position relative to the bounding box of the specimen does not allow this. The putative spot is marked by a red arrow that can be toggled on or off. Initially, the large image contains the slice of the focal maximum. A toggle button below the image switches to a maximum merge across slices. Provided the mRNAs are not too dense, a true spot should show up in the maximum merge as well as in its own slice. A slider below the image allows the user to zoom from 1× to 6×.

Three surface plots in the middle of the window show the spot box and the 7×7 pixel squares above and below it. A toggle button allows the user to flag a specimen as bad, although bad specimens were probably flagged earlier in the pipeline. The window has text fields reporting the number of accepted and rejected spots, the number and direction of any corrections, and some identifiers of the focal maximum. A checkbox in the lower right indicates whether the image stack has already been reviewed or not.

Three buttons in the middle of the window help the user review and correct the classification. If the classification for the focal maximum is incorrect, the user can correct it from bad to good by clicking *Good Spot* and from good to bad by clicking *Not a Spot*. When the user changes a spot from bad to good, the yellow boundary changes to cyan, the numbers are updated, the local maximum is added to the training set, and the focus shifts to the next spot box. The same is true for the converse except that the boundary changes from blue to orange. A third button, *Add to trainingSet*, allows the user to add a local maximum to the training set without changing the machine classification. This option is useful for adding marginal, but correctly classified, examples to the training set.

At the bottom of the right-hand side of the window lies a button called *Redo classifySpots*. Clicking this button retrains the classifier on the training set, which has been augmented by any corrections or additions, and then reruns the classification on the current image stack. The GUI images will be updated to reflect this latest classification. The user can repeat this process until satisfied with the performance of the machine learning classifier. However, unless the user manually reviews each image stack in a dataset (making the user the final classifier), it is important to use the same iteration of the classifier on all the images in the dataset to avoid artifacts introduced by improvements in the training set.

All corrections are stored in the worms data structure. Final classifications are stored in the classification field of spotInfo (Table 3). The user can write a MATLAB script to cycle through them and collect absolute counts of single molecules or use the locations field to perform a spatial analysis.

## 4. Notes

1. In mathematical morphology, opening is an erosion followed by a dilation of an image by a smaller set of pixels called a structuring element (for example, a square of area 25 pixels or a disk of radius 7 pixels). The process can be pictured as follows: Imagine that the image is a landscape where the height above sea level reflects the pixel intensity. Opening an image is the equivalent of taking the structuring element, holding it horizontally, and running it along the underside of the landscape and recording the maximum height achieved by the structuring element at each pixel location. A small structuring element will track the surface with good fidelity, only lowering tiny bumps that are smaller than it is. A large structuring element will be too big to be pressed up into most hills and will end up razing the landscape. A structuring element that is larger, but not too much larger, than the real features of the image will do a decent job of capturing the varied local background of the features. The program then subtracts this background estimate from the actual image and uses the pixel values of the result to rank local maxima.

2. For ranking purposes, most systematic differences in the raw intensities of the slices will be removed by the local background correction. However, because the machine learning algorithm works with the raw data, large differences in intensity between slices could reduce the usefulness of intensity as a diagnostic statistic. Normally, intensity is one of the most important statistics. For this reason, it may be a good idea to adjust the raw intensities to remove any systematic, noninformative differences between slices.
3. Because of the slice-based normalization, out-of-focus slices and slices without any spots will usually appear bright even if their average raw intensities are low. Because the intensity of these slices comes from noise, the average pixel intensity will fall around 0.5. Slices that contain true spots would ideally have bright pixels around spots and very low pixel intensities elsewhere.
4. If the ranking algorithm works as designed, it should be rarely necessary to change a gray pixel to blue, thereby designating a nonlocal maximum as a spot. This could happen if molecules are close together and their coronas overlap such that one obscures the other. Usually, though, each will be a local maximum, but they will be closer than 7 pixels from each other. The machine learning algorithm does a surprisingly good job of identifying such pairs or triplets as individual spots even if no such overlapping spots are contained in the training set. Because local maxima are identified in three dimensions, there will be bright pixels that clearly radiate intensity that are not marked with blue. In these cases, the surface plots of the neighboring slices will show that this pixel belongs to a local maximum from a neighboring slice.
5. The goodness-of-fit statistic is calculated as follows. First one-dimensional Gaussian parameters are estimated from the (by default) 7 pixel horizontal and vertical slices through the maximum intensity pixel. The mean squared error of each of these slices from an ideal Gaussian distribution is calculated, and the goodness-of-fit statistic is the square root of their average mean squared error.
6. There is a crucial distinction between the cutoffs here and the cutoffs used in threshold-based procedures for identifying spots (1). Spot classification is done by the machine learning algorithm. Evaluating all local maxima would certainly be possible, but it would be overkill. The cutoffs here are designed to preselect a set of local maxima that is empirically guaranteed to contain all true spots. There are two cutoffs in this procedure: the 60th percentile and the 0.9 threshold for the statistic. These only determine the lowest ranked local maximum that

will be evaluated by the classifier. These cutoffs were empirically chosen such that they will never exclude any potential spot. Because they are so conservative, the software will include many more maxima than will be true spots. To modify the values of these parameters, change the values for cutoffPercentile and cutoffStatisticValue in the file evaluateFISHImageStack.m.

## References


1. Raj A, van den Bogaard P, Rifkin SA et al (2008) Imaging individual mRNA molecules using multiple singly labeled probes. Nature Methods **5**:877–879
2. Paré A, Lemons D, Kosman D et al (2009) Visualization of individual Scr mRNAs during drosophila embryogenesis yields evidence for transcriptional bursting. Curr Biol **19**: 2037–2042
3. Lu J, Tsourkas A (2009) Imaging individual microRNAs in single mammalian cells in situ. Nucleic Acids Res **37**:e100
4. Femino AM, Fay FS, Fogarty K et al (1998) Visualization of single RNA transcripts in situ. Science **280**:585–590
5. Rodriguez AJ, Condeelis J, Singer RH et al (2007) Imaging mRNA movement from transcription sites to translation sites. Seminars Cell Dev Biol **18**:202–208
6. Betzig E, Patterson GH, Sougrat R et al (2006) Imaging intracellular fluorescent proteins at nanometer resolution. Science **313**:1642–1645
7. Rust MJ, Bates M, Zhuang X (2006) Sub-diffraction-limit imaging by stochastic optical reconstruction microscopy (STORM). Nature Methods **3**:793–796
8. Fusco D, Accornero N, Lavoie B et al (2003) Single mRNA molecules demonstrate probabilistic movement in living mammalian cells. Curr Biol **13**:161–167
9. MathWorks (2010) MATLAB. Retrieved from http://www.mathworks.com
10. Rifkin SA (2010). *spotFinding Suite*. http://www.biology.ucsd.edu/labs/rifkin/software.html
11. Raj A, Tyagi S (2010) Detection of individual endogenous RNA transcripts in situ using multiple singly labeled probes. In: Walter NG (ed), Single Molecule Tools: Fluorescence Based Approaches, Part A. Academic Press
12. Liaw A, Wiener M (2002) Classification and regression by randomForest. R News **2**: 18–22
13. Breiman L (2001) Random forests. Machine Learning **45**:5–32
14. Breiman L, Cutler A (2001) Random Forests. http://www.stat.berkeley.edu/~breiman/RandomForests/cc_home.htm

# Part VI

## Testing Candidate Genes and Candidate Mutations

# Chapter 21

# Experimental Approaches to Evaluate the Contributions of Candidate *Cis*-regulatory Mutations to Phenotypic Evolution

**Mark Rebeiz and Thomas M. Williams**


## Abstract

Elucidating the molecular bases by which phenotypic traits have evolved provides a glimpse into the past, allowing the characterization of genetic changes that cumulatively contribute to evolutionary innovations. Historically, much of the experimental attention has been focused on changes in protein-coding regions that can readily be identified by the genetic code for translating gene coding sequences into proteins. Resultantly, the role of noncoding sequences in trait evolution has remained more mysterious. In recent years, several studies have reached an unprecedented level of detail in describing how noncoding mutations in gene *cis*-regulatory elements contribute to morphological evolution. Based on these and other studies, we describe an experimental framework and some of the genetic and molecular methods to connect a particular *cis*-regulatory mutation to the evolution of any phenotypic trait.


**Key words:** *Cis*-regulatory elements, CRE, Morphological evolution, Enhancers, Pleiotropy, Noncoding sequences, Modularity, Gene expression

## 1. Introduction

A central aim of evolutionary research is to identify the genetic changes that have contributed to the evolutionary diversification of phenotypic traits – more specifically, which genes, and what regions of these genes, have been modified? The answers to these questions allow us to trace the history of genetic changes that collectively have enabled organisms to phenotypically adapt to their environment, and to determine which gene components are tolerant to change. Furthermore, as we learn more about the mutations that cause different phenotypes, certain classes of genetic and molecular modifications may turn out to be favored evolutionarily.

Virginie Orgogozo and Matthew V. Rockman (eds.), *Molecular Methods for Evolutionary Genetics*,
Methods in Molecular Biology, vol. 772, DOI 10.1007/978-1-61779-228-1_21, © Springer Science+Business Media, LLC 2011

At the most fundamental genetic level, new traits arise either by the evolution of new genes or through the modification of preexisting genes. Although genome content has certainly changed over eons, much of the evolutionary diversification of animals has occurred with a common set of regulatory, or "toolkit", genes (1). Hence, a large portion of the evolutionary narrative involves the modification of preexisting genes. For such cases, the evolution of gene function can be due to either changes in the attributes of the encoded proteins, via mutations in coding sequences, or changes in the noncoding regions of the gene. Although the relative contribution of coding and noncoding mutations to phenotypic variation has been hotly debated, several recent studies have shown how noncoding sequences play an important role (2), and must be considered when trying to understand the genetic basis of an evolved phenotype.

There are several types of *cis*-regulatory mutations that alter a variety of gene components including the following: the core-promoter region, which recruits the basal transcription machinery during transcriptional initiation; introns, which can alter how the primary RNA transcripts are spliced to make processed mRNAs; and the 5′ and 3′ untranslated regions (UTRs), where changes can alter mRNA stability or the rate at which mRNA transcripts are translated into proteins. Lastly, mutations in sequences here referred to as *cis*-regulatory elements (CREs), but also known as enhancers or *cis*-regulatory modules, can alter when, where, and how many mRNA transcripts are made for a given gene. For example, the gene *Sonic hedgehog* (*Shh*) encodes a signaling molecule deployed in a complex pattern that extends over multiple tissues during development (Fig. 1a). This complex gene expression profile is subject to individual regulation of specific subpatterns. Each subpattern is controlled by a relatively short segment of DNA that is bound by multiple transcription factors that temporally, spatially, and quantitatively restrict expression (Fig. 1b).

With so many mechanisms by which *cis*-regulatory sequences contribute to a gene's function, and given the relative difficulty in identifying important noncoding regions by DNA sequence inspection, it appears to be a daunting challenge to determine which *cis*-regulatory changes alter a gene's function. Fortunately, the tools and methods are now available to implicate and identify *cis*-regulatory mutations. In this chapter, we present a general experimental approach to determine whether a *cis*-regulatory mutation in a candidate gene is responsible for an evolutionary change.

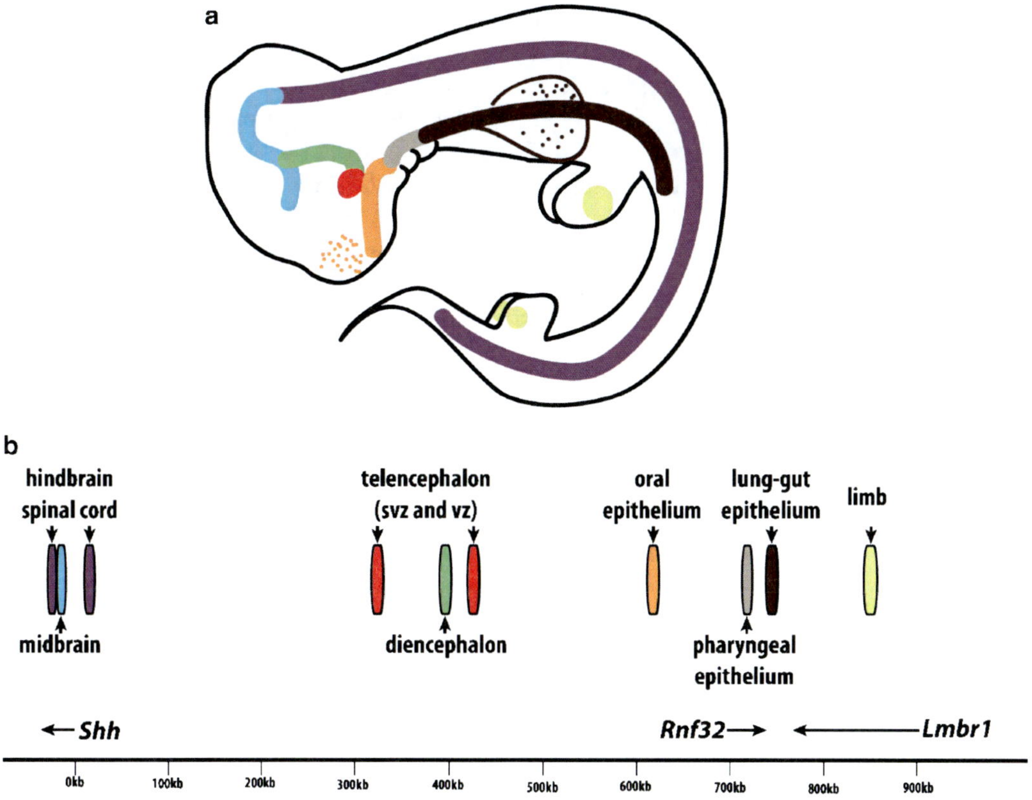


Fig. 1. A modular array of *cis*-regulatory elements controls the expression of many of the genes that pattern development. (**a**) In the developing mouse embryo, the signaling molecule sonic hedgehog (SHH) is deployed in a complex pattern that includes a variety of tissues. (**b**) This overall pattern is controlled by CREs spread across the surrounding genomic region of approximately a million base pairs. Each CRE controls a specific aspect of the *Shh* gene's expression pattern, such that all CREs combined will add up to the full profile of SHH deployment. Adapted from refs. 30, 54.

## 2. Up Close and Far Away: Tracing Evolution at the Micro and Macroevolutionary Levels

Typically, studies investigating the genetic and molecular bases for animal phenotypic variation have operated at different taxonomic scales of comparison. By analyzing traits that arise between closely related species or populations within a species, so-called microevolutionary comparisons, one can identify candidate genes for an evolutionary change through genetic mapping. For example, such comparisons have been employed to find the genes that contribute to regressive traits in cave-dwelling fish (3), stickleback fish body armor and melanism (4–6), and *Drosophila* trichomes and pigmentation (7, 8), among others. By contrast, macroevolutionary comparisons identify how evolutionary processes give rise to differences between more distantly related species. These comparisons involve species that cannot be crossed, and therefore, candidate genes are typically identified by the knowledge of their developmental function in a given reference species. For example, such comparisons have been successfully applied to study the evolution of pigmentation, bristle and trichome patterns in fruit flies (9–11), limblessness in snakes (12), and the morphologies of crustacean appendages (13), vertebrate axes (14), and bat digits (15).

Microevolutionary comparisons are often, but not exclusively, of relatively modest changes in morphology or function compared to macroevolutionary traits. What is lost in glamor is offset by the ability to precisely and confidently identify the causative gene and mutations. Furthermore, these studies provide the opportunity to find new genes and types of mutations that contribute to a trait's development and evolution. Macroevolutionary comparisons are desirable as they probe deeper into evolutionary history, delving into how elaborate traits and novelties were forged. However, these studies do not allow the causative gene to be identified with the same degree of certainty as microevolutionary studies, and the genetic differences can be so numerous that the exact causative mutations cannot be resolved. By embracing the application of both approaches, the full spectrum of evolutionary innovations can be appreciated, generating a more comprehensive perspective of how traits evolve.

Over the past several years, both microevolutionary and macroevolutionary studies have revealed mechanistic insights about the evolution of phenotypic traits via the modification of gene CREs through *cis*-regulatory mutations. From these studies, a general experimental approach can be distilled to determine whether a trait stems from *cis*-regulatory mutations, and if so, which ones. In this chapter we draw from studies that have used both microevolutionary and macroevolutionary approaches to explore the genetic and molecular bases for the evolution of fruit fly pigmentation traits to detail the key steps to determine whether a *cis*-regulatory mutation in a candidate gene region is responsible for an evolutionary change. The general concepts and experimental progression detailed here can, in principle, be extended to any trait in any species group being compared.

### 2.1. Obtaining and Evaluating Candidate Genes

All studies of phenotypic evolution eventually zero in on candidate genes that may or may not contribute to the trait in question. Microevolutionary comparisons often initiate by means of genetic mapping to delineate a genomic interval in which the causative mutations reside, the ultimate goal being to identify the gene and the particular genetic changes causing the evolved trait. However, QTL intervals often include a large number of genes (16), and even when the genetic changes responsible for a trait are narrowly circumscribed to a small region, the affected gene may lie outside of the interval. Thus, the candidate gene approach is an almost inevitable tactic in identifying the causative locus.

For example, the gene *ovo/shaven-baby* (*ovo/svb*) was implicated by genetic mapping to possess the genetic changes causing an evolutionary shift in larval trichome pattern between *Drosophila sechellia* and its sister species *D. simulans* (7). Using a deficiency mapping approach, the causative locus was restricted to a ~40 kb region containing about 20 genes. Among these genes, *ovo/svb* was a natural candidate due to its known role in trichome formation. Further investigation of this candidate clearly demonstrated that it was the gene responsible for the evolved phenotype. The demonstrated role for *ovo/svb* in this microevolutionary change subsequently facilitated its use as a candidate gene in a macroevolutionary study of convergent trichome patterns (9).

Often a candidate gene is suspected from the outset. In such cases, the suspected gene's role in the evolved trait can be validated by testing for a genetic association in hybrid offspring between a particular molecular marker genotype for the candidate gene and the presence of the evolved phenotype. For example, by sequencing the progeny of a cross between strains of wild-derived deer mice, a genotype–phenotype association was found for certain diagnostic haplotypes in the *agouti* gene, which correlated with cryptic coloration (17).

For macroevolutionary comparisons, candidate genes cannot be implicated using genetic mapping approaches, as the extant organisms cannot be intercrossed. Candidate genes emerge from an understanding of a gene, or a network of genes, that functions during a trait's development, often in a reference species evolutionarily diverged from the species under study. For example, a genetic study in mice had shown that the *Prx1* gene, which encodes a transcription factor, promotes skeletal elongation including the digits (18). Based on this knowledge, the RNA expression of the orthologous gene in a bat species was shown to be upregulated compared to the mouse gene. This increased expression evolved by the modification of a bat *Prx1* gene CRE, which is sufficient to account for a significant degree of the elongated bat forelimb digits (15).

For any candidate gene, it is useful to consider the function of the encoded protein, and the extent of its use. If the gene is used in multiple contexts (a so-called pleiotropic gene) and is controlled by multiple CREs, *cis*-regulatory mutations are a likely path for evolutionary change (19). On the contrary, if the gene is dedicated to a single function (not pleiotropic) and hence, is expressed in a single tissue under the control of a single CRE, this candidate gene may have evolved by a *cis*-regulatory change though it would not be predicted a priori. In this case, a change in gene expression is just as pleiotropic as a change to the protein-coding sequence. Irrespective of the degree of gene pleiotropy, to determine whether a *cis*-regulatory mutation is the causative change, the next step is to examine the gene's expression in relation to the divergent trait.

### 2.2. Determine Whether a Candidate Gene's Expression Pattern Has Changed

The strongest indication that a candidate gene might possess a relevant *cis*-regulatory change is the demonstration that its expression pattern has changed. By comparing the state of gene expression in several species, one can determine whether a change in the candidate gene's expression correlates with the evolved trait in question. There are two primary levels at which to assess gene expression: the mRNA transcript and protein abundance levels. A variety of suitable methods exist for assessing a gene's expression pattern/level, ranging from the quantitative (such as quantitative RT-PCR (see Chapter 17), microarray (see Chapter 13), and mass spectrometry) to the qualitative (RNA in situ hybridization (see Chapters 19 and 20) and protein immunohistochemistry).

Detecting gene expression at the RNA transcript level measures the abundance of a gene's mRNA, which generally reflects the rate of gene transcription as well as the stability of the gene's mRNA. In eukaryotes, assays of transcript abundance can also detect differences in gene splicing which may impinge on the gene's function; for example, the sexually dimorphic alternative splicing of the *D. melanogaster doublesex* (*dsx*) gene results in the production of sex-specific DSX protein isoforms and hence, sex-specific traits (20). Protein abundance is additionally influenced by posttranscriptional gene regulatory mechanisms that can be encoded in *cis* to a gene (on the same DNA molecule as the encoded protein) to control the level of transcription or the subsequent rate of translation. The complementary binding of miRNAs to mRNA transcripts represents a major mechanism that exerts posttranscriptional control. For example, developmental timing in *Caenorhabditis elegans* is controlled by the *let-7* miRNA, which binds to the mRNAs of target genes and ultimately results in their reduced expression and hence, function (21, 22). A second posttranscriptional mechanism operates through translational repression caused by the binding of mRNA transcripts by RNA-binding proteins. For example, binding of *glp-1* gene mRNAs by the RNA-binding protein GLD-1 results in the repression of GLP-1 translation during *C. elegans* embryonic asymmetry establishment (23).

The analysis of gene expression at the RNA or protein level respectively presents both advantages and disadvantages (see Note 1). Quantitative RT-PCR (see Chapter 17) provides a precise determination of the amount of transcript present in a particular cell or tissue type, but can only coarsely identify a spatial change in gene expression. On the contrary, RNA in situ hybridization (see Chapters 19 and 20) and immunohistochemistry are best suited to reveal spatial changes in RNA and protein levels, respectively, though some quantitative and semiquantitative approaches exist (24, 25). Thus, it may be pragmatic to employ both a quantitative and qualitative approach to validate a potential expression difference for a candidate gene.

Analyses of gene expression by RNA in situ hybridization (see Note 2) and protein immunohistochemistry (see Note 3) have been a part of the armament of developmental biologists for several decades, and as a result protocols are widely available. In recent years, these methods have been employed to demonstrate evolutionary changes in gene expression. For example, RNA in situ hybridization demonstrated that fruit flies with different degrees of body pigmentation (Fig. 2a, b) differ in the level and pattern of *ebony* gene expression (Fig. 2c, d) (25), a gene that was

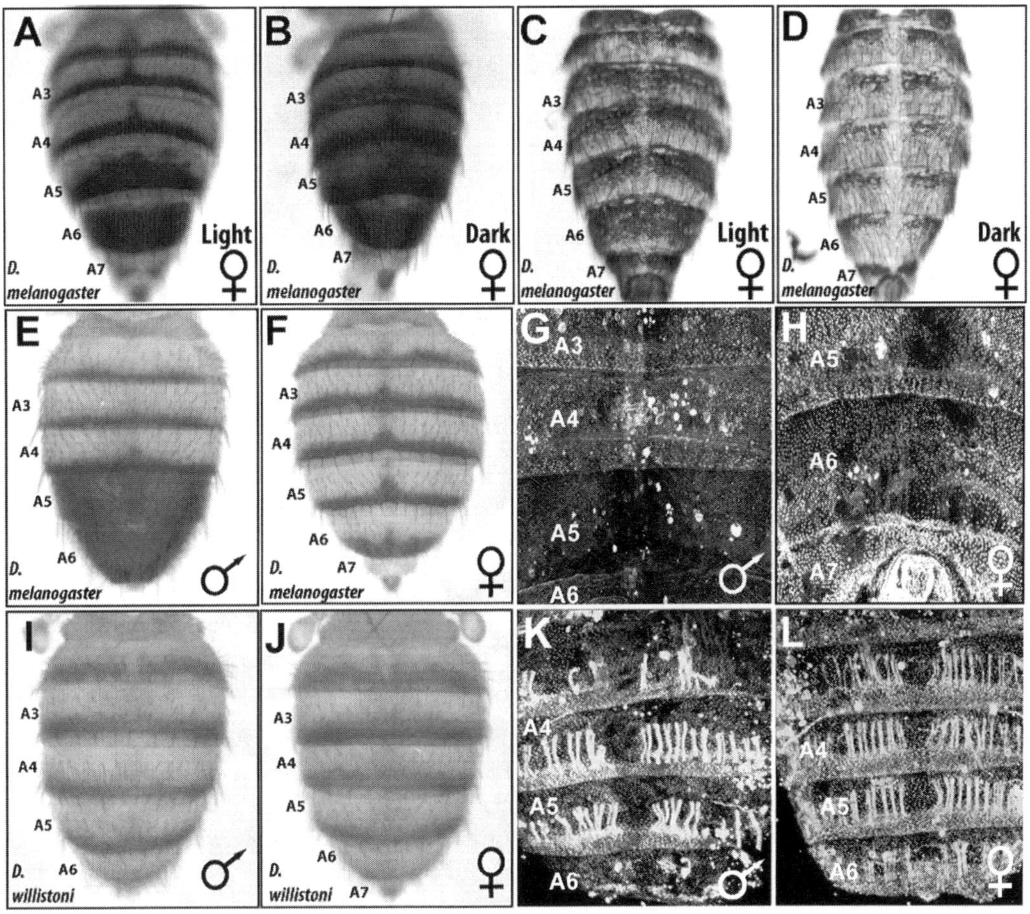


Fig. 2. Detection of gene expression differences at the RNA transcript and protein abundance level. RNA in situ hybridization and protein immunohistochemistry are two techniques for the visualization of gene expression patterns and differences. *Drosophila melanogaster* fruit flies can differ in the degree of abdominal pigmentation with some individuals being lightly (**a**) or darkly pigmented (**b**). This phenotypic difference results from differential expression of the *ebony* gene. RNA in situ hybridization demonstrates the high level of *ebony* expression in flies with lighter pigmentation (**c**), compared to those with darker abdomens (**d**). Abdominal pigmentation of *D. melanogaster* is sexually dimorphic, where males (**e**) are more fully pigmented than females (**f**). This trait is derived from a sexually monomorphic ancestor with light pigmentation similar to that of the extant species *D. willistoni* (**i** and **j**). A key gene expression difference, here, revealed by protein immunohistochemistry was the transition from the monomorphic expression of the Bab1 protein throughout the abdomen (**k** and **l**), to a sexually dimorphic pattern where Bab1 expression is now absent from the posterior segments A5 and A6 of males (**g**), and yet expression persists in these segments in females (**h**). (**a**–**d**) is adapted from ref. 25 and (**e**–**l**) from ref. 27.

formerly implicated by genotype–phenotype association to underlie this adaptive trait variation (26). Elsewhere, immunohistochemical analysis revealed an interspecific difference in Bab1 protein expression (compare Fig. 2g, h with k, l). This difference correlates with the evolved sexually dimorphic pigmentation pattern (compare Fig. 2e, f with i, j), and the known developmental function of the Bab1 protein (27). In addition to spatial changes in gene expression, it is also important to consider the dimension of time (see Note 4).

The case that an expression change is relevant to the trait rests heavily upon both the correlation of the expression change with the trait difference and what is known about the gene. For example, the *Pitx1* gene is expressed in and required for limb development in diverse vertebrates. Thus, the correlation of a loss of *Pitx1* gene expression in the regions where hindlimbs normally develop with the absence of hindlimbs would suggest that this expression change underlies the evolved trait. A priori though, such an expression change can be due to changes in the *Pitx1* gene itself or in another gene regulating *Pitx1*. In a comparison of stickleback fish populations differing in the size of pelvic fins, genetic mapping first implicated *Pitx1* as a candidate gene to underlie the phenotypic difference and subsequently, a correlated change in *Pitx1* gene expression was found (6). Recently, the reduced pelvic fin phenotype was shown to stem from a *cis*-regulatory change at the *Pitx1* locus that eliminated *Pitx1* gene expression in pelvic fin precursors (28). In cases where the molecular functions of a candidate gene are not known, the correlation between a change in gene expression and the trait's phenotype may be considered a strong enough impetus to further characterize the gene for a relevant *cis*-regulatory change (see Subheading 2.4).

### 2.3. Demonstrating a Cis-regulatory Change in Hybrids

For microevolutionary comparisons, if the two strains or species can be crossed, one can obtain definitive evidence that the gene expression change is encoded in *cis* by measuring allele-specific gene expression in hybrid organisms that contain a copy of each allele. Since the two alleles are in the exact same genetic background, if the alleles differ in expression, then the sole interpretation is that a *cis*-regulatory change contributes to the expression change. On the contrary, if both alleles are expressed similarly in the hybrid genetic background, then one can infer that the observed change in expression stems from either change outside of the gene locus in question (so-called *trans*-change) or a mix of *cis* and *trans* changes. Allele-specific gene expression can be measured by pyrosequencing cDNA from hybrid animals (see Chapter 18), in which the relative abundance of mRNA transcripts derived from each allele for a gene (distinguished by DNA sequence polymorphisms) is proportional to the number of times an allele is sequenced in a reaction (29). Alternately, if mRNA sequences are sufficiently different, in situ hybridization using probes that can distinguish both alleles can be performed in hybrids (see Chapter 19).

### 2.4. Identifying the Functional Mutations in a Cis-regulatory Element

Techniques such as RNA in situ hybridization and protein immunohistochemistry can reveal an expression difference for the candidate gene underlying an evolved trait. However, the observation of an expression difference does not prove that the difference is the result of a *cis*-regulatory change in the candidate gene. Rather the expression change may be due to changes at another gene or genes that function in *trans*. Such "*trans*" changes would result in differing transcriptional outputs without any functional divergence in a *cis*-regulatory element (CRE) for the candidate gene. This scenario may be dismissed through genetic mapping, or by demonstrating the existence of a functional *cis*-regulatory change in a CRE or CREs that controls the candidate gene's expression. In the later case though, one must often first identify the relevant CRE(s).

#### 2.4.1. Identify the Relevant CRE(s)

To establish that a *cis*-regulatory change caused a certain gene expression change, one must first identify the CRE(s) responsible for generating the pattern of expression in the cell or tissue under scrutiny. This can be an onerous task, as unlike protein-coding sequences, which typically are composed of several hundred to several thousand base pairs, the scope of gene noncoding sequences can be an order to several orders of magnitude larger in size. For example, in the gene *Sonic hedgehog* (*Shh*), a CRE that controls *Shh* gene expression in the developing limbs resides roughly a million base pairs upstream of the first exon of *Shh* and within a second gene, *Lmbr1* (Fig. 1b) (30). Hence, not only was this CRE difficult to find, but if this CRE was the root of an evolved limb morphology trait, *Shh* might not even lie in the genetically identified interval for the variable trait!

By comparing orthologous DNA sequences from several species, functionally important noncoding sequences can often be identified as DNA sequences that remain relatively unchanged throughout evolution (so-called "conserved sequences"). However, the utility of such sequence conservation is limited, as not all evolutionarily conserved noncoding sequences are CREs. Even if a conserved sequence is indeed a CRE, it remains unknown whether the sequence controls the candidate gene and the expression pattern of interest. Thus, when the CRE content of a locus is unknown, it is often necessary to map the CRE content by the production of transgenic organisms that possess "reporter genes". Here, a reporter gene includes both a noncoding sequence from a candidate gene, which is fused to a minimal gene promoter, and the coding sequence for a gene that produces an easily observable product (see Chapter 23). Commonly employed reporter genes are the *lacZ* and *GFP* genes (see Note 5) that respectively encode the β-galactosidase enzyme and green fluorescent protein (Fig. 4a, b).

Before initiating a survey to identify a relevant CRE or CREs for a candidate gene, one must decide which species' gene locus to evaluate and what species will serve as the host for the reporter transgenes. If the candidate gene for an evolved trait is expressed in the cells or tissue responsible for the derived phenotype, then it is advantageous to investigate the locus from this species. However, if the candidate gene is not expressed, and it appears that its expression was lost, it would then be pointless to perform the CRE survey using this species gene locus. In this case, it would be beneficial to survey the CREs from a species that has the ancestral expression pattern. Regarding the choice of host species for transgenes, typically it is either the species under investigation (derived trait) or a surrogate genetic model organism (see Note 6 regarding host choice). Depending on the nature of the transgene system, reporter genes are either incorporated extra-chromosomally, hence transiently, or into the genome, for long term propagation. *D. melanogaster* and the mouse are convenient hosts as protocols are both well-established and readily available (see Note 7), and the work can be outsourced (see Note 12). Any CRE activity can then be identified by assessing where and when during development the reporter gene's protein product is observed, and this CRE activity can be compared to the endogenous pattern of gene expression.

For example, the CREs that control the sexually dimorphic expression pattern of the *D. melanogaster* tandem duplicate *bric-à-brac* (*bab*) genes were identified by systematic transgenic inspection of the noncoding sequences for this locus (Fig. 3a; see Note 8 for a general strategy) (27). This screen resulted in the identification of several CREs within this locus that collectively contribute to the composite *bab* gene expression pattern (Fig. 3c–g). In recent years, recombination-based methods have been developed for use in various model organisms to aid in the analysis of very large loci (see Note 9 and Chapters 24 and 26).

Once a noncoding sequence possessing the relevant CRE activity has been located, for two reasons it is wise to determine the minimal sequence necessary to confer the expression pattern. First, with the ultimate goal being the identification of the precise mutation or mutations that cause the gene expression change, the larger the noncoding sequence under study the more mutational differences will exist between the sequences being compared. Secondly, a relatively large noncoding sequence may contain more than one CRE. In the aforementioned study of the *bab* locus, a noncoding sequence was found that activated sexually dimorphic expression in male and female fruit fly pupae (compare Fig. 3f, g). After the analysis of numerous truncated versions of this large noncoding sequence (Fig. 3b), it was found that the originally observed dimorphic expression pattern was the product of the activity of two separate CREs (Fig. 3h, i).

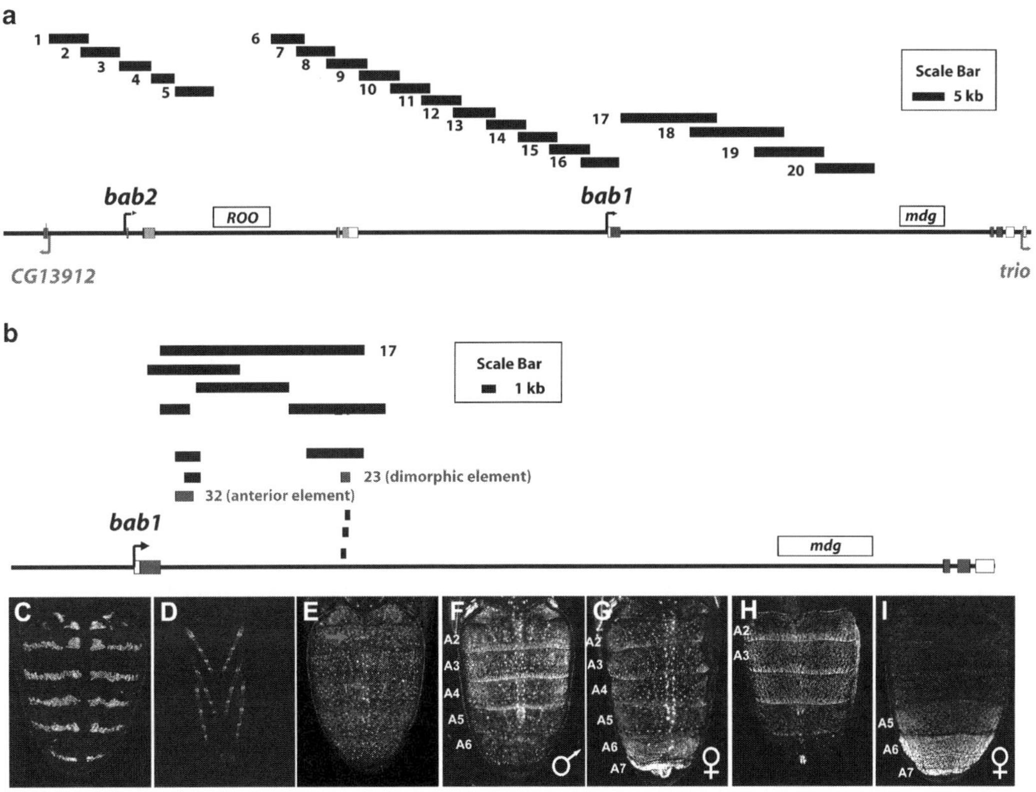


Fig. 3. A systematic screen of the noncoding sequences for a gene locus reveals the CRE content. For many genes where the expression pattern has evolved through mutations in noncoding sequences, the relevant CRE(s) remain unidentified. Here, for the *bab* locus (**a**) an initial screen of 20 noncoding sequences (ranging between 5 and 15 kb of sequence) were evaluated for the ability to activate GFP reporter gene expression in transgenic pupae. The sequences from the regions indicated *ROO* and *mdg* were not tested for CRE activity, as they are derived from transposable elements. Regulatory sequences were identified that individually control part of the overall *bab* gene expression pattern (**c**–**g**), including the sexually dimorphic expression in the abdominal epidermis (**f** and **g**). Further analysis of the large sequence found to control the sexually dimorphic pattern of expression, fragment 17, by a series of nested sequences (**b**) determined that this expression pattern is conferred by the action of two separate CREs (**h**, fragment 32; and **i**, fragment 23). Adapted from ref. 27.

#### *2.4.2. Do the Orthologous CRE Sequences Possess Differing Gene-Regulatory Capabilities?*

When a candidate CRE has been found, the next step is to determine whether its activity has changed in a way consistent with and explaining the RNA transcript or protein expression difference observed. One simple approach is to separately test the orthologous sequences derived from multiple species, or individuals under comparison, for the capability to regulate reporter gene expression in transgenic animals. If a difference is observed in the developmental timing, spatial pattern, and/or level of reporter gene expression that is consistent with what was observed for the endogenous gene, then it can be concluded that genetic changes within the CRE have caused the evolutionary transition in CRE activity. Comparable methods have successfully been employed to uncover the regulatory basis of evolutionary changes amongst diverse traits and taxa including tetrapod axial morphology (14), nematode excretory system (31), fruit fly pigmentation traits (11, 32, 33), fruit fly dorsocentral bristles (10), and stickleback fish pelvic reduction (28).

The aforementioned pioneering studies relied on the random nature by which transgenes generally integrate into the genome, which introduces a considerable degree of variation in transgene activity due to the site of integration and imposes technical difficulties and experimental limitations (see Note 10). In recent years, new site-specific integration technologies have been adapted to model organism systems to allow the incorporation of transgenes into the same genomic location, allowing a quantitative comparison of CRE activity (see Note 11). For example, the phiC31-integrase system (34, 35) has enabled the quantitative study of CRE evolution of *Drosophila* pheromone (36) and pigmentation (25, 27) traits. In a comparison of orthologous abdominal CREs from the *bab* locus (27), it was demonstrated that a female-specific CRE activity had evolved a qualitatively expanded domain of regulatory activity (Fig. 4a, b). By incorporating the reporter transgenes into

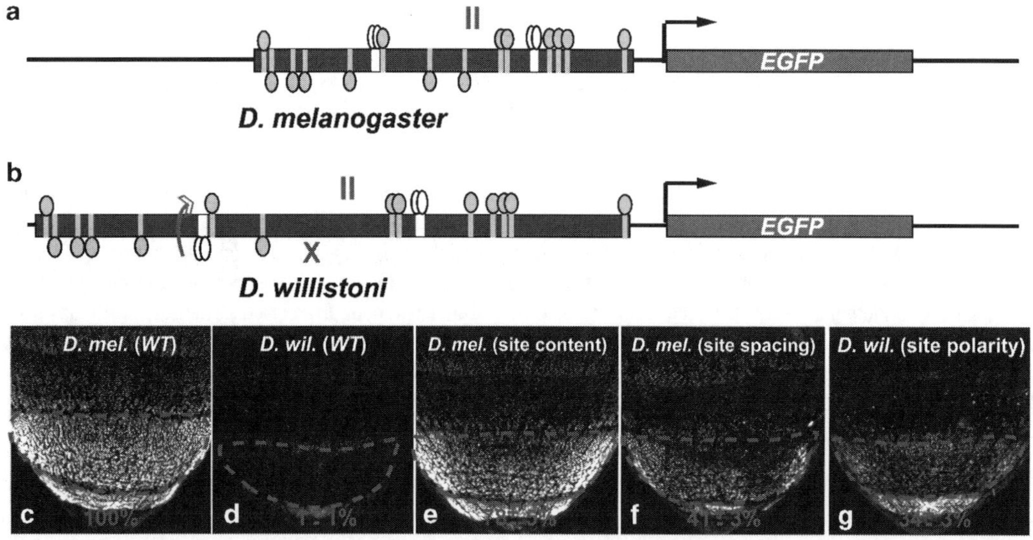


Fig. 4. Elucidation of key genetic changes that underlie a macroevolutionary transition in orthologous CRE activity using reporter transgenes. (**a**–**b**) Schematic of reporter transgenes possessing the orthologous fruit fly *bab* gene CREs upstream of a heterologous gene promoter (*arrow*) and *EGFP* gene. These CREs share many of the same transcription factor binding sites due to common descent but differ in the number (X marks a lost site), topology (II indicates a region where the spacing between conserved binding sites is expanded in *D. willistoni*), and polarity (*curved arrow* indicates a site with reversed polarity) of binding sites between the related species. The wild-type *D. willistoni* CRE's activity is both spatially and quantitatively reduced compared to that of *D. melanogaster* (compare **c** and **d**). Candidate mutations can be introduced into CREs and evaluated for an effect on reporter gene expression in transgenic animals. Here, both the removal of a binding site (**e**) and the alteration of the spacing between adjacent binding sites (**f**) of the *D. melanogaster* CRE, which are characteristic of the other species, result in the CRE activity becoming more like that of the *D. willistoni* CRE. Reciprocally, reversing the polarity of a binding site in the *D. willistoni* CRE (**g**), a characteristic of *D. melanogaster*, causes the activity to increase towards the level of the *D. melanogaster* CRE. Here, CRE activity measurements are represented as the percent of the *D. melanogaster* female activity ± SEM. Adapted from ref. 27.

the same genomic position, a quantitatively measurable difference in regulatory capability was identified for the orthologous CREs (compare Fig. 4c, d).

In this section, we have detailed an experimental approach to both identify the CRE content for a candidate gene implicated to underlie an evolutionary change, and to demonstrate whether two orthologous CREs possess divergent activity. At this juncture, it is now imperative to address which of the often numerous sequence differences are responsible for the evolutionary difference.

#### 2.4.3. Identify the Causative Mutation(s)

Which and how many mutations were necessary to cause the relevant change in gene expression? The difficulty in answering this question in large part depends upon the amount of sequence divergence between the two orthologous CREs being compared. CRE sequences are notorious for evolving rapidly, such that even when the transcriptional output remains unchanged, the number and location of transcription factor binding sites can change markedly (37, 38). In general, for microevolutionary comparisons the degree of the sequence difference between orthologous CREs is often reduced compared to macroevolutionary comparisons, as the number of mutations (both neutral and functionally relevant) increases with the time since species divergence. This simplifying feature of microevolutionary comparisons makes the identification of the nucleotide change(s) responsible for the trait change more feasible. An effective approach to pinpoint the causative mutations is to generate so-called chimeric CREs that introduce sequences or combine features of the "evolved" CRE into or with the "ancestral" CRE (or vice versa). Subsequently these chimeric CREs are tested in a transgenic reporter gene assay to determine whether the modifications convert the activity to the likeness of the orthologous CRE. Modified CREs can be assembled by PCR-stitching (see Chapter 27) to assemble a nonredundant subset of sequences from the compared CREs into a chimeric CRE, or by replacing the sequence of one CRE with the sequence present in the other by site-directed mutagenesis. For example, modified CREs led to the identification of a series of mutations that cause reduced *ebony* gene expression and pigmentation in a *D. melanogaster* population (25).

Another approach available to microevolutionary comparisons is to genetically map at a high resolution the sequences causing an evolutionary transition in gene expression between interfertile species or populations. For example, it was shown by high-resolution interspecific genetic mapping that genetic differences within three separate CREs at the *svb* gene locus are necessary and sufficient to account for the evolutionary transition in larval trichome pattern between *D. mauritiana* and its sister species *D. sechellia* (39). Impressively, besides locating where the *cis*-regulatory mutations reside, this approach produced definitive proof that these genetic changes are responsible for the evolutionary modification of this trait.

For macroevolutionary comparisons, it is often more difficult to determine the mutations responsible for evolved CRE activity, as sequence differences between the compared CREs are typically more numerous. In such cases, it may be beneficial to focus on one of the orthologous CREs and determine key sequences within it that are essential to generate the relevant gene expression pattern. This can be done by mutating particular sequence motifs and testing whether the introduced mutations alter CRE activity in a transgenic reporter gene assay. Upon successful identification of key sequences, the next step is to inspect the orthologous CRE with divergent activity for any differences in the content or quality of the key sequences. Any differences are candidates for mutations that underlie or contribute to the evolved gene regulatory difference. Candidate differences can be validated or invalidated through the production and transgenic analysis of modified CREs as described above. For example, the prior elucidation of the key transcription factor binding sites for a CRE within the *bab* locus led to the determination that the evolved CRE activity was due to the cumulative changes in transcription factor binding site number, polarity, and topology (Fig. 4c–g) (27).

In this section we outlined an experimental approach to identify which mutations cause orthologous CREs to differ in gene-regulatory activity. Traditionally, the execution of this experimental sequence is stymied by the requisite time and expense to generate derivations of an altered CRE sequence by methods such as PCR-stitching (see Chapter 27) or site-directed mutagenesis, which is a significant obstacle when many candidate mutational changes must be considered and tested in transgenic assays. However, recent developments in gene synthesis technologies have allowed investigators to obtain altered CREs by emailing the desired sequence to vendors to synthesize de novo, and the production of transgenic organisms can often be outsourced as well (see Note 12).

#### 2.4.4. What if a Modified CRE Is Not Found?

In the event that experiments yield no CRE that explains the observed change in gene expression, there are several explanations: Is CRE activity being assayed in the correct species background? Could the expression change stem from a change in *trans*, such as a mutation in an upstream regulator of the candidate gene? Could the observed change in expression be explained by a change in some other gene regulatory mechanism, for example, regulation by a distantly acting CRE, or alteration in either RNA splicing, mRNA stability, or yet a posttranscriptional mechanism such as regulation by either a miRNA or RNA-binding protein?

The most direct way to distinguish between these other mechanisms is to first demonstrate that the gene indeed contributes to the trait, e.g., by transgenically introducing the candidate gene into a surrogate species (expanded upon in Subheading 2.5). Once it has been demonstrated that the gene contributes, then the possibility of a *trans*-change has been eliminated, and the causative mutations lie somewhere in the transgenic construct used.

The location of such causative mutations can be pinpointed through the generation of chimeric constructs that map the phenotypically relevant variation down to a successively smaller area. If the variation maps to the 3′UTR, one might suspect that a binding site for either miRNAs or RNA-binding proteins has changed. If the variation maps to the protein coding region of a gene, perhaps a relevant coding sequence change occurred. If the variation maps to a noncoding region, it is possible that it is part of a more complex gene expression regulatory architecture. For example, the *ebony* gene contains separate noncoding sequences that function as repressive elements that are essential to produce the endogenous *ebony* abdominal expression pattern (25). In cases like this, negative regulatory elements will not show up in a reporter assay, unless properly situated in the context of positively acting elements. If the variation maps to an intronic location, it is entirely possible that splicing has changed, and as such, the abundance of mRNA splice variants can be compared to the total RNA abundance of the gene through the careful design of riboprobes or RT-PCR primers (see Note 13). With the numerous types of gene regulatory mechanisms, it is a possibility that other types of *cis*-regulatory change can be overlooked if our preconceptions of what is possible are incorrect. Therefore, the use of transgenic assays represents a powerful approach for functionally mapping causative changes, regardless of the mechanism of change.

### 2.5. Demonstrate that a Particular Cis-regulatory Change Contributes to the Evolved Trait

Thus far, we have given a perspective of how to determine whether *cis*-regulatory mutations are likely (via gene expression analysis), and whether they are responsible for expression differences (reporter gene analysis). Yet the experiments detailed thus far do not directly connect the changes in gene expression to a particular phenotypic effect. The clearest demonstration that an evolutionary change modified a phenotypic trait is to show the repercussions of making such a gene modification in vivo. This can be done in a variety of ways, which vary depending on the circumstances of the trait. If a gene expression pattern was lost in a particular context, the phenotypic outcome of restoring this expression pattern could be assessed. If gene expression was gained, then the effects of the relevant expression specificity should be assessed in a background that doesn't have this derived expression pattern.

When undertaking the functional validation of a *cis*-change, an important consideration is in what species to perform the genetic manipulation. One must ask how feasible is such a transgenic analysis in the species being studied? For many applications, transgenic manipulation of a closely related model organism might be the best bet for simplicity. For example, in studying the role of *Prx1* gene in bat wing evolution, transgenic mice were generated expressing

*Prx1* gene under the control of a bat CRE (15). This resulted in elevated *Prx1 gene* expression, and increased limb length compared to the mouse *Prx1* CRE. However, the most clear-cut case studies are those where gene activity is directly demonstrated in the species in question, since this eliminates confounding effects from working in a heterologous genetic background. For example, to demonstrate a role for the *ebony* gene in the evolution of abdominal pigmentation in *D. melanogaster*, transgenic complementation tests were performed with *ebony* transgenes derived from high-expressing (lightly pigmented) and low-expressing (darkly pigmented) fly lines (Fig. 5) (25). The differing transgenes were assayed in an *ebony* null mutant background, to compare phenotypic effect of replacing different *ebony* gene alleles. In this experiment, the *ebony* allele from darker flies resulted in a darker phenotype, compared to flies with the lighter animal's *ebony* allele, demonstrating that variation at the *ebony* gene contributes to variation in the adaptive pigmentation phenotype.

There are two additional benefits to the transgenic construct approach of functionally validating gene effects: (1) demonstrating the target gene of a *cis*-change and (2) eliminating coding sequence changes. As exemplified by the case of *Shh* gene (Fig. 1), a CRE can exist far away from its target gene. Even if one could engineer a *cis*-change of a single nucleotide at a locus, the target of this *cis*-regulatory mutation remains to be determined. This typically can be resolved by selectively including only a single gene and its CREs in a transgenic assay. An additional advantage of transgenic rescue constructs is that they can be used to eliminate the possible contribution of protein-coding sequence differences (see Note 14). By generating chimeric transgenes that separated the *ebony* gene CREs from the *ebony*-coding region, it was demonstrated that an abdominal CRE was the source of genetic variation causing the abdominal pigmentation phenotype (Fig. 5) (25).

Often, macroevolutionary studies on the evolution of pleiotropic genes disregard differences in the protein-coding sequence content between orthologous genes, as a vast body of experimental literature has demonstrated cases of functional equivalence between orthologous genes over long stretches of evolutionary divergence (2). The habit of reasoning away the impact of coding sequence changes instead of more definitive experiments largely stems from the difficulty in conducting gain- and loss-of-function experiments in nonmodel organisms. However, with the emergence of RNA interference (RNAi, see Chapter 28), it has become more routine to perform loss-of function experiments for gene function in non-model organisms (40–42). Additionally, improved transgenesis methods (43) have better facilitated gain-of-function experiments in an organism whether it is a canonical model or not. Thus, with the increased capabilities to manipulate genes in many organisms, the standard of experimental evidence should increase as well.

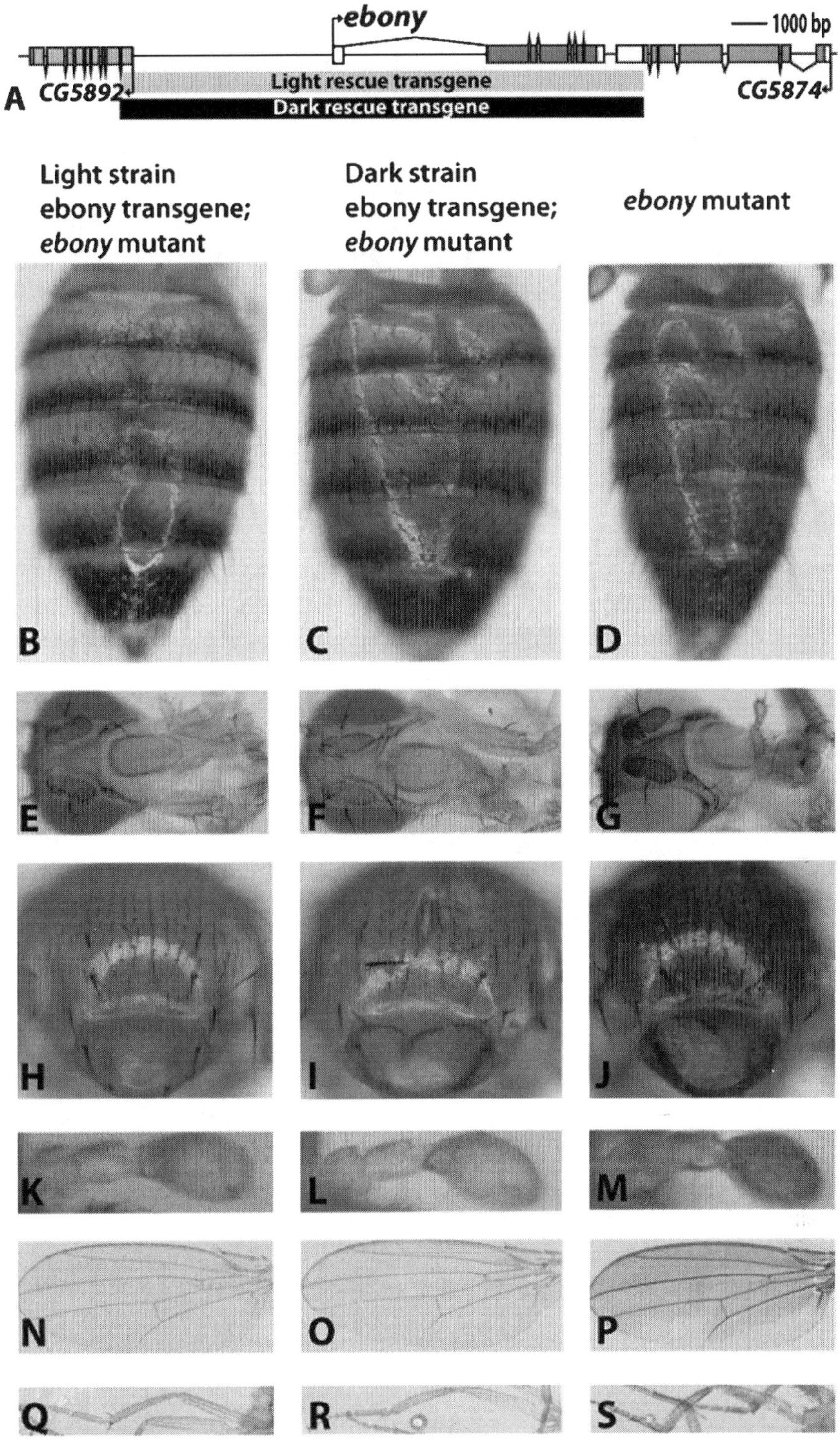


Fig. 5. The use of transgenic assays to directly connect allelic variation to phenotypic outcome. (**a**) Schematic of the *ebony* locus, and encompassing transgenes, derived from lightly and darkly pigmented fly lines from Uganda. When tested in an *ebony* null mutant background (**d**, **g**, **j**, **m**, **p**, **s**), the *ebony* gene from the *lightly colored line* can rescue all of the *ebony* mutant phenotypes (**b**, **e**, **h**, **k**, **n**, **r**). However, when the *ebony* mutant is rescued by a *dark line's ebony* gene, a dark abdomen phenotype results (**c**), while the other phenotypes are indistinguishable from the light line (**f**, **i**, **l**, **o**, **r**). Tissues shown are Abdomen (**b**, **c**, **d**), Head (**e**, **f**, **g**), Thorax (**h**, **i**, **j**), Haltere (**k**, **l**, **m**), Wing (**n**, **o**, **p**), and T2 Legs (**q**, **r**, **s**). Adapted from ref. 25.

## 3. Moving Forward

### *3.1. What Is Sufficient Evidence?*

Studies revealing the genetic changes causing phenotypic traits to evolve due to alterations of noncoding or *cis*-regulatory sequences were slow to emerge as suitable methods were lacking. Over the past several decades, these methodological limitations have been remediated, and as a result numerous examples of *cis*-regulatory mutations underlying evolutionary change have been detailed. Here, we present the key steps to rigorously demonstrate that a *cis*-regulatory change in a candidate gene is responsible for a trait's evolution and which particular mutation or mutations has caused this change. These steps are to (1) determine whether the candidate gene's expression has been altered in the cells or tissues producing the phenotype, (2) identify the relevant *cis*-regulatory element(s), (3) determine which mutational differences are responsible for the change in gene-regulatory activity and if possible, (4) validate the phenotypic significance of such, changes using in vivo assays. For every trait and candidate gene under study, all steps may not be feasible or even possible. However, each and every case must be evaluated by taking into consideration the body of evidence. If the candidate gene has an expression change, and if that change maps to mutations in a CRE, it is clear that some or all of the differences in expression are inscribed in some functional component of the CRE. The level of confidence in the phenotypic consequences of such *cis*-regulatory mutations can range from extremely high (the allele with divergent expression has been shown transgenically to confer a direct difference in phenotype) to moderate (the repercussions of manipulating the orthologous gene in a related species have been shown), to suggestive (an aspect of the gene's expression pattern is often associated with the trait across many species). As technologies develop, standards of evidence are expected to steadily rise over time. With advances in gene manipulation technologies, the previous roadblocks should less often be encountered, and hence, studies should aim for results providing high confidence in their conclusions.

### *3.2. Where Do We Go from Here?*

In the past several years numerous studies in diverse taxonomic comparisons have detailed how traits evolved due to changes in gene CREs. These studies have emboldened the argument that CREs have prominently contributed to the evolution of animal morphology (2, 44, 45), but they have additionally shown complexity both in the type and number of mutations needed to cause an evolutionary change in gene expression. Additional case studies documenting CRE evolution will emerge and add to the growing list, but how are the questions advancing as other instances of a more general phenomenon are reported? The evolution of phenotypic traits by alterations of gene CREs now rests upon a sufficient scientific foundation opening up a new cohort of questions to address. How pervasive is variation in CRE activity within and between species? How many sequences of CRE mutations – "mutational paths" – lead to the same evolved activity? What are the molecular alterations by which CRE genotypic variation is translated into gene expression variation? How do new CRE activities evolve to deploy old genes in new ways?

Moving forward, a major obstacle in our understanding of this important facet of phenotypic evolution is the elucidation of the so-called "regulatory logic" that underlies evolved CRE activities. Prominently, what are the transcription factor proteins that bind to CREs, do these factors activate or repress gene expression, and if so where? How have the CRE sequences to which these factors bind been modified? It is relatively straightforward now to test whether a *cis*-regulatory mutation in a candidate gene contributes to a given trait. Yet it remains prohibitively difficult to understand at a molecular level how such mutations alter the regulatory logic for a CRE. The major obstacles to an understanding of regulatory logic are (1) the permissive binding of transcription factors to many short simple sequences, (2) the lack of knowledge of what preference particular transcription factors have for particular binding sequences, and (3) the dearth of techniques available to identify factors that bind to a particular sequence with high confidence. Currently, techniques such as yeast one-hybrid or biochemical selection from nuclear extracts have a reputation for finding many false positives, and the validation of candidates from such approaches is a lengthy and laborious task. As new technologies facilitate a better understanding of the regulatory logic controlling gene expression, a whole new array of biological problems and mechanisms will be open for investigation.

The past several decades have been an exciting time in the field of evolutionary genetics, as we have witnessed first the emergence of genetic data suggesting the importance of gene regulatory sequence evolution and subsequently the emergence of case studies demonstrating its past evolutionary application. However, the excitement of *cis*-regulatory mutations and CRE evolution has not passed, but rather we are now prepared for a new series of questions to be answered.

## 4. Notes

1. From a practical standpoint, the visualization of RNA transcript abundance is simpler, as both quantitative RT-PCR and RNA in situ hybridization protocols utilize DNA primers, which are cheaply and quickly synthesized. These primers are used to amplify by PCR a sequence for a given gene directly

from the species being studied. By contrast, generating an antibody specific to the protein under investigation for immunohistochemical analysis of protein abundance is a relatively long and expensive process. The added time and expense to generate an antibody may be worth it, however, as assessing the level and pattern of protein expression surveys all potential *cis*-regulatory changes altering a gene's function. It is also worth noting that many antibodies, particularly polyclonal antibodies, are cross-reactive to distantly related species, and so, it is worth investigating whether an antibody exists to the protein of interest or developing one de novo.

2. A protocol for RNA in situ hybridization can be obtained at: http://www.molbio.wisc.edu/carroll/methods/abdomen_insitu.pdf.
3. A detailed protocol for carrying out protein immunohistochemistry on the epidermis of *Drosophila* pupae can be obtained at: http://www.ibdml.univ-mrs.fr/equipes/BP_NG/Methods-files/pupal_epidermis.pdf.
4. Gene expression comparisons between strains or species must be performed during the developmental time when a candidate gene is expressed and in age-matched individuals. Evolutionary modifications in the timing of gene expression (heterochrony) may underlie the phenotype, and traditionally, these types of changes are relatively difficult to pinpoint. In general, a suitable time point to compare gene expression can be determined by assessing gene expression over a broad range of times during development. Even so, a drastic change in expression over a short timeframe may be missed, and could yet be the cause of the change. It is important to note that because of the perdurability of protein compared to mRNA, antibody stains and reporter constructs may prove easier for detecting expression differences irrespective of the subtleties of developmental time.
5. Expression of the bacterial enzyme β-galactosidase can be observed by exposing a transgenic organism or tissue to the colorless substrate X-gal, which is converted to a colored precipitate that stains the cells at an intensity that is proportional to the amount of LacZ enzyme present. The *EGFP* gene is modified version of the *GFP* gene that was originally isolated from the jellyfish species *Aequorea victoria*. It encodes the EGFP protein whose expression is revealed by its emission of light at a wavelength of 509 nm when excited by light at a wavelength of 488 nm. Variants of the *EGFP* gene have been derived that are optimized to be excited by and emit light of different wavelengths (*EBFP*, *ECFP*, and *EYFP*). Additionally, the reporter gene *DsRed*, discovered in the anthozoan genus

*Discosoma*, is also used, as it encodes a red fluorescent protein, DsRed, which is excited by and emits light at 558 nm and 583 nm, respectively.

6. In reporter assays, the choice of host species for transgenes is an important parameter. In the best case, the CRE can be tested in one (or better yet, both) of the species being compared. However, this is not always convenient, or possible. Many studies utilize the nearest convenient model organism in which to conduct reporter assays. For example, human and bat CREs have been tested in the mouse (15, 46). Various insect CREs have been shown to work in *D. melanogaster*, including beetle (47), honeybee (48), mosquito (49), and sepsid (38) CREs. With increasing evolutionary divergence time between host species and that from which the CRE under investigation is derived, the level of faithful recapitulation tends to decrease. For example, the nematode *C. elegans* generally failed as a host for *D. melanogaster* CREs (50).
7. These transgenes were introduced into *D. melanogaster* by P-element based germ-line transformation. A detailed protocol for *Drosophila* germ-line transformation is available at: http://www.ibdml.univ-mrs.fr/equipes/BP_NG/Methods-files/injection.pdf. This protocol has also been adapted for use with other transposon systems (25, 27, 36).
8. An effective approach to indentify the CRE content for a gene typically begins with a coarse survey of the entire locus by a set of reporter genes, each possessing a relatively large noncoding sequence. The large noncoding sequence size serves two purposes: to minimize the number of transgenic organisms to be developed to screen the entire locus; and to enable the identification of CREs that are more diffuse in composition than those typically published (100–1,000 base pairs is a commonly observed CRE size). It is also advantageous to design contiguous noncoding sequences to overlap by 500–1,000 base pairs. The analysis of partially overlapping noncoding sequences protects your initial screen from the unfortunate event that arbitrarily assigned start and end points for noncoding sequences divides a functional CRE into two nonfunctional pieces. When a CRE activity of interest is identified to be within a noncoding sequence, it is typically worthwhile to perform a second transgenic screen that tests smaller portions of the larger noncoding sequence as a set of overlapping but truncated sequences. This second transgenic screen will refine both the DNA sequence that encodes a particular CRE activity and where the causative CRE changes are likely to occur.
9. A recombination-based method was developed to assess very large regions of genomic DNA for CRE activity in transgenic *Drosophila* (51). This P(acman) method allows the modification

of a bacterial artificial chromosome (BAC) sequence in bacteria to contain a reporter gene. This large fragment of genomic DNA with an incorporated reporter gene can be inserted into the genome of *D. melanogaster* using phiC31-mediated transgenesis. In the manuscript describing this technology a 133-kb sequence was successfully inserted into the genome of *D. melanogaster* (51). This fruit fly technology is comparable to a method routinely used is mouse genetic studies to investigate the regulatory content of a locus (52). Although technically more challenging than working with small transgenes, these methods are suitable when the candidate interval for a *cis*-regulatory mutation remains quite large.

10. In order to control for variation caused by the random insertion of transgenes, studies typically assess numerous independent integrations for each transgene being evaluated, often around 6–10. Even after this substantial amount of work, the conclusions drawn regarding CRE activity is restricted to qualitative differences and not quantitative differences.

11. In *D. melanogaster*, transgenes can be site-specifically integrated by either the use of a Cre recombinase- (53) or phiC31-integrase- (34, 35) derived system. These methods allow the comparisons of transgenes with different or modified CRE sequences when placed in the same genomic environment. This removes the complication of position effects, and allows the identification of qualitative and quantitative differences in gene regulatory activity.

12. A time- and cost-effective way to generate mutant CRE sequences, compared to the more traditional method of site-directed mutagenesis, is to have the sequence synthesized de novo commercially by vendors such as GenScript (http://www.genscript.com/). Additionally, for labs not set up for the production of transgenic animals, the procedure can be outsourced to vendors such as Best Gene (http://www.thebestgene.com/) or Genetic Services (http://www.geneticservices.com/) for fruit flies and genOway (http://www.genoway.com/) for mice.

13. When designing a probe for in situ hybridization or RT-PCR, it is important to carefully choose the portion of the gene to assay. A common practice is to start with a portion of the gene that would be expressed in most or all contexts (i.e., a domain that is common to all of the alternate transcripts). That way, a change in gene expression can be detected regardless of which promoter or splice variant is being used in the tissue being studied. However, as one's confidence in a gene increases, the possibility of splice variants should be considered: are there sequenced cDNAs that show an alternate pattern of splicing? If so, the alternates can be visualized by generating short in situ

hybridization probes that are specific for alternate exons (traditional probes can be as small as ~100 bp). RT-PCR primers that flank alternatively spliced introns (to discern bona fide mRNA signal from genomic contamination) can be strategically designed to monitor which alternate transcripts are being produced in a tissue.

14. In the best-case scenarios, there are no coding sequence differences in the orthologous genes. More likely though, there will exist some sequence differences within the coding sequences, a fraction of which do not alter the amino acid specified, referred to as synonymous changes. Often, such sequence differences are dismissed as neutral mutations that do not explain the evolved phenotype; however, these sequence changes may indeed be causative and should be considered. Changes that substantially alter the encoded protein, such as frameshift or nonsense mutations due to insertion or deletion events, are more decisive indicators that the coding sequence function has changed. Point mutations that result in the specification of a different amino acid, so-called nonsynonymous mutations, are more ambiguous and may or may not contribute to the trait (see Chapter 22).

## Acknowledgments

We are eternally grateful for the mentorship and nurturing research environment provided by Sean B. Carroll. This environment allowed us to delve into the functional basis for gene regulatory evolution that serves as the methodological foundation for this chapter. We thank Héloïse Dufour, Matt Rockman, and Virginie Orgogozo for critical comments on this chapter. Mark Rebeiz is supported by start-up funds from the University of Pittsburgh. Thomas Williams is supported by start-up funding from the Department of Biology at the University of Dayton and the University of Dayton Research Institute (UDRI).

### References

1. Carroll SB, Grenier JK, Weatherbee SD (2001) From DNA to Diversity. Blackwell Science, Malden
2. Carroll SB (2008) Evo-devo and an expanding evolutionary synthesis: a genetic theory of morphological evolution. Cell **134**:25–36
3. Protas ME, Hersey C, Kochanek D et al (2006) Genetic analysis of cavefish reveals molecular convergence in the evolution of albinism. Nat Genet **38**:107–111
4. Colosimo PF, Hosemann KE, Balabhadra S et al (2005) Widespread parallel evolution in sticklebacks by repeated fixation of Ectodysplasin alleles. Science **307**:1928–1933
5. Miller CT, Beleza S, Pollen AA et al (2007) cis-Regulatory changes in Kit ligand expression and parallel evolution of pigmentation in sticklebacks and humans. Cell **131**:1179–1189
6. Shapiro MD, Marks ME, Peichel CL et al (2004) Genetic and developmental basis of

evolutionary pelvic reduction in threespine sticklebacks. Nature **428**:717–723

7. Sucena E, Stern DL (2000) Divergence of larval morphology between *Drosophila sechellia* and its sibling species caused by cis-regulatory evolution of ovo/shaven-baby. Proc Natl Acad Sci USA **97**:4530–4534
8. Wittkopp PJ, Williams BL, Selegue JE et al (2003) *Drosophila* pigmentation evolution: divergent genotypes underlying convergent phenotypes. Proc Natl Acad Sci USA **100**:1808–1813
9. Sucena E, Delon I, Jones I et al (2003) Regulatory evolution of shavenbaby/ovo underlies multiple cases of morphological parallelism. Nature **424**:935–938
10. Marcellini S, Simpson P (2006) Two or four bristles: functional evolution of an enhancer of scute in Drosophilidae. PLoS Biol. doi: 10.1371/journal.pbio.0040386
11. Gompel N, Prud'homme B, Wittkopp PJ et al (2005) Chance caught on the wing: cis-regulatory evolution and the origin of pigment patterns in *Drosophila*. Nature **433**:481–487
12. Cohn MJ, Tickle C (1999) Developmental basis of limblessness and axial patterning in snakes. Nature **399**:474–479
13. Averof M, Patel NH (1997) Crustacean appendage evolution associated with changes in Hox gene expression. Nature **388**:682–686
14. Belting HG, Shashikant CS, Ruddle FH (1998) Modification of expression and cis-regulation of Hoxc8 in the evolution of diverged axial morphology. Proc Natl Acad Sci USA **95**:2355–2360
15. Cretekos CJ, Wang Y, Green ED et al (2008) Regulatory divergence modifies limb length between mammals. Genes Dev **22**:141–151
16. Abiola O, Angel JM, Avner P et al (2003) The nature and identification of quantitative trait loci: a community's view. Nat Rev Genet **4**:911–916
17. Linnen CR, Kingsley EP, Jensen JD et al (2009) On the origin and spread of an adaptive allele in deer mice. Science **325**:1095–1098
18. Martin JF, Bradley A, Olson EN (1995) The paired-like homeo box gene MHox is required for early events of skeletogenesis in multiple lineages. Genes Dev **9**:1237–1249
19. Carroll SB (2005) Evolution at two levels: on genes and form. PLoS Biol. doi:10.1371/journal.pbio.0030245
20. Baker BS, Burtis K, Goralski T et al (1989) Molecular genetic aspects of sex determination in *Drosophila melanogaster*. Genome **31**: 638–645
21. Reinhart BJ, Slack FJ, Basson M et al (2000) The 21-nucleotide let-7 RNA regulates developmental timing in *Caenorhabditis elegans*. Nature **403**:901–906
22. Vella MC, Choi EY, Lin SY et al (2004) The *C. elegans* microRNA let-7 binds to imperfect let-7 complementary sites from the lin-41 3′UTR. Genes Dev **18**:132–137
23. Marin VA, Evans TC (2003) Translational repression of a *C. elegans* Notch mRNA by the STAR/KH domain protein GLD-1. Development **130**:2623–2632
24. Pare A, Lemons D, Kosman D et al (2009) Visualization of Individual Scr mRNAs during *Drosophila* Embryogenesis Yields Evidence for Transcriptional Bursting. Curr Biol **19**: 2037–2042
25. Rebeiz M, Pool JE, Kassner VA et al (2009) Stepwise modification of a modular enhancer underlies adaptation in a *Drosophila* population. Science **326**:1663–1667
26. Pool JE, Aquadro CF (2007) The genetic basis of adaptive pigmentation variation in *Drosophila melanogaster*. Mol Ecol **16**:2844–2851
27. Williams TM, Selegue JE, Werner T et al (2008) The regulation and evolution of a genetic switch controlling sexually dimorphic traits in *Drosophila*. Cell **134**:610–623
28. Chan YF, Marks ME, Jones FC et al (2010) Adaptive Evolution of Pelvic Reduction in Sticklebacks by Recurrent Deletion of a Pitx1 Enhancer. Science **327**:302–305
29. Wittkopp PJ, Haerum BK, Clark AG (2004) Evolutionary changes in cis and trans gene regulation. Nature **430**:85–88
30. Lettice LA, Heaney SJ, Purdie LA et al (2003) A long-range Shh enhancer regulates expression in the developing limb and fin and is associated with preaxial polydactyly. Hum Mol Genet **12**:1725–1735
31. Wang X, Chamberlin HM (2002) Multiple regulatory changes contribute to the evolution of the Caenorhabditis lin-48 ovo gene. Genes Dev **16**:2345–2349
32. Jeong S, Rokas A, Carroll SB (2006) Regulation of body pigmentation by the Abdominal-B Hox protein and its gain and loss in *Drosophila* evolution. Cell **125**:1387–1399
33. Prud'homme B, Gompel N, Rokas A et al (2006) Repeated morphological evolution through cis-regulatory changes in a pleiotropic gene. Nature **440**:1050–1053
34. Bischof J, Maeda RK, Hediger M et al (2007) An optimized transgenesis system for *Drosophila* using germ-line-specific phiC31 integrases. Proc Natl Acad Sci USA **104**:3312–3317

35. Groth AC, Fish M, Nusse R et al (2004) Construction of transgenic *Drosophila* by using the site-specific integrase from phage phiC31. Genetics **166**:1775–1782
36. Shirangi TR, Dufour HD, Williams TM et al (2009) Rapid evolution of sex pheromone-producing enzyme expression in *Drosophila*. PLoS Biol. doi:10.1371/journal.pbio.1000168
37. Ludwig MZ, Bergman C, Patel NH et al (2000) Evidence for stabilizing selection in a eukaryotic enhancer element. Nature **403**:564–567
38. Hare EE, Peterson BK, Iyer VN et al (2008) Sepsid even-skipped enhancers are functionally conserved in *Drosophila* despite lack of sequence conservation. PLoS Genet. doi:10.1371/journal.pgen.1000106
39. McGregor AP, Orgogozo V, Delon I et al (2007) Morphological evolution through multiple cis-regulatory mutations at a single gene. Nature **448**:587–590
40. Tomoyasu Y, Wheeler SR, Denell RE et al (2005) Ultrabithorax is required for membranous wing identity in the beetle *Tribolium castaneum*. Nature **433**:643–647
41. Tomoyasu Y, Arakane Y, Kramer KJ et al (2009) Repeated Co-options of Exoskeleton Formation during Wing-to-Elytron Evolution in Beetles. Curr Biol **19**:2057–2065
42. Moczek AP, Rose DJ (2009) Differential recruitment of limb patterning genes during development and diversification of beetle horns. Proc Natl Acad Sci USA **106**:8992–8997
43. Horn C, Wimmer EA (2000) A versatile vector set for animal transgenesis. Dev Genes Evol **210**:630–637
44. Wray GA (2007) The evolutionary significance of cis-regulatory mutations. Nat Rev Genet **8**:206–216
45. Stern DL, Orgogozo V (2008) The loci of evolution: how predictable is genetic evolution?. Evolution **62**:2155–2177
46. Prabhakar S, Visel A, Akiyama JA et al (2008) Human-specific gain of function in a developmental enhancer. Science **321**:1346–1350
47. Cande J, Goltsev Y, Levine MS et al (2009) Conservation of enhancer location in divergent insects. Proc Natl Acad Sci USA **106**: 14414–14419
48. Zinzen RP, Cande J, Ronshaugen M et al (2006) Evolution of the ventral midline in insect embryos. Dev Cell **11**:895–902
49. Erives A, Levine M (2004) Coordinate enhancers share common organizational features in the *Drosophila* genome. Proc Natl Acad Sci USA **101**:3851–3856
50. Ruvinsky I, Ruvkun G (2003) Functional tests of enhancer conservation between distantly related species. Development **130**: 5133–5142
51. Venken K J, He Y, Hoskins RA et al (2006) a BAC transgenic platform for targeted insertion of large DNA fragments in *D. melanogaster*. Science **314**:1747–1751
52. Lehoczky JA, Innis JW (2008) BAC transgenic analysis reveals enhancers sufficient for Hoxa13 and neighborhood gene expression in mouse embryonic distal limbs and genital bud. Evol Dev **10**:421–432
53. Oberstein A, Pare A, Kaplan L et al (2005) Site-specific transgenesis by Cre-mediated recombination in *Drosophila*. Nat Methods **2**: 583–585
54. Sagai T, Amano T, Tamura M et al (2009) A cluster of three long-range enhancers directs regional Shh expression in the epithelial linings. Development **136**:1665–16674

# Chapter 22

# Experimental Approaches to Evaluate the Contributions of Candidate Protein-Coding Mutations to Phenotypic Evolution

Jay F. Storz and Anthony J. Zera

## Abstract

Identifying mechanisms of molecular adaptation can provide important insights into the process of phenotypic evolution, but it can be exceedingly difficult to quantify the phenotypic effects of specific mutational changes. To verify the adaptive significance of genetically based changes in protein function, it is necessary to document functional differences between the products of derived and wild-type alleles and to demonstrate that such differences impinge on higher-level physiological processes (and ultimately, fitness). In the case of metabolic enzymes, this requires documenting in vivo differences in reaction rate that give rise to differences in flux through the pathway in which the enzymes function. These measured differences in pathway flux should then give rise to differences in cellular or systemic physiology that affect fitness-related variation in whole-organism performance. Efforts to establish these causal connections between genotype, phenotype, and fitness require experiments that carefully control for environmental variation and background genetic variation. Here, we discuss experimental approaches to evaluate the contributions of amino-acid mutations to adaptive phenotypic change. We discuss conceptual and methodological issues associated with in vitro and in vivo studies of protein function, and the evolutionary insights that can be gleaned from such studies. We also discuss the importance of isolating the effects of individual mutations to distinguish between positively selected substitutions that directly contribute to improvements in protein function versus positively selected, compensatory substitutions that mitigate negative pleiotropic effects of antecedent changes.

**Key words:** Adaptation, Biochemical adaptation, Compensatory evolution, Enzyme kinetics, Enzyme polymorphism, Metabolic adaptation, Molecular adaptation

## 1. Introduction

To assess whether a given protein-coding mutation has contributed to adaptive phenotypic change, it is ultimately necessary to document and explain the mechanistic basis of fitness variation among

Virginie Orgogozo and Matthew V. Rockman (eds.), *Molecular Methods for Evolutionary Genetics*, Methods in Molecular Biology, vol. 772, DOI 10.1007/978-1-61779-228-1_22, © Springer Science+Business Media, LLC 2011

alternative single-locus genotypes. This is a tall order because adaptive changes in many phenotypic traits may be attributable to fitness differentials that fall well below the resolving power of "real-time" observational studies. As stated by Gillespie (1), "Selection coefficients for single amino acid substitutions as small as $10^{-4}$ to $10^{-3}$ are large enough to dominate genetic drift, yet are refractory to direct experimental investigations. In other words, most of protein evolution could be due to strong natural selection, yet we have no experimental protocol capable of measuring the selective differences." However, fitness differences among alternative genotypes ultimately stem from allelic differences in the concentration and/or biochemical properties of the encoded protein. It will often be possible to measure these allelic differences in protein concentration or protein function even in cases where the net effects on fitness lie below the threshold of experimental detection (2). At the most proximal level of trait variation, in vitro tests of protein function can provide mechanistic insights into the causal link between genotype and biochemical phenotype. After establishing this link – and after confirming that experimental results obtained in vitro are also manifest in vivo – the next challenge is to assess whether the observed change in biochemical phenotype impinges on whole-organism performance in a way that affects fitness.

Identifying the mechanisms by which allelic protein variants contribute to adaptation is a difficult task that requires multiple types of information, at multiple levels of biological organization. For example, adaptive changes in enzyme function can involve modifications of any one of several enzymatic properties such as catalytic efficiency, concentration, stability, and sensitivity to metabolic regulators, and each aspect can be altered in a number of different ways (Fig. 1). Moreover, changes in enzyme function do not necessarily affect higher-level physiological phenotypes (e.g., pathway flux).

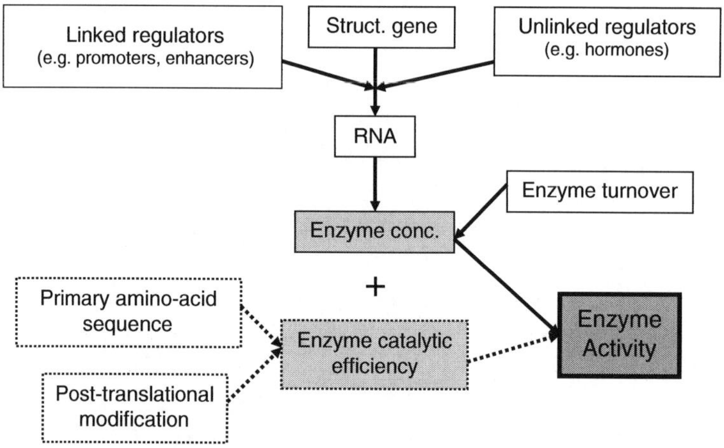


Fig. 1. Various factors affecting enzyme activity via influence on enzyme concentration or catalytic efficiency. Modified from ref. 45.

Population-genetic studies of protein polymorphism have traditionally focused on kinetic and thermodynamic properties of metabolic enzymes – parameters that had been identified as key aspects of enzyme adaptation by comparative biochemists (3) and enzymologists (4, 5). This field of study eventually expanded to include investigations into regulatory changes in enzyme concentration as well as enzyme function (6, 7). The importance of experimentally confirming the physiological consequences of protein polymorphism (8–13) came into especially sharp focus with the development of Metabolic Control Analysis, which predicts that change in the catalytic activity of an individual enzyme can often have negligible effects on steady-state pathway flux (14, 15). More recently, advances in molecular biology have permitted more detailed investigations into the regulation of protein-coding genes (e.g., measurement of transcript abundance) and the relationship between protein structure and function.

### 1.1. The Importance of Elucidating Mechanism in Studies of Adaptation

Once a given protein-coding gene has been implicated in adaptive phenotypic change, why is it important to identify the biochemical/physiological mechanisms by which the encoded protein exerts its effects on organismal performance? Beyond the obvious point that such information enriches our basic understanding of the biology of adaptation, insights into the mechanistic basis of genetic adaptation can also shed light on why particular genes or particular types of mutations make disproportionate contributions to phenotypic evolution. For example, an understanding of how variation in enzyme activity maps onto fitness can potentially explain why regulatory and structural mutations differ in their relative contributions to adaptive change in flux-based phenotypes, and may also explain why the two classes of mutation have different fixation probabilities at different time points in multistep evolutionary pathways. The stepwise acquisition of cefotaxime resistance in *Escherichia coli* involves a combination of coding and noncoding substitutions in the β-lactamase gene, and the initial steps are consistently attributable to amino-acid substitutions that enhance the catalytic efficiency of the enzyme (16, 17). Regulatory mutants are typically incorporated later in the evolutionary pathway because an increased expression of the enzyme only becomes advantageous once its catalytic efficiency has been optimized by the antecedent structural changes (17). In contrast to the evolution of antibiotic resistance, in the evolution of flux-limited metabolic pathways, mutations that increase gene expression may often be fixed early because an increased enzyme concentration can have a large effect on fitness (18).

Mechanistic studies of genetic adaptation can also provide insights into features of adaptive mutations – such as dominance, epistatic interactions, and pleiotropic effects – that exert a strong influence on trajectories of evolutionary change. A good example is provided by recent studies on the mechanistic basis of adaptive crypsis in lizards from the Chihuahuan desert (19). In several codistributed species of lizards that inhabit the white gypsum dunes of White Sands, New Mexico, the convergent evolution of blanched, substrate-matching coloration has involved different loss-of-function mutations in the melanocortin-1 receptor gene (*Mc1r*). In the little striped whiptail lizard, *Aspidoscelis inornata*, the blanched phenotype is associated with an amino-acid mutation in *Mc1r* that impairs receptor signaling, and in the eastern fence lizard, *Sceloporus undulatus*, the same phenotype is associated with a different amino-acid mutation in *Mc1r* that prevents the receptor from integrating into the melanocyte membrane. Both loss-of-function mutations produce the same blanched phenotype, but the mutation in *A. inornata* is recessive (because the disruption in receptor signaling is compensated by the wild-type allele), whereas the mutation in *S. undulatus* is dominant (because in heterozygotes, cell-surface expression of the wild-type receptor is suppressed as a result of dimerization with the mutant copy). Although both lizard species are presumably subject to similar selection regimes (mediated by visually oriented predators), the differences in dominance of the adaptive mutations are reflected by different spatial patterns of allele frequency variation across ecotonal transitions in substrate color. In these two lizard species, observed differences in the geographic patterning of *Mc1r* allele frequency variation only make sense in light of experimental findings that revealed differences in the penetrance of independently derived, loss-of-function mutations that impair different aspects of receptor function.

As the above examples illustrate, identifying mechanisms of molecular adaptation can provide key insights into the process of phenotypic evolution. Here, we discuss experimental approaches to evaluate the contributions of protein-coding mutations to adaptive phenotypic change. We discuss conceptual and methodological issues associated with in vitro and in vivo studies of protein function, and the evolutionary insights that can be gleaned from such studies. We focus largely on enzymes of intermediary metabolism, as this class of proteins has figured prominently in research efforts to establish causal connections between genotype, phenotype, and fitness in ecologically relevant contexts (9–12, 20). Although we focus primarily on the contributions of amino-acid mutations to adaptive phenotypic evolution, the issues and experimental approaches that we discuss are also applicable to assessments of nonadaptive or maladaptive change.

## 2. In Vitro Studies of Protein Function: Linking Genotype to Biochemical Phenotype

The main function of an enzyme is to catalyze (increase) the rate of a chemical reaction. Thus, the biochemical phenotypes of interest in evolutionary studies of enzyme polymorphism include catalytic efficiency and enzyme concentration, the two most important factors that influence the rate of an enzyme-catalyzed reaction. Catalytic efficiency, which is an intrinsic kinetic property of an enzyme, can be broadly defined as the rate at which substrate is converted into product per active site of an enzyme molecule under a specified set of conditions. It is important to keep in mind that noncatalytic aspects of enzyme function, such as inhibition or activation by various metabolic regulators, may also contribute to enzymatic adaptation independent of catalytic efficiency (e.g., (21)).

### *2.1. Enzyme Kinetics*

The proper interpretation and measurement of kinetic parameters are best considered in the context of the Michaelis–Menten equation, the basic equation of enzyme kinetics (5, 22, 23). In its simplest form, this equation describes the velocity of an enzyme-catalyzed reaction involving a single substrate that is irreversibly converted into product as a function of two experimentally measurable enzymatic parameters, $V_{max}$ and $K_M$:

$$v = \frac{V_{max}[S]}{K_M + [S]} \tag{1}$$

where $V_{max}$ = maximal velocity, [S] = substrate concentration, $K_M$ = the Michaelis constant, defined as the substrate concentration that results in half-maximal velocity, and $v$ = reaction rate. In addition, $V_{max} = [E] \times k_{cat}$; that is, maximal velocity consists of two components: enzyme concentration ([E]), and the kinetic constant, $k_{cat}$, or turnover number (i.e., the maximum number of substrate molecules converted to product per active site of an enzyme per unit time). The right-hand side of the above equation can be decomposed into separate components that reflect (a) enzyme concentration [E] and (b) intrinsic kinetic properties of the enzyme (terms on the right-hand side of the equation below):

$$v = [E] \times \frac{k_{cat} \times [S]}{K_M + [S]} \tag{2}$$

The most thorough in vitro kinetic comparisons of allelic enzyme variants (allozymes) have measured and standardized [E]. By controlling for variation in [E], it is then possible to quantify kinetic differences between alternative allozymes. What are the functional meanings of the kinetic parameters in Eq. 2? The answer is a bit complex for $K_M$, which has often been incorrectly interpreted as a measure of an enzyme's affinity for its substrate. This may or may not be the case depending upon the specific enzyme and substrate under consideration (5, 22–24). In the absence of direct data on substrate binding, $K_M$ is best considered a kinetic component of catalytic efficiency, the other kinetic component being $k_{cat}$. The relative contribution of $k_{cat}$ and $K_M$ to the catalytic rate is determined by the substrate concentration [S]. When [S] is very low ($<0.1\,K_M$), then [S] in the denominator of Eq. 2 can be ignored, and the kinetic part of the equation reduces to $v=(k_{cat}/K_M)\times[S]$. As [S] increases to intermediate levels (i.e., $[S]=K_M$), both $k_{cat}/K_M$ and $k_{cat}$ contribute to the rate of catalysis. Because [S] is thought to range from 1.0 to 0.1 $K_M$ in vivo for most enzymes of intermediary metabolism (5), the main kinetic contributor to catalytic efficiency is $k_{cat}/K_M$ alone or some combination of $k_{cat}/K_M$ and $k_{cat}$. The most thorough kinetic analyses of allozymes have focused on these kinetic constants (25–28).

Many enzymes catalyze complex reactions that cannot be adequately described by Eq. 1. For example, dehydrogenase enzymes bind more than one substrate (e.g., a cofactor such as $NAD^+$ or $NADP^+$, as well as a substrate specific for the particular enzyme). Although the rate equations for such enzymes contain additional terms, simplifying assumptions often have been used to reduce these more complex equations to the form of Eq. 1 (e.g., (25)). Many enzymes also catalyze reversible reactions, but again, the analyses have often been simplified by considering the reaction in only one direction.

A more comprehensive and realistic analysis of enzyme catalytic efficiency has been formulated by Albery and Knowles (4), which does not require any simplifying assumptions regarding the relative magnitude of $K_M$ and [S]. Rather than focusing on $k_{cat}/K_M$ alone, estimated values for $k_{cat}$ and $K_M$ are used in the full Michaelis–Mention equation to compare reaction velocities of enzymes across a range of substrate concentrations that occur in vivo. In addition, the approach of Albery and Knowles (4) considers the reaction velocity in both directions, and the primary focus is the net conversion of substrate to product in one direction. This more comprehensive type of analysis was used in a pioneering study of the PGI (phosphoglucose isomerase) polymorphism in *Mytilus edulis* (26, 29).

Finally, it is important to understand the limitations associated with measures of $V_{max}/K_M$. Standard steady-state kinetic analysis provides estimates of $K_M$ and $V_{max}$, from which $k_{cat}$ is estimated using the relationship: $k_{cat}=V_{max}/[E]$ (see above). However, estimation of $k_{cat}$ requires knowledge of enzyme concentration [E], which in turn requires completely purified enzyme. Since the purification of enzymes to homogeneity is often nontrivial, some studies have focused on allelic differences in $V_{max}/K_M$ in the absence of information on $k_{cat}/K_M$ (30, 31). The problem with this approach is that allelic differences in $V_{max}/K_M$ do not necessarily reflect intrinsic functional differences between the alternative allozymes. As discussed above, $V_{max}$ is a composite parameter that reflects kinetic properties of the enzyme ($k_{cat}$) as well as enzyme concentration [E]. Furthermore, genetic variation in [E] can be caused by background genetic variation independent of the structural locus that encodes the allozyme (e.g., *cis-* or *trans*-acting regulatory factors; (32)). Thus, while allelic differences in $k_{cat}/K_M$ are due to intrinsic kinetic differences between the allozymes, the same is not necessarily true for measured differences in $V_{max}/K_M$. Although measures of $V_{max}/K_M$ are important for understanding the relative catalytic power of allozymes in vivo due to the combined effects of enzyme kinetics and enzyme concentration, it is important to quantify the relative contributions of [E] and $k_{cat}/K_M$ to variation in $V_{max}/K_M$.

A discussion of experimental methods for estimating enzymatic parameters is beyond the scope of this article (for more detailed treatments, see refs. 22 and 29). A key aspect of in vitro kinetic measurements is that assay conditions should mimic in vivo conditions as much as possible with respect to pH, temperature-pH relations, ionic strength, the presence of various osmolytes, etc. (3, 23, 29). In addition to catalytic aspects of enzyme function, regulatory properties (e.g., inhibition by various metabolites) may often represent key factors in enzyme adaptation. For example, PGI allozymes of the sea anemone *Metridium senile* are differentially inhibited by the pentose-shunt metabolite 6-phosphogluconate (21). This allozyme-dependent inhibition results in differential diversion of carbon through the pentose shunt versus glycolysis, possibly playing a role in allozyme-dependent lipid biosynthesis. Finally, it is important to make biochemical comparisons between enzyme variants of known amino-acid sequence. Allozymes were originally characterized by their electrophoretic mobility, and it is now widely appreciated that electromorphs often contain a substantial amount of amino-acid sequence heterogeneity that could have functional consequences (20, 33). Failure to adequately deal with "cryptic variation" can result in erroneous conclusions regarding adaptive biochemical differences between allozymes and the geographic patterning of allele frequency variation (34, 35). Many classic studies of allozyme polymorphism have involved kinetic characterizations of PGI electromorphs of unknown amino-acid sequence (21, 26, 30, 31), and subsequent DNA-based studies of PGI polymorphism in a number of different animal taxa have revealed substantial levels of cryptic amino-acid variation within the previously characterized electromorphs (20, 33).

A number of studies of enzyme kinetics have been motivated by the results of electrophoretic surveys that revealed striking, locus-specific patterns of clinal variation or correlations with particular environmental variables (9, 20, 36, 37). In particular, latitudinal clines in allele frequency suggest the hypothesis that adaptive modifications of enzyme function are mediated by factors that are directly or indirectly related to temperature. Of these studies, the best examples involve kinetic analyses in which the products of alternative alleles were purified to homogeneity: ADH and G6PD in *Drosophila melanogaster*, LDH-B in *Fundulus heteroclitus*, and PGI in the blue mussel, *M. edulis* (25–27, 38). In each of these polymorphisms, significant allelic differences in $k_{cat}/K_M$ and its components were identified. These kinetic data provided the motivation for tests of specific physiological hypotheses regarding allozyme-dependent in vivo function (see below). In the case of the ADH and G6PD polymorphisms, functional characterizations were performed on allozymes that were known to differ by a single amino acid. The ADH-F allozyme exhibited a higher $k_{cat}$ for ethanol than the ADH-S allozyme (38), implicating an enhanced ability of the ADH-F allozyme to metabolize alcohol. Relative to G6PD-A, the G6PD-B allozyme exhibited a reduced $K_M$ for glucose-6-phosphate, which is expected to result in a 40% higher $k_{cat}/K_M$ in vivo, and greater flux through the pentose shunt, the pathway in which this enzyme functions. For the *Mytilus* PGI and *Fundulus* LDH polymorphisms, significant temperature-dependent differences in $k_{cat}/K_M$ or overall catalytic efficiency could be interpreted in light of the observed latitudinal clines in allele frequency.

### 2.2. Enzyme Concentration

As discussed previously, in vivo measures of enzyme activity (e.g., $V_{max}/K_M$) may reflect differences in enzyme kinetics ($k_{cat}/K_M$), differences in enzyme concentration ([E]), or both. In addition, regulatory variation in enzyme concentration can result from *cis*- and/or *trans*-acting factors, which also need to be distinguished (see Chapter 18). Studies of the ADH and G6PD polymorphisms in *D. melanogaster* and the LDH polymorphism in *F. heteroclitus* involved especially thorough examinations of variation in [E] and its underlying causes.

In the case of the G6PD polymorphism in *D. melanogaster*, activity differences between the two main allozymes were not attributable to differences in [E] or $k_{cat}$ (27, 39). In the case of the ADH polymorphism in *D. melanogaster*, the consensus of many studies is that a significantly higher concentration of ADH protein occurs in *Adh*$^{FF}$ compared with *Adh*$^{SS}$ genotypes, and this difference accounts for most of the difference in allozyme-specific activity (6). Site-directed mutagenesis studies indicated that the fast/slow amino-acid change responsible for the difference in $k_{cat}$ between the ADH-F and ADH-S allozymes does not affect enzyme concentration (32, 40). Instead, allelic differences in enzyme concentration appear to be largely attributable to a small insertion–deletion polymorphism in the first intron that is in strong linkage disequilibrium with the fast/slow amino-acid polymorphism (41).

Thus, variation in ADH activity among genotypes appears to be attributable to epistatic interaction between a single amino-acid polymorphism and one or more closely linked noncoding polymorphisms. Stam and Laurie (42) suggested that multiple polymorphic sites within the *Adh* gene may be targets of selection. Interestingly, no differences in mRNA transcript abundance or in vivo rates of enzyme degradation were observed between the $Adh^{FF}$ and $Adh^{SS}$ genotypes (6, 43), so the mechanistic basis of the observed variation in ADH enzyme concentration remains unknown.

In the case of the LDH polymorphism in *Fundulus*, allozyme-associated differences in transcript abundance and enzyme concentration stem from allelic differences at one or more closely linked *cis*-regulatory elements (7, 44). The difference in LDH enzyme concentration makes a much greater contribution to the in vivo rate of catalysis than does the difference in $k_{cat}/K_M$. Finally, in an analogous study involving crickets (*Gryllus firmus*), the activity of the lipogenic enzyme $NADP^+$-isocitrate dehydrogenase differs dramatically between alternative genotypes that differ in life history and lipid biosynthesis. In this case, in vivo differences in enzyme activity appear to be produced solely by genetic differences in transcript abundance and [E], but not $k_{cat}/K_M$ (45, 46).

## 3. In Vivo Studies of Protein Function: Linking Genotype to Whole-Organism Physiological Performance

To verify the adaptive significance of an enzyme polymorphism, it is necessary to demonstrate that biochemical differences between the products of alternative alleles give rise to differences in higher-level physiological processes (and ultimately, fitness) (2, 8, 9, 11). It is important that these studies be conducted in vivo under ecologically relevant conditions. There are two reasons why such investigations are especially important. First, the seminal studies of Kacser and Burns (14, 15) and subsequent studies (reviewed in refs. 10, 13, 47, 48) have demonstrated that enzyme activity often exhibits a highly nonlinear (hyperbolic) relationship to pathway flux (Fig. 2). Thus, even large changes in enzyme activity often result in only minimal changes in flux. For this reason, the effect of allozyme variation on pathway flux needs to be demonstrated experimentally.

Another reason to carefully consider the physiological context of gene function relates to recent discoveries that enzymes and other types of proteins, such as receptors and transmembrane channels, often have unexpected functions that are distinct from their "traditional" roles, a phenomenon termed "moonlighting" (49, 50). For example, several enzymes involved in intermediary metabolism

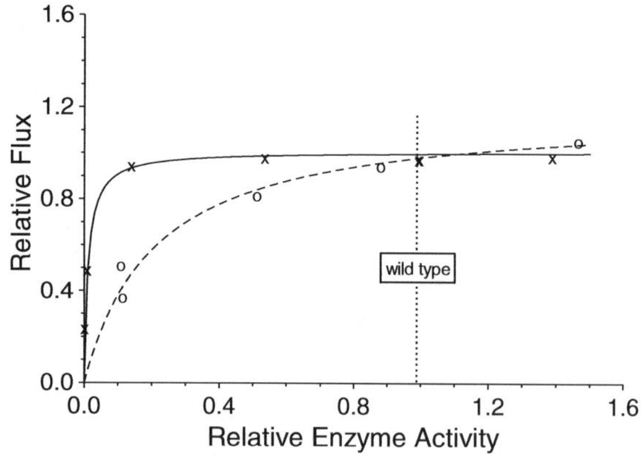


Fig. 2. Relationships between activity and pathway flux for components of lactose catabolism in *E. coli*. *Solid line*=β-galactosidase, *dashed line*=permease. In the case of β-galactosidase, a 50% decrease in activity results in a negligible (0.5%) decrease in pathway flux. In the case of permease, by contrast, the same decrement in enzyme activity results in a 13% decrease in pathway flux. Modified from ref. 10.

also function as secreted regulators of various processes such as growth or differentiation (e.g., PGI, cytochrome C). This phenomenon underscores the importance of examining the physiological consequences of protein variation and keeping an open mind with respect to the specific aspects of physiology that are chosen for investigation. For example, consider a polymorphic enzyme that is known to function in a particular metabolic pathway. If allelic variation in enzyme function is associated with some fitness-related measure of organismal performance in the absence of any detectable effects on pathway flux, then it is probably worth investigating whether the fitness effects stem from some unanticipated structural or functional role of the enzyme that is independent of the enzyme's known role in metabolism. These considerations are also relevant to cases where indirect evidence for the locus-specific effects of positive selection (based on comparisons of polymorphism and/or divergence at synonymous and nonsynonymous nucleotide positions) is not associated with detectable differences in protein function (e.g., (51)). Such cases suggest the possibility that the apparent effects on fitness stem from unexamined protein functions that are only tangentially related to the experimentally assayed properties.

### 3.1. Effects of Allelic Enzyme Variants on Pathway Flux and Higher Level Physiological Processes

What higher-level physiological effects do we need to document to draw firm conclusions about the adaptive significance of a given enzyme polymorphism? Ideally, we would like to verify that the products of alternative alleles exhibit in vivo differences in reaction rate and that this difference, in turn, results in a physiologically significant difference in flux through the pathway in which the enzyme functions. Moreover, measured differences in pathway flux should be consistent with the allelic differences in enzyme kinetics that are measured in vitro (9–11). Differences in pathway function should then give rise to differences in cellular or systemic physiology that can ultimately be traced to some fitness-related measure of whole-organism performance.

In an experimental study of the G6PD polymorphism in *D. melanogaster*, Eanes (52) used an ingenious genetic manipulation to unveil allelic differences in enzyme activity between lines that were coisogenic for 98% of the genome. A number of radioisotopic studies have demonstrated flux differences through various pathways in metabolism caused by allelic variation in the G6PD and ADH enzymes of *D. melanogaster*. For example, the higher activity of the G6PD-B allozyme is associated with greater pentose shunt flux relative to the lower activity G6PD-A allozyme (39, 53). For ADH in *D. melanogaster*, no flux differences were observed between ADH-F and ADH-S allozymes in the overall conversion of ethanol to triglyceride (energy storage) or $CO_2$ (energy utilization) in adults (54). However, significant differences were observed in the conversion of ethanol to triglyceride and a variety of other metabolites in juveniles (55, 56). These results suggest that the main fitness effects of the ADH polymorphism are manifest in the juvenile life stage and may result from the enhanced ability of the $Adh^{FF}$ genoptype to convert alcohol to triglyceride.

The relationship between enzyme activity and pathway flux has been most thoroughly studied by Dykhuizen, Dean, and colleagues in *E. coli*, focusing on polymorphic genes of lactose metabolism in chemostats (10, 13). In this single-celled organism, flux through the metabolically simple (3 enzymes/proteins) lactose catabolic pathway is proportional to growth (cell division) and fitness under lactose-limiting conditions. Thus, these studies simultaneously characterize the effect of allozyme variation on pathway flux and fitness, using lines that controlled for genetic background. In their landmark studies, Dykhuizen and Dean (10, 13) found that naturally occurring allozymes of β-galactosidase exhibit almost no effect on pathway flux (Fig. 2), thus indicating that these allozymes are selectively neutral.

## 4. The Chain of Causation Linking Genotype, Phenotype, and Fitness

To isolate the phenotypic effects of a specific gene, it is necessary to control for environmental variation as well as background genetic variation. Even at the most proximal level of phenotypic variation, the functional effects of specific proteins can be modulated by changes in the intracellular environment (e.g., temperature, pH, and the presence of cofactor molecules).

In vertebrates, fine-tuned adjustments in blood–oxygen affinity can play a key role in matching cellular oxygen supply and demand. These adjustments may be mediated by changes in the intrinsic oxygen affinity of hemoglobin, changes in the responsiveness of hemoglobin to allosteric cofactors that modulate oxygen affinity (organic phosphates, $H^+$ and $Cl^-$ ions), and/or changes in the concentrations of these various cofactors within the erythrocyte (57). Allosteric ligands preferentially bind and stabilize the deoxy conformation of the hemoglobin tetramer, thereby decreasing blood–oxygen affinity by shifting the allosteric equilibrium in favor of the low-affinity, deoxy quaternary structure. In hypoxia-tolerant animals that have evolved elevated blood–oxygen affinities, a common mechanism of hemoglobin adaptation involves structural changes that suppress sensitivity to the inhibitory effects of allosteric cofactors (58–60). For example, deer mice (*Peromyscus maniculatus*) that are native to high altitude are characterized by an elevated blood–oxygen affinity that helps safeguard arterial oxygen saturation under hypoxia. Experimental studies of purified hemoglobin revealed that the elevated blood–oxygen affinity of high-altitude mice is largely attributable to structural modifications of hemoglobin that suppress sensitivity to 2,3-diphosphoglycerate (a metabolite of glycolysis) and $Cl^-$ ions (61, 62). The important point is that insights into the mechanistic basis of the adaptive blood phenotype required oxygen-binding experiments on purified hemoglobin. Measuring the oxygen affinity of whole blood can yield physiologically relevant information, but such measures by themselves cannot be related to changes in hemoglobin structure because they are confounded by environmental effects as well as possible genotype–environment interaction effects (Fig. 3). This echoes the point made earlier about the importance of disentangling genetic and environmental components of variance when comparing in vivo measures of $V_{max}/K_M$ among enzyme variants.

It becomes especially challenging to control for environmental variation and background genetic variation when investigating the effects of specific genes on higher-level physiological processes (as discussed above for studies of pathway flux). In practice, the functional effects of protein-coding genes can be isolated by means of forward genetics (i.e., controlled crosses, including the construction of recombinant inbred lines [RILs] or nearly isogenic lines [NILs]) or reverse genetics (the direct manipulation of gene sequence [e.g., targeted gene replacement] or manipulation of gene expression [e.g., RNAi and gene insertion]). In many cases, isolating the effects of individual genes is not sufficient to identify the specific mechanism of molecular adaptation. As discussed below, it is often necessary to isolate the effects of individual mutations. It is also necessary to measure the functional effects of individual mutations – singly and in different multisite combinations – to address questions about the dynamics of adaptive walks (e.g., What

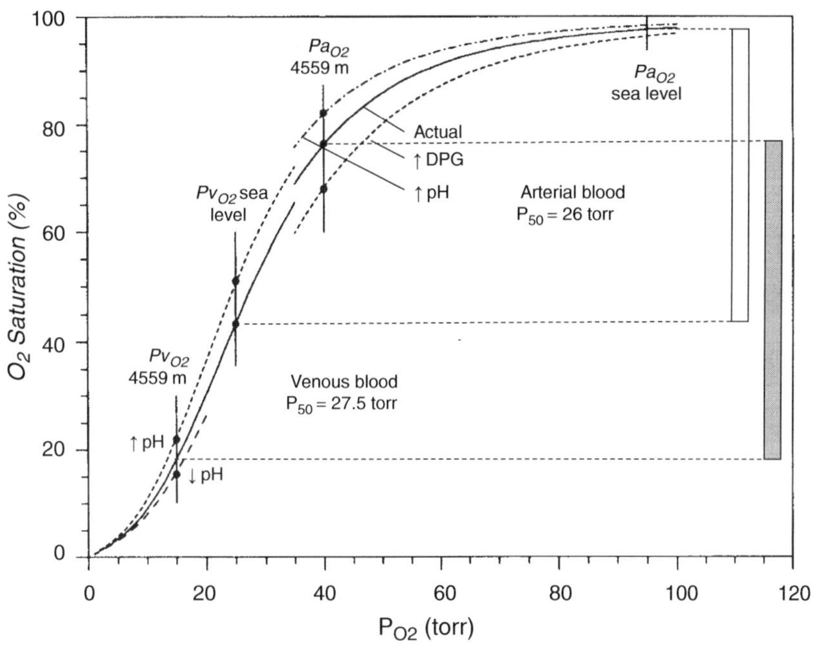


Fig. 3. Oxygen-equilibrium curves of human blood and environmentally induced changes in blood–oxygen affinity under hypoxic conditions at high altitude (4,559 m). *Solid curves* represent measured values for arterial blood ($P_{50}$ (the partial pressure of oxygen [$PO_2$] at which hemoglobin is 50% saturated) = 26 torr, upper section) and venous blood ($P_{50}$ = 27.5 torr). The *broken curves* depict the effects of increased DPG concentration (↑DPG) at unchanged pH, increased pH (↑pH) at unchanged DPG, and the decreased tissue pH (↓pH) that results from metabolic acidosis in the tissues. *Open and shaded vertical columns* denote the oxygen unloaded at sea level (venous $PO_2$ = 25 torr) and at high altitude (4,559 m; venous $PO_2$ = 15 torr), respectively. Displacements of the oxygen-equilibrium curve are attributable to environmentally induced changes in DPG and pH in red blood cells. For example, at high altitude, the increased red cell concentration of DPG produces a rightward shift of the curve (i.e., reduced oxygen affinity), and this may be partly counteracted by the effects of respiratory alkalosis (↑pH). Modified from ref. 58.

is the distribution of phenotypic effect sizes among adaptive substitutions? What is the role of epistasis in constraining the selective accessibility of mutational pathways to high-fitness genotypes?).

#### *4.1. Isolating the Effects of Individual Mutations*

In cases where specific protein-coding genes are known to contribute to adaptive variation in a particular trait, the products of alternative protein alleles are often distinguished from one another by multiple amino-acid substitutions. To cite just a few examples, in the malaria parasite *Plasmodium falciparum*, derived alleles at the dihydrofolate reductase gene that confer pyrimethamine resistance are distinguished from the wild-type susceptible allele by four amino-acid substitutions (63). In *E. coli*, derived alleles at the β-lactamase gene that confer cefotaxime resistance are distinguished from the wild-type susceptible allele by a combination of four amino-acid substitutions and one noncoding substitution (16). In the sheep blowfly *Lucilia cuprina*, a derived allele at the

*E3* esterase gene that confers diazinon resistance is distinguished from the wild type, susceptible allele by five amino-acid substitutions (64). In deer mice, differences in hemoglobin–oxygen affinity between high- and low-altitude populations are attributable to the independent or joint effects of eight amino-acid mutations in the α-chain subunits of the hemoglobin tetramer and four mutations in the β-chain subunits (61, 62, 65, 66). Such cases prompt an obvious question: Are allelic differences in protein function typically attributable to one or two causative mutations, or do the differences in biochemical phenotype depend critically upon the additive or epistatic effects of all mutations in combination? More generally: Are adaptive modifications of protein function typically attributable to a small number of mutations at key positions, or many minor mutations of individually small effect? To answer such questions, it is necessary to isolate the functional effects of individual mutations.

In some cases, the history of recombination in a given population sample may provide a number of naturally occurring sequence variants in which the mutations of interest are essentially randomized against different genetic backgrounds. By judiciously choosing which specimens to use as a source of purified protein for in vitro studies (on the basis of genotypic data), it may be possible to isolate and test a subset of the most important multisite combinations of mutations. In cases where recombination has not provided a sufficient number of naturally occurring sequence variants to make the comparisons of interest, it is necessary to use a protein-engineering approach to isolate the functional effects of individual mutations. This can be accomplished by means of site-directed mutagenesis, followed by in vitro expression and purification of recombinant protein for experimental studies. This experimental approach opens up exciting possibilities for reconstructive inference in studies of protein evolution. For example, it is possible to produce recombinant proteins with primary structures that represent inferred ancestral states (67) or unobserved, intermediate mutational steps in evolutionary pathways (16, 63).

#### *4.2. Epistasis and Compensatory Substitutions: When Adaptive Walks Take Two Steps Forward and One Step Back*

Even if an advantageous change in protein function can be attained by means of a single substitution at a key position in the active site, such changes may often require additional compensatory substitutions to offset negative pleiotropic effects of the original change. These compensatory mutations may be neutral or deleterious by themselves – they are only advantageous when preceded by the initial, function-altering substitution. By definition, the fitness effects of compensatory mutations vary as a function of the genetic background in which they appear. This context-dependence, therefore, represents a special form of epistasis that can influence the selective accessibility of mutational pathways through sequence space (68–70). If compensatory substitutions are pervasive, then in comparisons between the products of alternative alleles – or in comparisons between the products of orthologous genes in different species – it may often be exceedingly difficult to determine which substitutions were responsible for producing the primary adaptive improvements in protein function and which substitutions represent secondary compensatory changes. Experimental studies of protein function involving different multisite combinations of mutations will also be required to identify seemingly "compensated" genotypes that do not actually involve the correction of individually deleterious mutations (71, 72).

A number of recent comparative studies provide indirect evidence for the pervasiveness of compensatory substitutions by identifying cases where a pathogenic amino-acid mutation in one species appears as the wild-type amino acid at the same site in the orthologous proteins of other species. In order for potentially pathogenic mutations to become fixed, compensatory substitutions must have occurred at other sites in the same protein, or possibly even in different, interacting proteins (73–75). The former case seems to be more common, as evidence from a phylogenetically diverse array of organisms indicates that deleterious mutations and their associated compensatory mutations typically occur in the same gene and they also tend to be nonrandomly clustered in the tertiary structure of the encoded protein (76, 77).

The phenomenon of compensatory epistasis highlights the importance of considering structure–function relationships in multiple dimensions. In many cases, trade-offs between protein function and particular biophysical properties can be predicted based on principles of structural biology. Since catalytic activity requires mechanical flexibility, many aspects of protein function, protein stability, and aggregation propensity are intrinsically linked (78, 79). The latter two properties are interrelated because destabilizing mutations lead to a reduced ratio of folded and unfolded molecules, and the increased cellular concentration of unfolded molecules results in an increased rate of aggregation. The important implication is that evolutionary changes in catalytic activity will often have negative pleiotropic effects that require compensatory mutations to restore stability and/or resistance to aggregation. In bacterial pathogens, mutations that confer antibiotic resistance often have negative side effects on stability and aggregation. Thus, the evolution of drug-resistant bacteria often involves numerous compensatory substitutions that offset the destabilizing effects of substitutions at catalytic residues. In *E. coli*, for example, primary substitutions in the β-lactamase gene that increase cefotaximine resistance are typically coupled with stabilizing/aggregation-inhibiting substitutions at residues remote from the active site (78, 80).

Compensatory epistasis has important implications for the rate and mode of protein evolution, and it also poses interpretive challenges for microevolutionary studies of molecular adaptation. It may be that adaptive modifications of protein function (catalytic efficiency, ligand affinity, etc.) can often be achieved through a small number of substitutions at key residues, but the resultant perturbations of other biophysical properties may require numerous compensatory substitutions at remote sites. In such cases, both types of substitutions may be attributable to positive, directional selection, but substitutions of the latter type are only beneficial on specific genetic backgrounds. This highlights the important point that positive selection does not necessarily produce adaptive improvements in protein function – the conditionally beneficial compensatory substitutions may simply maintain the status quo with respect to structural stability or other biophysical properties. In comparative studies of sequence evolution, bursts of compensatory substitutions could produce an elevated level of protein divergence relative to neutral expectations, but most of the changes contributing to the elevated divergence may not have any direct effects on protein function. This point is seldom appreciated in comparative studies that seek to identify specific codons that have experienced an excess of nonsynonymous substitutions, as evidence for positive selection on coding sequence is often implicitly equated with evidence for adaptive evolution of protein function.

### 4.3. Future Prospects

Noteworthy successes in establishing causal connections between genotype, phenotype, and fitness come from studies of single-locus protein polymorphisms that have clearly defined effects on whole-organism physiological performance (2, 11, 12, 23, 81, 82). With the advent of genomic, transcriptomic, and proteomic technologies, efforts to dissect the mechanistic basis of fitness variation have expanded to focus more on adaptive changes at the level of whole pathways or networks, rather than functional properties of individual proteins (48, 56). Genomic analyses of sequence variation and expression variation in metabolic pathways can be expected to shed light on long-standing questions in evolutionary biology (e.g., What is the relative role of structural vs. regulatory changes in adaptive evolution?). Such studies can also be expected to push new questions to the forefront (e.g., How does the pathway position of a given protein influence its evolutionary dynamics?). Indeed, population genomic studies at the pathway or network level can be expected to make important contributions to the developing field of evolutionary systems biology. The simultaneous examination of multiple pathway components in a population-genetic framework should also provide important insights into the evolution of complex traits (e.g., floral pigmentation (83, 84); intermediary metabolism in insects (45, 85–90)).

## Acknowledgments

We thank Z. Cheviron, W. Eanes, V. Orgogozo, and M. Rockman for helpful comments, and we thank R. Weber for providing Fig. 3. The authors acknowledge grants from the National Science Foundation grants (DEB-0614342 and IOS-0949931 to JFS; IOS-0516973 to AJZ) and the National Institutes of Health (R01 HL087216 and HL087216-S1 to JFS).

### References

1. Gillespie JH (1991) The Causes of Molecular Evolution, Oxford University Press, New York
2. Storz JF, Wheat CW (2010) Integrating evolutionary and functional approaches to infer adaptation at specific loci, Evolution **64**: 2489–2509
3. Hochachka PW, Somero GN (2002) Biochemical Adaptation. Mechanism and Process in Physiological Evolution
4. Albery WJ, Knowles JR (1976) Evolution of enzyme function and the development of catalytic efficiency, Biochemistry **15**: 5631–5640
5. Fersht A (1999) Structure and Mechanism in Protein Science, W. H. Freeman and Co., New York
6. Laurie CC, Stam LF (1988) Quantitative analysis of RNA produced by slow and fast alleles of *Adh* in *Drosophila melanogaster*, Proc Natl Acad Sci USA **85**:5161–5165
7. Crawford DL, Powers DA (1989) Molecular basis of evolutionary adaptation at the lactate dehydrogenase-B locus in the fish *Fundulus heteroclitus*. Proc Natl Acad Sci USA **86**: 9365–9369
8. Clarke B (1975) The contribution of ecological genetics to evolutionary theory: detecting the direct effects of natural selection at particular polymorphic loci. Genetics **79**:101–113
9. Koehn RK, Zera AJ, Hall JG (1983) Enzyme polymorphism and natural selection. In: Nei M, Koehn RK, (eds.) Evolution of genes and proteins, Sinauer, Sunderland, MA
10. Dykhuizen DE, Dean AM (1990) Enzyme activity and fitness: evolution in solution. Trends Ecol Evol **5**:257–262
11. Watt WB, Dean AM (2000) Molecular-functional studies of adaptive genetic variation in prokaryotes and eukaryotes. Ann Rev Genet **34**:593–622
12. Dean AM, Thornton JW (2007) Mechanistic approaches to the study of evolution: the functional synthesis. Nat Rev Genet **8**:675–688
13. Dykhuizen DE, Dean AM (2009) Experimental evolution from the bottom up. In: Garland T, Rose MR (eds.) Experimental evolution: concepts, methods, and applications of selection experiments. Univ Calif Press, Berkeley
14. Kacser H, Burnes JA (1979) Molecular democracy: who shares the controls? Trans Biochem Soc 7:1149–1160
15. Kacser H, Burnes JA (1981) The molecular basis of dominance. Genetics **97**:639–666
16. Weinreich DM, Delaney NF, DePristo MA et al (2006) Darwinian evolution can follow only very few mutational paths to fitter proteins. Science **312**:111–114
17. Brown KM, DePristo MA, Weinreich DM et al (2009) Temporal constraints on the incorporation of regulatory mutants in evolutionary pathways. Mol Biol Evol **26**:2455–2462
18. Hall BG, Hauer B (1993) Acquisition of new metabolic activities by microbial populations. In: Abelson JN, Simon MI, Zimmer EA et al (eds.) Molecular evolution: producing the biochemical data. Academic Press Inc, San Diego
19. Rosenblum EB, Rompler H, Schoneberg T et al (2009) Molecular and functional basis of phenotypic convergence in white lizards at White Sands. Proc Natl Acad Sci USA **107**: 2113–2117
20. Eanes WF (1999) Analysis of selection on enzyme polymorphisms. Ann Rev Ecol Systemat **30**:301–326
21. Zamer WE, Hoffman RJ (1989) Allozymes of glucose-6-phosphate isomerase differentially modulate pentose-shunt metabolism in the sea anemone *Metridium senile*, Proc Natl Acad Sci USA **86**:2737–2741
22. Fromm HJ (1975) Initial rate enzyme kinetics. Springer, Berlin
23. Zera AJ, Koehn RK, Hall JG (1985) Allozymes and biochemical adaptation. In: Kerkut GA, Gilbert LI (eds.) Comprehensive insect physiology: biochemistry and pharmacology. Pergamon, Oxford

24. Greaney GS, Somero GN (1980) Contributions of binding and catalytic rate constants to evolutionary modifications in $K_m$ of NADH for muscle type ($M_4$) lactate dehydrogenase, J Comp Physiol B **137**:115–121
25. Place AR, Powers DA (1979) Genetic variation and relative catalytic efficiencies: lactate dehydrogenase-B allozymes of *Fundulus heteroclitus.* Proc Natl Acad Sci USA **76**: 2354–2358
26. Hall JG (1985) Temperature-related kinetic differentiation of glucosephosphate isomerase alleloenzymes isolated from the blue mussel, *Mytilus edulis* Biochem Genet **23**:705–728
27. Eanes W, Katona L, Longtine M (1990) Comparison of in vitro and in vivo activities associated with G6PD allozyme polymorphims in *Drosophila melanogaster*. Genetics **125**: 845–853
28. White MW, Mane SD, Richmond RC (1988) Studies of esterase 6 in *Drosophila melanogaster*. XVIII. Biochemical differences between the slow and fast allozymes. Mol Biol Evol **5**:41–62
29. Hall JG, Koehn RK (1983) The evolution of catalytic efficiency and adaptive inference from steady-state kinetic data. Evol Biol **16**:53–96
30. Watt WB (1983) Adaptation at specific loci. II. Demographic and biochemical elements in the maintenance of the *Colias* PGI polymorphism. Genetics **103**:691–724
31. Watt WB, Donohue K, Carter PA (1996) Adaptation at specific loci. VI. Divergence vs. parallelism of polymorphic allozymes in molecular function and fitness component effects among *Colias* species (Lepidoptera; Pieridae). Mol Biol Evol **13**:699–709
32. Chambers GK (1988) The Drosophila alcohol dehydrogenase gene-enzyme system, Advances Genet **25**:39–107
33. Wheat CW, Watt WB, Pollock DD et al (2006) From DNA to fitness differences: sequences and structures of adaptive variants of *Colias* phosphoglucose isomerase (PGI), Mol Biol Evol **23**:499–512
34. Verrelli BC, Eanes WF (2001) The functional impact of *Pgm* amino acid polymorphism on glycogen content in *Drosophila melanogaster*. Genetics **159**:201–210
35. Verrelli BC, Eanes WF (2001) Clinal variation for amino acid polymorphisms at the *Pgm* locus in *Drosophila melanogaster*. Genetics **157**:1649–1663
36. Powers DA, Lauerman T, Crawford D et al (1991) Genetic mechanisms for adapting to a changing environment. Ann Rev Genet **25**:629–659
37. Sezgin E, Duvernell D, Matzkin LM et al (2004) Single-locus latitudinal clines and relationship to temperate adaptation in metabolic genes and derived alleles in *Drosophila melanogaster*. Genetics **168**:923–931
38. Winberg JO, Hovik R, McKinley-McKee JS (1985) The alcohol dehydrogenase alleloenzymes $Adh^S$ and $Adh^F$ from the fruitfly *Drosophila melanogaster*: an enzymatic rate assay to determine the active-site concentration. Biochem Genet **23**:205–216
39. Labate J, Eanes WF (1992) Direct measurement of in vivo flux differences between electrophoretic variants of G6PD in *Drosophila melanogaster*. Genetics **132**:783–787
40. Laurie CC, Bridgham J, Choudhary M (1991) Associations between DNA sequence variation and variation in expression of the Adh gene in natural populations of *Drosophila melanogaster*. Genetics **129**:489–499
41. Laurie CC, Stam LF (1994) The effect of an intronic polymorphism on alcohol dehydrogenase expression in *Drosophila melanogaster*. Genetics **138**:379–385
42. Stam LF, Laurie CC (1996) Molecular dissection of a major gene effect on a quantitative trait: the level of alcohol dehydrogenase expression in *Drosophila melanogaster*. Genetics **144**:1559–1564
43. Anderson SM, McDonald JF (1983) Biochemical and molecular analysis of naturally occurring *Adh* variants in *Drosophila melanogaster*. Proc Natl Acad Sci USA **80**:4798–4802
44. Crawford DL, Powers DA (1992) Evolutionary adaptation to different thermal environments via transcriptional regulation. Mol Biol Evol **9**:806–813
45. Zera AJ, Harshman LG (2011) Intermediary metabolism and the biochemical-molecular basis of life history variation and trade-offs in two insect models. In: Flatt T, Heywood A, (eds.) Molecular mechanisms of life-history evolution. Oxford Univ Press, New York
46. Schilder RJ, Zera AJ, Black C et al (2011) The biochemical basis of life history adaptation: molecular and enzymological causes of $NADP^+$-isocitrate dehydrogenase activity differences between morphs of *Gryllus firmus* that differ in lipid biosynthesis and life history. In Press
47. Fell D (1997) Understanding the control of metabolism. Portland Press, London
48. Eanes WF (2011) Molecular population genetics and selection in the glycolytic pathway. J Exp Biol **214**:165–171
49. Jeffery C (1999) Moonlighting proteins. Trends Biochem Sci **24**:8–11

50. Copley S (2003) Enzymes with extra talents: moonlighting functions and catalytic promiscuity. Curr Opin Chem Biol 7:265–272
51. Runck AM, Weber RE, Fago A et al (2010) Evolutionary and functional properties of a two-locus β-globin polymorphism in Indian house mice. Genetics **184**:1121–1131
52. Eanes WF (1984) Viability interactions, *in vivo* activity and the G6PD polymorphism in *Drosophila melanogaster*. Genetics **106**: 95–107
53. Cavener DR, Clegg MT (1981) Evidence for biochemical and physiological differences between enzyme genotypes in *Drosophila melanogaster*. Proc Natl Acad Sci USA **78**: 11666–11670
54. Middleton RJ, Kacser H (1983) Enzyme variation, metabolic flux and fitness: alcohol dehydrogenase in *Drosophila melanogaster*. Genetics **105**:633–650
55. Freriksen A, de Ruiter BLA, Scharloo W et al (1994) *Drosophila* alcohol dehydrogenase polymorphism and carbon-13 fluxes: opportunities for epistasis and natural selection. Genetics **137**:1071–1078
56. Zera AJ (2011) Microevolution of intermediary metabolism: evolutionary genetics meets metabolic biochemistry. J Exp Biol **214**:179–190
57. Weber RE, Fago A (2004) Functional adaptation and its molecular basis in vertebrate hemoglobins, neuroglobins and cytoglobins. Respir Physiol Neurobiol **144**:141–159
58. Weber R E (2007) High-altitude adaptations in vertebrate hemoglobins. Respir Physiol Neurobiol **158**:132–142
59. Storz JF, Moriyama H (2008) Mechanisms of hemoglobin adaptation to high-altitude hypoxia. High Alt Med Biol **9**:148–157
60. Storz JF, Scott GR, Cheviron ZA (2010) Phenotypic plasticity and genetic adaptation to high-altitude hypoxia in vertebrates. J Exp Biol **213**:2565–2574
61. Storz JF, Runck AM, Sabatino SJ et al (2009) Evolutionary and functional insights into the mechanism underlying high-altitude adaptation of deer mouse hemoglobin. Proc Natl Acad Sci USA **106**:14450–14455
62. Storz JF, Runck AM, Moriyama H et al (2010) Genetic differences in hemoglobin function between highland and lowland deer mice. J Exp Biol **213**:2565–2574
63. Lozovsky E R, Chookajorn T, Brown KM et al (2009) Stepwise acquisition of pyrimethamine resistance in the malaria parasite. Proc Natl Acad Sci USA **106**:12025–12030
64. Newcomb RD, Campbell PM, Ollis DL et al (1997) A single amino acid substitution converts a carboxylesterase to an organophosphorus hydrolase and confers insecticide resistance on a blowfly. Proc Natl Acad Sci USA **94**: 7464–7468
65. Storz JF, Sabatino SJ, Hoffmann FG et al (2007) The molecular basis of high-altitude adaptation in deer mice. PloS Genet **3**:e45
66. Storz JF, Kelly JK (2008) Effects of spatially varying selection on nucleotide diversity and linkage disequilibrium: insights from deer mouse globin genes. Genetics **180**:367–379
67. Thornton JW (2004) Resurrecting ancient genes: experimental analysis of extinct molecules. Nat Rev Genet **5**:366–375
68. Weinreich DM, Watson RA, Chao L (2005) Sign epistasis and genetic constraint on evolutionary trajectories. Evolution **59**:1165–1174
69. Poelwijk FJ, Kiviet DJ, Weinreich DM et al (2007) Empirical fitness landscapes reveal accessible evolutionary paths. Nature **445**:383–386
70. Carneiro M, Hartl DL (2005) Adaptive landscapes and protein evolution. Proc Natl Acad Sci USA **107**:1747–1751
71. Haag ES, Molla MN (2005) Compensatory evolution of interacting gene products through multifunctional intermediates. Evolution **59**: 1620–1632
72. Haag ES (2007) Compensatory vs. pseudocompensatory evolution in molecular and developmental interactions. Genetica **129**:45–55
73. Kondrashov AS, Sunyaev S, Kondrashov FA (2002) Dobzhansky-Muller incompatibilities in protein evolution. Proc Natl Acad Sci USA **99**:14878–14883
74. Gao L, Zhang J (2003) Why are some human disease-associated mutations fixed in mice? Trends Genet **19**:678–681
75. Kulathinal RJ, Bettencourt BR, Hartl DL (2004) Compensated deleterious mutations in insect genomes. Science **306**:1553–1554
76. Poon A, Davis BH, Chao L (2005) The coupon collector and the suppressor mutation: estimating the number of compensatory mutations by maximum likelihood. Genetics **170**: 1323–1332
77. Davis BH, Poon AFY, Whitlock MC (2009) Compensatory mutations are repeatable and clustered within proteins. Proc Royal Soc B-Biol Sci **276**:1823–1827
78. Wang XJ, Minasov G, Shoichet BK (2002) Evolution of an antibiotic resistance enzyme constrained by stability and activity trade-offs. J Mol Biol **320**:85–95
79. DePristo MA, Weinreich DM, Hartl DL (2005) Missense meanderings in sequence space: a biophysical view of protein evolution, Nat Rev Genet **6**:678–687

80. Sideraki V, Huang WZ, Palzkill T et al (2001) A secondary drug resistance mutation of TEM-1 beta-lactamase that suppresses misfolding and aggregation. Proc Natl Acad Sci USA **98**:283–288
81. Feder ME, Watt WB (1992) Functional biology of adaptation. In: Berry RJ, Crawford TJ, Hewitt GM (eds.) Genes in ecology. Blackwell Scientific Publications, Oxford, UK
82. Dalziel AC, Rogers SM, Schulte PM (2009) Linking genotypes to phenotypes and fitness: how mechanistic biology can inform molecular ecology. Mol Ecol **18**:4997–5017
83. Rausher MD (2008) Evolutionary transitions in floral color. Int J Plant Sci **169**:7–21
84. Streisfeld MA, Rausher MD (2010) Population genetics, pleiotropy, and the preferential fixation of mutations during adaptive evolution. Evolution **65**:629–642
85. Eanes WF, Merritt TJS, Flowers JM et al (2006) Flux control and excess capacity in the enzymes of glycolysis and their relationship to flight metabolism in *Drosophila melanogaster*. Proc Natl Acad Sci USA **103**:19413–19418
86. Eanes WF, Merritt TJS, Flowers JM et al (2009) Direct evidence that genetic variation in glycerol-3-phosphate and malate dehydrogenase genes (*Gpdh* and *Mdh1*) affects adult ethanol tolerance in *Drosophila melanogaster*. Genetics **181**:607–614
87. Flowers JM, Sezgin E, Kumagai S et al (2007) Adaptive evolution of metabolic pathways in *Drosophila*. Mol Biol Evol **24**:1347–1354
88. Greenberg AJ, Stockwell SR, Clark AG (2008) Evolutionary constraint and adaptation in the metabolic network of *Drosophila*. Mol Biol Evol **25**:2537–2546
89. Merritt TJS., Kuczynski C, Sezgin E et al (2009) Quantifying interactions within the NADP(H) enzyme network in *Drosophila melanogaster*. Genetics **182**:565–574
90. Merritt TJS, Sezgin E, Zhu CT et al (2006) Triglyceride pools, flight and activity variation at the *Gpdh* locus in *Drosophila melanogaster*. Genetics **172**:293–304

# Chapter 23

# Making Reporter Gene Constructs to Analyze *Cis*-regulatory Elements

**José Bessa and José Luis Gómez-Skarmeta**

## Abstract

*Cis*-regulatory sequences control when, where, and how much genes are transcribed. A better understanding on these elements is a fundamental keystone to better understand development, cell differentiation, and morphogenesis. Several methods based on in silico analysis or ChIP-seq experiments have been developed to detect *cis*-acting sequences. Here, we describe a protocol to isolate such sequences from genomic DNA and to clone them into expression vectors for functional assays using the Gateway cloning technology.

**Key words:** Reporter construct, Transgenesis, Enhancers, *Cis*-regulatory elements, Gateway cloning technology

## 1. Introduction

In our days, considerable efforts are being devoted to understand transcriptional gene regulation, and methods have been developed to identify and test *cis*-regulatory sequences. Among several strategies to identify potential *cis*-regulatory sequences, we can underline genomic survey of histone methylation, chromatin organization, and protein distribution of specific factors that are commonly associated with enhancer activity such as p-300 (1–4). These studies, based on chromatin immunoprecipitation (ChIP), allow the identification of specific chromatin signatures that seem to be attributed to active enhancers and, therefore, are good methods to identify putative enhancers. An inexpensive alternative is phylogenetic footprinting (5–7), a technique based on genome comparison of phylogenetically related species, which allows identifying highly conserved noncoding regions (HCNR). High conservation is indicative of functional relevance, and therefore, these regions

Virginie Orgogozo and Matthew V. Rockman (eds.), *Molecular Methods for Evolutionary Genetics*, Methods in Molecular Biology, vol. 772, DOI 10.1007/978-1-61779-228-1_23, © Springer Science+Business Media, LLC 2011

are good candidates for *cis*-regulatory modules (8). Regardless of the method used to identify candidate *cis*-regulatory regions, functional validation of such sequences should be done by analyzing its ability to regulate transcription in specific tissues and developmental times. Therefore, for enhancer validation, the use of in vivo embryo transgenic experiments, rather than cell culture assays, is preferred.

The generation of transgenics with Bacterial Artificial Chromosomes (BACs), in which large DNA fragments are inserted by recombineering, is useful to test the *cis*-regulatory activity of large genomic regions (up to 200 kb) (9). Further recombineering can be done to specifically remove or modify different BAC regions to precisely identify the locations of the identified enhancers. These types of experiments have the strong advantage to analyze enhancers in their genomic context. However, the generation of transgenic animals with BACs (see for example ref. 10) is typically more demanding than with smaller DNA fragments. A recombineering protocol is described in Chapter 26 (see also (11)).

The use of short genomic elements (usually bellow 5 kb), which contain candidate enhancer regions, is a simpler alternative and is the focus of this chapter. Here, we describe a detailed protocol on how to isolate putative enhancers from genomic DNA by PCR and clone them in a desired reporter vector using the gateway cloning technology (12) (see Fig. 1). Ideally, reporter vectors should contain (a) a user friendly cloning site to insert the sequences of interest, (b) a minimal promoter with low endogenous expression that is able to read a broad range of different enhancers, and (c) a sensible reporter gene with high turnover rate, ideally which can be detected in vivo. These are common characteristics of most vectors used for enhancer analysis in model systems.

In zebrafish, *cis*-regulatory activity is usually assessed through transient expression or through stable transgenic lines. In the first case, the functional activity of the enhancers is analyzed at different developmental stages of embryos injected with the desired construct at one-cell stage. The DNA integration occurs in only some embryonic cells, allowing the detection of the enhancer activity in a mosaic manner. Therefore, this strategy, although faster, requires the analysis of a large number of embryos to define a consistent expression pattern. Automated imaging techniques have been developed to make this strategy feasible (13). Yet, automated systems tend to require an initial heavy investment that makes this kind of approach out of reach for many research groups. In addition, the precise expression pattern directed by the enhancer is never completely reproduced in these transient transgenic assays. The best alternative is to generate stable reporter transgenic lines. This requires the growing of injected embryos until adulthood and the screening in these fishes for DNA integration in their germ cells. This usually takes about 3 months. Nevertheless, the same

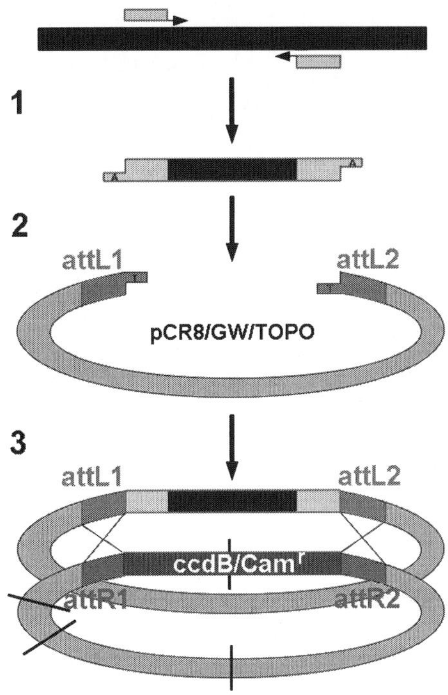


Fig. 1. Overview of the protocol. First, a putative enhancer is amplified from genomic DNA using specific primers (1). Then, the amplified DNA is cloned into the pCR8/GW/TOPO donor vector (2). Finally, the DNA fragment is recombined into a desired destination vector to test the enhancer activity of the amplified DNA (3). In (3) a destination vector similar to ZED is represented and *Bgl*II restriction sites are annotated as *black lines*.

injected embryos can be analyzed for transient expression and then for stable integration. Stable transgenesis might be performed using different shuttle vectors. Among the most efficient of them, we can find meganuclease, virus, or transposon-based vectors (14–16). Besides the characteristics described above, an ideal transgenesis vector should contain two important traits: (a) an internal control of transgenesis and (b) a system that decreases the noise generated by the position effect. This can be done by using insulators flanking the reporter cassette (17) or by site-specific integration (18). However, this last approach is only available for a limited number of model organisms so far.

## 2. Materials

### 2.1. Preparation of Genomic DNA

1. Extraction buffer (EB): 10 mM Tris–HCl, pH 8, 100 mM EDTA, pH 8, 0.5% SDS, and 200 μg/ml proteinase K (Roche).
2. Commercial phenol–chloroform mix: 25 Phenol: 24 Chloroform: 1 Isoamyl alcohol (Amresco).

3. 4 M NaCl stock solution.
4. Molecular grade absolute ethanol (Merck) is diluted in bidistilled water.
5. TE buffer with RNase: 10 mM Tris–HCl, pH 8, 1 mM EDTA, and 100 μg/ml RNase (Sigma).
6. Electrophoresis gel system.
7. TAE buffer stock (50×): 1 L of TAE buffer stock (50×) is prepared with 242 g of Tris, 57.1 ml of glacial acetic acid, and 100 ml of EDTA 0.5 M, pH 8.
8. Electrophoresis-grade agarose.
9. GelRed (Interchim).
10. DNA ladder, e.g., from Biolabs.
11. Loading Buffer (10×): 50% glycerol, 1 mM EDTA, and 0.25% bromophenol blue.

### 2.2. PCR Amplification of Putative Enhancers from Genomic DNA

1. Primers (Sigma-Aldrich).
2. Nucleotide Mix containing 10 mM adenine, 10 mM cytosine, 10 mM guanine, and 10 mM thymine nucleotides (SBS Genetch).
3. $HiFi^{Plus}$ Taq polymerase (Roche) and its corresponding buffer (10×; containing 15 mM $MgCl_2$).
4. A standard thermocycler with heated lid, e.g., MyCycler (Bio-Rad).

### 2.3. Subcloning of Putative Enhancers into pCR-GW-TOPO Vector

1. Electrophoresis gel material (items 6–11 in Subheading 2.1).
2. Scalpel.
3. Sterilized aquatic filter glass wool.
4. pCR8/GW/TOPO vector and its associated salt solution (1.2 M NaCl, 0.06 M $MgCl_2$) (Invitrogen).
5. pCR8/GW/TOPO dilution buffer: 50% glycerol, 50 mM Tris–HCl, pH 7.4, 1 mM EDTA, 1 mM DTT, 0.1% Triton X-100, and 100 μg/ml BSA.
6. Competent DH5α bacteria: 100-μl aliquots of competent DH5α bacteria are kept at −80°C. Previous to transformation, unfrozen aliquots are divided in two (50 μl each) and kept on ice.
7. LB and LB-Agar: 1 L of LB is prepared with 10 g of tryptone, 5 g of yeast extract, and 10 g of NaCl. 1 L of LB-Agar is prepared by adding 12.5 g of agar to LB.
8. Spectinomycin (Sigma).
9. Column-based plasmid DNA extraction kit (Favorgen).
10. *Eco*RI restriction enzyme and its 10× restriction buffer (Roche).

11. Sequencing primers: GW1 (5′-GTTGCAACAAATTGATGAG CAATGC-3′) and GW2 (5′-GTTGCAACAAATTGATGAGC AATTA-3′) primers.

#### 2.4. Recombination of the Putative Enhancer into the Test Vector

1. Gateway LR Clonase II: enzyme mix and its associated 2 µg/µl proteinase K solution (Invitrogen).
2. Top 10 or Mach1 highly efficient competent bacteria (Invitrogen).
3. LB and LB-Agar prepared as described in item 7 Subheading 2.3.
4. Ampicillin (Normon).
5. Column-based plasmid DNA extraction kit (Favorgen).
6. *Bgl*II restriction enzymes and its 10× restriction buffer (Roche).

## 3. Methods

#### 3.1. Preparation of Genomic DNA

This protocol reliably yields good-quality genomic DNA from any organism.

1. Fresh tissue is preferred. If tissue needs to be stored prior to DNA extraction, the best is to freeze it in liquid nitrogen and keep it at −80°C. Storage in 70% ethanol can also give satisfactory results.
2. Remove all solutions from the tissue. If tissues were stored in ethanol, evaporate residual ethanol for less than 2 min. Add extraction buffer (EB). The proportion of EB must be approximately 1 ml of EB per 100 mg of tissue. If the tissue was previously frozen, it must be smashed till dust and then EB is added. If the tissue is fresh, it must be homogenized directly in the EB with the help of a pestle for microcentrifuge tubes.
3. Incubate the homogenized tissue at 50°C for 3 h (minimum, it can be extended to overnight). During this incubation, the solution must be mixed by periodically inverting the tube several times.
4. Cool down the solution to room temperature. Afterward, three rounds of phenol–chloroform extraction are done as follows.
5. Add one volume of phenol–chloroform mix to the homogenized solution and mix gently until an emulsion is formed. Do not use vortex, since it shears DNA. Centrifuge at 13,226×$g$ for 10 min. All the centrifugation steps are done in a microcentrifuge. Collect the aqueous phase (upper phase) into a clean microcentrifuge tube. Repeat this step two additional times.

6. Measure the final collected volume using a micropipette and add NaCl to a final concentration of 200 mM. Gently add two volumes of 100% ethanol and mix well.
7. Centrifuge the solution for 15 min at 13,226 × *g*, remove supernatant, and wash the pellet with 70% ethanol.
8. Centrifuge once more for 5 min at 13,226 × *g* and discard supernatant. Air-dry the pellet for 3 min. Caution: if the DNA is too dry, it will be difficult to resuspend it.
9. Resuspend the pellet gently in 5–10 ml of TE buffer with RNase. The amount of buffer should be proportional to the amount of starting material: use about 5 ml of TE buffer for 1 g of starting material. Incubate the solution at 37°C for 45 min.
10. Proceed with another phenol–chloroform extraction (steps 5–8).
11. Resuspend the pellet gently in TE buffer (1 ml of TE per gram of tissue).
12. Examine 1 μl of the genomic DNA solution in a 1% agarose gel to check DNA purity and concentration (see Note 1).

### 3.2. PCR Amplification of Putative Enhancers from Genomic DNA

This step is necessary to isolate the candidate *cis*-regulatory region from genomic DNA.

1. Design primers to amplify the putative enhancer plus, approximately, 100–200 bp on each side of the target sequence. Ideally, the different set of primers should contain similar melting temperatures (*Tm*) to minimize the number of different thermocycler programs to use. In general, primers are designed with *Tm* of 65°C and are 22–25 bp long. Primer *Tm* is calculated using the following Web interface (http://www.sigma-genosys.com/calc/DNACalc.asp). Web interfaces for primer design are also freely available (e.g., Primer3, http://frodo.wi.mit.edu/primer3/). Optimal design of primers is described elsewhere (19).
2. For the PCR reaction, prepare two Master Mixes in 1.5-ml microcentrifuge tubes on ice. In Mix 1, add 1 μl of Nucleotide Mix, 100 ng of genomic DNA, and PCR-grade water up to a final volume of 20 μl. In Mix 2, add 19.5 μl of PCR-grade water, 5 μl of 10X PCR Buffer, and 0.5 μl of Taq polymerase (see Note 2). Dispense 20 μl of Mix1 for each reaction in different PCR tubes (on ice). Then, add 2.5 μl of each primer at 10 μM (5 μl total for each specific set of primers). Finally, 25 μl of Mix2 is added to each PCR tube. Mix the solution well and spin down.
3. Place samples in a thermocycler. Standard thermocycler conditions are as follows: initial denaturation at 94°C for 2 min,

30 cycles of (denaturation at 94°C for 15 s, annealing at *Tm* – 5°C for 30 s, elongation at 72°C for 1 min per kb), final elongation at 72°C for 5 min, keep at 4°C until samples are collected.

4. Examine 5 μl of each PCR on an agarose gel (1–2%, depending on the size of the expected band). If a single band is observed at the expected size, proceed to the next step. If several bands are observed, optimize PCR conditions or design new primers.

### 3.3. Subcloning of the Cis-regulatory Regions of Interest into pCR-GW-TOPO Vector

Once a DNA fragment is amplified, it must first be subcloned into pCR-GW-TOPO vector to confirm that the PCR fragment is the desired sequence and to then transfer this DNA to the destination vector.

1. Run 40 μl of the PCR product obtained in the previous step, together with an appropriated DNA size marker, in an agarose gel (1–2%, depending on the size of the expected band).
2. Visualize the gel in a UV transilluminator. Set it in its lowest intensity to avoid DNA damage. Before placing the gel in the transilluminator, it is advisable to clean the surface to avoid cross-contaminations with foreign DNA.
3. Excise the band from the rest of the gel using a clean scalpel by making four incisions tangential to the band. Pull out the band from its hole, tip it over in the transilluminator surface, and give a last cut to clear off the superficial agarose that does not contain DNA. This maximizes the proportion of DNA/agarose. If other bands are to be excised, the scalpel should be cleaned with ethanol and paper.
4. The excised bands are placed into handmade columns (see Note 3). Prepare these columns as follow: cut off the lid of a sterilized 1.5-ml microcentrifuge tube. This tube will collect the DNA. Inside, place a sterilized 0.5-ml microcentrifuge tube with its bottom perforated by a hypodermic needle. Fill the bottom of the 0.5-ml microcentrifuge tube with a small portion of sterilized aquatic filter glass wool with the help of a plastic micropipette tip. The glass wool, which should be well packed, should occupy the equivalent of 50 μl of volume. Place the band inside the 0.5-ml microcentrifuge tube and close the lid.
5. Centrifuge the column at 9,469 × *g* for 12 min.
6. After centrifugation, recover the flow-through and transfer it to new 1.5-ml microcentrifuge tubes (on ice). These tubes are later stored at –20°C.
7. Make an one-fifth dilution of the pCR8/GW/TOPO vector in its dilution buffer. This working solution can be stored at –20°C, together with the stock solution.
8. Add 1 μl of the pCR8/GW/TOPO vector working solution to a 1.5-ml microcentrifuge tube containing 4 μl of the

flow-through collected DNA from step 6 and 1 μl of salt solution. Incubate for 5 min at room temperature.

9. Add half of the volume of each pCR8/GW/TOPO reaction (3 μl) into 50 μl of DH5α competent cells previously unfrozen on ice. The other half of the reaction is stored at 4°C and might be used if transformation fails.
10. Incubate on ice for 30 min. During this incubation time, agar plates containing 100 mg/L of spectinomycin are taken from storage at 4°C and placed in an incubator at 37°C to dry.
11. Heat-shock DH5α cells at 42°C for 30 s in a water bath and place them back on ice for an additional 2 min.
12. Add 800 μl of sterile LB to the DH5α cells and place them in an incubator for 1 h at 37°C with agitation.
13. Centrifuge cells in a microcentrifuge for 4 min at 1,252 × *g* at room temperature. Discard most of the supernatant, leaving approximately 40 μl in the bottom of the tube. Resuspend the bacteria pellet in the remaining supernatant and plate them on spectinomycin plates. Place the plates in a 37°C incubator for 16 h or overnight.
14. Pick five colonies per plate using sterile pipette tips. Place each tip in a sterilized test tube containing 4 ml of LB with spectinomycin (100 mg/L). Incubate overnight (or at least 12 h) in a 37°C incubator under agitation.
15. Extract DNA using commercial available columns following the supplier protocol.
16. Confirm that the PCR product was successfully cloned in pCR8/GW/TOPO vector, by digesting the plasmid DNA with *Eco*RI. The digestion is performed using 3 μl of plasmid DNA, 2 μl of 10× restriction enzyme buffer, 14.5 μl of $ddH_2O$, and 0.5 μl of *Eco*RI in a 1.5-ml microcentrifuge tube incubated for 1.5 h at 37°C.
17. Run 10–20 ml of the digested DNA in a 1–2% agarose gel. If the PCR product was successfully cloned in pCR8/GW/TOPO, the vector band and another band with a size identical to the PCR product must be observed unless the predicted amplified sequence contains *Eco*RI restriction sites. If so, the number and sizes of the bands will depend on the number and positions of the *Eco*RI sites.
18. Send the cloned DNA for sequencing using GW1 and GW2 primers.

### 3.4. Recombination into the Test Vector

In this final step, the candidate *cis*-regulatory region is transferred to the destination vector.

1. Dilute the pCR8/GW/TOPO plasmid containing your insert and the destination vector in $ddH_2O$ to a final concentration of 30 ng/μl.

2. Mix in a PCR tube the following: 1 μl of the diluted pCR8/GW/TOPO, 1 μl of the diluted destination vector, and 0.5 μl of LR Clonase II. Incubate this mix in a thermocycler with a heated lid set at 25°C for 1 h (minimum). For large fragments (more than 2 kb), it is advisable to extend the recombination reaction to 2–3 h.
3. Add 0.25 μl of proteinase K solution to the mix and incubate it for 10 min at 37°C in the same thermocycler. The thermocycler should be programmed for one cycle of 10 min at 37°C and a cool-down step to 4°C till samples are collected.
4. Transform half of the volume of the recombination reaction (1.25 μl) in Match1 or TOP10 competent bacteria. Follow the protocol described in step 10 of Subheading 3.3, but use plates with an antibiotic compatible with the destination vector (it should not be spectinomycin). In our case, we use the Zebrafish Enhancer Detection ZED vector (16) that carries an ampicillin resistance gene; therefore, agar plates contain 100 mg/L ampicillin.
5. Pick two to four colonies as described in step 11 of Subheading 3.3. LB must contain the antibiotic used in the previous step.
6. Extract DNA using commercially available columns following the supplier protocol.
7. Confirm recombination either by PCR with the primers used to amplify the genomic sequence (template DNA should not be more than 10 ng) or by restriction enzyme digestion (see Fig. 2) (see Note 4). In our case, for ZED vector, *Bgl*II restriction enzyme is used (see Note 5). Digestion of the original ZED vector with *Bgl*II generates the following bands: 5,000 bp, 3,700 bp, 1,200 bp, and 500 bp. The 1,200 bp band is due to the presence of a restriction site in the gateway cassette and is lost when recombination occurs. Therefore, a ZED vector with a recombined insert has the following band profile: 4,300 bp + insert, 3,700 bp, 500 bp.

## 4. Notes

1. Agarose gel is prepared as follows. Add 1% of agarose to the desired volume of TAE buffer (1×). After homogeneous melting, the agarose solution is cooled down to approximately 65°C and GelRed is added to a final 1× concentration. The solution is then poured into a casting tray and allowed to solidify at room temperature. Gels must be stored at 4°C in darkness. Quantification is done by comparing the intensity of the genomic

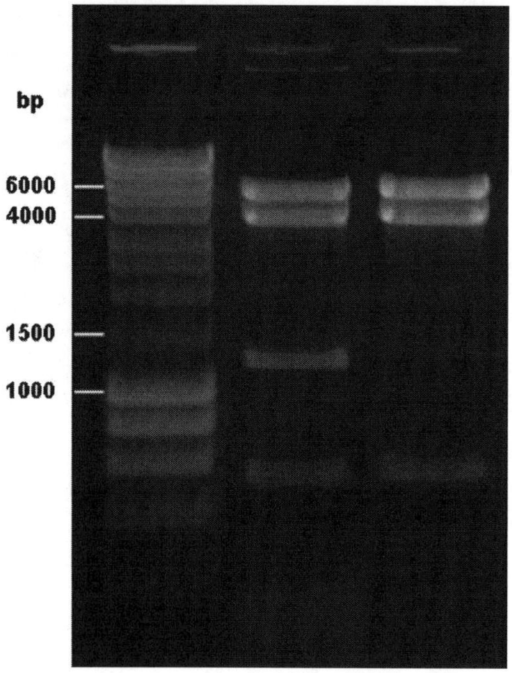


Fig. 2. Digestion of ZED vector with *Bgl*II to confirm Gateway recombination. The *first lane* shows a commercial 1-kb DNA ladder (HyperLadder I, Bioline). *Second lane* shows the empty ZED vector (no recombination) digested by *Bgl*II, generating the following bands: 5,184 bp, 3,754 bp, 1,196 bp, and 535 bp. The 1,196-bp band is due to the presence of a restriction site in the gateway cassette and is lost when recombination occurs. This is observed in the *third lane* that shows the ZED vector digested by *Bgl*II after recombining an insert of 588 bp. Samples were run in a 1% agarose, and relevant band sizes of the 1-kb ladder are indicated on the *left side* of the figure in base pairs.

DNA band and that of the DNA size marker. If the genomic DNA is extracted successfully, a clear heavy-weight band (at approximately 10 kb) is seen in a 1% agarose gel. If a large smear is detected, the genomic DNA quality is poor. This might be caused by endonuclease activity (DNases).

2. To minimize synthesis errors during PCR, a high-fidelity DNA polymerase mix with proofreading activity must be used. Different DNA polymerases have different specifications, so please follow manufacturer's instructions. Be sure that the polymerase produces PCR products compatible with T/A cloning.
3. Commercially available columns for DNA extraction from agarose gel are an alternative to the handmade columns.
4. The orientation of the cloned fragment in the destination vector can be predicted, since recombination is directional.
5. *Eco*RI can also be used to test successful recombination in the destination vector. The *Eco*RI sites that flank the insert in pCR8/GW/TOPO are also recombined to the destination

vector. Therefore, *Eco*RI will excise a band that corresponds to the recombined insert (or fragments of this band if *Eco*RI sites are present within the insert).

## Acknowledgments

We would like to thank R. Freitas, E. de la Calle-Mustienes, and J. Tena for comments on the manuscript. We also thank the Gomez-Skarmeta`s laboratory for the development and improvement of protocols. J.B. is a postdoctoral fellow of the Portuguese Fundação para a Ciência e a Tecnologia (POPH/FSE). This work was supported by grants from the Spanish Ministry of Education and Science (BFU2010-14839 and CSD2007-00008), Junta de Andalucía (CVI-3488) to JLG-S and by EFSD/Lilly to JB. CABD is institutionally supported by CSIC, Universidad Pablo de Olavide, and Junta de Andalucia.

### References

1. Visel A, Blow MJ, Li Z et al (2009) ChIP-seq accurately predicts tissue-specific activity of enhancers. Nature **457**:854–858
2. Heintzman ND, Stuart RK, Hon G et al (2007) Distinct and predictive chromatin signatures of transcriptional promoters and enhancers in the human genome. Nat Genet **39**:311–318
3. Barski A, Cuddapah S, Cui K et al (2007) High-resolution profiling of histone methylations in the human genome. Cell **129**: 823–837
4. Heintzman ND, Hon GC, Hawkins RD et al (2009) Histone modifications at human enhancers reflect global cell-type-specific gene expression. Nature **459**:108–112
5. Allende ML, Manzanares M, Tena JJ et al (2006) Cracking the genome's second code: enhancer detection by combined phylogenetic footprinting and transgenic fish and frog embryos. Methods **39**:212–219
6. Frazer KA, Elnitski L, Church DM et al (2003) Cross-species sequence comparisons: a review of methods and available resources. Genome Res **13**:1–12
7. Muller F, Blader P, Strahle U (2002) Search for enhancers: teleost models in comparative genomic and transgenic analysis of cis regulatory elements. Bioessays **24**:564–572
8. Blackwood EM, Kadonaga JT (1998) Going the distance: a current view of enhancer action. Science **281**:60–63
9. Jeong Y, El-Jaick K, Roessler E et al (2006) A functional screen for sonic hedgehog regulatory elements across a 1 Mb interval identifies long-range ventral forebrain enhancers. Development **133**:761–772
10. Suster ML, Sumiyama K and Kawakami K (2009) Transposon-mediated BAC transgenesis in zebrafish and mice. BMC Genomics **10**:477
11. Jeong Y and Epstein DJ (2005) Modification and production of BAC transgenes. Curr Protoc Mol Biol **Chapter 23**, Unit 23 11
12. Hartley JL, Temple GF, Brasch MA (2000) DNA cloning using in vitro site-specific recombination. Genome Res **10:**1788–1795Gehrig J, Reischl M, Kalmar E et al (2009) Automated high-throughput mapping of promoter-enhancer interactions in zebrafish embryos. Nat Methods **6**:911–916
13. Grabher C, Wittbrodt J (2007) Meganuclease and transposon mediated transgenesis in medaka. Genome Biol **8 Suppl 1**, S10
14. Ivics Z, Li MA, Mates L et al (2009) Transposon-mediated genome manipulation in vertebrates. Nat Methods **6**:415–422
15. Lin S, Gaiano N, Culp P et al (1994) Integration and germ-line transmission of a pseudotyped retroviral vector in zebrafish. Science **265**:666–669
16. Bessa J, Tena JJ, de la Calle-Mustienes E et al (2009) Zebrafish enhancer detection

(ZED) vector: a new tool to facilitate transgenesis and the functional analysis of cis-regulatory regions in zebrafish. Dev Dyn **238**:2409–2417

17. Fish MP, Groth AC, Calos MP et al (2007) Creating transgenic *Drosophila* by microinjecting the site-specific phiC31 integrase mRNA and a transgene-containing donor plasmid. Nat Protoc **2**:2325–2331
18. Sambrook J, Russell DW (2001) Molecular cloning, 3rd edn. CSHL Press, New York
19. Heery DM, Gannon F, Powell R (1990) A simple method for subcloning DNA fragments from gel slices. Trends Genet **6**:173

# Chapter 24

# PCR-Directed In Vivo Plasmid Construction Using Homologous Recombination in Baker's Yeast

**Erik C. Andersen**

## Abstract

A variety of applications require the creation of custom-designed plasmids, including transgenic reporters, heterologous gene fusions, and phenotypic rescue plasmids. These plasmids are created traditionally using restriction digests and in vitro ligation reactions, but these techniques are dependent on available restriction sites and can be laborious given the size and number of fragments to be ligated. The baker's yeast *Saccharomyces cerevisiae* provides a powerful platform to create nearly any plasmid through PCR-directed yeast-mediated ligation. This technique can ligate complex plasmids of up to 50 kilobasepairs (kb) in vivo to produce plasmids with precisely defined sequences.

**Key words:** Yeast, Homologous recombination, Tagging, Plasmid, Construct creation, Ligation cloning, Custom vectors

## 1. Introduction

The baker's yeast *Saccharomyces cerevisiae* efficiently recombines linear fragments of homologous DNA sequences (1). This observation quickly led to a variety of powerful techniques to manipulate the yeast genome, including precise gene knockouts, fusions, rearrangements, and allele replacements (2). In addition to direct modification of the yeast genome, homologous recombination can be used to make a variety of custom plasmids using yeast as the construction tool (3–6). The in vivo ligation reactions require only 30–40 basepairs (bp) of homology (7, 8) to efficiently combine DNA fragments generated by restriction digest (6), PCR (3–5), or both. Yeast-mediated ligations using PCR fragments can facilitate the construction of plasmids up to 50 kb for any molecular biology application, including transgenesis, gene expression determination

Virginie Orgogozo and Matthew V. Rockman (eds.), *Molecular Methods for Evolutionary Genetics*, Methods in Molecular Biology, vol. 772, DOI 10.1007/978-1-61779-228-1_24, © Springer Science+Business Media, LLC 2011

using reporters, and functional tests using heterologous gene fusions. Additionally, high-throughput construction of plasmids for gene knockouts in *Neurospora crassa* has been described using this technique (9).

This protocol employs inexpensive reagents to create custom plasmids using yeast as the construction tool. Because the endogenous homologous recombination machinery in the yeast ligates PCR fragments with homologous regions together, vectors are easily constructed by designing compatible primer sequences. There is no need for in vitro molecular biology steps, like ligation or repeated restriction digests, so yeast-mediated ligation offers a useful method to create plasmids for a variety of applications.

As alternatives to the yeast-mediated plasmid construction described here, bacterial recombineering or Invitrogen's Gateway recombinase system can be used to create plasmids for a variety of applications. Bacterial recombineering is similar to this technique except bacteria are the construction tools. Recombineering requires genomic clones (fosmids, cosmid, bacterial artificial chromosomes, etc.) to create chimeric plasmids, so unlike PCR-directed in vivo plasmid construction, specific clones must be created. Invitrogen's Gateway recombinase system uses bacteriophage integration enzymes to create plasmids. This system requires the creation of plasmids with enzyme recognition sites flanking the sequences to be combined. This technique is well suited for two different applications. First, because the Gateway system has a high success rate and uses in vitro reactions, it works well for high-throughput plasmid library construction. Second, when researchers want to focus on a specific gene, the Gateway system can be used to move a single gene into many individual target constructs. After the Gateway reaction, however, short recognition sequences (roughly 20 nucleotides) remain at the junctions between constructs. These sequences can interfere with gene functions.

To quickly and precisely create plasmids, PCR-directed in vivo homologous recombination in yeast works for most applications, especially in organisms without extensive genomic resources because only PCR of crude genomic DNA is required.

## 2. Materials

### 2.1. Plasmid Design and Linearized Shuttle Vector Preparation

1. Yeast YE-type shuttle vector pRS426 (ATCC, Manassas, VA).
2. *Bam*HI and *Xho*I restriction enzymes and Buffer 2 (New England Biolabs, Ipswich, MA).
3. Software to design primers (e.g., Primer3 (SourceForge.net)).

### 2.2. PCR Amplification of Vector Constituents

1. Proteinase K-digested genomic DNA or any other source of DNA.
2. Custom oligonucleotide primers (IDT, Coralville, IA).
3. 100 μM TE: 10 mM Tris–HCl pH 8.0, 1 mM EDTA.
4. Polymerase chain reaction (PCR) reagents: deoxynucleotide triphosphate solution mix (dNTP, 10 mM each, New England Biolabs, Ipswich, MA) and PrimeSTAR HS DNA polymerase and buffer (Takara, Shiga, Japan) or any other highly processive, high-fidelity polymerase.
5. Agarose gel electrophoresis equipment.
6. 1 kb Plus DNA Ladder (Invitrogen, Carlsbad, CA).

### 2.3. Yeast Transformation

1. *S. cerevisiae* strain FY2 (*MATalpha ura3-52*) (10) (ATCC, Manassas, VA).
2. Yeast liquid growth medium (YPD, Sigma-Aldrich), or 20 g/l bactopeptone, 10 g/l yeast extract, and 20 g/l glucose. Autoclave to sterilize.
3. Yeast solid growth medium (YPD, Sigma-Aldrich), or add 20 g/l bactopeptone, 10 g/l yeast extract, 20 g/l glucose, and 20 g/l agar, autoclave, and pour into 10 cm petri dishes (Fisher).
4. Transformation mix components: Prepare 50% polyethylene glycol 3350 (w/v, PEG, Sigma-Aldrich) freshly for each transformation. Unless PEG is stored anhydrously, use it immediately.
5. 1 M lithium acetate. This solution can be prepared and kept at room temperature.
6. 10 mg/ml sheared salmon sperm DNA (Invitrogen, Carlsbad, CA). This solution should be diluted to 2 mg/ml with water (see Note 1).
7. Yeast synthetic drop-out media without uracil (Sigma-Aldrich, Y1501). For plates, add 20 g/l agar, autoclave, and pour into 10 cm petri plates (Fisher).

### 2.4. Yeast DNA Isolation

1. Teflon cell scrapers, rubber policeman, or glass microscope slide (each available through Fisher).
2. Yeast lysis buffer: 2% Triton X100, 1% sodium dodecyl sulfate (SDS), 100 mM NaCl, 10 mM Tris–HCl pH 8.0, 1 mM EDTA.
3. Phenol:chloroform:isoamyl alcohol (25:24:1, v/v).
4. 0.45–0.5 mm glass beads (Sigma-Aldrich).

### 2.5. Electroporation of the Shuttle Vector into E. coli Bacteria

1. MegaX DH10B T1R Electrocomp *E. coli* cells (Invitrogen, Carlsbad, CA) or any other highly competent *E. coli* cell preparation.
2. Electroporator and electroporation cuvettes.
3. Recovery medium, usually SOC medium (Invitrogen, Carlsbad, CA).
4. Luria Broth (LB) agar plates with 75 μg/ml ampicillin (Sigma-Aldrich).

### 2.6. Determination of the Correct Ligated Plasmid

1. PCR reagents, as in Subheading 2.2, including gene-specific primers.
2. Agarose gel electrophoresis equipment.
3. 1 kb Plus DNA Ladder (Invitrogen, Carlsbad, CA).

## 3. Methods

Figure 1 shows an overview of each of the steps of the technique as applied to an example construct that combines three genomic fragments. This technique is also useful to create chimeric constructs, like fluorescent gene fusions. See ref. 4 for a good example of that application. For the first step, design primers that overlap the junctions to be ligated in the final plasmid. These primers will give the specificity for the homologous recombination that occurs in yeast. In the example, six primers will cover the genomic region to be amplified by PCR. Primers #1 and #6 have sequences homologous to the shuttle vector (11) and to the genomic region to be amplified. In the second step, high-fidelity polymerase with a minimum number of PCR cycles is used to create three DNA amplicons. These three amplicons and a restriction-digested shuttle vector are transformed into yeast and homologous recombination then combines the amplicons with each other and the shuttle vector in step three. The final three steps amplify the plasmids and identify the clone with the correct yeast-mediated ligation product. Plasmids up to 30 kb are readily made by in vivo ligation of up to ten PCR amplicons. The maximum size should only be limited by the transformation efficiency of a large number of individual amplicons into yeast and the transformation of a large final plasmid into *E. coli*. Plasmids larger than 30 kb might require optimizing these two steps.

### 3.1. Plasmid Design and Linearized Shuttle Vector Preparation

1. Prepare a large stock of 100 ng/μl restricted pRS426 shuttle vector to be used for many yeast-mediated ligations. Restriction enzyme digest 5 μg of pRS426 overnight in a 100 μl reaction containing 10 μl of 10× restriction buffer and 40 units each of *Bam*HI and *Xho*I at 37°C. Dilute this digested stock to 100 ng/μl. No cleanup of the restricted vector is required if

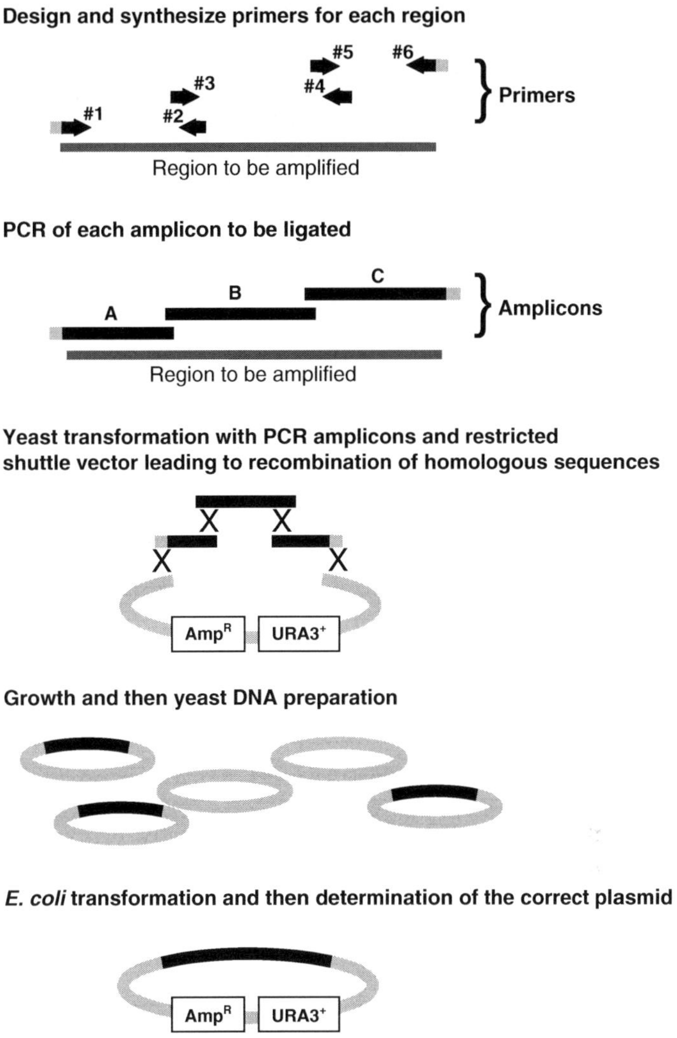


Fig. 1. *From top to bottom* this picture flowchart shows the five major steps in yeast-mediated ligation.

the yeast strain FY2 is used for the yeast-mediated ligation transformation.

2. For a depiction of how the yeast-mediated ligation is designed see Fig. 1. The region to be ligated into the shuttle vector should be tiled by PCR products of 2–4 kb. The PCR products are designed to be this length to ensure production of error-free amplicons using fewer PCR cycles. Design primers for the region(s) to be ligated into the shuttle vector. It is best to have overlap of at least 30 bp complementary between the different fragments (see Note 2). There are a variety of tools available for the design of oligonucleotides that optimize parameters such as melting temperature.

3. The outermost PCR products to be ligated to the shuttle vector require homology to the shuttle vector. For the 5′ (left-most) primer, add the 29-bp sequence shown below, 5′ to the approximately 20 bp of gene-specific sequence designed by the oligonucleotide design program.
   5′ – GTAACGCCAGGGTTTTCCCAGTCACGACG... 20 bp gene-specific sequence – 3′
4. For the 3′ (right-most primer), add the 29-bp sequence shown below 5′ to the approximately 20 bp of gene-specific sequence. Instruct the oligonucleotide production company to gel-purify these two longer primers in order to ensure that each primer is made up entirely of full-length product. This step ensures more successful ligations.
   5′ – GCGGATAACAATTTCACACAGGAAACAGC... 20 bp gene-specific sequence – 3′
5. The other primers are generated without the addition of any sequences, and they are short enough such that gel purification of the primers is not required.

### 3.2. PCR Amplification of Fragments to Be Combined with the Shuttle Vector

1. Prepare genomic DNA or any other source of DNA to be amplified for ligation into the yeast shuttle vector.
2. Resuspend oligonucleotide primers received from the production company in TE at a concentration of 100 μM. These freezer stocks of primers should be diluted with water to make 4 μM working primer stocks.
3. To prevent errors by the polymerase during PCR, it is best to use a high-fidelity polymerase in as few cycles as possible to get a product. Prepare enough master mix of PCR reagents to do an amplification of each fragment at three different cycle numbers. Most PCR amplifications using high-quality, high-fidelity polymerase produce error-free 2–3 kb amplicons after 25 cycles, but multiple numbers of cycles (e.g., 23, 25, and 27 cycles) should be tested. A final volume of 50 μl works well for most PCR amplifications. A recipe for 1× master mix without primers added is shown below. Prepare two more volumes of master mix than required (to reduce pipetting errors) and aliquot the master mix to the PCR tubes.

**Master mix recipe for 50 μl PCR**

| | |
|---|---|
| DNA template | 1 μl |
| PrimeSTAR HS DNA polymerase (2.5 units/μl) | 0.5 μl |
| 5× PrimeSTAR buffer | 10 μl |
| dNTP mixture (2.5 mM each) | 5 μl |
| Water | 23.5 μl |

4. To each reaction containing 40 μl of master mix, add 5 μl of each of the two 4 μM working primer solutions.
5. Run the PCR amplifications for the three different cycle conditions in a standard thermocycler.
6. Pour a 1% agarose TAE gel with ethidium bromide using a standard gel apparatus.
7. Remove 5 μl of each PCR amplification to a separate tube containing 10 μl of water.
8. Add 3 μl of 6× agarose gel loading dye to each reaction.
9. Separate the PCR products and 1 μg of 1 kb plus DNA ladder on a 1% TAE agarose gel with ethidium bromide at a constant 200 V for 20 min.
10. Visualize the PCR products on the gel using transmitted 365 nm ultraviolet light. The reaction that produces a band roughly equivalent to the intensity of the ladder 100 bp band or fainter should be used in the yeast transformation. If every reaction worked well, then repeat the PCR amplifications with fewer cycles. If no reaction worked, then repeat the PCR amplifications with more cycles.

### *3.3. Yeast Transformation (see Note 3)*

1. Obtain a culture of FY2 or other *ura3* mutant *S. cerevisiae* (see Note 4). The culture can be maintained for long term as a frozen stock at −80°C in 15% glycerol. A fresh culture can be streaked on a petri dish containing YPD from this frozen stock. Inoculate a test tube containing 5 ml of YPD with FY2. Put on a rolling drum and rotate overnight at 30°C.
2. The following day, check the optical density (O.D. at 600 nm) of the culture using a spectrophotometer. Make sure that the spectrophotometer reading is within the linear range for the device. It might be necessary to dilute the overnight culture to get an accurate reading.
3. Dilute the culture to an O.D. 600 of 0.2 in 50 ml of YPD. Grow with agitation for another 4 h at 30°C. Check the O.D. after this second growth to confirm that the yeast are in exponential growth phase. An O.D. of 0.8–1.0 will work well. Do not use a culture that has an O.D. greater than 2.0.
4. Pellet cells from the entire culture using a clinical centrifuge at approximately 2,000 × *g* for 2 min. Remove and discard the supernatant, retaining the cell pellet.
5. Resuspend the cells in 25 ml of water and pellet again as above. Remove and discard the supernatant, retaining the cell pellet.
6. Resuspend the cells in 1 ml of 100 mM lithium acetate.
7. Transfer to a microfuge tube and pellet cells at top speed in a microcentrifuge for 15 s.

8. Remove and discard the supernatant, retaining the cell pellet.
9. Resuspend the cells in 400 μl of 100 mM lithium acetate for each O.D. unit. For example, if after growth for 4 h the culture has an O.D. of 0.8, resuspend the cells in 320 μl of 100 mM lithium acetate.
10. Maintain cells at room temperature until ready to use but no longer than 1 h.
11. Boil the diluted 2 mg/ml salmon sperm DNA for 5 min and then cool on ice for 5 min. It is not necessary or desirable to boil the same carrier DNA for each transformation. Boil an aliquot of 2 mg/ml salmon sperm DNA and use for three consecutive transformations and then discard.
12. Vortex the yeast cells to mix and then pipette 50 μl of resuspended cells for each transformation into a new, labeled microfuge tube. Each yeast-mediated ligation should have three transformations:
    (a) FY2 without restricted plasmid or PCR amplicons to ensure that no growth occurs on the uracil drop-out media (this is to ensure that the yeast strain is behaving as expected).
    (b) FY2 with restricted plasmid but without PCR amplicons to determine how much shuttle vector is uncut.
    (c) FY2 with both restricted plasmid and PCR amplicons for production of the final ligated shuttle vector.
13. Centrifuge the transformation tubes for 15 s at full speed in a microcentrifuge. Remove and discard the supernatant.
14. To each transformation tube, add the transformation mix components in the following order: 240 μl 50% PEG 3350, 36 μl 1 M lithium acetate, 50 μl salmon sperm DNA (2 mg/ml, boiled and chilled on ice, see Note 5), 1 μl of restricted pRS426 plasmid (100 ng), 2 μl of each amplicon (see Note 6), and water to a final volume of 360 μl.
15. Vortex and invert to mix the transformation mixture until the cells are completely resuspended.
16. Incubate at 30°C for 30 min.
17. Invert to mix, and then heat shock in a 42°C water bath for 30 min.
18. After heat shock, pellet cells at full speed in a microcentrifuge for 15 s. Remove and discard the supernatant.
19. Rinse cells in 1 ml water by gently aspirating and dispensing solution until cells are fully resuspended, and then pellet the cells in a microcentrifuge for 15 s at full speed.
20. Remove and discard 800 μl of the supernatant, then resuspend cells in remaining supernatant by gently flicking the microfuge tube.

21. Pipette cells from each transformation onto separate drop-out uracil plates, and spread the cells using a cell spreader or large glass beads.
22. Put the plates at 30°C and grow for 3 days.
23. To determine whether the yeast-mediated ligation was successful, count the number of colonies from each of the three transformation plates for each ligation. The drop-out uracil plate with transformation (1) should have no colonies because there was no shuttle vector to provide the gene for growth in the absence of uracil. If this plate has any colonies, the strain used was either contaminated, the selection plates were wrong, or the strain is the wrong genotype. In this situation, do not proceed with the experiment. The drop-out uracil plate with transformation (2) likely will have some colonies from any incompletely restricted shuttle vector. The drop-out uracil plate with transformation (3) should have the most colonies. This plate will be used in the yeast DNA isolation (or scored for the correct plasmid by yeast colony PCR, as described in Subheading 4).

### *3.4. Yeast DNA Isolation*

1. Scrape off all of the yeast colonies using a Teflon cell scraper, rubber policeman, or glass microscope slide, being careful not to dig into the agar such that agar is scraped from the plate. Deposit the cells into a microfuge tube filled with 500 μl of water.
2. Pellet the cells for 15 s at full speed in a microcentrifuge. Remove and discard the supernatant.
3. To the pellet, add 200 μl of yeast lysis buffer, 200 μl of phenol:chloroform:isoamyl alcohol solution (see Note 7), and 300 g of 0.45–0.5 mm glass beads. These volumes assume that you have a yeast pellet equal to or less than 200 μl. Adjust volumes accordingly if there are more yeast cells. The beads can interfere with microfuge tube closure. Take care to ensure proper tube closure before proceeding to the next step.
4. Vortex for 5 min to break open the cells.
5. Centrifuge for 10 min at full speed, then remove 100 μl of the top aqueous phase to a new microfuge tube. Take care not to remove any of the interface or phenol layer.
6. Add 10 μl of 3 M sodium acetate pH 5.2 and 250 μl of 100% ethanol.
7. Centrifuge for 5 min at full speed in a microcentrifuge, then remove and discard the supernatant.
8. Rinse pellet with 500 μl of 70% ethanol, then centrifuge and remove residual ethanol by pipette.
9. Allow the pellet to dry for 5 min at room temperature and then resuspend in 50 μl of TE.

### *3.5. Electroporation of the Shuttle Vector into E. coli Bacteria*

1. Thaw 25 μl of MegaX DH10B T1R Electrocomp *E. coli* cells on ice.
2. Open an electroporation cuvette and chill on ice for 5 min.
3. Add 25 μl of electrocompetent cells and 1 μl of the yeast DNA preparation to the chilled cuvette.
4. Set the electroporator parameters recommended by the manufacturer for the competent cells. The parameters are often: resistance = 200 Ω, capacitance = 25 μF, volts = 2.5 kV (for a 0.2-cm cuvette).
5. Dry the outside of the cuvette, place it into the electroporator, and pulse the device using the manufacturer's instructions.
6. Return the cells to ice for 5 min, and then add 200 μl of SOC medium prewarmed to 37°C.
7. Pipette the cells in SOC medium to a test tube and incubate at 37°C for 1 h.
8. Pipette cells onto LB agar plates supplemented with 75 μg/ml ampicillin, and spread the cells using a cell spreader or large glass beads.
9. Incubate plates overnight at 37°C.

### *3.6. Determination of the Correct Ligated Plasmid (see Note 8)*

Each of the bacterial colonies that grow on LB plates with ampicillin has the shuttle vector. It must be determined which of the colonies also has the PCR amplicons ligated into the plasmid successfully. The successful construction of a ligated construct depends on the size of fragments ligated together and, ultimately, the size of the final shuttle vector. Smaller vectors transform more easily and grow faster. For vectors over 25 kb, it might be necessary to grow for an additional 12 h and score more independent colonies than described below. For plasmids over 10 kb, it is often better to avoid the largest colonies, as they often do not have ligated inserts.

1. Depending on the predicted size of the ligated shuttle vector, identify a number of colonies of different sizes and morphologies. As the length of the ligated inserts and the number of amplicons transformed into yeast increases, increase the number of colonies scored by PCR. Number each consecutively to aid in the identification of the bacterial colony after PCR.

| Size of final ligated vector | Recommended number of colonies to score |
|---|---|
| <10 kb | 22 |
| 10–25 kb | 46 |
| >25 kb | 94+ |

2. Select gene-specific primers that cover each junction of the ligated shuttle vector. For example, primers #2 and #3 in Fig. 1 were used to make two separate amplicons, but together they will amplify a shorter fragment from the junction of amplicons A and B.
3. Set up a PCR mix for each gene-specific junction without template DNA in PCR tubes.
4. Pick each bacterial colony to the PCR mix, placing the numbered colonies into the correct reaction tubes. Only a tiny fraction of the colony (less than 1 μl) needs to be transferred to each reaction tube. There will be plenty of cells in the colony, allowing each colony to be used in multiple reactions. For the positive control, add genomic DNA used for the initial reaction to a PCR tube, and for the negative control, add a colony from the drop-out uracil plate with only cut pRS426 shuttle vector added.
5. Perform the PCR amplification as above, except extend the initialization step of the PCR to 5 min at 95°C to heat lyse the bacteria.
6. Determine which colonies contained PCR products for each junction of the ligated shuttle vector by 2% agarose TAE gel with ethidium bromide, as described above. The genomic DNA positive control should have PCR products for each amplicon. The yeast shuttle vector negative control should have no PCR products for each amplicon. The size of each amplicon in the successfully ligated shuttle vector should be equal to the positive controls. Otherwise, rearrangements of the genomic DNA in the plasmid could have occurred.
7. Amplify and prepare plasmid DNA from the colony containing a successfully ligated shuttle vector. Standard kits for plasmid amplification are available from a variety of vendors; if the resultant vector is larger than 10 kb, be sure to check the manufacturer's instructions for any protocol modifications recommended for larger plasmids. If desired, determine the sequence of key regions of this vector.

## 4. Notes

1. All solutions should be prepared in water that has a total organic carbon of less than five parts per billion and a resistivity of 18.2 MΩ-cm. This standard is referred to as "water" in this text.
2. If the PCR amplicons have homologous sequences greater than 15 bp to the *S. cerevisiae* genome, these fragments could

be integrated into the yeast genome and not into the shuttle vector. This will result in shuttle vectors that do not contain the entire desired sequence. If repeated attempts at creating the vector are not successful, use a sequence comparison tool such as BLAST to compare your desired sequence to the yeast genome.

3. The yeast transformation protocol was modified based upon protocols from the laboratory of Dr. R. Daniel Geitz (University of Manitoba). His laboratory protocol website is an excellent resource for troubleshooting yeast transformations.
4. Some nonlaboratory strains of *S. cerevisiae* are sensitive to additional salts. Therefore, restricted DNA samples or PCR products require clean up before yeast-mediated ligation using these nonlaboratory strains. If the strain FY2 is used, no DNA cleanup is required.
5. One should avoid more than three freeze/thaw cycles of the salmon sperm DNA to avoid decreased quality. Aliquot the diluted salmon sperm and only use each aliquot three times.
6. Restriction digested products can be used instead of PCR products. The transformation will work effectively with any linearized double-stranded DNA substrate.
7. Appropriate personal protection should be worn when handling phenol. All procedures using phenol should be performed in a hood.
8. One could use yeast colony PCR (12) instead of bacteria colony PCR (13) to identify successful clones. After Subheading 3.3, score yeast colonies as described in Subheading 3.6. Once a successful clone has been identified, grow up an overnight culture in drop-out uracil liquid medium and follow Subheadings 3.4 and 3.5 to get the shuttle vector into *E. coli.*

## Acknowledgments

The author would like to thank Dr. Leonid Kruglyak for financial support and laboratory space. Additionally, Amy Caudy, Justin Gerke, and Robyn Tanny for many helpful comments. This protocol was adapted from one used by the laboratory of Dr. Jay Dunlap (Dartmouth Medical School) and communicated to the author by Dr. Allan Froelich. Many others have contributed to protocols and studies using yeast to create custom vectors and some of whom are referenced below. The author would like to apologize for any omissions of published works or protocols relevant to these studies. E.C.A. is supported by a Ruth L. Kirschstein National Research Service Award from the National Institutes of Health.

## References


1. Orr-Weaver TL, Szostak JW, Rothstein RJ (1981) Yeast transformation: a model system for the study of recombination. Proc Natl Acad Sci USA **78**:6354–6358
2. Rothstein R (1991) Targeting, disruption, replacement, and allele rescue: integrative DNA transformation in yeast. Methods Enzymol **194**:281–301
3. Raymond CK, Pownder TA, Sexson SL (1999) General method for plasmid construction using homologous recombination. Biotechniques **26**:134–138, 140–141
4. Oldenburg KR, Vo KT, Michaelis S et al (1997) Recombination-mediated PCR-directed plasmid construction in vivo in yeast. Nucleic Acids Res **25**:451–452
5. Nikawa J, Kawabata M (1998) PCR- and ligation-mediated synthesis of marker cassettes with long flanking homology regions for gene disruption in *Saccharomyces cerevisiae*. Nucleic Acids Res **26**:860–861
6. Ma H, Kunes S, Schatz PJ et al (1987) Plasmid construction by homologous recombination in yeast. Gene **58**:201–216
7. Manivasakam P, Weber SC, McElver J et al (1995) Micro-homology mediated PCR targeting in *Saccharomyces cerevisiae*. Nucleic Acids Res **23**:2799–2800
8. Baudin A, Ozier-Kalogeropoulos O, Denouel A et al (1993) A simple and efficient method for direct gene deletion in *Saccharomyces cerevisiae*. Nucleic Acids Res **21**:3329–3330
9. Collopy PD, Colot HV, Park G et al (2010) High-throughput construction of gene deletion cassettes for generation of *Neurospora crassa* knockout strains. Methods Mol Biol **638**:33–40
10. Winston F, Dollard C, Ricupero-Hovasse SL (1995) Construction of a set of convenient *Saccharomyces cerevisiae* strains that are isogenic to S288C. Yeast **11**:53–55
11. Sikorski RS, Hieter P (1989) A system of shuttle vectors and yeast host strains designed for efficient manipulation of DNA in *Saccharomyces cerevisiae*. Genetics **122**:19–27
12. Ling M, Merante F, Robinson BH (1995) A rapid and reliable DNA preparation method for screening a large number of yeast clones by polymerase chain reaction. Nucleic Acids Res **23**:4924–4925
13. Woodman ME (2008) Direct PCR of intact bacteria (colony PCR). Curr Protoc Microbiol **9**:A.3D.1-A.3D.6

# Chapter 25

# Production of Fosmid Genomic Libraries Optimized for Liquid Culture Recombineering and Cross-Species Transgenesis

Radoslaw Kamil Ejsmont, Maria Bogdanzaliewa, Kamil Andrzej Lipinski, and Pavel Tomancak

## Abstract

Genomic DNA libraries are a valuable source of large constructs that can contain all the regulatory elements necessary for recapitulating wild-type gene expression when introduced into animal genomes as a transgene. Such clones can be directly used in complementation studies. In combination with recombineering manipulation, the tagged genomic clones can serve as faithful *in vivo* gene activity reporters that enable studies of tissue specificity of gene expression, subcellular protein localization, and affinity purification of complexes. We present a detailed protocol for generating an unbiased genomic library in a custom pFlyFos vector that is optimized for liquid culture recombineering manipulation and site-specific transgenesis of fosmid-size *loci* across different *Drosophila* species. The cross-species properties of the library can be used, for example, to establish the specificity of RNAi phenotypes or to selectively introgress specific genomic *loci* among different *Drosophila* species making it an ideal tool for experimental evolutionary studies. The FlyFos system can be easily adapted to other organisms.

**Key words:** Fosmid, Genomic library, High molecular weight genomic DNA, FlyFos, Transgenesis

## 1. Introduction

Genomic DNA libraries have been widely used for gene cloning and whole genome sequencing (1). A whole new range of application for genomic libraries emerged recently in the fields of cell, developmental, and evolutionary biology. In these research areas, it is often desirable to monitor the behavior of modified transgenes re-introduced into the genome to assay tissue-specific gene expression, subcellular

Virginie Orgogozo and Matthew V. Rockman (eds.), *Molecular Methods for Evolutionary Genetics*,
Methods in Molecular Biology, vol. 772, DOI 10.1007/978-1-61779-228-1_25, © Springer Science+Business Media, LLC 2011

protein localization, or affinity purification of protein–protein or protein–DNA complexes. Traditional methods use tagged cDNA clones under the control of various tissue-specific or inducible promoters (2). However, these reporters typically do not recapitulate the wild-type gene expression specificity of the gene under study nor its expression levels. Unlike in cDNA constructs, large genomic clones can be selected in such a way that they likely include all the regulatory elements required to recapitulate the native gene expression, both qualitatively and quantitatively (3–5).

In tissue culture cells and in many model organisms, transformation techniques exists that allow the integration of large genomic constructs (like fosmids and BACs) into host genomes with ease (6). Moreover, new recombination systems enable precise and high-throughput modifications of BAC or fosmid-sized DNA fragments, and thus make them useful for creating reporter constructs (3–5, 7). The genomic clones can be in principle isolated from any species and re-introduced into any other species where large-clone transformation system is available, opening up new possibilities for functional evo-devo studies of partial hybrids. For instance, it has been shown that genomic clones from *Drosophila pseudoobscura*, a species moderately related to *Drosophila melanogaster*, can rescue RNAi phenotypes when introduced into *D. melanogaster* strain carrying RNAi hairpin constructs (8, 9). The divergence (estimated at 17% (10)) in the primary sequence of the orthologous *locus* in *D. pseudoobscura* is sufficient to render the heterospecific transgene immune to RNAi while complementing the endogenous gene function and providing a convenient proof or RNAi phenotype specificity. Tagged heterospecific transgenes can also be monitored in host species to assess the relative contribution of *cis*-regulatory sequences and *trans*-acting factors to the divergence of gene expression pattern among species, which is an important outstanding question in evolutionary developmental biology. All in all, genomic DNA libraries are a valuable source of rescue constructs and gene activity reporters that can be applied both within and across species.

Here, we present a method for creating a DNA library in a customized fosmid backbone (pFlyFos) designed to enable cross-species transgenesis within the genus *Drosophila*. From the library production stand-point, the fosmid packaging system ensures, in contrast to comparable BAC systems, strict size selection of the clones (on average 36 kb) and relatively low number of chimeric clones, which reduces the costs associated with mapping of the library by end-sequencing (3). The pFlyFos vector provides three features key for streamlining subsequent *in vivo* applications. First, it contains an inducible oriV origin of replication that allows maintenance of the construct in single copy state during recombineering manipulation and induction to high copy necessary for DNA isolation prior to transformation into flies. Second, pFlyFos contains attB sequences recognized by phiC31-integrase that can

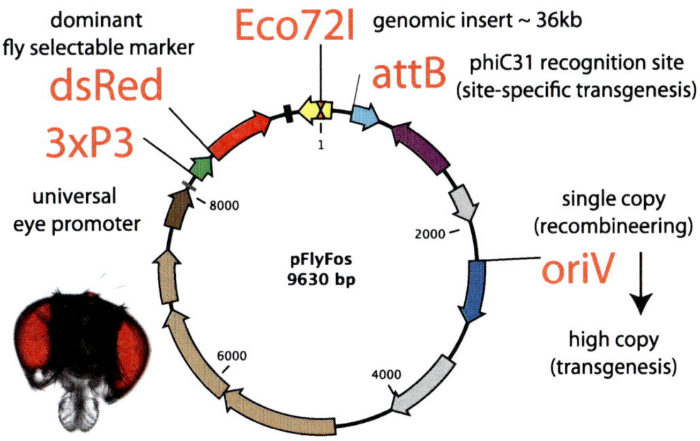


Fig. 1. Overview of the FlyFos vector. Genomic inserts of about 36 kb are cloned into the *Eco72I* site. An inducible origin of replication (oriV) ensures that the fosmid is maintained as single copy during recombineering, but as high copy number for isolation of the fosmid DNA for transgenesis. The attB sequence recognized by phiC31 integrase is used for site-specific integration into the *Drosophila* genome. The dsRed driven by an eye promoter functions as a dominant selectable marker for isolation of transformants.

catalyze site-specific integration into host genomes carrying attP sequence-containing landing sites (11). Third, for selection of transformants pFlyFos carries a dominant 3xP3-dsRed marker cassette that drives the expression of red fluorescent protein into eyes of many species (12, 13) (Fig. 1). The vector can be easily adapted to other model systems and thus the protocol presented here represents a universal approach to generate *in vivo* rescue construct libraries in species where such tools have not yet been introduced.

We describe all the steps required for generating and characterizing genomic fosmid library using the *D. melanogaster* source material as an example (see Note 1). We first describe a modified protocol for isolation of high molecular weight genomic DNA suitable for library production. This part of the procedure may have to be optimized for other model systems. We next proceed to DNA fragmentation by mechanical shearing, resulting in truly random DNA fragments. For efficient library production these fragments may have to be size selected to narrow down the range of fragment sizes and we provide detailed description on how to achieve that despite the fact that this step is not necessary for *Drosophila* genomic DNA. The actual library production by packaging into phages follows to the large extent the protocol developed by EPICENTRE (14) with minor modifications. Finally, we introduce a highly efficient, 96-well manual and 384-well robotic, protocol for miniprep scale fosmid DNA isolation suitable for end-sequencing and mapping of the clones. This protocol enables DNA isolation from tens of thousands of clones in a matter of days and has proved to be highly effective for relatively affordable mapping of fosmid libraries by end sequencing.

## 2. Materials

### 2.1. High Molecular Weight Genomic DNA Isolation

1. 1× PBS.
2. 1× PBT: 0.1% Tween 20 in 1× PBS.
3. 50% Household bleach (2.5% sodium hypochloride final concentration).
4. 100% *n*-Heptane.
5. 100% Methanol.
6. Lysis buffer: 50 mM Tris–HCl pH 8.0, 100 mM EDTA, 100 mM NaCl, 0.5% SDS, 50 μg/ml proteinase K, 100 μg/ml RNAse A.
7. Phenol:chloroform:isoamyl alcohol (25:24:1) pH 7.5.
8. Chloroform:isoamyl alcohol (24:1).
9. 3 M Potassium acetate (KAc), pH 5.2.
10. 100% Isopropanol.
11. 70% Ethanol.
12. 1× TE buffer, pH 8.0 (see Note 2).
13. Rotating wheel or nutator.

### 2.2. Shearing the Genomic DNA

1. Pulse Field Agarose (Bio-Rad).
2. 0.5× TBE.
3. MidRange II PFG Marker (NEB).
4. 10 mg/ml Ethidium bromide.
5. CopyControl™ HTP Fosmid Library Production Kit (EPICENTRE).
6. Hydroshear® DNA Shearing Device (DigiLab) with 4–40 kb shearing assembly.
7. A pulse-field gel electrophoresis (PFGE) system, e.g., CHEF Mapper XA (Bio-Rad).

### 2.3. Size-Selection of the Genomic DNA

1. Pulse Field Agarose (Bio-Rad).
2. 0.5× TBE.
3. MidRange II PFG Marker (NEB).
4. 10 mg/ml Ethidium bromide.
5. SeaPlaque LMP Agarose (LONZA).
6. CopyControl™ HTP Fosmid Library Production Kit (EPICENTRE).
7. A pulse-field gel electrophoresis (PFGE) system, e.g., CHEF Mapper XA (Bio-Rad).

***2.4. Final Purification of the Genomic DNA***

1. 3 M Potassium acetate (KAc), pH 7.0.
2. 100% Ethanol.
3. 70% Ethanol.
4. Nuclease-free water.
5. Millipore 0.025 μm VSWP membrane (Merck).

***2.5. Preparation of the Fosmid Vector***

1. LB + chloramphenicol (25 μg/ml).
2. LB + chloramphenicol (25 μg/ml) + arabinose (0.1%).
3. Plasmid Maxi Kit (QIAGEN).
4. Whatmann filter.
5. 50 ml Syringe.
6. 100% Isopropanol.
7. 70% Ethanol.
8. 1× TE buffer, pH 8.0.
9. *Pml*I (*Eco*72I) restriction enzyme (NEB).
10. NEBuffer 1 (NEB).
11. 10 mg/ml Bovine serum albumin (BSA) (NEB).
12. 0.8% Agarose gel.
13. Crystal violet (Sigma): use 1 μg per 1 ml of gel (optional).
14. QIAquick Gel Extraction Kit (QIAGEN).
15. Antarctic phosphatase (NEB).
16. Antarctic phosphatase buffer (NEB).
17. 5 M Lithium chloride (LiCl) solution.
18. Nuclease-free water.

***2.6. Ligation, Phage Packaging, and Infection***

1. LB.
2. T4 DNA Ligase (NEB).
3. 10× Ligase buffer (NEB).
4. LB + $MgSO_4$ (10 mM) + maltose (0.2%).
5. CopyControl™ HTP Fosmid Library Production Kit (EPICENTRE).
6. Phage dilution buffer (PDB): 10 mM Tris–HCl pH 8.3, 100 mM NaCl, 10 mM $MgCl_2$.
7. Chloroform.
8. Agar plates with LB + chloramphenicol (15 μM).

***2.7. DNA Isolation for Clone Mapping***

1. LB + chloramphenicol (25 μg/ml).
2. 50% Glycerol (sterilize the solution before use by passing it through 0.22 μm filter).

3. LB + chloramphenicol (25 μg/ml) + arabinose (0.1%).
4. Plasmid Maxi Kit (QIAGEN).
5. 100% Isopropanol.
6. 70% Ethanol.
7. Nuclease-free water.
8. 96-Well deep square well plates (2 ml) or 384-well deep square well plates (0.2 ml) (Genetix).
9. Air-permeable seal (Corning).
10. Shaker for deep well plates.
11. Centrifuge for deep well plates.
12. A liquid handling robot. The protocol described here uses Biomek FX (Beckman Coulter).
13. Sequencing primers: pCC2FOSfwd (GTA CAA CGA CAC CTA GAC) and pCC2FOSrev (CAG GAA ACA GCC TAG GAA).

## 3. Methods

### 3.1. High Molecular Weight Genomic DNA Isolation

Fosmid preparation requires exceptionally high quality, high molecular weight DNA. Our phenol–chloroform protocol for flies is applicable to other organisms, though modifications may be necessary.

1. Set up cages containing a total of about 1,000 adult flies.
2. Collect about 1 ml of embryos that are between 0 and 24 h old. Wash embryos thoroughly with tap water (see Note 3).
3. Dechorionate embryos for 2 min in bleach.
4. Wash embryos with 1× PBS.
5. Wash embryos with 1× PBT.
6. Transfer embryos into a bottle containing 1 volume of PBS and 1 volume of *n*-heptane. Use 20 ml of PBS per 1 ml of embryos. Mix by briefly shaking the bottle.
7. Remove PBS (lower phase). Leave the interphase intact.
8. Add 1 volume of methanol and shake vigorously by hand for 1 min. Embryos should sink to the bottom of the bottle.
9. Remove *n*-heptane and interphase.
10. Transfer embryos into a Falcon tube and wash twice with 1 volume of methanol.
11. Remove methanol completely.
12. Add 1 volume of lysis buffer. Lyse for 2–3 h at 55°C. Gently mix by inverting the tube every 15 min.

13. Centrifuge at 4,000× *g* for 30 min. Transfer supernatant to a new Falcon tube.
14. Add 1 volume of phenol:chloroform:isoamyl alcohol. Incubate on a rotating wheel or a nutator for 1 h at 4 °C.
15. Centrifuge at 4,000× *g* for 10 min. Transfer aqueous (upper) phase to a new Falcon tube.
16. Repeat steps 13–14.
17. Add 1 volume of chloroform:isoamyl alcohol. Incubate on a rotating wheel or a nutator for 1 h at 4 °C (see Note 4).
18. Centrifuge at 4,000× *g* for 10 min. Transfer aqueous (upper) phase to a new Falcon tube.
19. Add 0.05 volume of 3 M KAc. Mix by gently inverting the tube.
20. Add 0.7 volume of isopropanol. Incubate on a rotating wheel or a nutator for 30 min at 4 °C.
21. Centrifuge at 6,000× *g* for 15 min. Remove supernatant.
22. Wash the pellet twice with 1 volume of 70% ethanol.
23. Air-dry the pellet for 10 min at room temperature.
24. Dissolve the pellet in 1× TE prewarmed to 55 °C. Store DNA at 4 °C.

### 3.2. Shearing the Genomic DNA

The isolated genomic DNA has to be sheared to fragments of approximately 40 kb in order to be cloned in a fosmid vector. Fragments that are larger than 60 kb or smaller than 20 kb prevent phage assembly. Moreover, DNA fragments smaller than 20 kb that are included in the library production can lead to unwanted chimeric clones.

1. Dilute the genomic DNA to final concentration of 250 ng/μl with water (see Note 2).
2. Shear the DNA using the HydroShear device (DigiLab). Use 4–40 kb (large) shearing assembly. Since every shearing assembly has slightly different shearing properties, test different speedcodes by shearing about 5 μg of the DNA (minimal shearing volume is 50 μl – dilute the DNA accordingly). We have obtained the best results with the following parameters: speedcode 17, retraction speed 40, 25 shearing cycles, 200 μl sample volume.
3. Verify the shearing results by running a pulse-field gel electrophoresis (PFGE) with 1 μg of the sheared DNA. Include Fosmid Control DNA (100 ng) and MidRange II PFG Marker (500 ng) on the gel for reference. The following parameters are suggested for the Bio-Rad CHEF Mapper XA system. Use 0.8% Bio-Rad Pulse-Field Agarose in 0.5× TBE. Setup a two-state

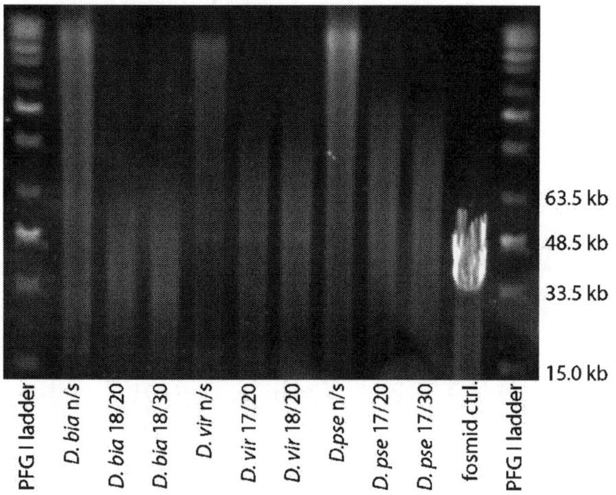


Fig. 2. Sample shearing results for *Drosophila biarmipes*, *Drosophila virilis*, and *D. pseudoobscura DNA*. Electrophoresis was run as described in the text. (n/s) – not sheared gDNA; first number represents speedcode, second shearing cycles, i.e., (18/20) means speedcode 18, 20 shearing cycles. The clear bands visible in the lower part of genomic DNA lanes are the fly mitochondrial DNA. The approximately 50 kb bands visible in *D. virilis* lanes are most likely the yeast mitochondrial DNA contamination (see Note 3).

program at 6.0 V/cm, initial switch at 1.5 s, final switch at 7.0 s, 120° angle, and linear ramping factor. Run the gel at 14°C for about 20 h. Figure 2 shows sample shearing results.

4. Stain the gel for 30 min with 0.5 μg/ml ethidium bromide in 0.5 ×TBE.
5. Destain the gel for 1 h in 0.5× TBE.
6. Visualize the sheared DNA in UV and determine the best shearing conditions. Choose the speedcode that produces maximal amount of DNA in the range of 30–60 kb and nearly no DNA below 20 kb. Including fragments smaller than 20 kb in the library production process may result in large number of chimeric clones. If shearing under a range of conditions fails to yield DNA that is directly suitable for library production, size-select the DNA as described in Subheading 3.3.
7. Shear 100 μg of the genomic DNA (2 ×200 μl) using the determined conditions. Use the newly sheared DNA for further processing.
8. Setup an end-repair reaction. If PFGE size-selection of the DNA in necessary, use 80 μg of sheared DNA in a 240-μl reaction. Otherwise set up an 80 μl reaction using 20 μg sheared DNA, 8 μl 10 ×End-Repair Buffer, 8 μl 2.5 mM dNTP Mix, 8 μl 10 mM ATP, 4 μl End-Repair Enzyme Mix, and water up to 80 μl.
9. Incubate the reaction at room temperature for 45 min.
10. Heat-inactivate the End-Repair Enzyme Mix at 55°C for 10 min. If PFGE size-selection is not needed, proceed directly to Subheading 3.4.

### 3.3. Size-Selection of the Genomic DNA (Optional) (See Note 5)

If shearing under a range of conditions fails to yield DNA that is directly suitable for library production, size-selection of the DNA by preparative pulse-field gel electrophoresis is required.

1. Load the end-repair reaction onto the 0.8% PFGE gel. Run the gel as in Subheading 3.2, step 3. Run both markers (Fosmid Control DNA and MidRange II PFG Marker) on both sides of the gel. In addition, include aliquots (1 μg) of the end-repaired DNA on both sides of the sample for reference (see Fig. 3a and Note 6).
2. Cut off the marker lanes from the gel, and stain them as described in Subheading 3.2. Mark the position between 24 and 73 kb bands of the MidRange II PFG Marker with a razor blade.
3. Reassemble the gel and excise a gel slice containing the sheared DNA between the marked positions. Excise the reference bands containing the sheared DNA as well. Do not expose sample DNA to UV light.
4. Embed the sample DNA gel slice flanked by reference gel slices in 1% SeaPlaque LMP Agarose in 0.5× TBE buffer. See Fig. 3b for reference.

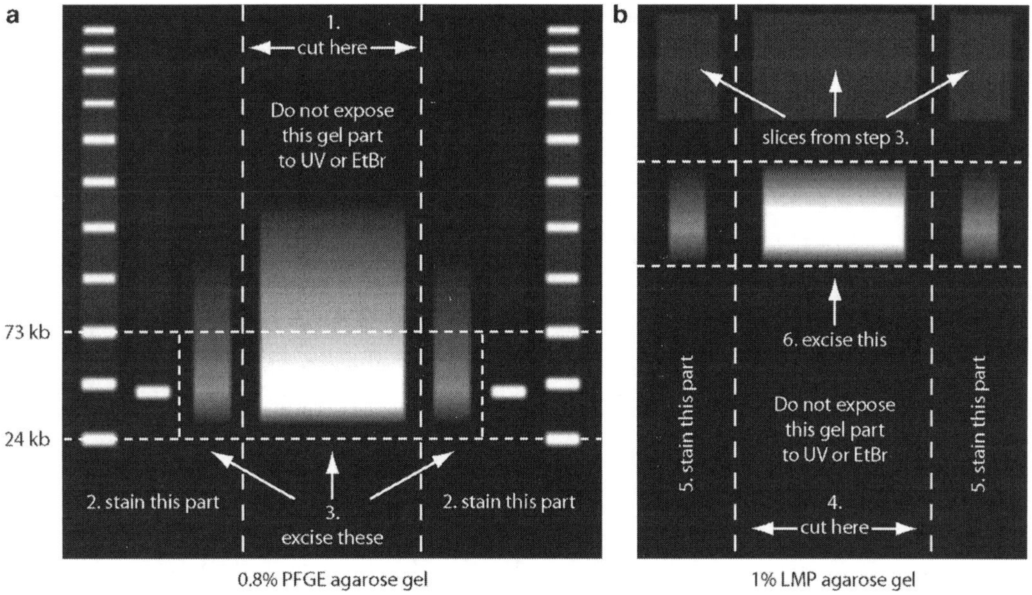


Fig. 3. Running and cutting the PFGE gel and LMP gel. The sheared DNA is run on a PFGE gel (**a**) together with markers (see text for details). After electrophoresis, the marker lanes are cut (*1*) and stained with ethidium bromide (*2*). The identified range is excised from not stained part of the gel containing sample DNA, together with reference lanes (*3*) and run on a LMP gel (**b**). Again, after electrophoresis, the marker lanes are cut (*4*), stained and visualized (*5*). The gel slice containing size-selected DNA in LMP agarose is finally excised (*6*).

5. Run the gel at 5 V/cm at 4 °C for 1.5–2 h to transfer DNA into the LMP agarose.
6. Cut off the reference bands and stain them as described previously. Mark the position of the DNA smear with a razor blade.
7. Reassemble the gel and excise a gel slice containing the sheared DNA between the marked positions. Do not expose sample DNA to UV light.
8. Weight the sample DNA slice in a tared tube.
9. Warm the GELase 50× Buffer to 45 °C. Melt the LMP agarose by incubating the tube at 70 °C for 10–15 min. Quickly transfer the tube to 45 °C.
10. Add the appropriate volume of warmed GELase 50× Buffer to 1× final concentration. Carefully add 2 U (2 μl) of GELase Enzyme Preparation to the tube for each 100 μl of melted agarose. Keep the melted agarose solution at 45 °C and gently mix the solution. Incubate the solution at 45 °C overnight.
11. Transfer the reaction to 70°C for 10 min to inactivate the GELase enzyme.
12. Remove 500 μl aliquots of the solution into sterile 1.5 ml microfuge tube(s).
13. Chill the tubes on ice for 5 min. Centrifuge the tubes in a microcentrifuge at ≥20,000× *g* for 20 min to pellet any insoluble oligosaccharides. Carefully remove the upper 90–95% of the supernatant, which contains the DNA, to a sterile 1.5-ml tube. Be careful to avoid the gelatinous pellet.

### 3.4. Final Purification of the Genomic DNA

In the following steps, the sheared (and optionally size-selected) genomic DNA is reprecipitated and dialyzed to remove residual oligosaccharides, protein, salt and to concentrate the DNA solution.

1. Add 0.1 volume of 3 M KAc (pH 7.0) to the end-repaired DNA (Subheading 3.2) or the DNA that has been purified from the LMP agarose gel (Subheading 3.4). Mix gently by inverting the tube.
2. Add 2.5 volumes of ethanol. Mix gently by inverting the tube.
3. Incubate sample at room temperature for 10 min and centrifuge at ≥20,000× *g* for 15 min. Remove the supernatant.
4. Wash DNA pellet with 1 ml room-temperature 70% ethanol, and centrifuge at ≥20,000× *g* for 5 min. Carefully decant the supernatant without disturbing the pellet.
5. Wash DNA pellet again with 1 ml room-temperature 70% ethanol, and centrifuge at ≥20,000× *g* for 5 min. Carefully decant the supernatant without disturbing the pellet. Use a pipet to completely remove the remaining ethanol.

6. Air-dry the pellet for 5–10 min, and redissolve the DNA in 10 μl of warm (55 °C) nuclease-free water.
7. Dialyze the DNA solution against water on the Millipore 0.025 μm VSWP membrane for 1 h. Pour about 20 ml of nuclease-free water into a 10-cm Petri dish. Float the membrane on the water surface (shiny side up) and let it hydrate for 5 min. Apply the DNA solution (10 μl) onto the middle of the membrane. Incubate for 1 h at room temperature. After incubation, recover the DNA into sterile 1.5 ml microfuge tube (see Note 7).
8. Use 1 μl of the solution to determine the DNA concentration by running it on a gel and using 100 ng of the Fosmid Control DNA as a reference. Store the prepared DNA at −20 °C or use it directly for ligation (recommended).

### 3.5. Preparation of the Fosmid Vector

The pFlyFos fosmid vector has to be amplified and isolated from bacteria. Isolated fosmid vector is then cut and dephosphorylated. Dephosphorylation of the vector prevents it from self-ligating and greatly increases the cloning efficiency.

1. Inoculate 50 ml of LB + Cm with a single colony of pFlyFos-transformed EPI300 bacteria. Culture overnight at 37 °C with vigorous shaking.
2. Use 2× 5 ml to inoculate 2× 500 ml LB + Cm + Ara in 2,500 ml flasks. Culture overnight at 37 °C. Shake cultures vigorously – at 250 rpm in a bare minimum.
3. Harvest the bacterial cells by centrifugation at 6,000× *g* for 15 min at 4 °C.
4. Resuspend the bacterial pellet from both flasks combined in 50 ml of Buffer P1.
5. Add 50 ml of Buffer P2, mix thoroughly by vigorously inverting 4–6 times, and incubate at room temperature for 5 min.
6. Add 50 ml of chilled Buffer P3, mix immediately and thoroughly by vigorously inverting 4–6 times, and incubate on ice for 30 min.
7. Centrifuge at ≥20,000× *g* for 30 min at 4 °C. Remove the supernatant containing fosmid DNA promptly.
8. Place folded Whatmann filter in a 50-ml syringe. Prewet and compress filter by passing water through the syringe. Use such prepared syringe for filtering supernatant.
9. Precipitate the DNA by adding 105 ml (0.7 volumes) of room temperature isopropanol to the lysate. Centrifuge at ≥15,000× *g* for 30 min at 4 °C, and carefully decant the supernatant.
10. Redissolve the DNA pellet in 500 μl warm (60 °C) TE buffer, pH 8.0, and add Buffer QBT to obtain a final volume of 12 ml.
11. Equilibrate a QIAGEN-tip 500 by applying 10 ml Buffer QBT, and allow the column to empty by gravity flow.

12. Apply the DNA solution from step 10 to the QIAGEN-tip and allow it to enter the resin by gravity flow.
13. Wash the QIAGEN-tip twice with 30 ml Buffer QC. Allow the QIAGEN-tip to empty by gravity flow.
14. Elute DNA with 15 ml Buffer QF.
15. Precipitate DNA by adding 10.5 ml (0.7 volumes) of room temperature isopropanol to the eluted DNA. Mix and centrifuge immediately at ≥15,000× *g* for 30 min at 4 °C. Carefully decant the supernatant.
16. Wash DNA pellet with 5 ml room-temperature 70% ethanol, and centrifuge at ≥15,000× *g* for 10 min. Carefully decant the supernatant without disturbing the pellet.
17. Wash DNA pellet again with 5 ml room-temperature 70% ethanol, and centrifuge at ≥15,000× *g* for 10 min. Carefully decant the supernatant without disturbing the pellet.
18. Air-dry the pellet for 5–10 min, and redissolve the DNA in a suitable volume (250 µl) of warm (55 °C) nulcease-free water. Store purified fosmid vector at 4 °C.
19. Set up a 100-µl restriction digest of the pFlyFos DNA. Use 10 µl NEBuffer 1; 1 µl BSA; 30 µg pFlyFos DNA; 5 µl *Pml*I; water to 100 µl. Incubate at 37 °C overnight.
20. Run the digested vector on a 0.8% agarose gel. Include undigested vector (500 ng) and an aliquot of digested vector (500 ng) as a reference.
21. Cut out the agarose slice containing digested DNA (the linear vector migrates slower than superhelical reference plasmid). Avoid UV exposure. Use undigested and digested vector reference samples to determine where agarose should be cut. As an alternative, crystal violet can be used for gel staining.
22. Weight the agarose slice and isolate DNA using QIAquick Gel Extraction Kit. Use two columns (each per 50 µg of restriction digest). Elute vector DNA from each column with 50 µl water. Combine the eluates.
23. Add 12 µl of antarctic phosphatase buffer and 5 µl of antarctic phosphatase to the eluate. Adjust the volume to 120 µl with water and incubate at 37 °C for 3 h. Heat inactivate enzyme at 65 °C for 15 min.
24. Precipitate DNA by adding 6 µl of 5 M LiCl and 90 µl of isopropanol. Mix by vortexing and centrifuge at ≥20,000× *g* for 15 min at 4 °C. Remove the supernatant.
25. Wash DNA pellet with 1 ml room-temperature 70% ethanol, and centrifuge at ≥20,000× *g* for 5 min. Carefully decant the supernatant without disturbing the pellet.
26. Wash DNA pellet again with 1 ml room-temperature 70% ethanol, and centrifuge at ≥20,000× *g* for 5 min. Carefully decant the

supernatant without disturbing the pellet. Use a pipet to completely remove the remaining ethanol.

27. Air-dry the pellet for 5–10 min, and redissolve the DNA in 10 μl of warm (55 °C) nuclease-free water.
28. Dialyze the DNA solution against water on the Millipore 0.025 μm VSWP membrane for 1 h (see Note 7).
29. Use 1 μl of the solution to measure the DNA concentration and adjust it to 500 ng/μl with nuclease-free water. Store the prepared vector at −20 °C or use it directly for ligation (recommended).

### 3.6. Ligation, Phage Packaging, and Infection

In the following steps, the genomic DNA library is constructed. Sheared genomic DNA is ligated with the vector and packaged into phage particles, which are used for infecting the bacteria. Upon infection, the fosmid gets injected into bacterial cells and maintained by them similarly to plasmids.

1. Inoculate 50 ml of LB with a single colony of EPI300-T1$^R$ cells. Culture overnight at 37 °C. Store culture at 4 °C for up to 48 h. This culture will be used in steps 3 and 13.
2. Set up a 10-μl ligation reaction with 500 ng of cut pFlyFos from Subheading 3.5, 250 ng to 5 μg of sheared genomic DNA, 1 μl of 10 ×Ligase Buffer, and 1 μl of T4 DNA Ligase. The optimal amount of genomic DNA can differ depending on DNA quality. For our ligations, it was 2 μg. Incubate ligation reaction overnight at 16 °C (see Notes 8 and 9).
3. Inoculate 50 ml of LB + $MgSO_4$ + Maltose with 0.5 ml of the EPI300-T1$^R$ overnight culture. Culture cells at 37 °C with vigorous shaking until OD(600) reaches 0.8–1.0.
4. Thaw on ice one tube of the MaxPlax Lambda Packaging Extract. When thawed, immediately transfer 25 μl of the packaging extract to a new tube. Keep the tube on ice. Return the remaining 25 μl of the packaging extract to −80 °C. Avoid exposing MaxPlax Lambda Packaging Extracts to any source of $CO_2$.
5. Add 10 μl of the ligation reaction to 25 μl of the packaging extract. Mix by pipetting, avoid introduction of air bubbles. Incubate at 30 °C for 2 h.
6. Add the remaining 25 μl of the packaging extract to the reaction tube. Incubate at 30 °C for 2 h.
7. Add 950 μl of the PDB to the packaging reaction. Mix gently by inverting the tube.
8. Add 25 μl of chloroform to precipitate unassembled phage proteins. Mix gently by inverting the tube.
9. Prepare 1:10, 1:100, and 1:1,000 serial dilutions of the phage particles in PDB.

10. Use 10 μl of each dilution and the undiluted phage individually to infect 100 μl of the EPI300-T1$^R$ cell culture (from step 3). Incubate each tube for 1 h at 37°C. Store the remaining phage dilutions and undiluted phage suspension at 4°C for up to 48 h.
11. Plate cells on plates with LB + Cm$^{15}$. Incubate plates overnight at 37°C. Sometimes longer incubation times (up to 36 h) are necessary to obtain large colonies.
12. Count colonies on the plates and determine the phage titer using the following formula:

$$\frac{(\text{Number of colonies}) \times (\text{dilution factor}) \times 1{,}000}{(\text{Volume of phage extract}[\mu l])} = x$$

(in colony-forming units per ml).

13. Inoculate 50 ml of LB + $MgSO_4$ + Maltose with 0.5 ml of the EPI300-T1$^R$ overnight culture (from step 3). Culture cells at 37°C with vigorous shaking until OD(600) reaches 0.8–1.0.
14. Dilute phages from step 8 accordingly to obtain 100 colonies from 100 μl of cells infected with 10 μl of phage particles. Infect EPI300-T1$^R$ cells for 1 h at 37°C.
15. Plate the library on plates with LB + Cm. During plating, keep the infected cells on ice to prevent the formation of duplicate clones. Incubate plates overnight at 37°C. Sometimes longer incubation times (up to 36 h) are necessary to obtain large colonies.

### 3.7. DNA Isolation for Clone Mapping (Manual 96-Well Protocol)

1. Pick fosmid clones into 96-well plates with LB + Cm. Seal plates with air-permeable seal and culture overnight at 37°C with vigorous shaking.
2. Aliquot cultures into backup plates, add 0.2 volume of 50% glycerol, mix, and freeze in −80°C.
3. Use 50 μl of the primary culture to inoculate 1,000 μl of LB + Cm + Ara. Seal plates with air-permeable seal and culture overnight at 37°C with vigorous shaking.
4. Harvest the bacterial cells by centrifugation at 6,000× *g* for 15 min at 4°C. Discard the supernatant by inverting plates over the sink and placing them on a stack of paper towels.
5. Transfer 350 μl of Buffer P1 to each well.
6. Vortex plates vigorously to resuspend bacteria.
7. Transfer 350 μl of Buffer P2. Mix by inverting sealed plate 4–6 times.
8. Incubate plates at room temperature for 5 min.
9. Transfer 350 μl of Buffer P3. Mix by vigorously inverting sealed plate 4–6 times.

10. Centrifuge plates at ≥6,000× *g* for 45 min at 4°C.
11. Transfer 900 μl of supernatant into the new plates. Be careful to avoid touching the precipitate. If transferred supernatant contains precipitate, repeat centrifugation (step 10) and transfer supernatant into the new plates.
12. Precipitate DNA by adding 600 μl (~0.7 volume) of isopropanol into each well.
13. Mix by vortexing and centrifuge plates at ≥6,000× *g* for 45 min at 4°C. Discard the supernatant by inverting plates over the sink and placing them on a stack of paper towels.
14. Wash DNA pellet with 1,000 μl of 70% ethanol, and centrifuge at ≥6,000× *g* for 15 min. Discard the supernatant by inverting plates over the sink and placing them on a stack of paper towels.
15. Wash DNA pellet again with 1,000 μl of 70% ethanol, and centrifuge at ≥6,000× *g* for 15 min. Discard the supernatant by inverting plates over the sink and placing them on a stack of paper towels.
16. Place inverted plates on a stack of paper towels. Allow the remaining ethanol to be completely absorbed through capillary forces. Replace towels when they become wet.
17. Air-dry the plates for 15–30 min.
18. Redissolve the DNA in 200 μl of nuclease-free water.
19. End-sequence clones using pCC2FOSfwd and pCC2FOSrev primers.

### 3.8. DNA Isolation for Clone Mapping (Automated 384-Well Protocol) (See Note 10)

1. Pick fosmid clones into 96-well plates with LB + Cm. Seal plates with air-permeable seal and culture overnight at 37°C with vigorous shaking.
2. Aliquot cultures into backup plates, add 0.2 volume of 50% glycerol, mix, and freeze in −80°C.
3. Use 5 μl of the primary culture to inoculate 100 μl of LB + Cm + Ara in 384-well plates. Array clones originating from four 96-well plates into each 384-well plate. Seal plates with air-permeable seal and culture overnight at 37°C with vigorous shaking.
4. Harvest the bacterial cells by centrifugation at 6,000× *g* for 15 min at 4°C. Remove the supernatant by aspirating 1 mm from the well bottom at speed of 10 μl/s, move within a well at 50% of speed. Discard the supernatant to the waste container. Wash tips in ethanol and the wash station after pipetting is finished.
5. Transfer 15 μl of Buffer P1 to each well. Wash tips in the wash station after pipetting is finished.

6. Vortex plates vigorously to resuspend bacteria.
7. Transfer 15 μl of Buffer P2. Wash tips in the wash station after pipetting is finished.
8. Incubate plates at room temperature for 5 min.
9. Transfer 15 μl of Buffer P3. Wash tips in the wash station after pipetting is finished.
10. Centrifuge plates at ≥6,000× *g* for 45 min at 4°C.
11. Transfer 40 μl of supernatant into the new plates. Wash tips in the wash station between each pipetting step. Aspirate 2 mm from the well bottom at speed of 10 μl/s, move within a well at 50% of speed.
12. Precipitate DNA by adding 25 μl (~0.7 volume) of isopropanol into each well.
13. Mix by vortexing and centrifuge plates at ≥6,000× *g* for 45 min at 4°C. Remove the supernatant by aspirating 2 mm from the well bottom at speed of 10 μl/s, move within a well at 50% of speed. Discard the supernatant to the waste container. Wash tips in the wash station after pipetting is finished.
14. Wash DNA pellet with 75 μl of 70% ethanol, and centrifuge at ≥6,000× *g* for 15 min. Remove the supernatant by aspirating 2 mm from the well bottom at speed of 10 μl/s, move within a well at 50% of speed. Discard the supernatant to the waste container. Wash tips in the wash station after pipetting is finished.
15. Wash DNA pellet again with 75 μl of 70% ethanol, and centrifuge at ≥6,000× *g* for 15 min. Remove the supernatant by aspirating 2 mm from the well bottom at speed of 10 μl/s, move within a well at 50% of speed. Discard the supernatant to the waste container. Wash tips in the wash station after pipetting is finished.
16. Place inverted plates on a stack of paper towels. Allow the remaining ethanol to be completely absorbed through capillary forces. Replace towels when they become wet.
17. Air-dry the plates for 15–30 min.
18. Redissolve the DNA in 20 μl of nuclease-free water.
19. End-sequence clones using pCC2FOSfwd and pCC2FOSrev primers (see Note 11).

## 4. Notes

1. In able hands, the production of the library takes about 2 weeks. The suggested timing schema is presented in Table 1. Protocols described here are partially based on EPICENTRE CopyControl™ HTP Fosmid Library Production Kit protocol (14), QIAGEN

**Table 1**
**Suggested timeline of the library production**

| | Genomic DNA preparation | Vector preparation |
|---|---|---|
| Tuesday | Embryo collection | Vector preculture (step 1 in Subheading 3.5) |
| Wednesday | Genomic DNA isolation(Subheading 3.1) | Vector induction (step 2 in Subheading 3.5) |
| Thursday | Testing DNA shearing conditions (steps 1–2 in Subheading 3.2 ) | Vector preparation (steps 3–18 in Subheading 3.5 ) |
| | Check PFGE (steps 3–6 in Subheading 3.2) | |
| Monday | Final DNA shearing (step 7 in Subheading 3.2 ) | |
| | Genomic DNA end-repair (steps 8–10 in Subheading 3.2) | |
| | Preparative PFGE (step 1 in Subheading 3.3) | |
| Tuesday | Isolation of genomic DNA from the gel (steps 2–13 in Subheading 3.3) | Vector digest (step 19 in Subheading 3.5) |
| Wednesday | Final purification of genomic DNA (Subheading 3.4) | Vector purification (steps 20–29 in Subheading 3.5) |
| | Preparation of EPI300 cells (steps 1 in Subheading 3.6) | |
| | Ligation (steps 2 in Subheading 3.6) | |
| Thursday | Phage packaging (steps 4–8 in Subheading 3.6) | |
| | Phage titering (steps 3 and 9–11 in Subheading 3.6) | |
| Friday | Final infection and plating (steps 12–15 in Subheading 3.6) | |
| Monday | Clone mapping (Subheading 3.7) | |

Plasmid Maxi Kit protocol (15), and GeneMachines HydroShear® DNA Shearing Device User Manual (16).

2. Use nuclease-free water to prepare DNA handling buffers and all enzymatic reactions.

3. Since embryos are collected on agar plates covered with yeast, the yeast DNA is a very common contaminant. To avoid yeast DNA contamination, wash embryos well with water or PBS. Make sure that yeast were removed completely. Yeast contamination can be fairly easily detected when genomic DNA is run on the pulse-field agarose gel. The ~85-kb superhelical yeast mitochondrial DNA migrates at the speed of ~50 kb linear DNA and can be seen as a distinct band on the gel (Fig. 2).

4. Any mechanical stress should be avoided during preparation of the high molecular weight genomic DNA. Mix DNA solutions only by slowly inverting the tube. When incubating DNA on a rotating wheel of a nutator use very low rpm settings.
5. We observed that the pulse-field agarose gel electrophoresis ensures good resolution of the genomic DNA fragments. However, the efficiency of the DNA isolation from such gel is extremely low. Therefore, the sheared genomic DNA has to be transferred from pulse-field agarose into a low melting point (LMP) agarose that allows for efficient DNA isolation, but gives poor resolution in pulse-field electrophoresis.
6. Exposure of the sheared genomic DNA to UV light leads to the formation of thymine dimers and as a result DNA lesions. Although moderate exposure to UV is usually acceptable for short DNA molecules, high molecular weight DNA is damaged even upon very short UV exposure. The UV damage occurs with a certain frequency per nucleotide. For short DNA molecules, the chance that majority of molecules will be damaged is low, but this is not the case for long DNA molecules. Therefore, it is crucial to avoid exposing genomic DNA to the UV light. All variations of the protocol presented here where the DNA was exposed to UV failed to produce any colonies after packaging and infection.
7. When placing the membrane on the water additional care should be taken to avoid any water droplets on the membrane's top (shiny) surface. Avoid pushing against the membrane with a pipette tip when applying and removing the DNA solution. Dialyze samples in a safe location, so that the dish does not get disturbed.
8. Always use fresh digested vector and fresh sheared genomic DNA for the ligation reaction. The ligation reaction works best when DNA added to the reaction is dissolved in water. Such DNA is not protected from damage by nucleases (storing DNA at $-20^{\circ}C$ decreases but does not completely eliminate the risk). Therefore, it is best to use fresh vector and insert for the ligation reactions.
9. We have found that ligation with NEB T4 Ligase at $16^{\circ}C$ overnight is more efficient than ligation with EPICENTRE Fast-Link Ligase for 2 h at room temperature, as suggested in the EPICENTRE protocol. Therefore, we suggest using the NEB T4 Ligase and an overnight incubation time instead of the kit-supplied enzyme.
10. We have evaluated several different variations of the robotic 384-well miniprep protocol by measuring the absorbance

spectra of the isolated fosmid DNA. In the simplest version of the procedure, we simply dump the supernatant after isopropanol precipitation and during ethanol washes by inverting the plate and pushing the liquid out (Fig. 4c). This version of the protocol results in relatively low yield of DNA template, but it was nevertheless successfully used to map about 15,000 clones of the *D. melanogaster* library. Subsequently, we optimized the robotic miniprep protocol to increase the yield and purity of the fosmid DNA. Removing the solvents robotically during DNA precipitation by transferring 25 μl of liquid from each well in each plate to a waste container improved the DNA yield significantly (Fig. 4b). We remove the solvents by placing the robotic tips 2 mm from the bottom of the plate and aspirating at speed of 10 μl/s while moving within a well at 50% of speed. Additionally, a second 70% ethanol wash dramatically reduced the salt contamination of the isolated DNA and produces very high quality template for sequencing (Fig. 4a).

11. The aim of the fosmid libraries described in this protocol is to achieve maximal coverage of the target genome so that most of the genes that can be covered by a fosmid are represented by at least one clone. In order to estimate the number of clones that have to be sequenced in order to achieve such complete coverage, we developed a computer simulation predicting the number of genes cloned in a library of a certain size. The program first randomly shears the DNA into fragments that match the distribution of sizes expected from the packaging step. Subsequently, it uses a random number generator to pick clones, maps them back to the target genome and evaluates the number of genes that are included in each simulated clone. The criteria for inclusion of a gene model into the clone are provided as parameters to the program. We usually require at least 10 kb of DNA upstream and 5 kb downstream of the gene model. By plotting the cumulative number of covered genes against the number of randomly selected clones one obtains an intuitive measure of how many clones need to be sequenced in order to achieve certain coverage of the genome. In our experiments, the actual sequencing of real fosmid clones very closely matched the results of the simulation, suggesting that the method can be used to optimize the library coverage (Fig. 5). The source code for the simulation program is available for download at http://transgeneome.mpi-cbg.de/downloads/shear.c. GNU C compiler (GCC) and GNU Scientific Library (GSL) are required to compile this program.

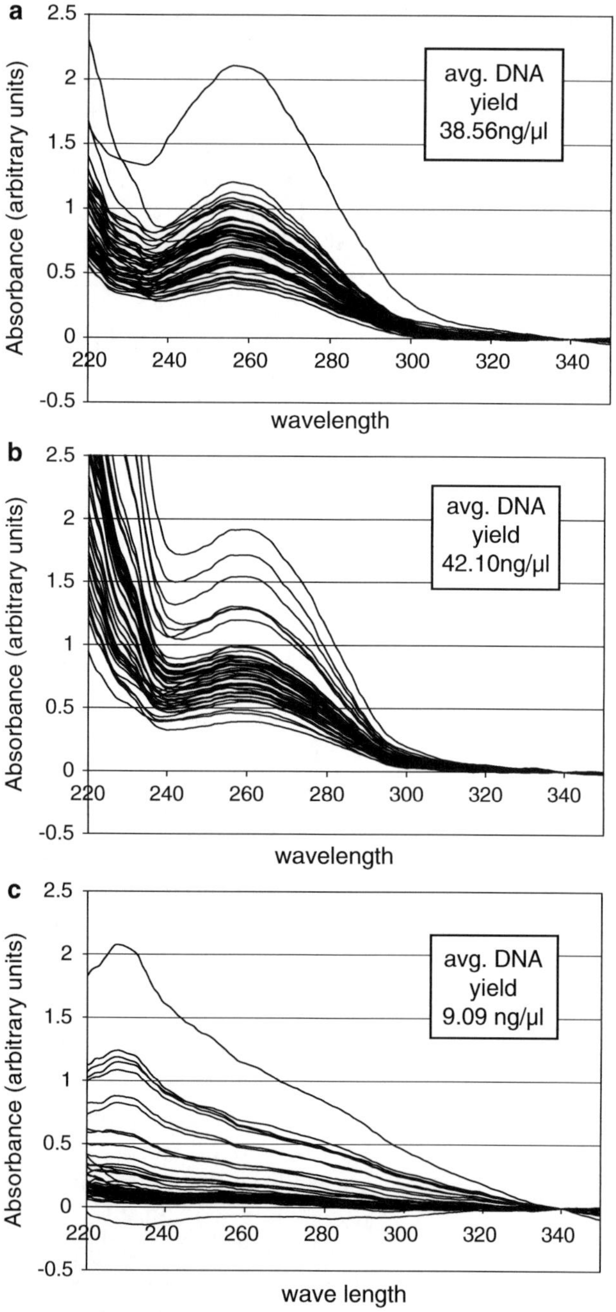


Fig. 4. DNA quality and quantity after high-throughput minipreps. Forty-eight absorbance profiles measured by Nanodrop sampled from a 384-well plate with fosmid DNA isolated using three different versions of the robotic miniprep protocol: robotic removal of the supernatant after protein precipitation step combined with two 70% ethanol washes (**a**), robotic removal of the supernatant combined with single 70% ethanol wash (**b**), and manual removal of the supernatant during a single ethanol wash (by simply tossing the liquid out of the plate) (**c**).

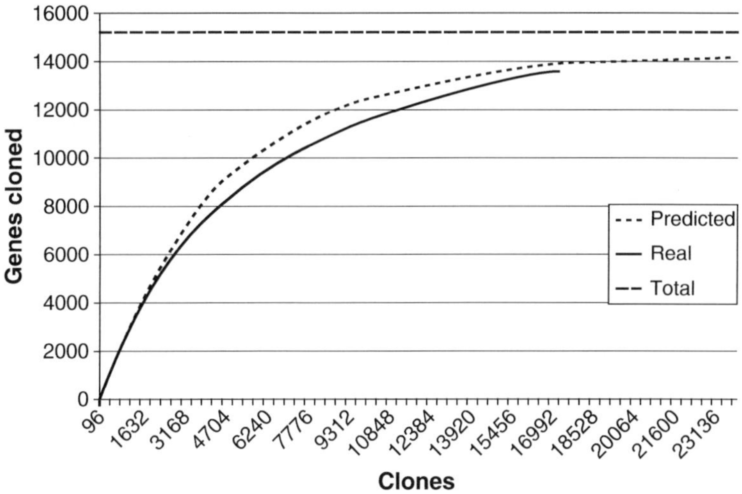


Fig. 5. Comparison of simulated and actual data on library mapping. *Dotted* (in printed version) line shows the cumulative number of genes included in simulated clones as a function of clones picked randomly from the pool of fragments. *Solid* (in printed version) line shows the number of genes included in actual clones as a function of number of clones that were end-sequenced. The *Dashed* (in printed version) line shows the total number of genes in the *Drosophila* genome. Note that about 7% of the genes are larger than a typical fosmid clone and thus cannot be cloned. Data shown for *D. melanogaster* FlyFos library, after Ejsmont et al. (3).

## References


1. Adams MD, Celniker SE, Holt RA et al (2000) The genome sequence of Drosophila melanogaster. Science **287**:2185–2195
2. Hunt-Newbury R, Viveiros R, Johnsen R et al (2007) High-throughput *in vivo* analysis of gene expression in Caenorhabditis elegans. PLoS Biol **5**:e237
3. Ejsmont RK, Sarov M, Winkler S et al (2009) A toolkit for highthroughput, cross-species gene engineering in Drosophila. Nat Methods **6**: 435–437
4. Venken KJT, Carlson JW, Schulze KL et al (2009) Versatile P[acman] BAC libraries for transgenesis studies in Drosophila melanogaster. Nat Methods **6**:431–434
5. Sarov M, Schneider S, Pozniakovski A et al (2006) A recombineering pipeline for functional genomics applied to Caenorhabditis elegans. Nat Methods **3**:839–844
6. Venken KJT, He Y, Hoskins RA et al (2006) P[acman]: a BAC transgenic platform for targeted insertion of large DNA fragments in D melanogaster. Science **314**:1747–1751
7. Poser I, Sarov M, Hutchins JRA et al (2008) BAC TransgeneOmics: a high-throughput method for exploration of protein function in mammals. Nat Methods **5**:409–415
8. Langer CCH, Ejsmont RK, Schönbauer C et al (2010) In vivo RNAi rescue in Drosophila melanogaster with genomic transgenes from Drosophila pseudoobscura. PLoS One **5**: e8928
9. Kondo S, Booker M, Perrimon N (2009) Cross-species RNAi rescue platform in Drosophila melanogaster. Genetics **183**: 1165–1173
10. Zdobnov EM, Bork P (2007) Quantification of insect genome divergence. Trends Genet **23**:16–20
11. Groth AC, Fish M, Nusse R et al (2004) Construction of transgenic Drosophila by using the site-specific integrase from phage phiC31. Genetics **166**:1775–1782
12. Horn C, Jaunich B, Wimmer EA (2000) Highly sensitive, fluorescent transformation marker for Drosophila transgenesis. Dev Genes Evol **210**:623–629
13. Horn C, Schmid BGM, Pogoda FS et al (2002) Fluorescent transformation markers for insect transgenesis. Insect Biochem Mol Biol **32**: 1221–1235
14. EPICENTRE (2010) CopyControl Fosmid Library Production Kit. EPICENTRE Biotechnologies
15. QIAGEN (2010) QIAGEN Plasmid Purification Handbook. QIAGEN
16. GeneMachines (2010) HydroShear DNA Shearing Device User Manual. GeneMachines

# Chapter 26

# Recombination-Mediated Genetic Engineering of Large Genomic DNA Transgenes

**Radoslaw Kamil Ejsmont, Peter Ahlfeld, Andrei Pozniakovsky, A. Francis Stewart, Pavel Tomancak, and Mihail Sarov**


## Abstract

Faithful gene activity reporters are a useful tool for evo-devo studies enabling selective introduction of specific loci between species and assaying the activity of large gene regulatory sequences. The use of large genomic constructs such as BACs and fosmids provides an efficient platform for exploration of gene function under endogenous regulatory control. Despite their large size they can be easily engineered using in vivo homologous recombination in *Escherichia coli* (recombineering). We have previously demonstrated that the efficiency and fidelity of recombineering are sufficient to allow high-throughput transgene engineering in liquid culture, and have successfully applied this approach in several model systems. Here, we present a detailed protocol for recombineering of BAC/fosmid transgenes for expression of fluorescent or affinity tagged proteins in *Drosophila* under endogenous in vivo regulatory control. The tag coding sequence is seamlessly recombineered into the genomic region contained in the BAC/fosmid clone, which is then integrated into the fly genome using φC31 recombination. This protocol can be easily adapted to other recombineering projects.


**Key words:** Red/ET, Recombineering, FlyFos

## 1. Introduction

Recombineering (recombination-mediated genetic engineering, also known as Red/ET cloning) is a technique for DNA engineering in *Escherichia coli*. Recombineering relies on the highly efficient homologous recombination activities mediated by the products of the RecE and RecT genes from*E. coli sbcA* strain (1) or Red alpha and Red beta genes originating from phage λ (2). In typical recombineering experiment, a linear fragment of DNA,

Virginie Orgogozo and Matthew V. Rockman (eds.), *Molecular Methods for Evolutionary Genetics*,
Methods in Molecular Biology, vol. 772, DOI 10.1007/978-1-61779-228-1_26, © Springer Science+Business Media, LLC 2011

usually containing an antibiotic resistance marker, flanked by short (30–50 bp) regions of homology is transformed into recombineering proficient *E. coli* cells containing the target sequence, which can be the bacterial genome itself or an episomal construct such as plasmid, fosmid, BAC, or PAC. The homologous recombination reaction then occurs within minutes, and the recombination product is selected for by overnight growth on selective media.

Since recombineering is not constrained by specific sequence requirements such as the presence of restriction sites, it provides a great freedom and flexibility and has been applied to broad range of DNA engineering tasks (3–5). Recently, we demonstrated that recombineering can be optimized for multistep engineering in liquid culture, without the need to isolate and verify the intermediate products. We have successfully applied this high-throughput approach for engineering of BAC/fosmid clones into transgenes for expression of fluorescent- and/or affinity-tagged proteins under their endogenous control in *Caenorhabditis elegans* (6), mammalian cells (7), and *Drosophila* (8). As fosmid/BAC library can be easily generated (see Chapter 25), this approach is generally applicable for any model organism of interest. Recently, we have created a fosmid library that can be used for straight-forward generation of transgenic fly lines using φC31 site-specific integration (8, 9). Here, we present the detailed protocol for engineering of *Drosophila* genomic fosmid clones into tagged transgenes (8) by combination of Red/ET recombineering and Flp/FRT site-specific recombination. The recombineering pipeline consists of three steps, where (1) host strain carrying targetted fosmid is transformed with recombineering helper, thus rendering bacteria recombineering-competent; (2) PCR-amplified recombineering cassette is introduced into induced bacteria expressing recombineering genes, and (3) selectable marker included in the recombineering cassette is removed using flipase (Fig. 1). The protocol allows for simultaneous processing of multiple samples in microcentrifuge tubes or in 96-well plate format. This protocol can be easily adapted to other recombineering projects.

## 2. Materials

### 2.1. Amplification of the Tagging Cassette

1. Phusion®; high-fidelity DNA polymerase (NEB).
2. 5× Phusion™ HF buffer.
3. 10 mM dNTPs.
4. 96-Well thermal cycler.
5. PureLink™ PCR purification kit (Invitrogen).
6. Nuclease-free water (see Note 1).

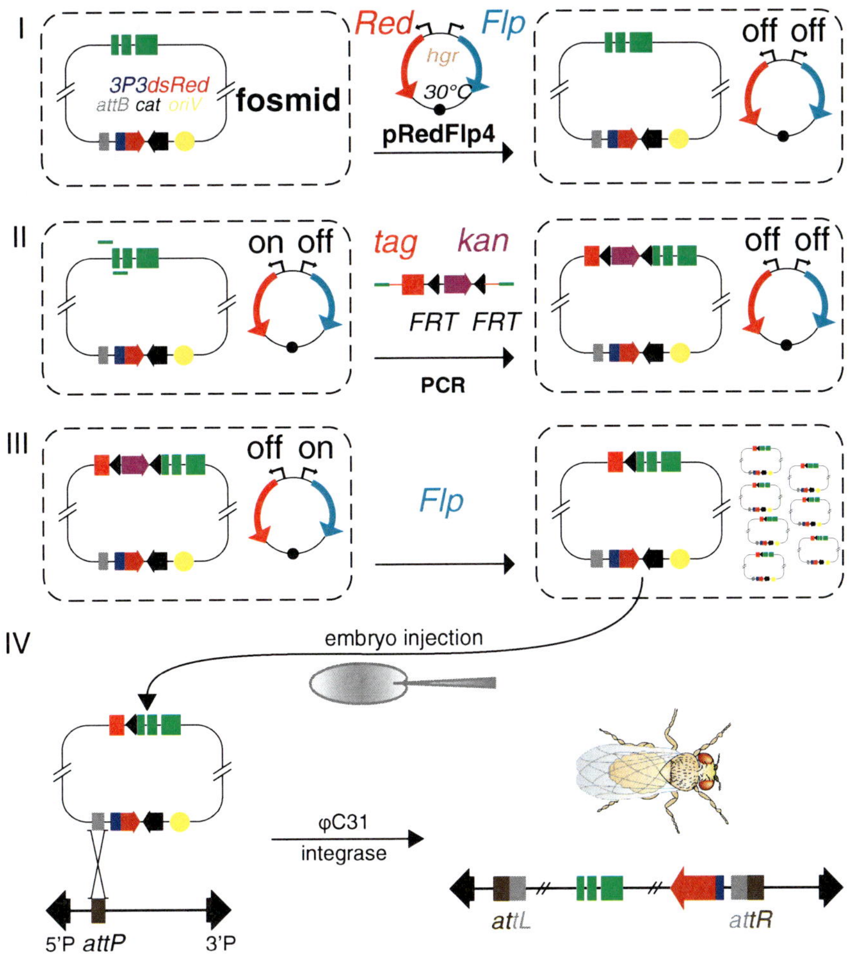


Fig. 1. The recombineering pipeline. *Escherichia coli* cultures containing a fosmid clone of interest are rendered recombineering proficient by transformation of the pRedFlp4 plasmid, which carries both the Red operon genes and the Flp recombinase under independently inducible promoters. (**a**) After L-rhamnose-induced Red operon expression, a PCR product carrying 50 bp homology arms surrounding the tag and the FRT-flanked kanamycin resistance gene (*kan*) is electroporated into the cells. Only recombinant fosmids are able to grow efficiently in the presence of kanamycin (**b**) The *kan* gene is removed by inducing Flp expression with anhydrotetracycline on the pRedFlp4 plasmid, leaving the tagged transgene with a residual FRT sequence on the gene–tag boundary. (**c**) Finally, the clone is induced to high copy and injected into flies carrying an *attP* landing site for targeted integration (**d**).

### *2.2. Transformation of pRedFlp4 Recombineering Helper*

1. 10% Glycerol in Milli-Q grade water (see Note 2).
2. SOC medium (see Note 3).
3. LB + chloramphenicol (25 μg/ml).
4. YENB (0.75% bacto yeast extract, 0.8% nutrient broth) + chloramphenicol (25 μg/ml) (see Note 4).
5. LB + chloramphenicol (25 μg/ml) + hygromycin (50 μg/ml) (see Note 5).

6. 96-Well deep square well plates (2 ml)/microcentrifuge tubes (2 ml).
7. Air-permeable seal.
8. Shaker for deep well plates/thermomixer (Eppendorf).
9. Centrifuge for deep well plates/microcentrifuge (Eppendorf).
10. 96-Well electroporator (Harvard Apparatus)/electroporator (BioRad).
11. 96-Well electroporation cuvette (Harvard Apparatus)/electroporation cuvette (BioRad).

***2.3. Tagging by Red/ET Recombination***

1. 10% Glycerol in Milli-Q grade water.
2. SOC medium.
3. YENB + chloramphenicol (25 μg/ml) + hygromycin (50 μg/ml).
4. LB + chloramphenicol (25 μg/ml) + hygromycin (50 μg/ml) + kanamycin (25 μg/ml).
5. 25% L-rhamnose in water.
6. 96-Well deep square well plates (2 ml)/microcentrifuge tubes (2 ml).
7. Air-permeable seal.
8. Shaker for deep well plates/thermomixer (Eppendorf).
9. Centrifuge for deep well plates/microcentrifuge (Eppendorf).
10. 96-Well electroporator (Harvard Apparatus)/electroporator (BioRad).
11. 96-Well electroporation cuvette (Harvard Apparatus)/electroporation cuvette (BioRad).

***2.4. Removal of the Selectable Marker and pRedFlp Helper***

1. LB + chloramphenicol (25 μg/ml).
2. LB + chloramphenicol (25 μg/ml) + hygromycin (50 μg/ml) + anhydrotetracycline (200 nM).
3. 96-Well deep square well plates (2 ml)/microcentrifuge tubes (2 ml).
4. Air-permeable seal.
5. Shaker for deep well plates/thermomixer (Eppendorf).

***2.5. Verification of the Tagging Result***

1. High-throughput miniprep kit (see Chapter 25).
2. DNA sequencing.

***2.6. DNA Purification and Fly Transformation***

1. LB + chloramphenicol (25 μg/ml).
2. LB + chloramphenicol (25 μg/ml) + l-arabinose (0.1%).
3. Plasmid Maxi Kit (QIAGEN).
4. Whatmann filter paper.

5. 100% Isopropanol.
6. 70% Ethanol.
7. 1× TE, pH 8.0.
8. Nuclease-free water.

## 3. Methods

Liquid culture recombineering can be preformed in both Eppendorf tubes and 96-well plates using the same protocol. Format-specific differences are indicated in the text below.

### 3.1. Amplification of the Tagging Cassette

In this step, the linear tagging cassette is amplified from the tagging vector (Fig. 2). The cassette is flanked by homology arms targeting it to the desired location.

1. Design recombineering primers for each sample. Primers include a priming part (20–25 bp) that is complementary to the ends of the tag sequence (forward and reverse) on 5′ end and 50 bp homology arms complementary to the target sequence (see Note 6). Verify the orientation of both primers.
2. Set up 50 μl PCRs to amplify the tagging cassettes (see Note 7). Use 25–50 ng of the tagging vector as a template. Use HPLC-purified recombineering primers at 10 nmol/μl final concentration. Run the PCR for 20–25 cycles (see Notes 1 and 8).
3. Verify the PCR by running 5 μl of the reaction on an agarose gel.
4. Purify the DNA with (96-well) PCR purification kit following the manufacturer's instructions (see Note 9). Elute DNA with 500 μl of nuclease-free water.
5. Store the amplified tagging cassettes at −20 °C.

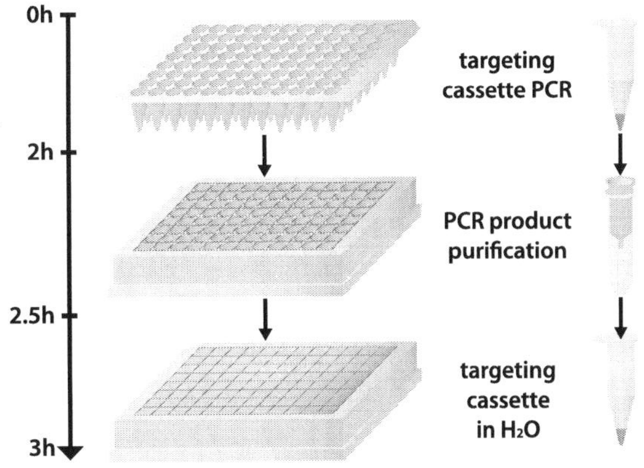


Fig. 2. Amplification of the tagging cassette.

### 3.2. Transformation of pRedFlp4 Recombineering Helper

In the following steps, the recombineering helper that encodes Red operon and flipase is introduced into the bacteria by electroporation (Figs. 1a and 3).

1. Use glycerol stocks to inoculate 1 ml of LB + Cm in a 96-well deep well plate/2 ml tube (see Note 10). Seal the plate with an air-permeable seal and culture overnight at 37°C with vigorous shaking. If using single tube, puncture the lids with a sterile needle.

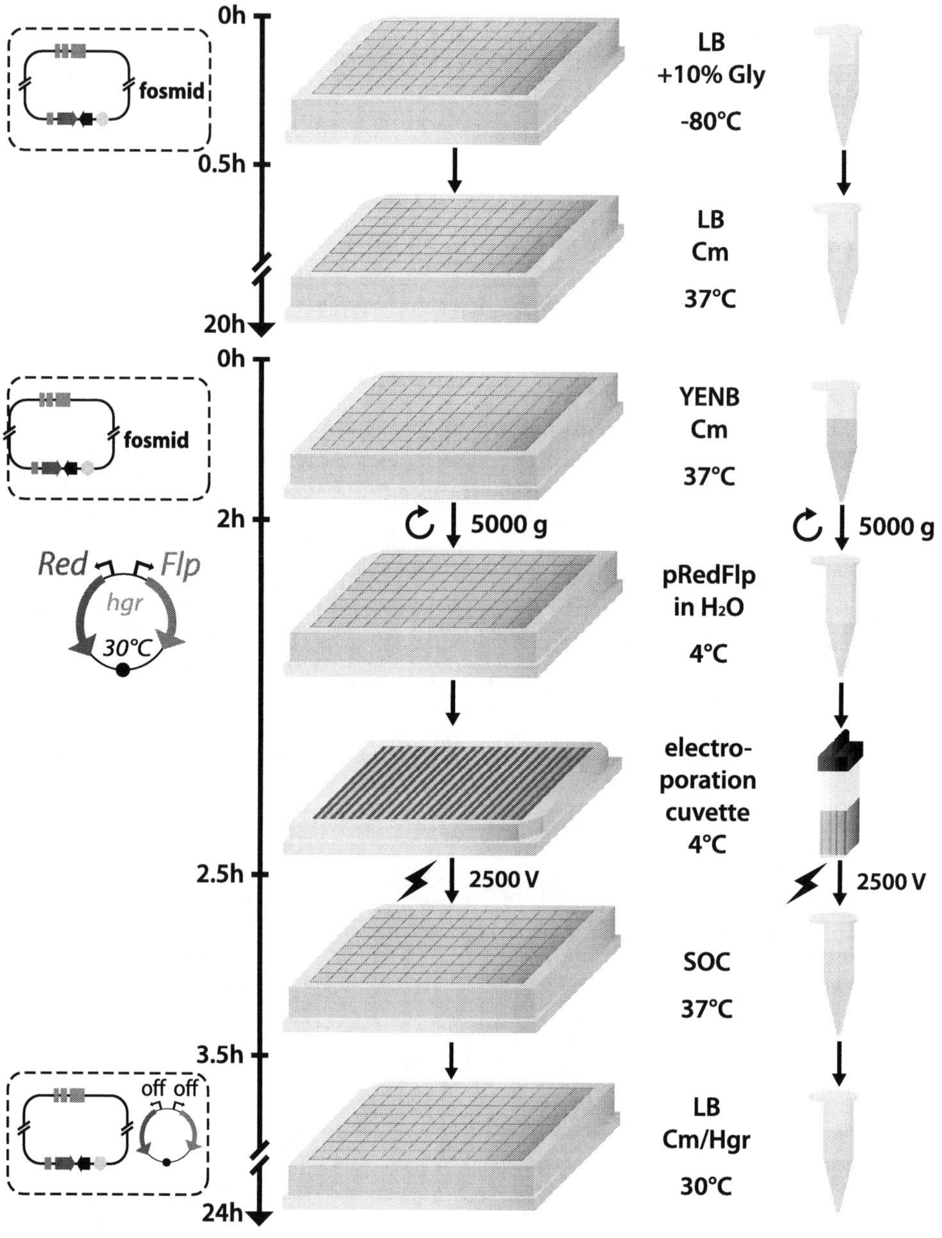


Fig. 3. Transformation of the recombineering helper.

2. Use 40 μl of the overnight cultures to inoculate 1 ml of YENB + Cm per well/tube. Seal the plate with an air-permeable seal and culture cells for 2 h at 37 °C with vigorous shaking. If using a single tube, puncture the lid with a sterile needle.
3. Centrifuge the plate/tube at 5,000 × *g* for 10 min at 2 °C. Discard the supernatant and blot any media residues on a stack of paper towels.
4. Add 1 ml of ice-cold 10% glycerol into each well/tube. Seal the plate with an aluminum or plastic seal.
5. Resuspend the bacteria by shaking the plate at 1,400 rpm for 1 min at 2 °C or by vortexing the tube.
6. Centrifuge the plate/tube at 5,000× *g* for 10 min at 2 °C. Discard the supernatant and blot any media residues on a stack of paper towels.
7. Add 100 μl of pRedFlp4 (0.1 ng/μl in ice-cold water) into each well/tube. Resuspend the bacteria by pipetting.
8. Transfer the cell suspension into a chilled (96-well) electroporation cuvette and electroporate at 2,500 V (see Note 11).
9. Immediately transfer the cell suspension into a new plate/tube with 1 ml of SOC per well/tube.
10. Seal the plate with an air-permeable seal and culture for 1 h at 37 °C (see Note 12) with vigorous shaking. If using a single tube, puncture the lid with a sterile needle.
11. Use 100 μl of the transformed bacteria to inoculate 1 ml of LB + Cm + Hgr per well/tube. Seal the plate with an air-permeable seal and culture overnight at 30 °C with vigorous shaking. If using a single tube, puncture the lid with a sterile needle.

### 3.3. Tagging by Red/ET Recombination

In the following steps, the Red-mediated homologous recombination is performed (Figs. 1b and 4). l-Rhamnose induces Red operon expression and thus homologous recombination. Then the PCR product is electroporated into the cells. This PCR product contains a kanamycin resistance gene. In the last step, recombinant fosmids are selected on kanamycin. Two controls can help in the evaluation of the success of each step prior to clone validation: a "no tagging cassette" control and a "no Red induction" control.

1. Use 40 μl of the overnight cultures to inoculate 1 ml of YENB + Cm + Hgr per well/tube.
2. Seal the plate with an air-permeable seal and culture cells for 2 h at 30 °C with vigorous shaking. If using a single tube, puncture the lid with a sterile needle.
3. Induce Red operon expression by adding 20 μl of 25% l-rhamnose into each well/tube.

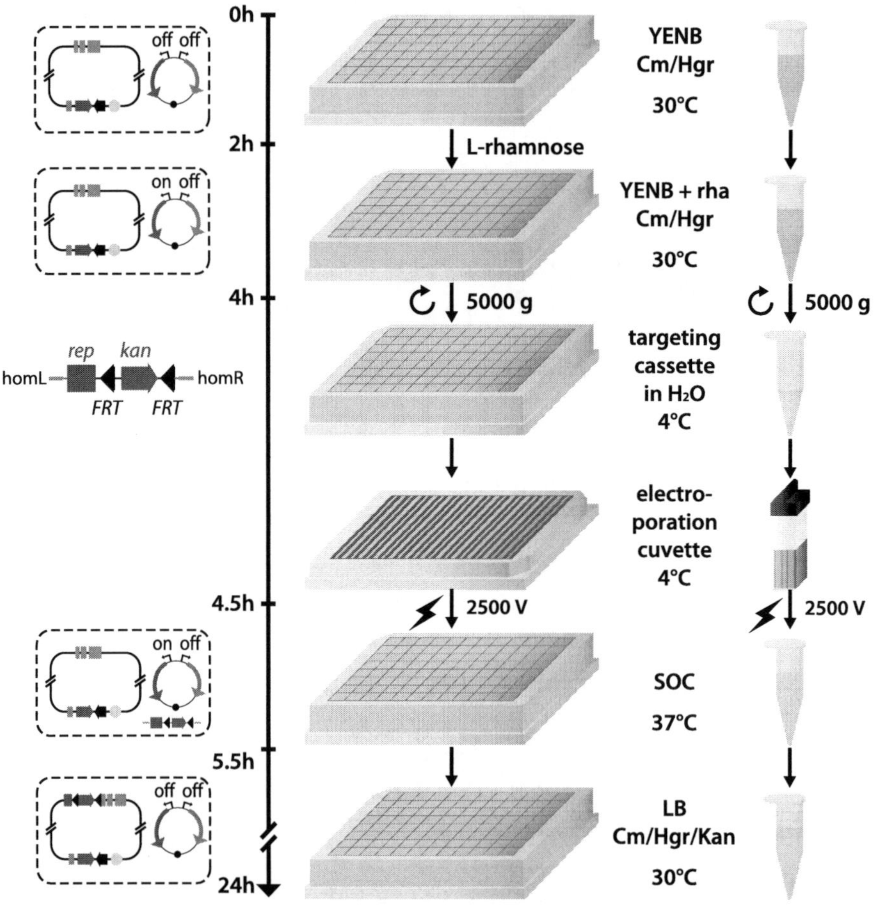


Fig. 4. Tagging by homologous recombination.

4. Seal the plate with an air-permeable seal and incubate plate/tube for 2 h at 30 °C with vigorous shaking. If using a single tube, puncture the lid with a sterile needle.
5. Centrifuge the plate/tube at 5,000× *g* for 10 min at 2 °C. Discard supernatant and blot any media residues on a stack of paper towels.
6. Add 1 ml of ice-cold 10% glycerol into each well/tube. Seal the plate with an aluminum or plastic seal.
7. Resuspend the bacteria by vigorously shaking the plate for 1 min at 2 °C or by vortexing the tube.
8. Centrifuge the plate/tube at 5,000× *g* for 10 min at 2 °C. Discard the supernatant and blot any media residues on a stack of paper towels.
9. Add 100 μl of the tagging cassette (5 ng/μl in ice-cold water) into each well/tube. Resuspend cells by pipetting.

10. Transfer the cell suspension into a chilled (96-well) electroporation cuvette and electroporate at 2,500 V.
11. Immediately transfer the cell suspension into a new plate/tube with 1 ml of SOC per well/tube.
12. Seal the plate with an air-permeable seal and culture for 1 h at 37 °C with vigorous shaking. If using a single tube, puncture the lid with a sterile needle.
13. Use 100 μl of the transformed bacteria to inoculate 1 ml of LB + Cm + Hgr + Kan per well/tube. Seal the plate with an air-permeable seal and culture overnight at 30 °C with vigorous shaking. If using a single tube, puncture the lid with a sterile needle (see Notes 13 and 14 for suitable efficiency controls at this step).

### 3.4. Removal of the Selectable Marker and pRedFlp Helper

In the following steps, the FRT-flanked selectable marker is removed (Figs. 1c and 5). Anhydrotetracyclin (AHT) induces Flippase (Flp) expression. This enzyme catalyzes recombination between Flippase Recognition Target (FRT) sites and thus removes the kan gene. The pRedFlp plasmid (6) has a temperature-sensitive origin of replication from pSC101 (1). In the last step, overnight growth at 37 °C instead of 30 °C removes pRedFlp plasmids from the cells.

1. Use 10 μl of the overnight cultures to inoculate 1 ml of LB + Cm + Hgr + AHT per well/tube.

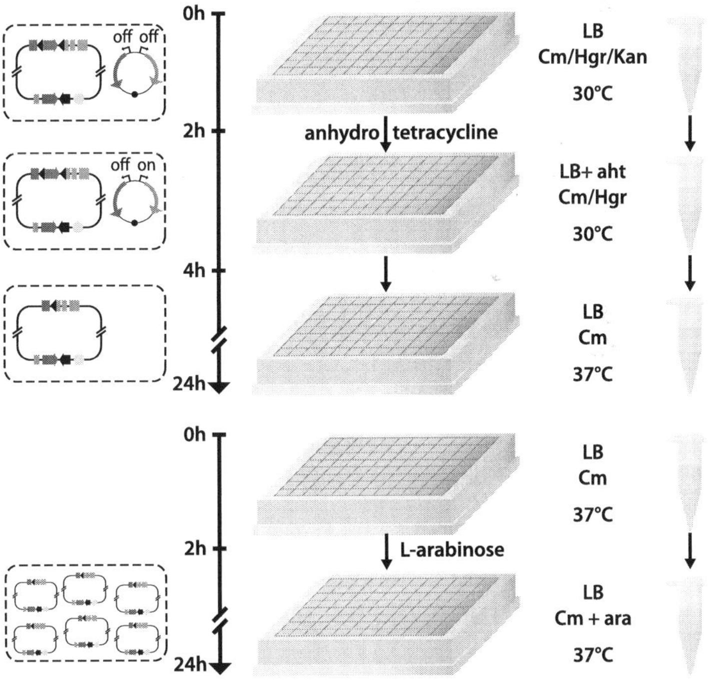


Fig. 5. Removal of selectable marker.

2. Seal the plate with an air-permeable seal and culture for 2 h at 30 °C with vigorous shaking. If using a single tube, puncture the lid with a sterile needle.
3. Use 100 µl of the cultures to inoculate 1 ml of LB + Cm per well/tube.
4. Seal the plate with an air-permeable seal and culture overnight at 37 °C with vigorous shaking. If using a single tube, puncture the lid with a sterile needle.

### 3.5. Verification of the Tagging Result

The recombinant clones are verified by sequencing (Fig. 6).

1. Design a pair of sequencing primers extending from within the tag toward the gene–tag junctions. If the recombineering cassette contains the FRT-flanked selectable marker, include the primer on the selectable cassette side before the first FRT.
2. Isolate the BAC/fosmid DNA from the modified clones. We suggest using the high-throughput miniprep protocol (see Chapter 25) or the Epicentre miniprep kit.
3. Sequence the modified clones using designed primers.
4. Verify the sequencing results. The sequencing reads should include the tag end-sequences and the homology arms. The FRT-flanked selectable marker should not be present.

### 3.6. DNA Purification and Fly Transformation

Fosmid DNA purified from the modified FlyFos clones can be directly used for fly transgenesis. l-Arabinose (Ara) is used to induce fosmids to high copy by activating oriV. This part of the protocol requires the Plasmid Maxi Kit (QIAGEN).

1. Inoculate 50 ml of LB + Cm with a single colony of FlyFos strain. Culture overnight at 37 °C with vigorous shaking.
2. Use 2 ×5 ml to inoculate 2 ×500 ml LB + Cm + Ara in 2,500 ml flasks. Culture overnight at 37 °C. Shake cultures vigorously.
3. Harvest the bacterial cells by centrifugation at 6,000× *g* for 15 min at 4 °C.
4. Resuspend the bacterial pellet from both flasks combined in 50 ml of Buffer P1.

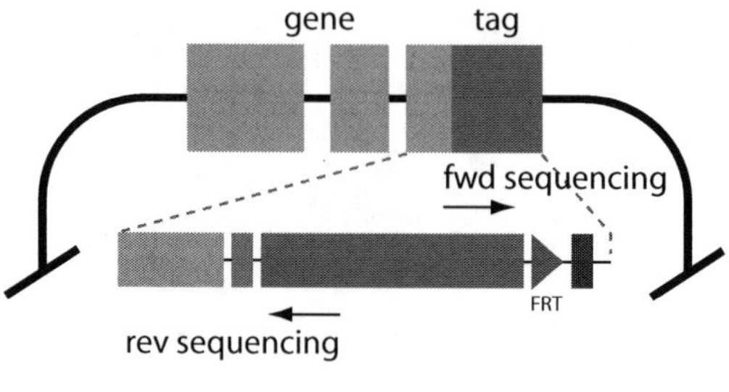


Fig. 6. Tagging verification.

5. Add 50 ml of Buffer P2, mix thoroughly by vigorously inverting 4–6 times, and incubate at room temperature for 5 min.
6. Add 50 ml of chilled Buffer P3, mix immediately and thoroughly by vigorously inverting 4–6 times, and incubate on ice for 30 min.
7. Centrifuge at ≥20,000× *g* for 30 min at 4°C. Remove supernatant containing fosmid DNA promptly.
8. Place folded Whatmann filter in a 50-ml syringe. Prewet and compress filter by passing water through the syringe. Use such prepared syringe for filtering supernatant.
9. Precipitate the DNA by adding 105 ml (0.7 volumes) of room temperature isopropanol to the lysate. Centrifuge at ≥15,000× *g* for 30 min at 4°C, and carefully decant the supernatant.
10. Redissolve the DNA pellet in 500 μl of warm (60°C) TE buffer, pH 8.0, and add Buffer QBT to obtain a final volume of 12 ml.
11. Equilibrate a QIAGEN-tip 500 by applying 10 ml of Buffer QBT, and allow the column to empty by gravity flow.
12. Apply the DNA solution from step 10 to the QIAGEN-tip and allow it to enter the resin by gravity flow.
13. Wash the QIAGEN-tip with 2 × 30 ml of Buffer QC.
14. Elute DNA with 15 ml of Buffer QF.
15. Precipitate DNA by adding 10.5 ml (0.7 volumes) of room temperature isopropanol to the eluted DNA. Mix and centrifuge immediately at ≥15,000× *g* for 30 min at 4°C. Carefully decant the supernatant.
16. Wash DNA pellet with 5 ml of room-temperature 70% ethanol, and centrifuge at ≥15,000× *g* for 10 min. Carefully decant the supernatant without disturbing the pellet.
17. Wash DNA pellet again with 5 ml of room-temperature 70% ethanol, and centrifuge at ≥15,000× *g* for 10 min. Carefully decant the supernatant without disturbing the pellet.
18. Air-dry the pellet for 5–10 min, and redissolve the DNA in a suitable volume (250 μl) of warm (60°C) nuclease-free water.
19. Use isolated fosmid DNA for injection into the *attP* landing line (see Note 15).

## 4. Notes

1. Use nuclease-free water to prepare DNA handling buffers and all enzymatic reactions.
2. Use Milli-Q or equivalent to minimize the salt concentration during electroporation.

3. Super Optimal broth with Catabolite repression (SOC) is a rich bacterial medium that greatly increases transformation efficiencies by facilitating cell survival after electroporation.
4. Yeast Extract, Nutrient Broth (YENB) medium is a rich, salt-free medium, optimal for preparation of the electrocompetent cells (10). While other media, like LB or SOC can be used for bacterial culture, two washing steps are required for optimal electroporation.
5. Active concentrations of hygromycin from different providers vary, test each batch to ensure that you are using the restrictive concentration and store it in single use aliquots at –20°C.
6. The recombineering efficiency is proportional to the length of the homology arms and reverse-proportional to the length of the insert. Therefore, it might be wise to extend the homology arms for long recombineering cassettes. Moreover, as it is suggested that recombineering of fragments longer than 3kb occurs in an alternate, low efficiency pathway (11), the recombineering cassette size should be kept below 3kb if possible. Longer fragments can still be used for recombineering, however, lower efficiencies should be expected. Therefore, we recommend plating bacteria on selective agar (LA+Cm+Kan+Hgr, culture ON at 30°C) and screening clones by PCR after the tagging step.
7. We have developed and tested dozens of tagging cassettes that include various fluorescent markers. Some examples are presented in Fig. 7. The tagging cassettes are cloned in a pR6K-based (5) vector that can be propagated in *pir-116 E. coli* strain (Epicentre) only. This greatly reduces background originating from trace amounts of the PCR template that transforms bacteria (6, 8). If other vectors are used for amplification of the tagging cassette, we suggest digesting the PCR product with *DpnI* (NEB), that cuts methylated DNA only.
8. Minimize the amount of PCR cycles to avoid point mutations introduced by the polymerase. Increase the amount of PCR template if necessary. Use a good proof-reading polymerase (we recommend Phusion from NEB/Finnzymes).
9. We recommend using a PCR purification kit with oligonucleotide cut-off over 100 bases, such as Invitrogen PureLink™ PCR purification Kit.
10. When preparing electrocompetent cells, work in a cold room. Avoid exposing cells to temperatures higher than 41°C. For best efficiencies work as fast as possible.
11. The presented voltage (2,500V) applies to cuvettes with 2mm electrode gap. For other types of cuvettes, use 1,250V/mm.

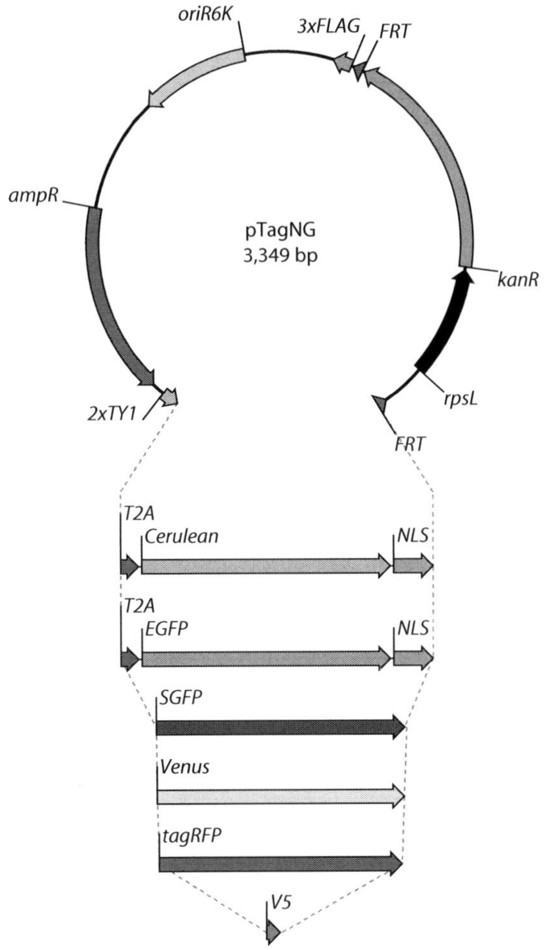


Fig. 7. Example recombineering vectors.

12. The pRedFlp plasmid (6) has a temperature-sensitive origin of replication from pSC101 (1). It has to be maintained at 30°C and can be removed from the cells by overnight growth at 37°C in the absence of hygromycin.
13. Plating on selective agar (LA + Cm + Kan) after the tagging step will give you an estimate of the success rate of recombineering. Expect between 10 and 100 cfu/reaction.
14. In our experiments, we have repeatedly obtained recombineering efficiencies (successfully validated out of attempted constructs) between 75 and 100%.
15. We strongly recommend using landing lines that express φC31 integrase in the posterior pole, such as *nanos* or *vasa* promoter-driven constructs (12). For best results, use the prepared DNA as soon as possible. Avoid freezing isolated fosmids.

## References


1. Zhang Y, Buchholz F, Muyrers JP et al (1998) A new logic for DNA engineering using recombination in Escherichia coli. Nat Genet **20**:123–128
2. Murphy KC (1998) Use of bacteriophage lambda recombination functions to promote gene replacement in Escherichia coli. J Bacteriol **180**:2063–2071
3. Muyrers JP, Zhang Y, Testa G et al (1999) Rapid modification of bacterial artificial chromosomes by ET-recombination. Nucleic Acids Res **27**:1555–1557
4. Testa G, Zhang Y, Vintersten K et al (2003) Engineering the mouse genome with bacterial artificial chromosomes to create multipurpose alleles. Nat Biotechnol **21**:443–447
5. Wang J, Sarov M, Rientjes J et al (2006) An improved recombineering approach by adding RecA to lambda Red recombination. Mol Biotechnol **32**:43–53
6. Sarov M, Schneider S, Pozniakovski A et al (2006) A recombineering pipeline for functional genomics applied to Caenorhabditis elegans. Nat Methods **3**:839–844
7. Poser I, Sarov M, Hutchins JRA et al (2008) BAC TransgeneOmics: a high-throughput method for exploration of protein function in mammals. Nat Methods **5**:409–415
8. Ejsmont RK, Sarov M, Winkler S et al (2009) A toolkit for high-throughput, cross-species gene engineering in Drosophila. Nat Methods **6**:435–437
9. Groth AC, Fish M, Nusse R et al (2004) Construction of transgenic Drosophila by using the site-specific integrase from phage phiC31. Genetics **166**:1775–1782
10. Sharma RC, Schimke RT (1996) Preparation of electrocompetent E coli using salt-free growth medium. Biotechniques **20**:42–44
11. Maresca M, Erler A, Fu J et al (2010) Single-stranded heteroduplex intermediates in lambda Red homologous recombination. BMC Mol Biol **11**:54
12. Bischof J, Maeda RK, Hediger M et al (2007) An optimized transgenesis system for Drosophila using germ-line-specific phiC31 integrases. Proc Natl Acad Sci USA **104**: 3312–3317

# Chapter 27

# Overlap Extension PCR: An Efficient Method for Transgene Construction

**Matthew D. Nelson and David H.A. Fitch**

## Abstract

Combining genes or regulatory elements to make hybrid genes is a widely used methodology throughout the biological sciences. Here, we describe an optimized approach for hybrid gene construction called overlap extension PCR. In this method, the polymerase chain reaction (PCR) is employed for efficient and reliable construction of hybrid genes. A PCR-based approach does not rely on available restriction sites or other specific sequences, an advantage over more conventional cloning or recombineering methods. With the use of high-fidelity DNA polymerase, this method can be used for making even very large constructs (>20 kb) with minimal unwanted mutations. Finally, overlap extension-PCR can be used as a means for site-directed mutagenesis, introducing desired mutations to the final hybrid gene.

**Key words:** PCR, Cloning, Hybrid genes, Transgenics, Site-directed mutagenesis, Gene expression

## 1. Introduction

Hybrid genes are powerful tools for the study of gene expression and function. Temporal and spatial expression of genes and gene products can be determined by fusing *cis*-regulatory elements and coding sequences of genes to the coding sequences of reporters, such as the green fluorescent protein (1). Gene regulation can be studied by subsequent mutagenesis of stretches of sequence within these hybrid genes. For example, mutating a functional transcription factor binding site within the promoter of a gene can result in altered expression of a reporter relative to its nonmutated form. Also, fusing variations of the coding sequence of a protein to a reporter can provide information about the localization and function of gene products. In addition, for a more detailed study of where and how a protein functions in vivo, one can misexpress or

Virginie Orgogozo and Matthew V. Rockman (eds.), *Molecular Methods for Evolutionary Genetics*,
Methods in Molecular Biology, vol. 772, DOI 10.1007/978-1-61779-228-1_27, © Springer Science+Business Media, LLC 2011

partially express a gene using the promoter of another gene. In the context of evolutionary investigations, fusion of genes can be used to create hypothetical ancestors, interspecific hybrids, or other such constructs. *Cis*-regulatory evolution can involve the reorganization and change in sequences of *cis*-regulatory elements (2), and specific hypotheses can be tested via the construction of reporters driven by various regulatory sequences. Also, directed evolution experiments to design thermostable enzymes (3) have used various gene fusion methods to study protein-coding sequence evolution.

For all of the above applications, one must combine multiple genes or portions of genes together to construct a hybrid gene. Hybrid gene construction has conventionally been accomplished by restriction enzyme-based cloning methods. The gene constructs can then be further manipulated via site-directed mutagenesis. Powerful as these methods are, conventional cloning usually requires multiple days to weeks of work and troubleshooting. Such cloning methods are dependent on particular sequences recognized by restriction enzymes. Recombineering methods, which utilize recombinase systems, are much faster and more versatile than traditional restriction enzyme-based methods but more costly and still require the incorporation of particular sequences.

Overlap-extension PCR (OE-PCR) provides a rapid and cost effective means for the creation of hybrid genes without the need for available enzyme recognition sequences (4–7). Furthermore, PCR-based methods have become increasingly reliable with the introduction of high-fidelity DNA polymerases, thus limiting the number of unwanted mutations in the final construct (8). This method has proven to be useful for the construction of even very large hybrid genes (>20 kb) (9). Not only does OE-PCR allow for combining genes; it can also be used to directly mutate sequences within the genes that are being fused together (10, 11). OE-PCR produces a linearized hybrid gene that can simply be cloned into a standard plasmid for bacterial propagation (or used directly, as in the case of *C. elegans* transgenics). This chapter describes the methodology of OE-PCR for the construction of hybrid genes and for the application of site-directed mutagenesis. The protocol described here has been adapted from previously published methods (9, 10) and optimized in our lab for making fluorescent protein fusions and gene expression reporters for *C. elegans* developmental genetics, as well as for creating hybrids from genes of different species. However, the method is generally applicable for genetic engineering.

## 2. Materials

### 2.1. PCR

1. DNA oligonucleotides (oligos) purified by desalting and manufactured at standard synthesis scale (0.025 μmol for oligos <50 bp, and 0.05 μmol for >50 bp). Oligos are dissolved in 1×

TE buffer (pH 8.0, 10 mM Tris–HCl, 1 mM EDTA) to 100 μM stocks and stored at −20°C. Working stocks are diluted in ultrapure water to 25 μM and stored at −20°C.

2. Herculase Hotstart DNA polymerase (Agilent Technologies), stored at −20°C. Any *Pfu* DNA polymerase can be used. A 10× stock of Herculase reaction buffer is provided with the enzyme. Importantly, a DNA polymerase such as that derived from *Pyrococcus furiosus* (*Pfu*) must be used, not an enzyme such as that derived from *Thermus aquaticus* (*Taq*). Taq enzymes leave A-overhangs at the 3′-end, which would disrupt the overlap steps (9).
3. Deoxyribonucleotide triphosphates (dNTPs) are diluted to a working solution of 10 mM each in ultrapure water.

### 2.2. DNA Purification and Agarose Gel Electrophoresis

1. Agarose is dissolved in 1× TAE buffer (40 mM Tris–acetate, 1 mM EDTA), heated to make an agarose gel, and supplemented with ethidium bromide (0.5 μg/mL). Electrophoresis is carried out in 1× TAE.
2. When a PCR reaction contains only a single fragment, visualized by gel electrophoresis as a single band, the PCR reaction can be purified directly over a column. We use the QIAquick PCR purification kit (Qiagen).
3. However, if the PCR product contains multiple fragments, the PCR products must be separated by gel electrophoresis and the appropriate bands cut out and purified. We use the Wizard® SV gel and PCR-purification system (Promega).
4. Concentration of PCR products is determined using a NanoDrop 2000c (Thermo Scientific).

## 3. Methods

The concept of OE-PCR is to combine fragments of DNA by using complementary 3′ or 5′ ends in a PCR reaction without primers (Fig. 1). The complementary sequence is introduced to one or both ends of a fragment through hybrid primers which match the template for approximately 20 nucleotides at the 3′ end and have a 5′ tail which matches the sequence of the fragment to be fused. This allows the complimentary ends of the fragments to act as priming sites for DNA polymerase so that the fragments are spliced together. Nested primers are added in a subsequent PCR reaction to amplify the desired hybrid gene.

### 3.1. Oligo Design

A crucial first step in OE-PCR is the design of oligonucleotides. Designing oligos that bind at the 5′ and 3′ ends of the desired hybrid gene is straightforward and does not require the addition of

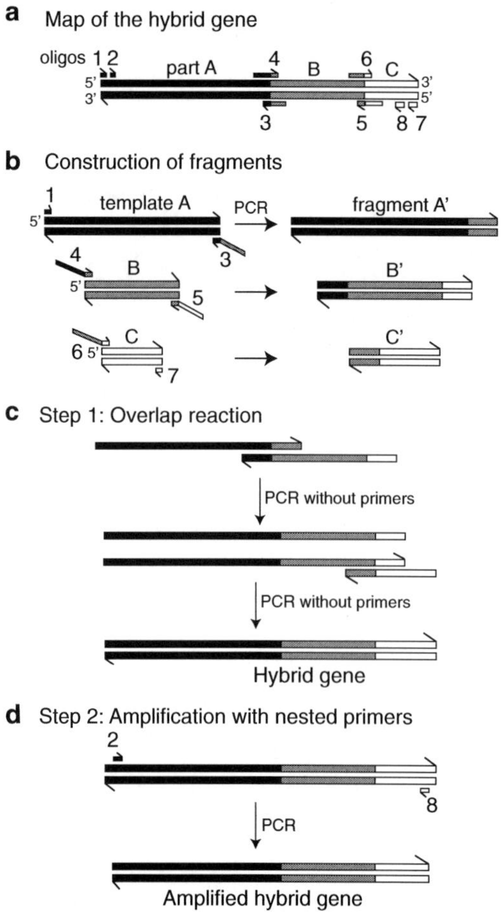


Fig. 1. The concept of OE-PCR. *Bars* represent single DNA strands; *different shades of the bars* represent the different sequences that will be fused. The 3′ end of the strand is indicated by a *small line like a half-arrowhead projecting from the end of each bar*. The 5′ end is sometimes indicated with a *label*. (**a**) Overall map of the oligo sequences to the final hybrid product. The hybrid consists of three parts: A, B, and C. In the example described in the text, A is the 5′-regulatory region of *C. elegans nhr-25*, B is the coding sequence for GFP, and C is the 3′-UTR of *nhr-25*. Sequences corresponding to the eight primers (*thin bars*) used to generate this hybrid gene are indicated adjacent to the strand from which the sequences come (*sense on top*, *antisense on bottom*). (**b**) Construction of the fragments. Oligo pairs (e.g., oligos 1 and 3) are shown that bind to a template sequence (e.g., template A) and are used to amplify a fragment (e.g., fragment A′). Only the 3′ end of each hybrid primer (here, oligos 3–6) binds to the template. The 5′ tails of the hybrid primers generate the portions of the fragment that overlap the sequence of a different template. (**c**) In step 1 of the overlap reaction (overlap extension), which occurs in the absence of primers, some of the reannealing strands will be from different fragments; they will anneal in the overlap regions created by the hybrid primers. Extension from the 3′ ends of the overlapping fragments will result in "fused" products. This will actually occur in at least two steps. In the example shown, fragment A′ and B′ combine first and, in a subsequent step, an A′ + B′ strand anneals with a C′ strand; extension will then result in the final tripartite hybrid product. (**d**) In step 2 of the overlap reaction (amplification), the hybrid gene is specifically amplified by using nested primers (oligos 2 and 8).

any noncomplementary sequences to the ends (Fig. 1, oligos 1, 2, 7, 8). However, the internal oligos that connect different stretches of DNA require the addition of nucleotides to the 5′end (Fig. 1, oligos 3–6). The additional sequence is not complementary to the template sequence but is complementary to the sequence to which the PCR product will be fused. The specifics for the design of oligos are as follows (see Fig. 1a, b):

1. The number of oligos needed for a given gene construct can be determined by the formula: $2N+2$, where $N$ is the number of unique PCR amplified sequences to be fused together. Figure 1 shows a hybrid gene composed of three parts and thus requires 8 oligos. Theoretically, however, this technique can be used to fuse as many fragments as desired.
2. Oligos 1, 2, 7, and 8 should be >21 bp in length to prevent nonspecific binding and thus unwanted products that will interfere with the overlap steps. In this example, oligos 1 and 2 are "forward" primers (contain sequence from the "sense" strand) and oligos 7 and 8 are "reverse" primers (i.e., contain sequence from the "antisense" strand). That is, oligos 7 and 8 must be antiparallel to the orientation of oligos 1 and 2. Also, it should be noted that oligos 2 and 8 are nested with respect to oligos 1 and 7. The distance between oligos 1 and 2 or between 2 and 8 is arbitrary (see Note 1).
3. Oligos 1 (sense) and 3 (antisense) are the primer pair used to produce and amplify fragment A′. The 3′ portion of oligo 3 which binds to template A should be 21–30 bp in length. The 5′ portion of oligo 3 that is not complementary to template A should be as long as possible (>20 bp) without significant secondary structure and should be complementary to template B. If fusing two coding sequences, make sure the sequences maintain the correct reading frame. Also, ensure that the orientation of the fusion is correct (i.e., for oligo 3, the 5′ end of the antisense sequence from template A is linked to the 3′ end of the antisense sequence from template B).
4. Oligos 4 (sense) and 5 (antisense) are the primer pair for amplifying fragment B′. Oligo 4 is essentially the reverse complement of oligo 3. However, the 3′ part that binds to template B should be adjusted to include 21–30 bp at the end of template B. Also, the 5′ tail of oligo 4 should be lengthened (relative to the corresponding portion of oligo 3) if possible to increase the amount of overlap. The 3′-end of oligo 5 is the antisense sequence of template B. The 5′ portion of oligo 5 contains sequence complementary to the beginning of template C.
5. Oligos 6 (sense) and 7 (antisense) are used to produce and amplify fragment C′. Oligo 6 is similar to, but the reverse complement of oligo 5. The 3′ portion of oligo 6 that binds to

template C should be 21–30 bp long and the 5′ tail that overlaps with B sequence should be as long as possible.

A general principle in designing the overlap primers is that the 3′ portion that is complementary to the template should range 21–30 bp in length and the 5′ tail with the "overlap sequence" should be as long as possible so as to maximize the chances of overlap in subsequent steps. This requires the design of relatively long oligos (50–90 bp), and optimization of sequences to limit homo- and heterodimer formation is necessary. Tools useful for estimating the properties of the designed oligos are listed below. However, other online or downloadable tools are also available.

To check for homodimers and to estimate the melting temperature ($T_m$), we use the Sigma DNA Calculator (http://www.sigma-genosys.com/calc/DNACalc.asp).

To determine the nature of interactions between oligo pairs (i.e. heterodimers), we use the Finnzyme Multiple primer analyzer (http://www.finnzymes.com/java_applets/multiple_primer_analyzer.html). The default settings are sufficiently stringent to design useful oligos, and the "value for sensitivity of dimer detection" has been adjusted as high as 5 (scale 1–10) with success.

### 3.2. Amplification of Fragments and Purification

While OE-PCR can be used to create a broad spectrum of different types of hybrid genes, one very useful application is the construction of GFP (green fluorescent protein) transgenes. We use this application as an example for the remainder of this chapter. In this example, the hybrid gene is composed of three fragments: A′, B′, and C′, which are amplified from templates A, B, and C, respectively. Both the A′ fragment and C′ fragment are amplified from genomic DNA, while the B′ fragment is amplified from a gfp-containing plasmid, pPD95.75 (Addgene) (12). Fragment A′ is the 5′-*cis*-regulatory region and promoter of the *nhr-25* gene of *C. elegans*; fragment B′ is the coding sequence, containing synthetic introns, of GFP; and fragment C′ is the 3′-UTR (untranslated region) of *nhr-25* (Fig. 1a).

1. Reaction mix for fragment A′:

   38.5 μl Ultrapure water

   5 μl 10× Herculase Buffer

   1 μl 10 mM dNTPs

   2 μl oligo 1 (25 μM)

   2 μl oligo 3 (25 μM)

   1 μl purified genomic DNA at 50 ng/μl (see Notes 2 and 3)

   0.5 μl (2.5 U) Herculase Hotstart DNA Polymerase

   In our example, fragment A′ should be ′9.1 kb in length, which is confirmed by the presence of a single band on a 1% agarose gel (Fig. 2a, lane 2).

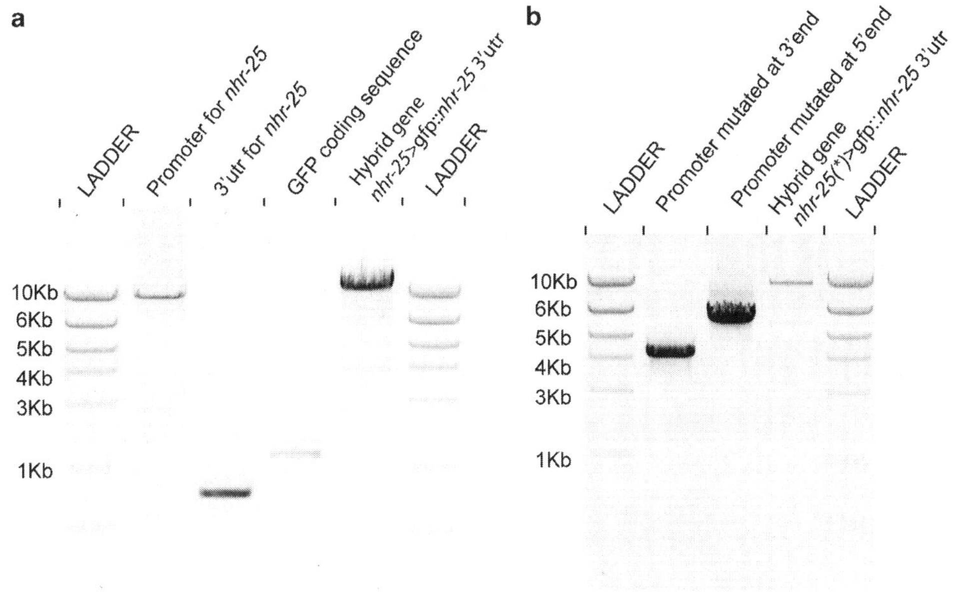


Fig. 2. 1% Agarose gels showing products of the PCR reactions to generate the fragments for OE-PCR and successful amplification of the hybrid genes *nhr-25*> *gfp::nhr-25* 3′utr (**a**) and *nhr-25*(*) > *gfp::nhr-25* 3′utr, which is mutated in the 5′-regulatory region (**b**). (**a**) *Lanes 2–4* show the three fragments A′, C′, and B′, and *lane 5* contains the hybrid gene. (**b**) *Lanes 2* and *3* show the two fragments for the mutated 5′-regulatory region of the gene. *Lane 4* shows the final hybrid gene after amplification. The hybrid was made by combining the two mutated promoter fragments, the GFP-coding fragment and the *nhr-25* 3′ UTR fragment. For this example, each fragment and the hybrid gene were column purified.

2. Reaction mix for fragment B′:

   39.4 μl Ultrapure water

   5 μl 10× Herculase Buffer

   1 μl 10 mM dNTPs

   2 μl oligo 4 (25 μM)

   2 μl oligo 5 (25 μM)

   0.1 μl pPD95.75 at 200 ng/μl

   0.5 μl Herculase Hotstart DNA Polymerase

   Fragment B′, in our example, is the coding sequence for GFP, and is approx. 1.1 kb (Fig. 2a, lane 4).

3. Reaction mix for fragment C′:

   38.5 μl Ultrapure water

   5 μl 10× Herculase Buffer

   1 μl 10 mM dNTPs

   2 μl oligo 6 (25 μM)

   2 μl oligo 7 (25 μM)

   1 μl purified genomic DNA

   0.5 μl Herculase Hotstart DNA Polymerase

The 3′UTR, which is ′420 bp, is fragment C′, and is verified on the gel (Fig. 2a, lane 3).

4. Thermocycler settings for all reactions:

| | |
|---|---|
| Initial denaturation | 92°C, 1 min |
| Amplification (37 cycles) | 92°C, 10 s (denaturation)<br>$T_m$-5°C, 30 s (annealing) (Note: for our example, we used an annealing temperature of 59°C)<br>68°C, 1 min/kb of fragment (extension) |
| Final extension | 72°C, 1 min/kb of fragment + 5 min |

5. 2 μl of the PCR product should be run on a 1% agarose gel to check whether more than one fragment was made.
6. Fragments can be purified using the QIAquick PCR purification kit and the clean products eluted in 50 μl of elution buffer. Go to Subheading 3.3.
7. If there is evidence of contaminating bands, the fragment should be gel purified (see Note 4).

### 3.3. Step 1 of the Overlap PCR Reaction: Overlap-Extension

The next step of the protocol is to combine the purified fragments in a PCR reaction that does not contain oligos for priming the reaction. The priming in this reaction will be facilitated by the overlapping ends of the fragments (Fig. 1c). In order for OE-PCR to work optimally, it is crucial that the fragments are combined at equimolar ratios (9).

1. Concentrations of each fragment must be determined. We use the Nanodrop 2000c, which determines concentrations in ng/μl. For our example, the concentrations of fragments A′, B′, and C′ are 65, 43, and 81 ng/μl, respectively.
2. The concentration of each fragment must then be converted to pmol/μl. Conversion tools are available online. Our lab uses the eBioInfogen Biotools micrograms to picomole calculator, www.ebioinfogen.com/biotools/micrograms-picomoles.htm. In our example, the concentrations of fragments A′, B′, and C′ are 0.011, 0.059, and 0.292 pmol/μl, respectively.
3. An equimolar amount of each fragment is combined in the reaction mix for a total concentration of 0.1 pmol for each fragment (the volume of each fragment solution required is calculated as 0.1/μl). The reaction mix (50 μl total volume) is as follows:

   to 50 μl with ultrapure water

   5 μl 10× Herculase Buffer

   1 μl 10 mM dNTPs

   0.1 pmol/μl of each fragment

   0.5 μl Herculase Hotstart DNA polymerase

Using our example, we would need the following reaction mix:

32.36 μl ultrapure water

5 μl 10× Herculase Buffer

1 μl 10 mM dNTPs

9.1 μl fragment A

1.7 μl fragment B

0.34 μl fragment C

0.5 μl Herculase Hotstart DNA polymerase

4. Thermocycler settings for this reaction is as follows:

| | |
|---|---|
| Initial denaturation | 92°C, 1 min |
| Amplification (13 cycles) | 92°C, 10 s (denaturation)<br>60°C, 1 min (annealing of fragments)<br>68°C, 1 min/kb of final hybrid gene size (extension) |
| Final elongation | 72°C, 1 min/kb of final hybrid gene size + 5 min |

In our example, the hybrid gene should be 9.1 kb + 1.1 kb + 420 bp, or approximately 10.6 kb in length. Thus, we used extension times of 11 min.

5. The products of this PCR reaction should not be visualized on a gel but should be purified directly using the QIAquick PCR purification kit, eluted in 30 μL of elution buffer.

### 3.4. Step 2 of the Overlap PCR: Amplification and Purification of the Final Product

The final step of the OE-PCR reaction is to amplify the desired hybrid genes. This is accomplished by using the purified product from step 1 as a template and the nested primers, oligos 2 and 8 (Fig. 1c). Using the nested primers instead of primers 1 and 7 ensures that only the desired fusion product is amplified.

Reaction Mix for Step 2:

29.5 μl ultrapure water

5 μl 10× polymerase buffer

1 μl 10 mM dNTPs

2 μl oligo 2 (25 μM)

2 μl oligo 8 (25 μM)

10 μl purified reaction products from step 1 above

0.5 μl DNA polymerase (We usually use Herculase for this amplification, as in the other PCR reactions described above. However, if the final product is to be cloned into a TA-cloning vector, an enzyme that adds an adenosine residue should be used.)

The final hybrid gene in our example is 10.6 kb in length (Fig. 2a, lane 5).

### 3.5. Using OE-PCR for Site-Directed Mutagenesis

OE-PCR can be used as a quick and efficient means to introduce mutations to specific positions of the hybrid gene (10, 11). The protocol for this application is the same as described above, except for modifications to the oligo design (Fig. 3a). As an example, we use the same hybrid gene described above, but we incorporate a mutation into the 5′ regulatory region of *nhr-25*. This requires the initial A′ fragment to be amplified as two fragments, A* and A**.

1. Mutations in the hybrid gene product are introduced using the primers. In our example, the 5′ tails of oligos 3a (antisense) and 3b (sense) carry the mutation (Fig. 3a, b). Oligo 3a and oligo 1 are the primer pair used to amplify fragment A*. The 3′ portion of oligo 3a that binds to the template should be directly adjacent to the sequence to be mutated and 21–30 bp in length. The 5′ tail of oligo 3a carries the mutation (but in this case is only noncomplementary to the template in the region of the mutation but not the surrounding sequences; Fig. 3b). The 5′ tail of oligo 3a should be as long as possible to increase the chances of overlap.
2. Oligo 3b (sense) and oligo 3 (antisense) are used to amplify fragment A**. Oligo 3b is essentially the reverse complement

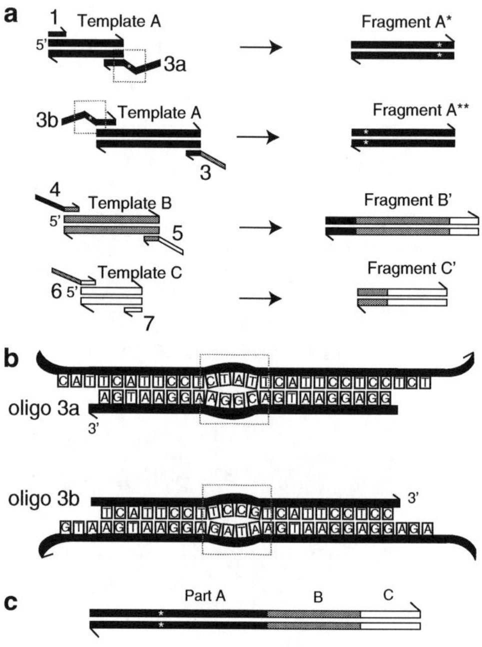


Fig. 3. Site-directed mutagenesis using OE-PCR. (**a**) Fragment A* is constructed using oligos 1 and 3a and fragment A** is made with oligos 3b and 3. Fragments B′ and C′ are made as described in Fig. 1. (**b**) Oligos 3a and 3b are complementary to the template but introduce a mutation (*indicated as an asterisk*). In this example, primers 3a and 3b are reverse complements of each other. (**c**) The result of the overlap reaction is a hybrid gene with a mutation in part A.

of oligo 3a (Fig. 27.3b). However, the 3′ portion of the oligo that binds to the template should be 21–30 bp, and the 5′ tail should be as long as possible.

3. Reaction mix for amplification of fragment A*:

   38.5 μl Ultrapure water

   5 μl 10× Herculase Buffer

   1 μl 10 mM dNTPs

   2 μl oligo 1 (25 μM)

   2 μl oligo 3a (25 μM)

   1 μl purified genomic DNA

   0.5 μl Herculase Hotstart DNA Polymerase

   In our example, fragment A* is 3.6 kb in length (Fig. 2b, lane 2).

4. Reaction mix for amplification of fragment A**:

   38.5 μl Ultrapure water

   5 μl 10× Herculase Buffer

   1 μl 10 mM dNTPs

   2 μl oligo 3b (25 μM)

   2 μl oligo 3 (25 μM)

   1 μl purified genomic DNA

   0.5 μl Herculase Hotstart DNA Polymerase

   This results in the amplification of fragment A**, which in our example is 5.5 kb (Fig. 2b, lane 3).

5. See Subheadings 3.2, steps 2 and 3 for the amplification of fragments B′ and C′, respectively.
6. Thermocycler settings are the same as above, Subheading 3.2, step 4.
7. For purification of fragments, see Subheading 3.2 steps 5–7.
8. OE-PCR is carried out in the same way as described above, Subheadings 3.3 and 3.4.
   In our example, we combine four fragments, A*, A**, B′, and C′ to make a 10.6-kb hybrid gene which carries a mutation in a specific region of the 5′-regulatory region (Fig. 3c).

## 4. Notes

1. Oligos 2 and 8 can also be designed with noncomplementary tails. Any restriction enzyme site can be incorporated for cloning into a circular plasmid for propagation of the hybrid gene in a bacterial strain. If such a site is to be engineered, it is often important to include additional nucleotides beyond the

restriction recognition site to allow the enzyme to cut the DNA. Manufacturers of restriction enzymes (e.g., New England Biolabs) generally provide information about how many or what additional nucleotides are required.

2. Cell lysates can be used in place of isolated genomic DNA as a template in the amplification of the initial fragments.
3. It is best to not use the same plasmid for generating the fragments for both ends of the hybrid gene. In such a case, the nested primers for amplifying the overlap product will also bind to the plasmid. Even small amounts of plasmid carried over from the initial PCR reactions will preferentially act as template in the amplification reaction instead of the hybrid gene. To eliminate this problem, gel purification can be used at all steps of the protocol.
4. An alternative to gel purifying the fragments, which we have found to work equally well, is to skip gel purification and purify the PCR product directly with the QIAquick PCR purification kit (Qiagen, Valencia, CA), leaving the contaminating fragments in with the desired fragments. The OE-PCR steps can be carried out with the contaminating fragments, resulting in a final desired product with multiple undesirable byproducts. Only one gel purification step is then required at the end.

## References


1. Chalfie M, Tu Y, Euskirchen G et al (1994) Green fluorescent protein as a marker for gene expression. Science **263**:802–805
2. Crocker J, Tamori Y, Erives A (2008) Evolution acts on enhancer organization to fine-tune gradient threshold readouts. PLoS Biol **6**:e263
3. Hamamatsu N, Aita T, Nomiya Y et al (2005) Biased mutation-assembling: an efficient method for rapid directed evolution through simultaneous mutation accumulation. Protein Eng Des Sel **18**:265–271
4. Mullis K, Faloona F, Scharf S et al (1986) Specific enzymatic amplification of DNA in vitro: the polymerase chain reaction. Cold Spring Harb Symp Quant Biol **51**:263–273
5. Horton RM, Hunt HD, Ho SN et al (1989) Engineering hybrid genes without the use of restriction enzymes: gene splicing by overlap extension. Gene 77:61–68
6. Yon J, Fried M (1989) Precise gene fusion by PCR. Nucleic Acids Res **17**:4895
7. Yolov AA, Shabarova ZA (1990) Constructing DNA by polymerase recombination. Nucleic Acids Res **18**:3983–3986
8. Lundberg KS, Shoemaker DD, Adams MW et al (1991) High-fidelity amplification using a thermostable DNA polymerase isolated from *Pyrococcus furiosus*. Gene **108**:1–6
9. Shevchuk NA, Bryksin AV, Nusinovich YA et al (2004) Construction of long DNA molecules using long PCR-based fusion of several fragments simultaneously. Nucleic Acids Res **32**:e19
10. Heckman KL, Pease LR (2007) Gene splicing and mutagenesis by PCR-driven overlap extension. Nat Protoc **2**:924–932
11. Ho SN, Hunt HD, Horton RM et al (1989) Site-directed mutagenesis by overlap extension using the polymerase chain reaction. Gene 77:51–59
12. Fire A, Harrison SW, Dixon D (1990) A modular set of lacZ fusion vectors for studying gene expression in *Caenorhabditis elegans*. Gene **93**:189–198

# Chapter 28

# Gene Knockdown Analysis by Double-Stranded RNA Injection


## Benjamin N. Philip and Yoshinori Tomoyasu



## Abstract

The discovery of RNAi, in which double-stranded RNA (dsRNA) suppresses the translation of homologous mRNA, has had a huge impact on evolutionary genetics by enabling the analysis of loss-of-function phenotypes in organisms in which classical genetic analysis is laborious or impossible.

In this chapter, we discuss an RNAi method via simple dsRNA injection in the red flour beetle, *Tribolium castaneum*. *Tribolium* is gaining popularity in evolutionary genetics due in part to the ease of RNAi application. We describe procedures for dsRNA synthesis and injection and provide a description of the injection apparatus. In addition, we detail two methods to validate the efficacy of RNAi (real-time PCR and western blot analyses). Although this chapter focuses mainly on *Tribolium*, many of the molecular biology and injection procedures described here are applicable to other organisms with some modifications. A few notes regarding dsRNA injection in other species are also included.



**Key words:** RNA interference, Double-stranded RNA, Injection, Real-time PCR, Western blot


## 1. Introduction

RNAi is an evolutionarily conserved gene silencing pathway found in diverse eukaryotic species (1–3). This biological process enables the analysis of loss-of-function phenotypes in organisms in which classical genetic analysis is laborious or impossible. The ease of RNAi application in the red flour beetle, *Tribolium castaneum*, has, thus, made this species a popular and powerful model in evolutionary genetics (4, 5).

In brief, RNAi is triggered by dsRNA molecules, which are processed into small interfering RNAs (siRNAs) by a dsRNase, Dicer. siRNA then binds to several proteins including Argonaute, forming a complex called RISC (RNA-Induced Silencing Complex). RISC binds to the target mRNA using complementarity between the


Virginie Orgogozo and Matthew V. Rockman (eds.), *Molecular Methods for Evolutionary Genetics*, Methods in Molecular Biology, vol. 772, DOI 10.1007/978-1-61779-228-1_28, © Springer Science+Business Media, LLC 2011

target sequence and the siRNA sequence and cleaves the mRNA through the action of the catalytic Argonaute protein. This intracellular RNAi machinery is well conserved among eukaryotes; therefore, RNAi can be triggered in many organisms once dsRNA (or siRNA) molecules are delivered inside the cell.

In contrast to the intracellular RNAi response, the mechanism by which the dsRNA enters a cell appears to be less conserved. This cellular dsRNA uptake process, sometimes called "systemic RNAi" (see Note 1), has an important implication for the application of RNAi to an organism of interest, as dsRNA molecules injected at a multicellular stage need to be taken up by cells to trigger an RNAi response. The degree of systemic RNAi effectiveness differs greatly among organisms (6–9), presumably in part because of the less conserved dsRNA cellular uptake machinery. Unfortunately, to date, it has been very difficult to predict whether an organism shows a robust systemic RNAi response without actually testing RNAi in the organism. A multi-transmembrane protein Sid-1 is an essential factor for systemic RNAi found in the nematode *Caenorhabditis elegans* (10, 11) and is suggested to be a determinant for the presence of systemic RNAi in some organisms (11). However, this view is currently under debate because of inconsistencies between the presence of *sid-1* homologs and the efficacy of systemic RNAi in some organisms, as well as the question whether *sid-1* homologs found outside nematodes are true orthologs of the *C. elegans sid-1* (8). Therefore, it is important to assess the efficacy of systemic RNAi carefully in an organism of interest before utilizing RNAi as a genetic tool in the organism.

*Tribolium* is found to show a robust systemic RNAi response throughout development, which makes it possible to perform RNAi at the postembryonic stage by injecting dsRNA into larval body cavities (larval RNAi) (12), or trigger an RNAi response in offspring embryos by injecting dsRNA into the mother's body cavity (parental RNAi) (13). As such, RNAi phenotypes in *Tribolium* are easy to obtain, highly reproducible, and are able to phenocopy the genetically null phenotypes (for example, *see* (13–15)). In addition, virtually all *Tribolium* tissues can respond to extracellular dsRNA (6). These traits allow researchers to create loss-of-function phenotypes at any desired stage in *Tribolium* by simple larval or pupal injection, making *Tribolium* a good alternative model organism to study gene function outside classic model organisms.

## 2. Materials

### 2.1. dsRNA Synthesis

1. A fragment of gene cloned into a plasmid. TOPO TA Cloning Kit for Sequence (Invitrogen) should be used in the case TOPO-RNAi primer is used for dsRNA template synthesis (see Subheading 3.1.1).

2. Go Taq DNA polymerase (Promega).
3. dNTP mixture (Takara Bio).
4. Thermal cycler (e.g., Bio-Rad).
5. DNA loading dye (Promega).
6. 100 bp DNA ladder 6× (Promega).
7. QIAquick PCR purification kit (QIAGEN).
8. DNA/RNA/Genetic analysis-grade agarose.
9. Spectrophotometer (e.g., NanoDrop 2000, Fisher Thermo Science).
10. Heating block (37°C and 70°C).
11. MEGAscript T7 Kit (Ambion). This kit contains TURBO DNase I.
12. MEGAclear (Ambion).
13. 100% ethanol.
14. 70% ethanol (diluted with $ddH_2O$) (stored at −20°C).

### 2.2. dsRNA Injection

Items 1–7 describe materials for *Tribolium* culturing (Fig. 1). Injection buffer requires items 8–14. Items 27–32 describe the injection apparatus (two examples of injection settings are shown

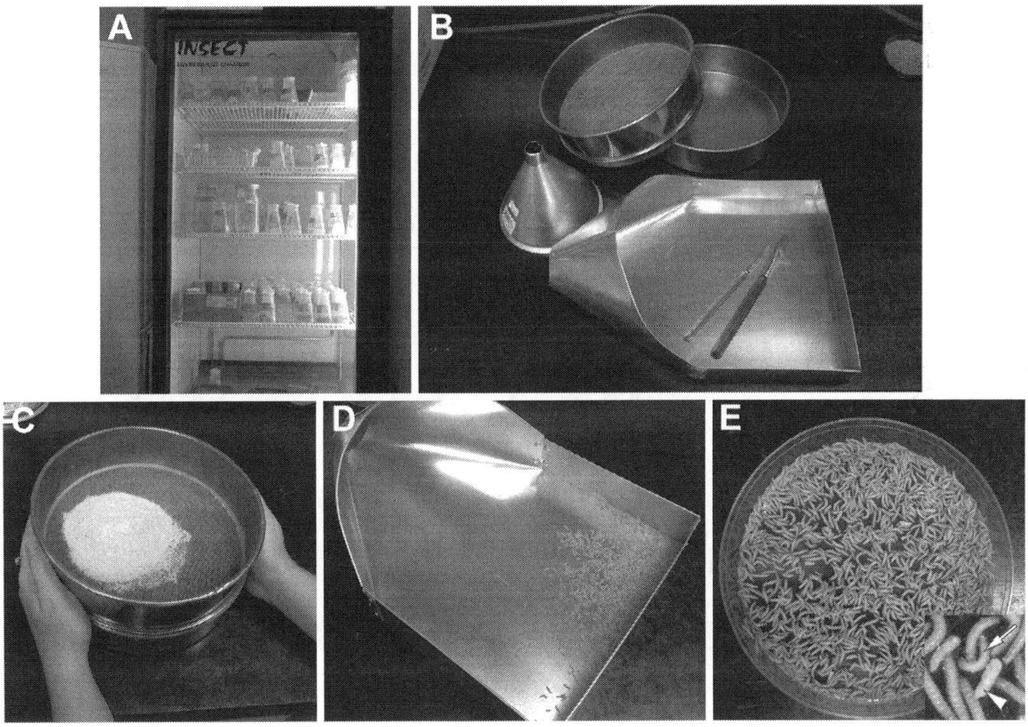


Fig. 1. *Tribolium* culturing and manipulation. (**a**) A beetle incubator. (**b**) Typical beetle equipment. (**c**, **d**) Isolating beetles from culture flour using a sieve (**c**) and a seed pan (**d**). (**e**) Isolated beetles (larvae and pupae) in a plastic Petri dish. A larva and pupa are indicated by *arrow* and *arrowhead* in inset, respectively.

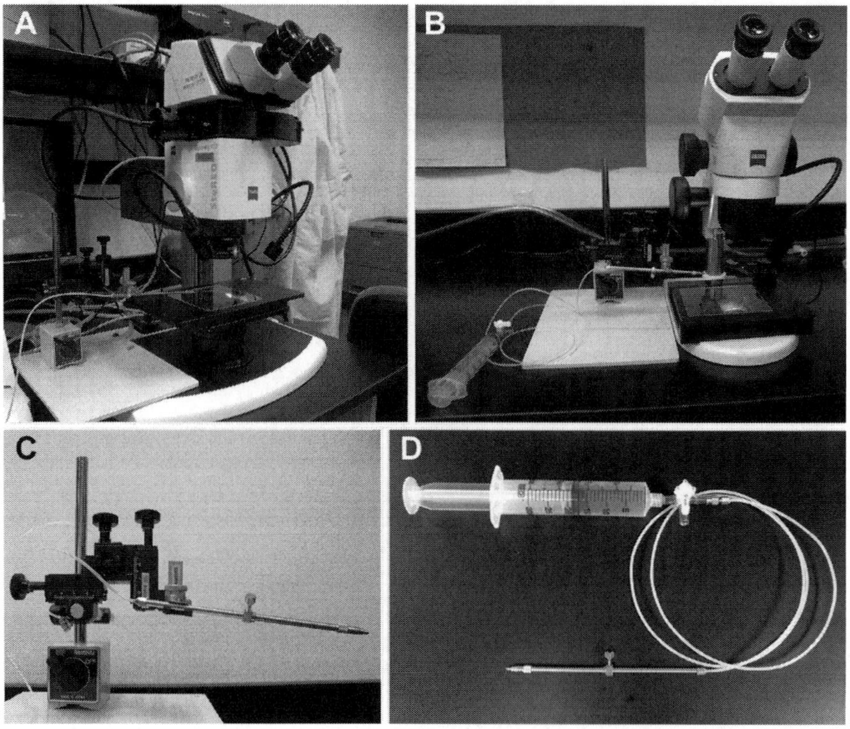

Fig. 2. Injection apparatus. (**a**, **b**) Two injection setups. (**c**) Typical manipulator orientation. (**d**) Injection syringe with a needle holder.

in Fig. 2a, b), and items 33–35 describe the etherization apparatus (Fig. 3c–e).

1. Flour: Organic whole wheat flour (e.g., Golden Buffalo Flour. Heartland Mill Inc. Kansas).
2. Brewer's Yeast (MP Biomedicals).
3. Culture Flour: Add 5% (by weight) of yeast to flour for nutrition supplement. Store at −20°C.
4. Culture bottles (Fig. 1a): 6 oz plastic *Drosophila* stock bottles (Flystuff.com).
5. Sieves: 8 in. diameter sieve (Fig. 1b, c) (#25 for larvae, pupae, and adults, #50 for embryos) (Fisher).
6. Beetle collection pan (Fig. 1b, d): 1.5 quart spouted sample pan (Seedburo Equipment Co.).
7. Incubator (Fig. 1a): A humidity-controlled incubator is preferable, e.g., Insect Chamber (BioCold Environmental Inc). *Tribolium* can be cultured at 30°C with 50% humidity. A lower temperature (20–25°C) can be used for long-term stock maintenance. Detailed *Tribolium* husbandry information can be found at the USDA *Tribolium* home page (16).

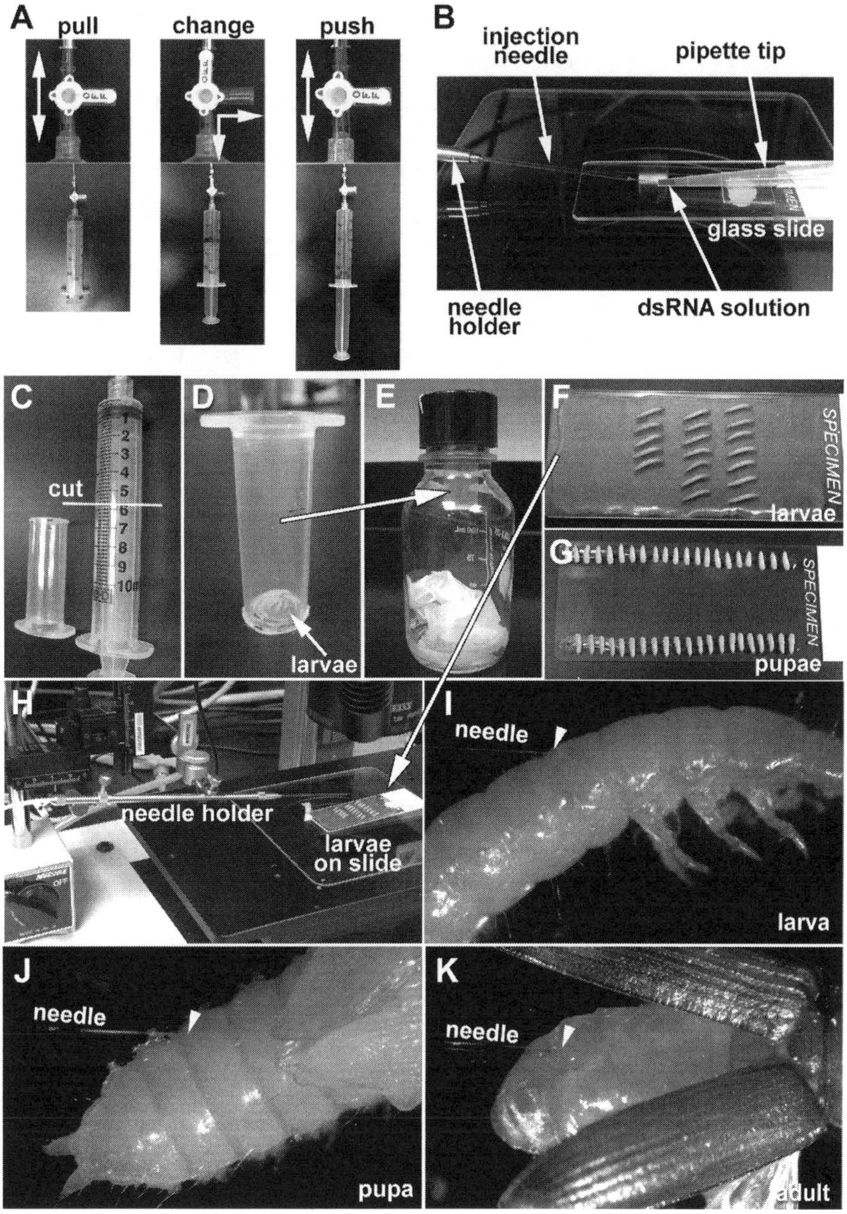


Fig. 3. Injection procedures. (**a**) Injection syringe with different stopcock positions. The air-flow direction is indicated by *arrows*. (**b**) Front loading the injection needle. (**c–e**) Etherization apparatus. (**f**, **g**) larvae (**f**) and pupae (**g**) on a sticky glass slide. (**h**) Injection setting. (**i–k**) Injection points for a larva (**i**), pupa (**j**), and adult (**k**). *Arrowheads* indicate injection points.

8. 1 M $Na_2HPO_4$.
9. 1 M $NaH_2PO_4$.
10. 0.1 M sodium phosphate buffer, pH 7.6 at 25°C: Mix 8.5 ml of 1 M $Na_2HPO_4$ with 1.5 ml of 1 M $NaH_2PO_4$ to obtain 10 ml of 0.1 M sodium phosphate buffer. Check the pH with a pH indicator strip and adjust accordingly.

11. 0.5 M KCl.
12. Food dye (green, blue, or red preferable) (Kroger).
13. 10× injection buffer (1 ml): 0.1 M sodium phosphate buffer (10 μl), 0.5 M KCl (100 μl), food dye (100 μl), and double-distilled water (dd$H_2O$) (790 μl).
14. 2× injection buffer (1 ml): 10× injection buffer (200 μl) and dd$H_2O$ (800 μl). Store at 4°C.
15. Glass slide (Fisher).
16. Repositionable Glue (e.g., Aleen's TACK-IT Over&Over).
17. Plastic CD case (10 mm thick) (Amazon.com).
18. Glass capillary: O.D. 1 mm, I.D. 0.5 mm, without filament (Sutter Instrument).
19. Needle puller: P-87 or P97 Micropipette Puller (Sutter Instrument).
20. Injection needle: Use a needle puller to pull glass capillaries. "Pipette Cookbook" downloadable from the Sutter Instrument Web site (17) is an excellent reference to determine the needle pulling condition. "Adherent Cell, *C. elegans*, *Drosophila*, & Zebrafish – Recommended Programs" described in the cookbook is recommended for *Tribolium* injection. Store pulled needles in a plastic CD case. A strip of removable mounting putty can be used to hold needles in the CD case.
21. Removable mounting putty (e.g., LockTite Fun-Tak, Henkel Consumer Adhesives).
22. Compressed gas duster.
23. Forceps: INOX #1 and #5 (Fine Science Tool or ROBOZ Surgical Instrument).
24. Ethyl ether, anhydrous (Fisher).
25. Nylon mesh: 120-μm pore size/49% open area (Flystuff.com). Nylon mesh available at a fabric store can also be used.
26. Narrow-mouth 250-ml glass bottle (e.g., KIMAX).
27. Stereomicroscope: A stereomicroscope with a magnification range of 10–50× and a working distance of about 5–10 cm will suit the injection procedure (e.g., Stemi2000 or SteREO Discovery V12, Zeiss. Fig. 2a, b).
28. X-Y mechanical stage for stereomicroscopes (see Note 3).
29. Manipulator: M-152 (Fig. 2C) (Narishige).
30. Magnetic stand: GJ-1 (Narishige).
31. Glass capillary holder: IM-H1 Injection Holder Set (Narishige).
32. Injection syringe (Fig. 2d): A 30-ml disposable syringe (e.g., BD syringe) and a four-way stopcock (e.g., Stopcocks with Luer Connections; 4-way; male slip, EW-30600-03,

Cole-Parmer Instrument Co.) connected to a glass capillary holder. The stopcock allows you to change the position of the syringe plunger without applying pressure to the injection needle (see Fig. 3a for stopcock usage).

33. A fume hood for handling ether.
34. Etherization bottle (Fig. 3e): Place two pieces of tissue papers (e.g., Kimberly-Clark Wipes) in a 250-ml narrow-mouth glass bottle and pour about 70 ml of ether onto the paper.
35. Etherization basket (Fig. 3c, d): Remove the syringe plunger from a 10-ml disposable syringe and carefully cut in half along the 6 ml line. Discard the tip. Briefly heat the cut surface with a gas burner until plastic becomes soft and quickly place the heated syringe onto a piece of nylon mesh (the mesh will be glued onto the syringe). Trim off the edge with scissors to make the edge smooth and round. This "basket" will fit on a 250-ml narrow-mouth glass bottle (Fig. 3e).
36. Sticky glass slide: apply repositionable glue on a glass slide. Cover the entire slide for larval injections or make two thin strips along the longer edges for pupal and adult injection (Fig. 3f, g).

### 2.3. RNA Isolation and Real-Time PCR

1. RNeasy Mini Kit (QIAGEN).
2. RNase Away Spray Bottle (Molecular BioProducts/Thermo Fisher).
3. 20-gauge needle.
4. 1-ml syringe.
5. Disposable pestles for 1.5-ml microcentrifuge tubes (Fisher).
6. Liquid nitrogen.
7. Spectrophotometer, e.g., NanoDrop 2000 (Fisher Thermo Science).
8. 0.5 M EDTA: Add 93.05 g of EDTA to 400 ml of $ddH_2O$. Mix briefly on a stir plate, then carefully add 8 g of NaOH pellet. Mix until the solution becomes clear. Adjust pH to 8.0 with NaOH if necessary. Adjust the final volume to 500 ml with $ddH_2O$.
9. RNase-free recombinant DNase I (Roche).
10. Protector RNase Inhibitor (Roche).
11. iScript One-Step RT-PCR Kit with SYBR Green (Bio-Rad).
12. Optically clear PCR tubes.
13. Real-time PCR thermal cycler (e.g., iCycler, Bio-Rad).

### 2.4. Protein Extraction and Western Blot

#### 2.4.1. Total Protein Extraction

1. Protein extraction buffer: 150 mM NaCl, 10 mM Tris–HCl, 0.1% (w/v) sodium deoxycholate, pH 7.2. To make 100 ml of this buffer, add 0.876 g of NaCl and 0.156 g of Tris–HCl to 100 ml of $ddH_2O$. Bring the solution to pH 7.2 with NaOH and add 0.1 g of sodium deoxycholate.
2. Protease Inhibitor Cocktail (e.g., Sigma # P8340).
3. Disposable pestles for 1.5-ml microcentrifuge tubes (Fisher).

#### 2.4.2. Electrophoresis and Transfer

1. 10× TGS buffer: 10× Tris/Glycine/SDS stock solution (Bio-Rad).
2. Transfer buffer: mix 100 ml of 10× TGS, 700 ml of $ddH_2O$ and 200 ml of methanol (see Note 5).
3. Methanol.
4. β-Mercaptoethanol, 14.2 M stock solution (Bio-Rad).
5. Laemmli Sample Buffer (Bio-Rad).
6. Protein loading buffer: Laemmli + 5% β-mercaptoethanol (95 μl Laemmli + 5 μl β-mercaptoethanol).
7. Protein standard: MagicMark XP (Invitrogen).
8. Ready Gel Tris–HCl Gel: precast 4–15% linear gradient polyacrylamide gel (Bio-Rad).
9. Hybond ECL Nitrocellulose Membrane (GE Healthcare).
10. Power supply: PowerPac 1000 (Fig. 4c) (Bio-Rad).

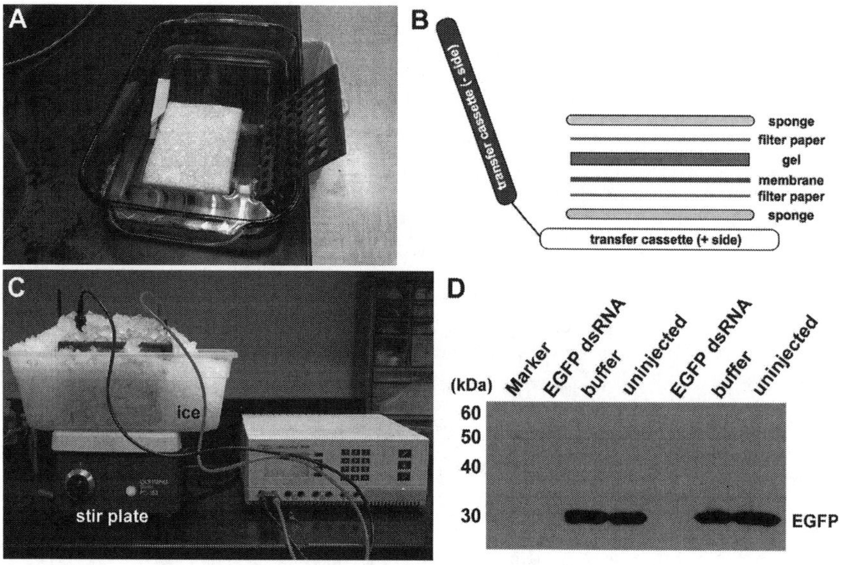


Fig. 4. Monitoring EGFP RNAi efficacy by Western blot. (**a**) A transfer cassette in a large shallow dish filled with transfer buffer. (**b**) A scheme of transfer cassette assembly. (**c**) A typical western blot setup. (**d**) Reduction of EGFP protein by EGFP RNAi shown by western blot. dsRNA for EGFP (500 ng/μl) was injected into last-instar *Pu11* larvae. Injection buffer was used for a control group. Another set of larvae was isolated for an uninjected control. Total proteins were isolated 7 days after injection from the three experimental groups. One pupa was used from each experimental group (experiments were triplicated). GFP antibody (1:500, ab6673, abcam) and HRP-conjugated Donkey anti-Goat antibody (1:50,000) were used for immunoblotting.

11. Bio-Rad Mini-PROTEAN vertical gel electrophoresis and blotting system. Other suitable systems can be substituted.
12. Gel loading tips.
13. Blot absorbent filter paper (Bio-Rad).
14. Stir plate.
15. Rocking platform.

#### 2.4.3. Immunoblotting

1. 10× Tris-buffered saline (10× TBS): 100 mM Tris, 1 M NaCl, pH 7.5. To make 2 L of 10× TBS, add 24 g of Tris and 116 g of NaCl to 2 L of $ddH_2O$. Adjust the pH to 7.5 with HCl.
2. Tris-buffered saline with Tween (TBS-T): 10 mM Tris, 100 mM NaCl, pH 7.5, with 0.1% Tween20. To make 1 l of TBS-T, mix 100 ml of 10× TBS, 899 ml of $ddH_2O$, and 1 ml of Tween-20.
3. Nonfat dry milk (available in a grocery store).
4. Blocking buffer: 10% (w/v) nonfat dry milk in TBS-T (10 g of nonfat dry milk in 100 ml of TBS-T).
5. Antibodies buffer: 5% (w/v) nonfat dry milk in TBS-T (5 g of nonfat dry milk in 100 ml of TBS-T).
6. Primary antibodies.
7. Horseradish peroxidase (HRP)-labeled secondary antibodies.
8. Enhanced Chemiluminescence (ECL) Detection kit (GE Healthcare).
9. Blue Basic Autoradiography Film (ISC BioExpress).
10. Autoradiography film processing equipment.

## 3. Methods

### 3.1. dsRNA Synthesis

A summary of the dsRNA synthesis process is shown in Fig. 5. Initially, a gene fragment with the T7 polymerase promoter site at both ends is amplified by PCR with primers that have T7 sequence at their 5′ ends (T7 tail) (see Fig. 5a and the next section). This PCR product will be used as a template in an in vitro transcription (Fig. 5b). Sense and antisense strands of RNA are synthesized and annealed together in an in vitro transcription process. dsRNA is then purified using an RNA purification kit for subsequent injection procedures.

#### 3.1.1. Primer Design for dsRNA Synthesis

1. Prepare gene-specific primers with the T7 sequence (taatacgactcactatagggg) at their 5′ ends. About 15 mer sequence should be sufficient for the gene specific portion of the primers. These primers amplify a gene fragment with the T7 polymerase

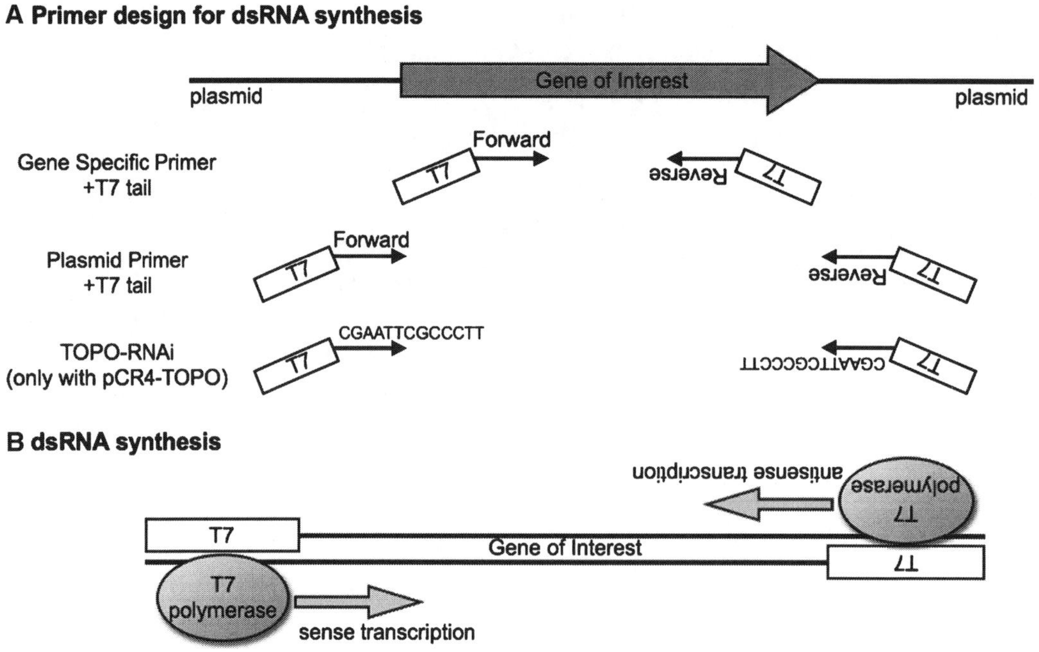


Fig. 5. An outline of dsRNA synthesis (**a**) Primer design for dsRNA synthesis, and (**b**) dsRNA synthesis scheme.

promoter site at both ends (see Note 2 for the primers used here to knock down EGFP).

5′-taatacgactcactataggg----------------------------- -3′

T7 ~15 mer gene-specific sequence

2. Alternatively, primers designed to prime on two plasmid regions that flank the inserted gene fragment can also be used, which eliminates the process of ordering gene-specific primers with T7 tail for each gene.

3. Only one primer is necessary if TOPO TA Cloning Kit for Sequence (pCR4-TOPO vector, Invitrogen) is used. This primer is designed to prime on two pCR4-TOPO vector regions that flank the inserted gene fragment (8) (Fig. 5a).

   TOPO_RNAi_T7 primer: 5′-taatacgactcactatagggcgaattcgccctt-3′

   T7

4. The dsRNA length coincides with the gene fragment amplified with the primers described above. dsRNA shorter than 100 bp appears to have weaker effect (Tomoyasu et al., manuscript in preparation), so dsRNA longer than 100 bp is recommended. A dsRNA length of 400–1,000 bp is routinely reported in the *Tribolium* literature.

5. Off-target effect (OTE) is a major concern in RNAi experiments (18). Targeting several nonoverlapping portions of a gene in separate experiments helps evaluate whether an observed phenotype is caused by depletion of the targeted gene or by an OTE. Phenotypes caused by depleting the target should be observed regardless of the region of the mRNA targeted, while phenotypes caused by an OTE are likely to be seen only when a certain sequence within the target mRNA is targeted.

#### 3.1.2. Template Preparation for dsRNA Synthesis

In the following procedures, the DNA template for dsRNA synthesis is synthesized by PCR. After specificity of the PCR is confirmed on an agarose gel, the DNA template is then purified using the QIAGEN QIAquick PCR purification kit.

1. Prepare a gene of interest (either a full-length or a partial fragment) cloned into a plasmid (see Note 6).
2. Adjust the plasmid concentration to 10 ng/µl using $ddH_2O$.
3. Set up the PCR reaction as follows:

| | |
|---|---|
| $ddH_2O$ | 102 µl |
| 5× GoTaq buffer with $Mg^{2+}$ | 40 µl |
| dNTP mix (2.5 mM stock) | 16 µl (0.2 M) |
| primer 1 (10 M stock)* | 15 µl (0.75 M) |
| primer 2 (10 M stock)* | 15 µl (0.75 M) |
| plasmid DNA (10 ng/µl) | 10 µl |
| Go Taq polymerase (5 U/µl) | 2.5 µl |
| Total | 200 µl |

*Both primers can be replaced with 30 µl of TOPO-RNAi primer (10 M stock) when the template fragment is cloned into pCR4-TOPO plasmid.

4. Split the PCR reaction mix into eight tubes of 25 µl for heat transfer efficiency.
5. Run the following program.

| | | |
|---|---|---|
| | Denature: | 94°C×2 min |
| | Denature: | 94°C×30 s |
| 35 cycles | Annealing: | 57°C×30 s |
| | Extension: | 72°C×__min/s* |
| | Extension: | 72°C×5 min |
| | Hold: | 4°C |

*depends on the length of the PCR product (60 s/1,000 bp).

6. Take 1 µl from one of the tubes and mix with 4 µl $ddH_2O$ and 1 µl 6× DNA loading dye.

7. Run a gel to confirm the specificity of the PCR reaction (see Note 7).
8. Combine the PCR reactions into a 1.5-ml microcentrifuge tube.
9. Add 1 ml of buffer PBI (5 volumes of the sample) and mix well by vortexing.
10. Place a QIAquick spin column in a provided 2-ml collection tube.
11. Apply half of the sample (600 μl) to the QIAquick column and centrifuge for 1 min at 8,000 rpm. All the centrifugation steps are done in a microcentrifuge (the *g*-force value for 8,000 rpm and 12,000 rpm is 5,000 × *g* and 11,000 × *g*, respectively).
12. Discard the flow-through and place the QIAquick column back into the same tube.
13. Apply the other half of the sample to the QIAquick column and repeat steps 11 and 12.
14. Add 750 μl of buffer PE to the column and centrifuge for 1 min at 8,000 rpm.
15. Discard flow-through and place the QIAquick column back in the same tube.
16. Centrifuge the column for 1 min at 12,000 rpm to completely remove the residual buffer PE.
17. Place QIAquick column in a clean 1.5-ml microcentrifuge tube.
18. Add 30 μl of buffer EB to the center of the QIAquick membrane and allow it to stand for 1 min.
19. Centrifuge the column for 1 min at 12,000 rpm to collect the template DNA sample.
20. Quantitate the amount of DNA with a Spectrophotometer . A minimum of 125 ng/μl is required for the next step (see Note 8). Usually, a concentration of 300–500 ng/μl is obtained.
21. The sample can be stored at –20°C for at least several months.

#### 3.1.3. In Vitro Transcription

The following protocol uses Ambion MEGAscript T7.

1. Prepare the reaction mix as follows:

| | |
|---|---|
| NTP mix solution | 8 μl |
| 10× Reaction buffer | 2 μl |
| Enzyme mix | 2 μl |
| Template | μl (1.5 μg) |
| Add nuclease-free water to | 20 μl |

The nucleoside triphosphate solutions (ATP, CTP, GTP, and UTP) come separately in the MEGAscript T7 kit. They can be premixed (1:1:1:1) and stored at −20°C (NTP mix solution). Vortex the 10× Reaction Buffer well, as it is very viscous, and keep it at room temperature while assembling the reaction.

2. Incubate the reaction mix at 37°C for 5–6 h. Although a shorter incubation time is recommended in the MEGAscript manual, a longer incubation appears to give a higher dsRNA yield.
3. Add 1 μl of TURBO DNase I. Mix well by pipetting.
4. Incubate at 37°C for 30 min.
5. Turn on a heat block and set the temperature at 70°C for subsequent procedures.

#### 3.1.4. dsRNA Purification

1. Bring the dsRNA sample to 100 μl with 79 μl of elution solution. Mix gently but thoroughly.
2. Add 350 μl of Binding Solution Concentrate to the sample and mix gently by pipetting.
3. Add 250 μl of 100% ethanol to the sample and mix gently by pipetting.
4. Insert the Filter Cartridge into the Collection Tube provided.
5. Pipette the sample mixture (700 μl) onto the Filter Cartridge.
6. Centrifuge for 1 min at 12,000 rpm.
7. Discard the flow-through and place the Filter Cartridge back in the same tube.
8. Apply 500 μl of Wash Solution Concentrate (make sure ethanol has been added).
9. Centrifuge for 1 min at 12,000 rpm.
10. Discard the flow-through and place the Filter Cartridge back in the same tube.
11. Repeat steps 8–10 with a second 500-μl aliquot of Wash Solution Concentrate.
12. Centrifuge again for 1 min at 12,000 rpm to make sure that the Filter Cartridge is dry.
13. dsRNA elution:
    (a) Place the Filter Cartridge in a new Collection Tube.
    (b) Apply 50 μl of Elution Solution to the center of the Filter Cartridge.
    (c) Close the cap of the Collection Tube and incubate in a heat block at 70°C for 10 min.
    (d) Recover eluted dsRNA by centrifuging for 1 min at room temperature at 12,000 rpm. Keep the collected dsRNA solution in the Collection Tube.

(e) Repeat steps b–d with another 50-μl aliquot of Elution Solution.

(f) Discard the Filter Cartridge.

14. Ethanol precipitation:

(a) Add 10 μl of 5 M Ammonium Acetate (provided) and 275 μl of 100% ethanol to the sample.

(b) Mix well by vortexing and incubate at −80°C overnight.

(c) After overnight incubation, centrifuge the sample at 12,000 rpm for 15 min at 4°C.

(d) Carefully remove the supernatant and discard it (do not disturb the dsRNA pellet).

(e) Wash the pellet by adding 500 μl of 70% cold ethanol (stored at −20°C) and gently inverting the sample tube several times (but it is not necessary to disturb the dsRNA pellet).

(f) Centrifuge at 12,000 rpm for 10 min at 4°C.

(g) Carefully remove the 70% ethanol and discard it (do not disturb the dsRNA pellet).

(h) Air-dry the pellet briefly by leaving the tube lid open for 15 min at room temperature (do not overdry the pellet, as it may be difficult to get dissolved).

15. Resuspend the pellet in 16 μl of nuclease-free water (provided in the MEGAscript T7 kit).

16. Take 0.5 μl from the purified dsRNA sample and mix with 9.5 μl of $ddH_2O$ in a new 1.5-μl microcentrifuge tube (20× diluted sample).

17. Run 5 μl of the 20× diluted sample mixed with 1 μl of 6× DNA loading dye on gel electrophoresis. A regular agarose gel for DNA is sufficient for this step.

18. Use the rest of the 20× diluted sample for sample quantification by a Spectrophotometer. Usually, a concentration of 150–300 ng/μl (therefore, the sample concentration is 3,000–6,000 ng/μl) is obtained.

## 3.2. dsRNA Injection

### 3.2.1. dsRNA Preparation for Injection

1. Various concentrations of dsRNA can be used to achieve different degrees of gene knockdown (from close to null to very week hypomorphic) (see Supplemental Data of ref. 19 for example). 1 g/μl (final concentration after mixing with injection buffer) is a reasonable starting concentration. RNAi with dsRNA concentration of as high as 7–8 g/l, and as low as 5 pg/l have been tested, producing various degrees of phenotypes in *Tribolium* ((12, 19), and Tomoyasu Y., unpublished data).

2. Adjust the concentration of the dsRNA solution to the desired concentration (e.g., 2 g/l to obtain 1 g/l final concentration) and mix the dsRNA solution 1:1 with 2× injection buffer. Keep the sample on ice during the injection procedures.

*3.2.2. Needle Preparation*

1. Break the tip of an injection needle with sharp forceps #5 under a stereomicroscope to create a sharp and stiff tip.
2. Place the needle in the needle holder and place the needle holder onto the manipulator (Fig. 2c). Adjust the angle of the needle close to horizontal (Fig. 2c).
3. Adjust the position of the injection needle by changing the position of the manipulator to place the tip of the injection needle at the center of the stereomicroscope field.
4. Cut the tip of a 20-μl disposable micropipette tip using scissors.
5. Pipette 10 μl of dsRNA solution into the micropipette tip prepared above using a micropipettor. Carefully remove the tip from the micropipettor so that the dsRNA solution remains.
6. Place the micropipette tip horizontally on a glass slide using a piece of removable mounting putty (Fig. 3b).
7. Set the injection syringe to the pulling position (Fig. 3a).
8. Under a stereomicroscope, carefully insert the injection needle into the dsRNA solution in the micropipette tip (Fig. 3b).
9. Slowly pull the injection syringe plunger to load the dsRNA solution into the injection needle. Do not overload the injection needle to avoid possible contamination of the needle holder (see Note 9).
10. Control the filling by gently pushing the injection syringe plunger to neutralize the pulling pressure.
11. Carefully remove the injection needle from the micropipette tip. Raise the position of the injection needle using the *z*-axis of the manipulator to avoid any accidental contact to the injection needle.
12. Remove the glass slide with the micropipette tip from the microscope stage (see Note 10 for alternative injection settings for other organisms).

*3.2.3. Beetle Preparation*

1. Isolate beetles of the desired stage (such as larvae, pupae, or adults) using a #25 sieve and a collecting pan (Fig. 1c–e).
2. Place beetles in the etherization basket and then place the basket in the etherization bottle (Fig. 3d, e). Close the bottle lid and etherize beetles for about 4 min (see Note 11). Do not let beetles touch ether, as it will kill beetles. A fume hood must be used when handling ether.

3. There is no need to etherize pupae. Pupae can be laid on a sticky slide (Fig. 3g) prior to all of the above injection procedures (or even a day before).
4. Lay the etherized beetles on a sticky slide under a separate stereomicroscope using forceps #1 (Fig. 3f). This procedure should be performed as quickly as possible (preferably less than 5 min) to avoid beetles awakening during the following injection process. You may have to reduce the stickiness of the glue by briefly touching the glue several times with your finger (see Note 12 for dipteran larvae).

#### *3.2.4. Injection*

1. Place the sticky glass slide with beetles under the injection microscope (Fig. 3h).
2. Switch the position of the injection syringe to the pushing position (Fig. 3a).
3. Carefully insert the injection needle into a beetle. Injection points for a larva, pupa, and adult are shown in Fig. 3i–k; however, the injection point does not appear to significantly affect RNAi efficiency; the circulatory system in the beetle allows the dsRNA solution to quickly spread out within the entire beetle body, causing a systemic effect.
4. Gently apply pressure onto the injection syringe plunger to inject dsRNA solution into the beetle. Approximately 0.5–0.8 μl of the dsRNA solution can be injected into one last-instar larva, pupa, or adult (see Note 13).
5. Slowly remove the injection needle from the beetle. Briefly pull the plunger to counter the pushing pressure as you pull out the needle from the beetle (see Note 9).
6. Repeat steps 3–5 until all the beetles on the sticky slide are injected. Make sure to remove beetles that were unable to be injected.
7. Leave the beetles on the sticky slide until the beetles wake up.
8. For larvae and adults, carefully remove the injected beetles from the slide using forceps #1 under a stereomicroscope. Leave the beetles in a plastic Petri dish without culture flour for 15 min to let the injection wound dry and then place the beetles in a culture bottle.
9. For pupae, leave the injected pupae on the sticky slide. Flip the slide upside down and place it on culture flour in a large plastic Petri dish (100 mm diameter).
10. Culture the beetles in an incubator at 30°C with 50% humidity until the desired stage for phenotype analysis (see Note 14 regarding the survival rate).

11. For parental RNAi, let the injected pupae close to adults. Culture adults for several days for sexual maturation. Analyze phenotypes in offspring embryos.
12. Alternatively, adults can also be used for parental RNAi. Injection at the adult stage allows to bypass the RNAi effect on oogenesis, as some oocytes have already matured at the time of injection. Adult injection is ideal when knocking down the gene of interest at the pupal stage has a drastic effect on oogenesis and prevents the production of embryos.

### 3.3. RNA Isolation and Real-Time RT-PCR

There are several methods available to monitor RNAi efficacy. Real-time PCR is one way to validate RNAi effect by directly measuring the amount of targeted mRNA molecules. First, total RNA needs to be isolated from beetles. Then, the total RNA is used as a template for one-step reverse-transcription (RT) real-time PCR to monitor the amount of target mRNAs. The following protocol describes a total RNA isolation method as well as one of the quantification methods using real-time PCR, comparative Ct method. See Chapter 17 for additional information.

#### 3.3.1. Primer Design for Real-Time RT-PCR

1. Two sets of primers are required for quantitative real-time PCR. The first set is designed against the gene of interest. The second set should be designed against an internal control gene (reference) that maintains a relatively uniform expression level throughout development (such as housekeeping genes). *Polyubiquitin* and ribosomal protein genes have been used as internal controls in *Tribolium* (20, 21) (see Note 4 for example primers).
2. Assuming that the injected dsRNA corresponds to a portion of the gene of interest, at least one of the primers used for real-time PCR should complement an area of the gene that is outside the dsRNA sequence. This prevents real-time PCR from inadvertently measuring the dsRNA as endogenous gene expression.
3. PCR amplicons shorter than 100 bp are preferable to minimize the effect on amplification efficiency.
4. Primer design programs exist that assist users in developing primers of high quality (e.g., Integrated DNA Technologies Web site (22)).

#### 3.3.2. Total RNA Isolation

The following protocol uses QIAGEN RNeasy Mini Kit (see Note 15). Also, see Note 16 about RNA work in general.

1. Place individual or groups of larvae, pupae, or adults (see Note 17) in a 1.5-ml microcentrifuge tube.
2. Freeze the sample in liquid nitrogen and grind the sample thoroughly using a disposable pestle. Freeze the pestle in liquid nitrogen before use.

3. Add 350 μl of buffer RLT.
4. Homogenize the sample by passing lysate 20 times through a 20-gauge needle with a 1-ml disposable syringe. This step is essential to avoid genomic DNA contamination.
5. Centrifuge for 3 min at 12,000 rpm at room temperature to pellet debris.
6. Transfer the supernatant to a new 1.5-ml microcentrifuge tube.
7. Add 350 μl of 70% EtOH and mix well by pipetting.
8. Transfer the whole solution (~700 μl) to an RNeasy Mini Column.
9. Centrifuge for 30 s at 12,000 rpm at room temperature. Discard flow-through.
10. Add 700 μl of buffer RW1 to the RNeasy Mini Column.
11. Centrifuge for 30 s at 12,000 rpm at room temperature.
12. Transfer the RNeasy Mini Column to a new 2-ml Collection Tube (supplied). Do not allow the RNeasy Mini Column to touch the flow-through.
13. Add 500 μl of RPE to the RNeasy Mini Column.
14. Centrifuge for 30 s at 12,000 rpm at room temperature. Discard flow-through.
15. Add 500 μl of RPE to the RNeasy Mini Column.
16. Centrifuge for 2 min at 12,000 rpm at room temperature.
17. Transfer the RNeasy Mini Column to a new 1.5-ml tube (supplied).
18. Apply 30 μl of RNase-free water (supplied) directly to the column membrane.
19. Centrifuge for 1 min at 12,000 rpm at room temperature to collect the total RNA solution.
20. Measure RNA concentration in the sample with a spectrophotometer. Usually, a concentration of 200–500 ng/μl is obtained.
21. DNase treatment (optional. See Notes 15 and 18). Prepare the reaction mix as follows:

| | |
|---|---|
| RNA solution | μl (corresponding to 3 g) |
| 10× DNase buffer | 5 μl |
| DNase | 1 μl |
| RNase inhibitor | 1 μl |
| Add Nuclease-free water to | 50 μl |

Incubate the reaction mix at 37°C for 20 min. Then, add 1 µl of 0.5 M EDTA and inactivate DNase by incubating the reaction mix at 75°C for 10 min.

22. Proceed to the next step or store the sample at –80°C.

*3.3.3. Real-Time RT-PCR*

Real-time PCR uses a fluorescence molecule to monitor the amplification of PCR products in real time. One way to monitor the amount of PCR products is to use a DNA binding dye (DNA intercalator such as SYBR Green), which emits fluorescence upon excitation only when it binds to DNA. The intensity of the fluorescence corresponds to the amount of DNA molecules, allowing quantification of PCR products during PCR. Regular PCR primers can be used in this Intercalation method, making this method relatively easy and inexpensive. However, caution must be taken, as a DNA intercalator binds to any DNA molecules in the reaction, emitting fluorescence even when it binds to DNA amplified nonspecifically. A melt curve analysis allows one to assess the specificity of the PCR (multiple $T_m$ may indicate the amplification of more than one kind of PCR products). An alternative to the Intercalation method is the Fluorescence probe method, in which a fluorescence probe is used to detect PCR products in a sequence specific manner. This method has an advantage over the intercalation method, as it monitors the amount of target PCR products specifically, excluding other DNA molecules amplified nonspecifically. However, it requires a specific fluorescence probe, making this method more expensive to perform.

The following protocol details the Intercalation method using SYBR Green as a reporter dye. There are several different methods to quantitate DNA or RNA using Real-time PCR. The following protocol uses the comparative Ct (Threshold Cycle) method, which is able to determine the relative amount of target RNA molecules in samples. A guide for the comparative Ct and other methods is detailed in the *User Bulletin #2: ABI PRISM 7700 Sequence Detection System* manual (23).

The comparative Ct method requires that the amplification efficiencies of the two sets of primers (for the target and reference) are relatively equal; otherwise, the results are uninterpretable. Therefore, a standard curve analysis should first be performed to validate that the two sets of primers show similar amplification efficiency.

1. Assay validation. Primer concentrations should be empirically tested to determine which concentration is used for the standard curve measurements (between 50 and 300 nM concentration is recommended).
2. The standard curves are made for both the target and reference by diluting total RNA over a range of concentrations (at minimum 100-fold) with the primer concentration determined above.

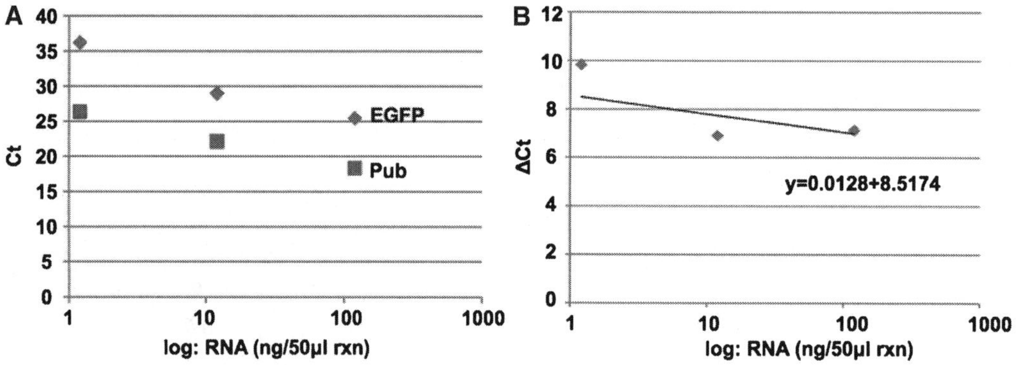


C

| | average Ct for EGFP (target) | average Ct for Pub (reference) | ΔCt Ct(target)-Ct(ref) | ΔΔCt ΔCt-ΔCt(ref) | $2^{-\Delta\Delta Ct}$ | relative expression % |
|---|---|---|---|---|---|---|
| uninjected | 31.30 | 18.60 | 31.3-18.6=12.7 | 12.7-12.7=0 | 1 | 100 |
| EGFP dsRNA | 34.00 | 17.95 | 34-17.95=16.05 | 16.05-12.7=3.35 | 0.098 | 9.8 |

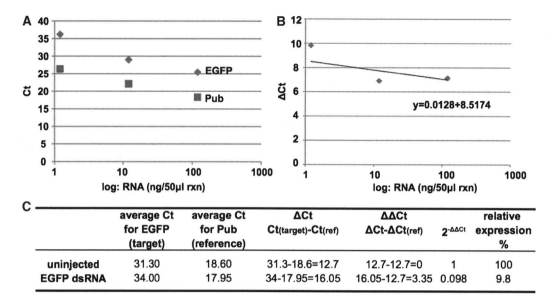

Fig. 6. Monitoring EGFP RNAi efficacy by real-time PCR in a *Tribolium* strain that expresses EGFP (Enhanced Green Fluorescence Protein) in the eyes and the future wing-related tissues (*Pu11*) (12). dsRNA for EGFP (500 ng/μl) was injected into last-instar *Pu11* larvae. Total RNA was isolated 7 days after the injection from both injected and uninjected groups of three pupae. (**a**) Ct values for *EGFP* and *Tc-polyubiquitin* (*pub*, internal control) with three different RNA concentrations (1.2 ng, 12 ng, and 120 ng/50 μl reaction mix: rxn) plotted against the log input RNA. (**b**) The difference between Ct values of *EGFP* and *pub* PCR (ΔCt) plotted against the log input RNA. The slope of the linear regression line is 0.013, indicating that the amplification of both products is approximately equal. (**c**) ΔCt and ΔΔCt calculated from the Ct values obtained from *EGFP* and *pub* PCR using RNA isolated from uninjected or dsRNA injected beetles. The EGFP dsRNA injected group shows a 90.2% reduction in EGFP mRNA expression compared to the uninjected group.

3. The difference between the Ct of both target and reference (ΔCt) within each input amount of total RNA is plotted against the log input RNA (see Fig. 6a as an example). The slope of the line should be inferior to 0.1, which ensures the amplification of the products is approximately equal (Fig. 6b).
4. Once this is verified, the experimental samples can be tested with these primer sets.
5. *Quantification.* Run one-step real-time PCR with the total RNA isolated from the experimental samples, using the primer sets validated above. The concentration of total RNA can be determined based on the standard curve analysis above (e.g., the RNA concentration that gives a Ct value between 15 and 30). The reactions should be run in triplicate.
6. A master mix of all the components, except the input RNA, should be assembled to minimize pipetting errors.
7. Additional samples should be run with no reverse transcriptase to verify if the RNA is free of genomic DNA contamination (see Note 18).

8. An example reaction protocol for one-step real-time PCR is as follows:

| | |
|---|---|
| cDNA synthesis | 10 min at 50°C |
| RT inactivation | 5 min at 95°C |
| PCR (45 cycles) | 10 s at 95°C<br>30 s at 60°C (data collection) |
| Melt curve analysis | 1 min at 95°C<br>1 min at 55°C<br>10 s at 55°C (80 cycles, increasing by 0.5°C each cycle) |

9. The relative quantity of target, normalized to a reference, is calculated by $2^{-\Delta\Delta Ct}$ (see Note 19). The ΔCt is the difference between the Ct of the target and reference for each sample. Once this is determined, a "calibrator" group is identified (such as uninjected control), which will serve as the group to which all other measurements are compared (see Fig. 5c as an example).

### 3.4. Protein Extraction and Western Blot

Another way to validate RNAi efficacy is to monitor the amount of the protein products of the targeted gene by Western blot. The following protocol details a protein isolation method and western blot using *Tribolium*.

#### 3.4.1. Total Protein Isolation

1. Place individual or groups of larvae, pupae, or adults on ice in a 1.5-ml microcentrifuge tube.
2. Homogenize samples in the protein extraction buffer with Protease Inhibitor Cocktail (1:100 dilution) with a disposable pestle. Use approximately 8–10 μl of protein extraction buffer per 1 mg of tissue. For one *Tribolium* pupa, we typically use 100 μl of protein extraction buffer.
3. Centrifuge the protein extract in a microcentrifuge for 10 min at 1,000 ×*g* at 4°C.
4. Take out the supernatant, containing the protein fraction, and make aliquots of approximately 90 μl. The aliquots can be used immediately in downstream applications, including gel electrophoresis, or should be frozen at –80°C for future use.

#### 3.4.2. Electrophoresis and Transfer

1. Prepare the 1× Electrophoresis running buffer and the transfer buffer. Store at 4°C.
2. Assemble the Bio-Rad Mini-PROTEAN gel apparatus with the lanes of the gel facing inward and lock into place. Verify that there are no leaks in the electrode assembly by placing running buffer between the gel and buffer dam (or two gels). Once

confirmed, place the electrode assembly into the buffer tank and fill with the remainder of electrophoresis running buffer.

3. Determine the total amount of protein to be added to the lane and mix 1:1 with protein loading buffer. It is important to verify that the volume of the sample and loading buffer does not exceed the capacity of the well.
4. Denature proteins by incubating the samples at 95°C for 3 min and briefly centrifuge tubes to recover sample.
5. Load samples and standards (see Note 20) into wells using gel loading tips and place the lid onto the buffer reservoir, ensuring that the correct terminals are connected.
6. Run the gel at 120 V for 5 min and then at 180 V for 45 min.
7. Equilibrate the sponges, filter paper, and nitrocellulose membrane for transfer in a large shallow dish filled with transfer buffer.
8. Once the electrophoresis is completed, remove the electrode assembly from the buffer reservoir and carefully place the gel into the transfer cassette, which should contain, in the following order, sponge, filter paper, nitrocellulose membrane, gel, filter paper, and sponge (Fig. 4a, b). It is important to remove bubbles from spaces between the different layers, as they prevent proper transfer of proteins to the nitrocellulose membrane. Place the membrane between the gel and the anode to ensure proper transfer.
9. Place the transfer cell into the buffer reservoir, which contains the remaining transfer buffer. Add a magnetic stir bar into the reservoir and place the reservoir on a stir plate, surrounded with ice (Fig. 4c). Alternatively, perform the transfer at 4°C.
10. Let the proteins transfer to the nitrocellulose membrane over 1.5–2 h at 80 V.

#### 3.4.3. Immunoblotting

1. Remove the membrane from the transfer cassette and place it into blocking buffer overnight at 4°C, with gentle agitation on a rocking platform.
2. Dilute primary antibodies in the antibody buffer and add the antibodies solution onto the membrane in a shallow dish (see Notes 21 and 22). The dish can be placed into a larger container with a lid to prevent evaporation. Incubate for 1.5–2 h at 21°C with gentle agitation.
3. Remove the antibodies solution and wash the membrane in copious amounts of TBS-T four times for over 45 min.
4. Repeat step 2 with HRP-conjugated secondary antibodies.
5. Remove the secondary antibodies solution from the membrane and wash the membrane in TBS-T four times for over 45 min.

6. Mix the two components of the ECL kit (1:1). Place the membrane into a shallow dish and cover with the ECL reagent for 2 min.
7. Remove excess reagent and wrap the membrane with plastic wrap. Place the membrane inside a film cassette, expose to autoradiography film in a dark room, and develop using the autoradiography film processing equipment of choice (see Fig. 4d as an example).

## 4. Notes

1. Systemic RNAi was initially described in plants as spread of posttranscriptional gene silencing (24–26). *Caenorhabditis elegans* was the first animal in which RNAi was shown to work systemically (1, 11). The phenomenon can be subdivided into at least three distinct (but overlapping) processes: uptake of dsRNA by cells (cellular dsRNA uptake), systemic spreading of the RNAi effect (RNAi spreading), and uptake of dsRNA from the outside environment (feeding RNAi or environmental RNAi). For reviews of systemic RNAi, see (8, 9, 27–31).
2. The following primers were used to create an EGFP dsRNA template (520 bp). GFPiF2: taatacgactcactatagggcgatgccacct, GFPiR5: taatacgactcactatagggcggactgggtg (the T7 site is underlined) (8, 12).
3. An X-Y Mechanical stage for stereomicroscopes can be purchased from major microscope companies. However, an inexpensive mechanical stage (e.g., A512, MicroscopeNet.com), which is compatible with most stereomicroscopes (some modifications might be necessary), can also be used for injection (Fig. 2b).
4. The following primers were used for real-time PCR (EGFP and *Tc-polyubiquitin*). EGFPqF2: gacaaccactacctgagcac, EGFPqR2: caggaccatgtgatcgcg, PUBqF1: ggccgtactctttccgatta, PUBqR1: tgtctgagggttctacttcc.
5. 10× Tris/Glycine/SDS stock solution should be diluted down to 1× before adding methanol.
6. Uncloned PCR products can be used as an alternative source to make templates for the subsequent in vitro transcription, but this method is not recommended. A possible contamination of undesired PCR products in the PCR sample could produce dsRNA molecules that are unrelated to the targeted gene, causing unintended genes to be knocked down. However, uncloned PCR products may be ideal when a significant number of genes are required to be assayed (such as in a high-throughput screening), as it can bypass the cloning step.

7. It is critical to observe a single specific PCR band, as any nonspecific PCR products in this step will lead to the contamination of nonspecific dsRNA in the final product.
8. If the concentration is lower than 125 ng/μl, an additional PCR can be run with a regular T7 primer using the dsRNA produced as a template.
9. The needle holder should be thoroughly cleaned out if the RNA solution is sucked into the holder. Remove the needle holder from the teflon tube by carefully unscrewing the back screw. Prepare two wash bottles, one with water and the other with 100% ethanol. Place the nozzle of the water wash bottle to the backside of the needle holder, and squeeze the wash bottle to let the water run through the holder. Be careful not to suck in the liquid in the holder into the wash bottle. Repeat the same procedure with ethanol. After the needle holder is thoroughly washed, a compressed gas duster can be used to remove any residual ethanol in the holder.
10. Instead of using the injection needle (and the needle holder/injection apparatus) described in this protocol, a Hamilton syringe (e.g., Hamilton Syringe 1800 Series Gastight) or auto-nanoliter injector (e.g., Nanoject, Drummond) can be used for a bigger organism (such as bigger coleopteran larvae or cricket nymphs) (32, 33).
11. A time ranging between 3.5 and 4.5 min is recommended at a regular room temperature (~23°C). However, the optimal duration for etherization varies depending on temperature and humidity.
12. For dipteran larvae, a slide with a piece of double-sided sticky tape works better than the sticky glass slide. Larvae without etherization can be placed onto a piece of double-stick tape on a glass slide. Let the larva crawl on the tape until they stick themselves on the tape. Adding a drop of water will easily detach them from the tape after injection.
13. An approximate amount of RNA solution injected in each beetle can be estimated by dividing the total amount of the solution loaded in the injection needle by the number of beetles injected.
14. Injection procedures do not significantly affect the survival rate of *Tribolium* (survival rate with injection buffer is usually above 90%). The following possibilities should be considered if a lower survival rate is observed.
    (a) Inappropriate culture condition (such as overcrowded condition or lower humidity) might be causing lethality.
    (b) Injection buffer might be too old. Injection buffer older than 6 months should not be used.

(c) The needle tip might be too blunt or too big, making a big wound. Make sure to use a needle with a sharp tip.

(d) The sticky glass slide might be too sticky, causing damage upon removing larvae from the slide. You may have to reduce the stickiness of the glue by briefly touching the glue several times with your finger.

15. Different techniques can be used to isolate RNA from samples; however, the yield should be free of genomic DNA. Therefore, it is often advantageous to treat RNA extracts with Dnase.

16. For RNA work, always wear disposable gloves while handling samples and reagents. Avoid touching your skin or hair during the procedures. Decontaminate the bench area, pipette and tube stands with RNase Away Spray Bottle (Molecular BioProducts/Thermo Fisher). Use RNase-free, filtered pipette tips. Maintaining a separate area for RNA work with its own set of pipettes and tube stands is recommended.

17. As few as two beetles (last-instar larvae, pupae, or adults) are sufficient for total RNA isolation using QIAGEN RNeasy Mini kit.

18. The reactions without reverse transcriptase should not result in a measurable amount of product. If there is a measurable Ct, the sample is probably contaminated with genomic DNA, which is being amplified in the reaction. Therefore, all of the experimental reactions for that sample are contaminated, and the Ct values are influenced by the genomic DNA. In this case, it is advisable to treat the RNA samples with DNase.

19. For a detailed description of the theory behind $2^{-\Delta\Delta CT}$, or the alternative standard curve method, see Chapter 17 or consult the Applied Biosystems User Bulletin #2 (23).

20. The MagicMark XP standard, which reacts to the secondary antibody, is only visible on the developed film. Therefore, other prestained standards can be used if visible bands are desired on the membrane.

21. Shallow dishes are required to incubate the antibody and membrane. It is desirable for the dish to be flat-bottomed and slightly larger than the membrane, to reduce the amount of antibodies needed for incubation. Depending on the size of the blot, slide or coverslip box lids can be used.

22. Primary antibodies require different dilutions to be effective in immunoblots. Therefore, one can run multiple lanes of the same protein, cut the membrane into strips and empirically determine which concentration of antibody is most effective. It is easiest to cut the membrane when the transfer is finished and the gel is still on the membrane. Small notches in the corners can be used to track gels and their proper orientation.

## References


1. Fire A, Xu S, Montgomery MK et al (1998) Potent and specific genetic interference by double-stranded RNA in *Caenorhabditis elegans*. Nature **391**:806–811
2. Meister G, Tuschl T (2004) Mechanisms of gene silencing by double-stranded RNA. Nature **431**:343–349
3. Mello CC, Conte D Jr (2004) Revealing the world of RNA interference. Nature **431**: 338–342
4. Denell R (2008) Establishment of tribolium as a genetic model system and its early contributions to evo-devo. Genetics **180**:1779–1786
5. Klingler M (2004) Tribolium. Curr Biol **14**:R639–640
6. Miller SC, Brown SJ, Tomoyasu Y (2008) Larval RNAi in *Drosophila*? Dev Genes Evol **218**:505–510
7. Belles X (2010) Beyond *Drosophila*: RNAi in vivo and functional genomics in insects. Annu Rev Entomol **55**:111–128
8. Tomoyasu Y, Miller SC, Tomita S et al (2008) Exploring systemic RNA interference in insects: a genome-wide survey for RNAi genes in *Tribolium*. Genome Biol **9**:R10
9. Huvenne H, Smagghe G (2010) Mechanisms of dsRNA uptake in insects and potential of RNAi for pest control: a review. J Insect Physiol **56**:227–235
10. Feinberg EH, Hunter CP (2003) Transport of dsRNA into cells by the transmembrane protein SID-1. Science **301**:1545–1547
11. Winston, W. M., Molodowitch, C., and Hunter, C. P. (2002) Systemic RNAi in *C. elegans* requires the putative transmembrane protein SID-1. Science **295,** 2456–2459.
12. Tomoyasu Y, Denell RE (2004) Larval RNAi in *Tribolium* (Coleoptera) for analyzing adult development. Dev Genes Evol **214**: 575–578
13. Bucher G, Scholten J, Klingler M (2002) Parental RNAi in *Tribolium* (Coleoptera). Curr Biol **12**:R85–86
14. Brown S, Holtzman S, Kaufman T et al (1999) Characterization of the *Tribolium* Deformed ortholog and its ability to directly regulate Deformed target genes in the rescue of a *Drosophila* Deformed null mutant. Dev Genes Evol **209**:389–398
15. Cerny AC, Bucher G, Schroder R et al (2005) Breakdown of abdominal patterning in the Tribolium Kruppel mutant jaws. Development **132**:5353–5363
16. Tribolium Home page. http://bru.usgmrl.ksu.edu/proj/tribolium/index.html
17. Sutter Instrument Technical Support. http://www.sutter.com/contact/technical_support.html
18. Ma Y, Creanga A, Lum L et al (2006) Prevalence of off-target effects in *Drosophila* RNA interference screens. Nature **443**: 359–363
19. Tomoyasu Y, Arakane Y, Kramer KJ et al (2009) Repeated co-options of exoskeleton formation during wing-to-elytron evolution in beetles. Curr Biol **19**:2057–2065
20. Arakane Y, Lomakin J, Beeman RW et al (2009) Molecular and functional analyses of amino acid decarboxylases involved in cuticle tanning in *Tribolium castaneum*. J Biol Chem **284**:16584–16594
21. Arakane Y, Muthukrishnan S, Beeman RW et al (2005) Laccase 2 is the phenoloxidase gene required for beetle cuticle tanning. Proc Natl Acad Sci USA **102**:11337–11342
22. Integrated DNA Technologies https://www.idtdna.com/Home/Home.aspx
23. ABI PRISM 7700 Sequence Detection System, User Bulletin #2. http://www3.appliedbiosystems.com/cms/groups/mcb_support/documents/generaldocuments/cms_040980.pdf
24. Palauqui JC, Elmayan T, Pollien JM et al (1997) Systemic acquired silencing: transgene-specific post-transcriptional silencing is transmitted by grafting from silenced stocks to non-silenced scions. Embo J **16**:4738–4745
25. Voinnet O, and Baulcombe DC (1997) Systemic signalling in gene silencing. Nature **389**:553
26. Voinnet O, Vain P, Angell S et al (1998) Systemic spread of sequence-specific transgene RNA degradation in plants is initiated by localized introduction of ectopic promoterless DNA. Cell **95**:177–187
27. May RC, Plasterk RH (2005) RNA interference spreading in *C. elegans*. Methods Enzymol **392**:308–315
28. Mlotshwa S, Voinnet O, Mette MF et al (2002) RNA silencing and the mobile silencing signal. Plant Cell **14 Suppl**:S289–301
29. Voinnet O (2005) Non-cell autonomous RNA silencing. FEBS Lett **579**:5858–5871
30. Xie Q, Guo HS (2006) Systemic antiviral silencing in plants. Virus Res **118**:1–6
31. Hunter CP, Winston WM, Molodowitch C et al (2006) Systemic RNAi in *Caenorhabditis*

*elegans*. Cold Spring Harb Symp Quant Biol **71**:95–100

32. Moczek AP, Rose DJ (2009) Differential recruitment of limb patterning genes during development and diversification of beetle horns. Proc Natl Acad Sci USA **106**:8992–8997

33. Nakamura T, Mito T, Tanaka Yet al (2007) Involvement of canonical Wnt/Wingless signaling in the determination of the positional values within the leg segment of the cricket *Gryllus bimaculatus*. Dev Growth Differ **49**:79–88

# Index




Virginie Orgogozo and Matthew V. Rockman (eds.), *Molecular Methods for Evolutionary Genetics*,
Methods in Molecular Biology, vol. 772, DOI 10.1007/978-1-61779-228-1, 

## Q



## R



## S



## T



## U

## V



## X



## Y



## Z